DATE DUE

Everyone's Guide to

CANCER THERAPY

*W*hat must I do to be saved?

ACTS 16, 30

*I*t is knowledge that ultimately gives salvation.

MOHANDAS GANDHI

Everyone's Guide to
CANCER
THERAPY

MALIN DOLLINGER MD
ERNEST H. ROSENBAUM MD
AND GREG CABLE

A Somerville House Book

♦

Andrews and McMeel
A Universal Press Syndicate Company
Kansas City • New York

For information, please write to: Andrews and McMeel, a Universal Press
Syndicate Company, 4900 Main Street, Kansas City, Missouri 64112.

Produced by Somerville House Books Limited.
1 Eglinton Ave. East, Suite 305
Toronto, Ontario
Canada
M4P 3A1

Interior design of book: Falcom Design and Communications Inc.

Medical illustrations: Kam Yu

Library of Congress Cataloging-in-Publication Data
Dollinger, Malin.

    Everyone's guide to cancer therapy: how cancer is diagnosed, treated, and
managed day-to-day/by Malin Dollinger and Ernest H. Rosenbaum with Greg Cable;
preface by Samuel Broder.
    p.   cm.
    Includes index.
    ISBN 0-8362-2418-3 (hd): $29.95. — ISBN 0-8362-2417-5 (ppb): $19.95
    1. Cancer—Popular works.   I. Rosenbaum, Ernest H.   II. Cable,
Greg, 1946- .   III Title.
RC263.D59 1991
616.99'406—dc20
    91-8397
    CIP

To our wives, Lenore and Isadora

and

*To Vincent DeVita, Jr., MD, Susan Molloy Hubbard, RN,
and Richard A. Bloch for their vision, ingenuity and dedication
in creating PDQ – The Physicians Data Query.*
MD and EHR

*To Diana Darroch, a kind-hearted, loving, compassionate nurse who
knows the challenge and the victory.*
GC

To Agnes Thomson (Tommie) Somerville.
JS

CONTENTS

◇

PART I: DIAGNOSIS AND TREATMENT

PART IV: TREATING THE COMMON CANCERS

ACKNOWLEDGMENTS

The successful completion of such a complex and comprehensive book depends upon the support, assistance and help of a great number of people.

A very special word of gratitude goes first and foremost to our editor and co-writer Greg Cable. We wish to acknowledge the hard work, dedication and enormous effort he put into making highly complex medical information comprehensible to the general public. His contribution was essential in the successful completion of this book.

We are especially indebted to Jane Somerville, whose creative instincts and dedication to addressing an important need in our society have been singularly important in the creation of *Everyone's Guide to Cancer Therapy*. Her able and effective co-workers, including Patrick Crean, Keith Dundas, Kathy Legris, Dawn Arnold, Vivien Clark and Elizabeth Sherman have been of invaluable assistance. Thanks are warmly extended as well to Shaun Oakey for his skillful copyediting, Fortunato Aglialoro for designing this book, and Voirrey Broe, RN for her editorial comments. We are also grateful for the skill and artistic talent of medical illustrator Kam Yu.

We extend warm thanks to our American publisher Tom Thornton of Andrews and McMeel, and his Editorial Director Donna Martin and Promotion Director Kathy Massman for their tremendous support and enthusiasm.

Our contributing authors generously gave to the project the extremely important gifts of their time and energies, sharing with us their expertise in their particular fields. Their contributions were critical to ensuring that the information presented here would be as complete, comprehensive and up-to-date as possible. We hereby acknowledge and express our gratitude to them all for their excellent work, especially Carlos A. Pellegrini, MD (Surgical Oncology), T. Stanley Meyler, MD, and Lawrence Margolis, MD (Radiation Oncology), for their comprehensive review of chapters dealing with specific tumors. John Hayward, MD, reviewed the entire book and offered invaluable advice and criticism.

In medicine, as in any scientific endeavor, peer review of published material is not only valuable but essential. Many people expert in the treatment of cancer and the care of cancer patients reviewed the manuscript and gave us the benefit of their knowledge and insights. We would like to express our thanks to:

Arthur Ablin, MD, Frederick Aronson, MD, Orlo Clark, MD, Lloyd Damon, MD, Jerry Finklestein, MD , Bruce Friedman, MD, Gary Friedman, MD, Anthony Giorgio, MD, William Goodson, MD, Francine Holberg, MD, Robert Ignoffo, MD, Phil Kivitz, MD, Benjamin Landau, MD, Stephen Lemkin, MD, Kenneth McCormick, MD, Eugene Morita, MD, Joyce O'Shaughnessy, MD, Jacob Rajfer, MD, Arthur Rosenbaum, MD, J.C. Rosenberg, MD, PhD, Gene Sherman, MD, Thomas Simko, MD, James Tamkin, MD, Frank Valone, MD, Kenneth A. Woeber, MD.

We owe our special thanks for valuable assistance to:

Mary Arnold, Tina Anderson, Jeanine Bernet, Denise Boland, Barry Bowman, Sharon Buckeridge, David Chan, MD, Paula Chung, Carmel Finigan, Lowell Greenberg, MD, Chester Gottlieb, MD, Sue Harmon, Jean Jenkins, Melinda Johnson, Liz Jorgensen, Anita Klecker, Diane McElhiney, Dottie Miller, Patty Mullins, Carol Richardson, Brett Ringler, Elaine

Ryan, Beth Silverstein, Carolyn Small, Gail Sorrough, Teresa Squires, Jill Sternthal, William Sundbeck, Kathleen M. Thompson, Celeste Torrens, Ted Wilden, Arthur Wisot, MD, Gloria Won and Stuart Wong, MD.

A very special acknowledgment is due the National Cancer Institute Information Center for providing the Physicians Data Query (PDQ) database and literature updates. This book is a knowledge link to PDQ, since much of the information in it is taken from PDQ sources. We want to express our appreciation and thanks to the National Cancer Institute for the concept of carrying the message of modern comprehensive cancer care to the practicing physician and the public, and to the staff of the Institute's PDQ Section for their cooperation in making the database available and for the time and attention they devoted to our needs. In so many ways they facilitated our use and understanding of the PDQ material, which was of great help in preparing the manuscript in a format suitable and useful to the general reader.

We thank David Bull, publisher of Bull Publishing Co. for drug and nutritional data. We would also like to express our appreciation to Mt. Zion Medical Center of the University of California, San Francisco, specifically Louis Giancola, COO, Martin Diamond, President and CEO, the Arseny Olga Koushar Memorial Foundation and the Ernest H. Rosenbaum Research Fund for support of this endeavor. We are equally indebted to American Medical International, Inc., South Bay Hospital, Redondo Beach, California, and its CEO, Dennis Bruns, for major support and assistance, and the Better Health Programs, a project of the Regional Cancer Foundation.

We owe a tremendous personal debt to our teachers, David Karnofsky, MD, Joseph Burchenal, MD, Irwin Krakoff, MD, William Dameshek, MD, Harris Fishban, MD, John J. Sampson, MD, and Russell Tat, MD, who cared about the advance of knowledge, about their patients and about us.

We also now understand why authors thank their spouses. Their acceptance and tolerance of the many hours, days, weeks and months of time devoted to "The Book" is an all-important ingredient in any manuscript's completion.

In our case, there is an even more important contribution. Our professional lives have been devoted to the care of seriously ill patients who often seemed like "family" too. Our wives, Lenore Dollinger and Isadora Rosenbaum, have understood and accepted the many demands created by our professional relationships, and they have freely given us the support, the time and the inspiration to continue.

Finally, we are grateful to our patients who have shared with us some of the most important and difficult struggles of their lives. They have allowed us to play a part in their struggle and in many cases to feel like one of the family. We have learned much from them over the years, not only about cancer and its treatment but about hope, courage and the indomitable human spirit.

In a larger sense, we want to express our appreciation to all cancer patients. Most of the current research on cancer treatment has been obtained through the clinical trial programs where promising new treatments can be compared with either a standard treatment or another promising treatment. Virtually all advances in cancer therapy have emerged from these extremely important clinical investigations and literally thousands of patients have consented to participate in them. We, and society, owe them a great debt and thanks.

Malin Dollinger, MD
Ernest H. Rosenbaum, MD
California, 1991

PREFACE

by Samuel Broder, MD, Director, National Cancer Institute, Bethesda, Maryland

◇

If people with cancer are to become full partners with their doctors and health care teams in their recovery from the disease, then it is critical that they have an understanding of the illness and of the kinds of treatments that might be recommended.

Everyone's Guide to Cancer Therapy offers an excellent step-by-step approach to this process. It explains what is currently known about the early detection of cancer, how a malignancy develops, how and why the correct stage of the cancer is determined and how each tumor is best treated. The book explains the basis for the many tests all cancer patients must undergo. It explains clearly and simply what to expect from the various forms of therapy and outlines the many ways individuals can cope and contribute to their own well-being during the period of recovery.

I would like to highlight one critical aspect of this book that I especially applaud—the central role that clinical trials play in cancer care. The National Cancer Institute (NCI) in the United States sponsors clinical trials all over the country aimed at improving the best currently available therapy for each type of cancer.

This clinical research process is vital. It is the mechanism by which advances are made in the treatment of cancer. All NCI-sponsored clinical trials undergo vigorous scientific and ethical review so that all participants can be assured that the therapy they receive in a clinical trial is at least as good as—and perhaps better than—standard treatment. They are fully informed of all their options and are kept abreast of any developments in the treatment of their disease.

It is important for those with cancer and their families to understand that for a tumor for which no highly effective therapy exists, investigational therapy within the context of an NCI-sponsored clinical trial represents the very best therapy available. Clinical cancer research is first and foremost treatment. It is state-of-the-art therapy that defines and builds upon the standard of care.

FOREWORD

◇

In 1978, I was diagnosed with terminal lung cancer. I was given three months to live and told there were no treatments that could help me. The following week, I went to a major cancer center in another state where the doctor told me I could be cured.

Over the next three years, I learned a great deal about cancer. It is an extremely complex disease. There are hundreds of types and stages, with numerous treatment methods available. Progress in finding more effective treatments is being made at a staggering rate, and I soon came to realize there is no conceivable way any single human being could know the latest and most appropriate treatment for every kind of cancer. It is difficult to keep up with every current treatment for even one kind of cancer. Yet if cancer is to be beaten, it must be treated promptly, properly and thoroughly. There is often no second chance.

I also came to realize that if a doctor is unaware of the latest and best treatment for an individual patient, all the research—all the work done and all the money spent—is wasted as far as that patient is concerned. Many lives can be lost not because treatments to cure or control a cancer haven't been discovered, but because the physician may be unaware of them.

In 1981, I was Chairman of the Board of H & R Block, Inc., my family's income tax firm. We had acquired a computer service company in Columbus, Ohio, named CompuServe. One of its services was a network whereby anyone with a computer could call a local telephone number, be connected with the huge mainframes in Columbus and get all kinds of information instantly. One kind of information service offered was news.

When a newspaper is set today, it is done on a computer and CompuServe had arrangements with eleven major newspapers in the United States to have their articles fed into the company's mainframes as they were set. At night, I could contact CompuServe with my home computer and read the next morning's New York Times, Los Angeles Times, Washington Post or Chicago Tribune. I could read the front page, the editorial page, the sports, financial columns or whatever I selected. And I could read it before the people in those cities could get their paper locally.

It seemed obvious that, in the same way, a continually updated computer database of the latest cancer treatments could instantly deliver state-of-the-art information to any practicing physician in his or her own office.

The National Cancer Institute (NCI) had been working along similar lines. The Institute had the task of developing effective methods to prevent, diagnose and treat cancer, and was given additional resources by Congress to develop a program to disseminate cancer information.

First, an International Research Data Bank had been established, and in 1974 NCI began developing specialized systems to aid in collecting information to be made available to the scientific community. Mary Lasker, a member of the National Cancer Advisory Board at that time, requested that the NCI publish a book of treatment protocols to help practicing physicians find out about promising investigational therapies. She also asked that the book be updated every six months, but it wasn't feasible to prepare the equivalent of a textbook on clinical cancer research and change it semi-annually.

In response, Dr. Vincent T. DeVita, Jr., then the Director of NCI's Division of Cancer Treatment, decided to develop a computerized database called CLINPROT (Clinical Protocols) containing information on protocols supported by the Institute. By 1980, Dr. DeVita, now director of the NCI, had established a working group to expand the database with state-of-the-art treatment information and make it available to the growing number of physicians with personal computers.

In 1981, I communicated to Dr. DeVita my idea of having an easily accessible database of cancer therapies. He heartily agreed about how important it was to communicate fresh information directly to physicians and explained that NCI was developing such a database in two stages. The first stage involved adding a geographic matrix to CLINPROT, allowing physicians to identify investigational studies by area and other factors. This new file would be called PDQ1. The second stage involved adding state-of-the-art treatment information to PDQ1 and developing a comprehensive directory of physicians and treatment facilities that could be contacted for cancer care. This expanded database was named the Physicians Data Query system, but came to be known simply as PDQ.

I was so enthusiastic about this project that I assembled a group of donors to purchase a building just off the NIH campus to house these activities. And in 1982 I became a member of the National Cancer Advisory Board. Throughout my six-year term on the Board, I continued to support the development and refinement of the system.

PDQ is now available instantly to physicians in the United States as well as in many other parts of the world through their personal computers, their hospital computers or the facilities of any medical library. And it is available absolutely free to any individual by calling 1-800-4-CANCER.

Everyone's Guide to Cancer Therapy continues this important work in making the most up-to-date cancer information as widely available as possible. In its tumor treatment sections, it expands on the PDQ database and translates the information into clear, easily understood terms. It is hoped that the *Guide* will serve as a critical resource for cancer patients, their families and anyone else whose life has been or might be affected by this disease. It is also hoped that it will serve health professionals who want additional information about cancer and supportive care techniques for themselves and for their patients.

The NCI has stated that if physicians used the latest recommended therapy, cancer mortality would be reduced 10 percent, saving some 40,000 lives annually.

Considering that the proper information can now be had so rapidly and easily, can there be any excuse to lose lives by failing to get it for every patient?

Richard Bloch
Kansas City, 1991

TO THE READER

When your life has been touched or, rather, grabbed by cancer, many things change. Whether it has happened to you, a member of your family, or a friend, the impact of a cancer diagnosis is always the same. It's like being hit by a truck.

New emotions suddenly crop up, the greatest being the cold fear of a new and unknown disease. New questions arise. What can be done to cure me? What medical and psychological help is available? Will I suffer? Will there be pain? How can I live with this disease? Do I have to die?

Your life and the lives of those around you are affected in many significant ways. You have likely had no preparation for these sudden, drastic changes.

It is our wish and purpose to give you as thorough, as careful and as complete an understanding as possible of what you are facing and what you can expect. Our aim is to describe in easily understood language the details and consequences of the particular cancer you or someone close to you may be confronting. We'll explain what treatments are available, what they involve and what you should do to get the best treatment in the shortest time with the least worry, discomfort and uncertainty.

Cancer comes with its own vast vocabulary, most of it probably unfamiliar to you. Many new words and complicated descriptions will become part of your everyday thinking. The extensive glossary of medical terms will help you keep your bearings as you travel through this strange new world.

Important questions will arise. How should you choose a cancer physician or an appropriate hospital? What tests will be done and what is their significance? What treatment options are available?

What are their risks and side effects? Who is involved in the treatment plan? How can open and clear communication be maintained? We have included a general guide to the cancer treatment system that will help you find answers to these questions.

Cancer can also be an emotionally devastating issue, not only to you as a sufferer but to your family and friends. So we have included a section on living with cancer and how you can work to improve your physical and mental well-being.

Cancer treatments are continually changing, and this book is a guide to diagnosis and treatment, not a collection of definitive medical opinions suitable for everyone. Each person with cancer is a unique individual in a unique situation.

Your physician has the role and responsibility of making diagnostic and treatment decisions, discussing them with you, giving you the benefit of his or her medical opinion and devising together with you the treatment plan most appropriate to your situation.

We have attempted to present the most current and accurate information about cancer, but it is not possible to convey all possible approaches to diagnosis and therapy. Although we have tried to reflect the treatment guidelines listed by the information services of the National Cancer Institute, there may in some cases be alternative approaches or even newer methods of diagnosis and treatment that your physician may discuss with you.

This book is to help you get more out of these discussions by helping you understand the complex problems of cancer treatment, ask the right questions and search for and obtain the best medical care.

CONTRIBUTORS

Malin R. Dollinger, MD
Clinical Professor of Medicine, University of Southern California, Los Angeles, CA

Director, Cancer Risk Assessment Center, South Bay Hospital, Redondo Beach, CA

Member, Cancer Care Associates, Torrance, Redondo Beach, San Pedro and Gardena, CA

Malin Roy Dollinger's lifelong dedication to the field of oncology and patient education has included a research post at the Memorial Sloan Kettering Cancer Center for Cancer Research in New York and a post as Director of Medical Oncology at Harbor General Hospital/ UCLA Medical Center in Los Angeles. He has written over 50 articles about cancer and is a member of the editorial advisory board of "The Medical Letter" (New York), Patient Care Publications (San Francisco) and "The New England Journal of Medicine."

In addition to his extensive patient care activities, he teaches at the University of Southern California School of Medicine and has lectured extensively to medical professionals and the public. He is especially interested in improving communication with cancer patients and their families and in the emotional issues associated with the disease.

Ernest H. Rosenbaum, MD
Clinical Professor of Medicine, University of California, San Francisco, CA

Associate Chief of Medicine, Mt. Zion Medical Center of the University of California, San Francisco, CA

Founder of the Medical Oncology Service, Mt. Zion Medical Centre of the University of California, San Francisco, CA

Associate, Cancer Research Institute, University of California, San Francisco, CA

Director, Better Health Foundation for Preventive Medicine, San Francisco, CA

Ernest H. Rosenbaum's career has included a fellowship at the Blood Research Laboratory of Tufts University School of Medicine (New England Center Hospital) and MIT. He teaches at the Mount Zion Medical Centre and UCSF, and was the co-founder of the Northern California Academy of Clinical Oncology.

His passionate interest in good communication with patients and colleagues has led to over 50 articles on cancer and hematology, including some for the Journal of the American Medical Association. He has participated in many national radio and television programs and frequently lectures to medical and public groups.

He has co-authored *Nutrition for the Cancer Patient* and has written numerous books, including *Living With Cancer* and *A Comprehensive Guide for the Cancer Patients and their Families*. For the latter work, he received Honorable Mention from the American Medical Writers Association for Excellence in Medical Publications.

Greg Cable, BA
A writer and editor since 1970, Greg Cable has worked in publishing, television, film and education. For many years he was a senior editor with publishing houses in Toronto, editing over a hundred books. He has written a wide range of materials for many of the major arts organizations in Canada and has collaborated on several books in a variety of fields. His most recent co-authored work (1989) was *Catch: A Major League Life*, the best-selling autobiography of Toronto Blue Jays catcher Ernie Whitt.

Robert E. Allen, Jr., MD
[Surgical Oncologist]

Professor of Surgery, University of California School of Medicine, San Francisco, CA

James O. Armitage, MD
[Medical Oncologist]
Professor of Medicine, University of Nebraska School of Medicine
Director, Bone Marrow Transplantation Center, University of Nebraska

Kenneth A. Arndt, MD
[Dermatologist]
Professor of Dermatology, Harvard Medical School, Boston, MA
Chief of Dermatology, Beth Israel Hospital, Boston, MA

Josefa Azcueta, RN, OCN
[Nurse Oncologist]
Director, Oncology Nursing, Cancer Care Associates, Torrance, Redondo Beach, San Pedro, and Gardena, CA

Harold H. Benjamin, PHD
Founder and Executive Director, Wellness Community, Santa Monica, CA
Author: *From Victim to Victor*

Christopher Benz, MD
[Medical Oncologist]
Associate Professor of Medicine, University of California, School of Medicine, San Francisco, CA

Richard Bloch,
Founder H & R Block, Kansas City, Missouri

David G. Bullard, PhD
[Clinical Psychologist]
Associate Clinical Professor of Medicine and Medical Psychology [Psychiatry], University of California, San Francisco, CA

Barrie R. Cassileth, PhD
Director, Psychosocial Research Programs and Cancer Control Program, University of Pennsylvania Cancer Center
Associate Professor, Medical Sociology in Medicine, University of Pennsylvania School of Medicine, Philadelphia, PA

Raphael Catane, MD
[Medical Oncologist]
Acting Director, Sharett Institute,

Hadassah Hospital, Jerusalem, Israel
Associate Professor of Oncology, Hebrew University-Hadassah Medical School, Jerusalem, Israel

Vincent T. DeVita, Jr., MD
[Medical Oncologist]
Physician-in-Chief, Memorial Sloan-Kettering Cancer Center and Professor of Medicine, Cornell University Medical School, NY
Co-creator: PDQ

Lenore Dollinger, PhD, RN
Certified Health Consultant, Redondo Beach, CA

Lawrence Drew, MD , PhD
[Internist]
Associate Clinical Professor of Medicine and Laboratory Medicine, University of California, San Francisco, CA
Director of Microbiology and Infectious Disease, Mount Zion Medical Center of the University of California, San Francisco, CA

Frederick Eilber, MD
[Surgical Oncologist]
Professor of Surgery, University of California, Los Angeles, CA
Associate, Jonsson Comprehensive Cancer Center, Los Angeles, CA

Jerry Z. Finklestein, MD, CM
[Pediatric Oncologist]
Adjunct Professor of Pediatrics, University of California, Los Angeles, CA
Medical Director of Jonathan Jaques Children's Cancer Center, Miller Children's Hospital, Long Beach, CA

Timothy S. Gee, MD
[Medical Oncologist]
Associate Professor of Clinical Medicine, Cornell University Medical College, New York, NY
Attending Physician, Acting Chief, Leukemia Service, Memorial Hospital for Cancer and Allied Diseases, New York, NY
Clinical Member, Sloan-Kettering Insti-

tute for Cancer Research, New York, NY

Alan B. Glassberg, MD
[Medical Oncologist]
Clinical Professor of Medicine, University of California, San Francisco, CA
Chief of Oncology/Associate Chief of Medicine, Mount Zion Medical Center of the University of San Francisco, CA Associate, Cancer Research Institute, University of California, San Francisco, CA

Deborah Hamolsky, RN, MS, OCN
Nurse Oncologist, Mount Zion Medical Center of the University of California, San Francisco, CA

Russell Hardy, MD
[Medical Oncologist]
Fellow in Medicine, Stanford University School of Medicine, Stanford, CA

James T. Helsper, MD
[Surgical Oncologist]
Associate Clinical Professor of Surgery, University of Southern California School of Medicine, Los Angeles, CA
President, Society of Head and Neck Surgeons

Sandra Horning, MD
[Medical Oncologist]
Associate Professor of Medicine, Stanford University School of Medicine, Stanford, CA

Susan Molloy Hubbard, RN, BS
[Oncology Nurse, Co-creator of PDQ]
Director of International Cancer Information Center
Associate Director, National Cancer Institute, Bethesda, MD

Eliot S. Krames, MD
[Anesthesiologist]
Medical Director, San Francisco Center for Comprehensive Pain Management
Medical Director of Mount Zion Medical Center of the University of California, San Francisco, CA Pain Management Program

Robert A. Kyle, MD
[Medical Oncologist]
Professor of Medicine and Laboratory Medicine, Mayo Medical School
Chairman, Division of Hematololgy, Mayo Clinic, Rochester, MN

Kerry Anne McGinn, RN, BSN, MA
[Ostomy Nurse]
Nurse, Planetree Model Hospital Unit, Pacific Presbyterian Medical Center, San Francisco, CA

Lawrence W. Margolis, MD
[Radiation Oncologist]
Clinical Professor and Vice Chairman, Department of Radiation Oncology, University of California Medical Center, San Francisco, CA
Chief of Radiation Therapy, Zellerbach Saroni Tumor Institute, Mount Zion Medical Center of the University of California, San Francisco, CA

T. Stanley Meyler, MD
[Radiation Oncologist]
Clinical Professor of Radiotherapy, University of California, San Francisco, CA
Associate Chief of Radiation Therapy, Zellerbach Saroni Tumor Institute, Mount Zion Medical Center of the University of California, San Francisco, CA

Lawrence Mintz, MD
[Internist, Infectious Disease Specialist]
Co-Director of Microbiology and Infectious Disease, Mount Zion Medical Center of the University of California, San Francisco, CA
Associate Clinical Professor of Medicine and Laboratory Medicine, University of California School of Medicine, San Francisco, CA

Malcolm S. Mitchell, MD
[Medical Oncologist]
Professor of Medicine and Microbiology, University of Southern California, Los Angeles, CA
Head, Tumor Immunology and Immunotherapy, and formerly Chief of

Medical Oncology and Director for Clinical Investigations, USC Cancer Center, Los Angeles, CA

Guy Newell, MD
[Cancer Prevention Specialist/Internist]
Mesa Petroleum Co. Professor of Cancer Prevention, University of Texas, Houston, Texas
Chairman of the Department of Cancer Prevention and Control, M.D. Anderson Cancer Center, Houston, TX
Formerly, Interim Director, National Cancer Intstitute

Carlos Pellegrini, MD
[Surgical Oncologist]
Professor of Surgery, University of California, San Francisco, CA

Herbert A. Perkins, MD
[Hematologist]
Clinical Professor of Medicine, University of California, School of Medicine, San Francisco, CA
Director, Irwin Memorial Blood Centers, San Francisco, CA

Barbara F. Piper, RN, MS
[Oncology Nurse Specialist]
Oncology Nurse Specialist, Mount Zion Medical Center of the University of California, San Francisco, CA

Margaret Poscher, MD
[Internist]
Attending Physician, Mount Zion Medical Center of the University of California, San Francisco, CA

Isadora R. Rosenbaum, MA
Medical Assistant, San Francisco Hematology Oncology Medical Group

Ivan J. Silverberg, MD
[Medical Oncologist]
Associate Clinical Professor of Medicine, University of California, San Francisco, CA

Jill R. Slater-Freedberg, MD
[Dermatologist]
Resident in Medicine, Beth Israel Hospital, Boston, MA

Penny K. Sneed, MD
[Radiation Oncologist]
Assistant Professor, Department of Radiation Oncology, University of California Medical Center, San Francisco, CA

Jeffrey L. Stern, MD
[Gynecologic Oncologist]
Associate Professor of Obstetrics, Gynecology and Reproductive Sciences
Director of Gynecologic Oncology, University of California School of Medicine, San Francisco, CA

Jean M. Stoklosa, RN, MS
Formerly, Clinical Specialist, Veterans Administration Hospital, San Francisco, CA

Alan P. Venook, MD
[Medical Oncologist]
Assistant Clinical Professor of Medicine, University of California, San Francisco, CA
Director, Liver Tumor Treatment Group, Cancer Research Institute, University of California, San Francisco, CA

Alan Yagoda, MD
[Medical Oncologist]
Professor of Clinical Medicine and Professor of Clinical Surgery, Cornell University Medical College, New York, NY

Norman Zinner, MD
[Surgeon]
Adjunct Associate Professor of Surgery/Urology, University of California, Los Angeles, CA
Private Practice, Doctor's Urology Group, Torrance, CA
Formerly, Professor and Chairman, Department of Urology, Charles R. Drew Postgraduate Medical School, Los Angeles, CA
Formerly, Boorhaave Professor, University of Leiden, The Netherlands

PART I:
DIAGNOSIS AND TREATMENT

1
UNDERSTANDING CANCER

Malin Dollinger, MD, and Ernest H. Rosenbaum, MD

◇

Cancer is a general term for the abnormal growth of cells.

Our bodies are vast collections of cells, and every one of them contains 23 pairs of chromosomes. Winding through each pair is the double spiral of the DNA molecule, the genetic blueprint for life. DNA is the controller and transmitter of the genetic characteristics in the chromosomes we inherit from our parents and pass on to our children.

Our chromosomes contain millions of different messages that tell the body how it should grow, function and behave. One gene tells our stomachs how to make gastric juice; another tells the glands to secrete this juice when food lands in the stomach. Other genes determine the color of our eyes, tell injured tissues how to repair themselves and direct the female breasts to make milk after a baby is born. Most of the time these genes function properly and send the right messages. We remain in good health, with everything working as it should.

But there are an incredible number of genes and an unimaginable number of messages. And since the chromosomes reproduce themselves every time a cell divides, there are lots of opportunities for something to go wrong. Sometimes something does go wrong in the process of cell division—a mutation that alters one or more of the genes.

The altered gene starts sending the wrong message or at least a message different from the one it should give. A cell begins to grow rapidly. It multiplies again and again until it forms a lump that's called a malignant tumor. Or cancer.

Uncontrolled Growth Rapid cell growth is not the same as malignancy. We all experience two normal situations in which our body tissues grow much more rapidly than they usually do. We grow from a single cell to a perfectly formed human being in nine months. Then we grow into a normal-sized adult human being over the next 16 years or so. As well, when we are injured and need rapid repair, restoration and replacement of damaged tissues, our bodies can produce many new cells in a very short time.

When either of these processes—growth or healing—is completed, a set of genes tells the body that it is time to "switch off." We don't continue growing throughout our lives, and the scar we have after a cut has healed remains just that—a scar. Those are the rules.

But a cancer cell doesn't obey the rules. The change in its genetic code makes it "forget" to stop growing. Once growth is turned on, cancer cells continue to divide in an uncontrolled way. It's as though you set the thermostat in your house for a certain temperature, but no matter how hot your house gets the furnace keeps running. No matter what you do to turn it off, it produces heat as if it had a mind of its own.

Doubling Times Cancer starts with one abnormal cell. That cell becomes two abnormal cells that become four abnormal cells and so on. Cells divide at various rates, called doubling times. Fast-growing cancers may double over one to four weeks; slow-growing cancers may double over two to six months. It may take up to five years for the duplication process to happen 20 times. By then the tumor may contain a million cells yet still be only the size of a pinhead.

So there is a "silent" period after the cancer has started to grow. There is no lump or mass. It's too small to be detected by any means now known. What is not commonly appreciated is that the silent period is considerably longer than the period when we do know a tumor is present.

After many months, usually years, the doubling process has occurred 30 times or so. By then the lump may have reached a size that can be felt, seen on an x-ray or cause pressure symptoms such as pain or bleeding. To be able to see a tumor on an x-ray, it usually has to be about half an inch (1 cm) in diameter. At that stage, it will contain about 1 billion cells. When it is smaller, x-ray imaging techniques are not usually sensitive enough to detect it, although some newer imaging methods—especially computerized tomography (CT) and Magnetic Resonance Imaging (MRI)—may sometimes detect such small tumors.

Benign and Malignant Tumors Tumors are not always malignant. Benign tumors can appear in any part of the body. Many of us have them—freckles, moles, fatty lumps in the skin—but they don't cause any problems except (sometimes) cosmetic ones. They can be removed or left alone. However they are treated, they stay in one place. They do not invade or destroy surrounding tissues.

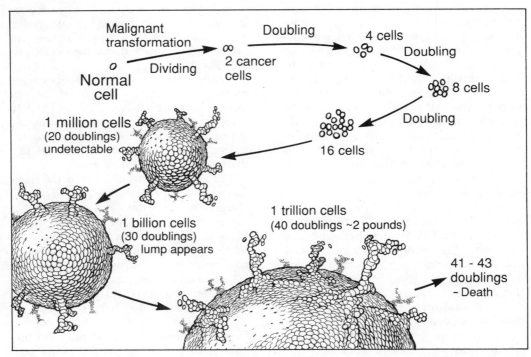

The malignant transformation of a normal cell and subsequent doublings. After 20 doublings (one million cancer cells) the cancer is still too small to detect.

Malignant tumors, on the other hand, have two significant characteristics:

♦ They have no "wall" or clear-cut border. They put down roots and directly invade surrounding tissues.

♦ They have the ability to spread to other parts of the body. Bits of malignant cells fall off the tumor, then travel like seeds to other tissues where they land and start similar growths. Fortunately, not all the many thousands of cancer cells that break off a tumor find a place to take root. Most die like seeds that go unplanted.

This spreading of cancer is called metastasis. And doctors are always concerned about whether the cancer has metastasized during the silent period. If it has, then the migrating cancer cells have begun to go through their own silent period. They too are too small to detect for many months or years.

Almost all cancers share these two properties, although cancers arising in various organs tend to behave differently. They spread to different parts of the body. They grow in very specific ways that are characteristic of that cancer. The consequence is that there is a specific method of diagnosis, staging and treatment for each kind of cancer. One set of principles governs diagnosis and treatment of breast cancer, for example, while the rules for lung or colon cancers are just as complex but somewhat different.

WHAT CAUSES CANCER

Although cancer is usually thought of as one disease, it is in fact more than 200 different diseases. For many of these cancers, no definite cause is known. There is no one single cause. In fact, cancer remains something of a mystery. But new clues and solid research are greatly increasing our understanding.

The Role of Oncogenes One of the most exciting and important developments has been the recent discovery that some nor-

mal genes may be transformed into genes that promote the growth of cancer. These have been called oncogenes, the prefix *onco* meaning tumor. This discovery has led to much research, better understanding of how cancer develops and insights into methods of prevention, detection and treatment.

What usually stops the normal genes from being transformed are other genes called suppressor genes. If they don't do their job properly or are missing altogether, the cancer-producing action of the oncogene may not be suppressed (*see* Chapter 30).

The Implications for Screening All this new information raises the possibility that we may soon be able to test individuals to discover whether a specific oncogene is present and if the suppressor gene is defective or absent. The presence of certain oncogenes may even give us information about how likely it is that a cancer will spread. We soon may be able to identify people with a higher risk for cancer and possibly carry out other intensive detection and screening methods. Techniques for testing for oncogenes have been developed recently and are beginning to be available for general use. This new knowledge is already used in the study of familial (inherited) polyps of the colon.

How the Process Works There are anywhere from 50,000 to 100,000 genes within a human cell. But research suggests that not more than a hundred regulate cell growth or division. It is now also thought that we all carry normal cells that contain oncogenes in the chromosomes but that these oncogenes are never activated. They simply lie dormant throughout our lives.

In other cases, a mutation may occur because of some assault on the cell structure. Some stimulus or chemical agent turns on a "switch," several oncogenes are activated, and they set to work together to

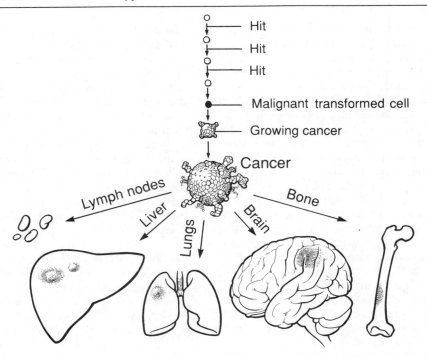

Hit

Hit

Hit

Malignant transformed cell

Growing cancer

Cancer

Lymph nodes

Liver

Lungs

Brain

Bone

After two or more "hits" a transformed malignant cell grows into a lump we call cancer. Cells may eventually break off and spread (metastasize) via lymph vessels or blood vessels.

transform a normal cell into a cancer cell. This is thought to be at least a two-step process. First, the DNA must go through an initial change that makes the cell receptive. Then a subsequent change or set of changes in the DNA transforms the receptive cell into a tumor cell.

The big question is, what causes these changes in cellular DNA in the first place? There are several theories. One focuses on viruses, which can insert their own DNA into a cell's DNA and make the cell produce more virus-containing cells. Viruses may insert a viral oncogene or they might simply act as a random mutating agent.

There is also some evidence that an assault by a "single carcinogenic bullet" hitting the cell at just the right spot can make a cell become cancerous. But the theory that has gained a lot of support focuses on multiple "hits."

The Multiple Hit Theory According to this theory, all cancers arise from at least two changes or "hits" to the genes in the cell. These hits build up and interact over time. Eventually, a breaking point is reached and cancerous growth is switched on.

The hits may come from chemical or foreign substances that cause cancer, called carcinogens. These initiate the cancer process. Or the hits may be promoters that accelerate the growth of abnormal cells. What is critical is the number and types of hits, their frequency and their intensity.

Initiators include:
♦ Tobacco and tobacco smoke carcinogens. Lung cancer was a rare disease before cigarette smoking became widespread.
♦ X-rays. It is well known that there is an increased incidence of leukemia among

atomic bomb survivors. This same increase has been noted in radiologists, the doctors who specialize in the use of x-rays. (It should be pointed out that the average diagnostic use of x-rays does not increase the chance of getting cancer enough to rule out their use as a valuable health care tool. The risk of not having an x-ray may far outweigh the risk of cancer being caused by the use of x-rays for diagnosis. Used properly, x-rays are of great benefit in finding cancer at an early, curable stage.)

♦ Certain hormones and drugs, such as DES, some estrogens (female hormones) and some immunosuppressive drugs.

♦ Excessive exposure to sunlight.

♦ Industrial agents or toxic substances in the environment, such as asbestos, coal tar products, benzene, cadmium, uranium and nickel.

♦ Excesses or deficiencies in diet, particularly high-fat and low-fiber diets.

♦ Obesity.

♦ Sexual practices, including the age of a woman when she first had intercourse and first becomes pregnant. Certain sexually transmitted viruses can cause cancers, and the risk of catching one of these viruses increases with unprotected sexual contact and with the number of sexual partners. This is particularly true for AIDS-related cancers such as Kaposi's sarcoma.

Promoters include:

♦ Alcohol, which is a factor in 4 percent of cancers, mainly in cancers of the head and neck and the liver.

♦ Stress, which may weaken the immune system. Stress is also relieved all too often with cigarettes, alcohol, rich food and drugs.

Miscellaneous Factors include:

♦ Heredity.

♦ Weaknesses of the immune system.

When two or more hits are combined—tobacco smoke and asbestos exposure, or cigarette smoking and alcohol, for exam-

ple—the chance of getting cancer is not the sum of the individual risks. Rather, the chances are multiplied. Cancer is an additive process with many different hits occurring and interacting over many, many years.

What it comes down to is that the risk of developing cancer depends on:

♦ who you are (genetic makeup);

♦ where you live (environmental and occupational exposures to carcinogens); and

♦ how you live (personal lifestyle).

Now that so many factors in our daily lives that affect the risk of getting cancer can be identified, cancer risk assessment has become increasingly vital to our continued good health. Risk assessment screening of apparently healthy people is now used in many cancer centers (*see* Chapter 29).

HOW CANCER SPREADS

Although tumors can start to grow in several places simultaneously, that is unusual. They usually grow at a single site. So if cancer spreads, it is usually because small bits of cancer cells are cast off the original, or primary, tumor and travel to other parts of the body. There are three ways for the cancer to spread (*see* Figure 1:2).

Direct Extension As the tumor mass grows, it invades the organs and tissues immediately next to it. It tends to form roots, growing into the layers of surrounding tissue like carrots growing into the earth.

Through the Blood (Hematogenous Spread) Tumors have a blood supply. Arteries pump blood into the malignant cells and veins take it away. Pieces of the tumor can grow through the walls of these blood vessels, enter the bloodstream and circulate around the body until they land in various organs. Fortunately, very few of these circulating cells actually find a place to grow.

CANCER RISK FACTORS, WITH PERCENTAGES

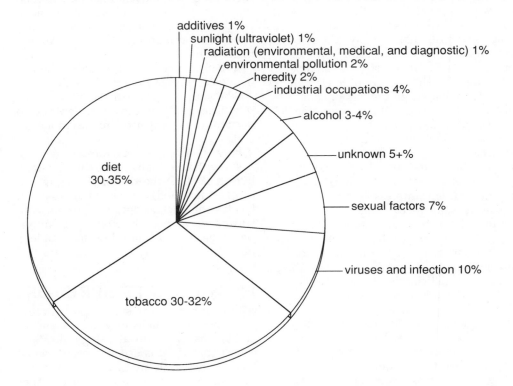

additives 1%
sunlight (ultraviolet) 1%
radiation (environmental, medical, and diagnostic) 1%
environmental pollution 2%
heredity 2%
industrial occupations 4%

alcohol 3-4%

unknown 5+%

sexual factors 7%

viruses and infection 10%

diet
30-35%

tobacco 30-32%

Through the Lymphatic System There are two blood vessel systems in the body. One consists of arteries that move blood to all parts of the body, veins that return the blood to the heart, and small capillaries around the organs and tissues that allow oxygen to be transferred.

The second is the lymphatic system. This is a separate system of tiny blood vessels—called lymphatics—under the skin and throughout the body. These vessels carry a liquid called lymph. The purpose of lymph is to drain waste products such as infectious, foreign or otherwise toxic materials.

Lymph Nodes Stations along these vessels, called lymph nodes, trap these materials.

Tonsils, for example, are lymph nodes. When you have tonsillitis you have a high temperature, you have trouble swallowing and you generally feel awful. But you feel that way because the tonsils are doing their job by trapping bacteria and preventing them from getting into your body. If they weren't doing their job, you might develop a bloodstream infection—"blood poisoning."

The lymph system begins with very small tubes that drain into lymph nodes at different levels of the body. Eventually the system feeds into the thoracic duct in the left side of the neck. That duct drains into the venous system, which returns the lymph fluid to the heart. From there it is pumped through the body.

Tumor cells can easily spread into the lymphatic system. Breast cancer, for example, often spreads initially via lymphatic vessels to the lymph nodes in the armpit (axillary nodes). If not stopped there, the cancer cells continue traveling in the lymphatics to other locations in the body. A doctor can sometimes feel the axillary nodes during a physical examination. But just to be sure, the nodes have to be examined under a microscope after they are surgically removed.

When breast cancer spreads to the lymph glands under the armpit, we hope the glands did their job and prevented the cells from spreading any farther. You might visualize these lymph glands as train stations and the lymph blood vessels as tracks. We hope the cells behave like a local train, stopping at the next lymph node station, and don't behave like an express, scooting past several nodes and getting directly into the body.

THE DIFFERENT KINDS OF TUMORS

Treating cancer properly depends on defining each and every tumor very precisely. All kinds of characteristics are taken into account when coming up with this definition, but all these characteristics essentially fit into three broad categories. The three key questions that have to be answered are: where is the tumor growing, how fast is it growing, and how big has it already grown?

The first of these questions is critical because, again, cancers that develop in different tissues tend to behave differently. There are generally three types of malignant tumors, which develop in the three kinds of tissues.

Carcinomas These develop in the tissues that cover the surface or line internal organs and passageways (epithelium). Most epithelial cancers—carcinomas— develop in an organ that secretes some-

thing. For example, lung tissue secretes mucus, breast tissue secretes milk, and the pancreas secretes digestive juices.

Sarcomas These are soft tissue or bone tumors. They develop in any supporting or connective tissues—muscles, bones, nerves, tendons or blood vessels. Since supporting or connective tissue is found throughout the body, sarcomas can be found anywhere.

The same organ that develops a carcinoma can also develop a sarcoma, since the organ also has connective tissue in it. There are blood vessels in the pancreas, for example, and if a cell in the wall of the blood vessel develops a tumor, the tumor is a sarcoma even though it's in the pancreas.

Lymphomas and Leukemias These tumors develop in the lymph glands or arise from the blood-forming cells in the bone marrow.

Lymphomas (lymphosarcomas) are the tumors that develop in the lymph glands, the small, round or bean-shaped structures found throughout the body. These tumors are almost always malignant. One specific kind of tumor in this broad class is called Hodgkin's disease, and all the other ones have come to be referred to as non-Hodgkin's lymphomas. To make things more complicated, there are many sub-varieties of both Hodgkin's disease and non-Hodgkin's lymphomas.

The leukemias are cancers of the white blood cells and are named after the type of white blood cell affected. Plasma cell myeloma (multiple myeloma) is a cancer of the plasma cells in the bone marrow.

Understanding Tumor Names There are many different names for the various cancers and it's easy to get confused. There are tumors in each of the three tumor categories that are named after the doctors who discovered them— Hodgkin's disease, Ewing's sarcoma of the bone, Kaposi's sarcoma or Wilms' tumor of the kidney. Tumors may also be named after the tissue of origin, such as a schwannoma, which is a tumor that develops in the Schwann cells surrounding nerves.

For the most part, there is a method to this confusing terminology. Every tissue or body part has a specific name. We all know these names in English. Bone is bone and fat is fat. But scientific medicine usually uses the Greek or Latin name for a body part and then adds a helpful tag onto the end of it. The rule for naming sarcomas, for example, is that if the tumor is benign, *oma* is usually added to the Greek or Latin name. If the tumor is malignant, *sarcoma* is added.

The term for bone, for example, is *osteo*, so a benign tumor in the bone is an osteoma and a malignant tumor is an osteosarcoma. The term for fat is *lipo*, so there are lipomas and liposarcomas.

There are also different names for some organs, so a carcinoma of the stomach may be called a gastric carcinoma and a carcinoma of the kidney may be referred to as renal carcinoma. There are also alternative designations. For example, since the glands in the lung usually line the air passage (bronchus), carcinomas of the lung are sometimes called bronchogenic carcinoma (*genic* being the Latin way of saying "formed from").

MEASURING THE RATE OF GROWTH

The second way to classify tumors is according to how fast they are growing. It would be nice if there were a simple way of doing this, like pointing a radar gun at the tumor and getting a read-out of the speed. But what usually has to happen is that a piece of the tumor is surgically removed and examined under a microscope, a process known as a biopsy. Its appearance and behavior can reveal a lot of information.

Well-Differentiated Tumors Under the microscope, some tumor cells look very much like the normal tissue they came from. If they do, they are called well-differentiated. A normal pancreas has a characteristic look, for example. A pathologist can look at a slide of tissue and see that it's a pancreas even if it is cancerous. Similarly, a follicular carcinoma of the thyroid resembles normal thyroid tissue rather well, so it is not difficult for a pathologist to know where that tumor comes from.

Undifferentiated Tumors Other tumors don't particularly look like the normal tissues they come from. They resemble the tissue of origin only slightly or not at all. They look more primitive or immature. Sometimes they don't really look like any specific tissue. These are called undifferentiated or poorly differentiated.

Looking at a piece of undifferentiated tissue under the microscope, a pathologist will probably not be able to tell where the tissue was taken from. An undifferentiated tumor of the pancreas may look the same as an undifferentiated tumor of the lung, so the pathologist has to rely on the surgeon to say what area the tissue is from.

Undifferentiated or poorly differentiated tumors tend to be more aggressive in their behavior. They grow faster, spread earlier and have a worse prognosis than well-differentiated tumors. But there are exceptions for both types of tumors. Some poorly differentiated tumors grow no faster than well-differentiated ones.

High-Grade and Low-Grade Tumors There is another classification system that sometimes overlaps with the system based on differentiation. This system refers to tumors as "high-grade" or "low-grade." A high-grade tumor is immature, poorly differentiated, fast growing and aggressive. A low-grade tumor is usually mature, well-differentiated, slow growing and less aggressive. The grading of tumors is used to help determine cancer prognosis.

DEFINING THE STAGE OF CANCER

The third classification used in cancer treatment is called the staging system. Staging has a number of purposes.

♦ It is a useful way of identifying the "extent" of the tumor—its size, the degree of growth and spread. Obviously, if a tumor is found in only one place it is in an early stage. If it has spread to some distant part of the body or is found in several places, it is in an advanced stage.

♦ It provides an estimate of the prognosis since the chance of cure decreases as you move across the categories into more advanced or extensive stages.

♦ It provides a common and uniformly agreed upon set of criteria against which doctors around the world can compare treatments for a specific stage of tumor. They can then know that if one treatment has better results than another, the difference is really due to the treatment and not to differences among patients or the stages of the disease.

♦ It is generally the most important factor in deciding on the appropriate treatment.

The TNM System All kinds of staging systems have been developed for different kinds of cancer. But in the past few years a lot of thought and effort has been going on around the world to develop a relatively uniform classification system.

This system is known as TNM. T stands for the size of the tumor, N for the degree of spread to lymph nodes, and M for the presence of metastasis. A number is added to each of these letters to indicate degrees of size and spread.

Greatly simplified:

♦ T0 means the tumor was completely removed by the biopsy used to establish the diagnosis. T1 indicates the smallest tumor. T2, T3 and T4 indicate larger tumors that may have grown into surrounding tissues.

♦ N0 means that the nearby lymph nodes are free of tumor. N1, N2 and N3 signify increasing degrees of involvement of these regional nodes. An N2 tumor is more serious than an N1 tumor.

♦ M0 means that no distant metastases (cancer cells) have been found. If there are metastases, the classification is M1.

This seems simple enough. But the system is actually quite complex. The classifications are defined differently for each kind of cancer and each stage can include variations to the basic TNM classification. Here are the staging categories and stage grouping for breast carcinoma, for example (*see* figure page 10).

A breast cancer might be classified as a T2 N1 M0 lesion. This could represent a tumor 1 inch (2.5 cm) in diameter removed from the breast with some involvement of lymph nodes in the armpit but with no evidence of metastasis.

The TNM system has two overlapping classifications, the second having to do with the stage of cancer that represents a composite of the TNM classification. You will see in the tumor section that each tumor is grouped in usually four stages. Since there are many possible further TNM subdivisions, these are lumped together. You have to refer to the specific table for each cancer to be sure of the specific stage. For example, the T2 N1 M0 breast cancer described above is a Stage IIB cancer. A T3 N2 M0 cancer is Stage IIIA.

Staging and Treatment The significance of this classification is that treatment depends on the stage of the disease as defined by the TNM system. Your doctor has to know the stage to decide on appropriate therapy and to interpret the always evolving guidelines for treatment produced by major cancer centers and research groups.

This system has to be understood precisely so that very critical decisions can be made. Some stages of cancer are best treated surgically, others with radiotherapy, still others with chemotherapy. It is also becoming more and more common to use two of these treatment methods together and sometimes all three. Occasionally, they are given in sequence.

All these decisions are closely correlated with the stage of the tumor. In treating colon cancer, for example, chemotherapy with the drugs 5-fluorouracil and levamisole is given for Stage III cancer, but not for Stages IA or IIB. Similarly, Stage I prostate cancer may be treated surgically. But surgery is not usually an option by Stage III, when the tumor has extended beyond the prostate.

Although the TNM system is not applicable to all cancers—it is not used with lymphomas, for example—it has now replaced earlier classification systems for tumors in the colon and rectum and is used to stage many other kinds of cancer. As of 1991, it is the recommended staging system for most cancers.

AMERICAN JOINT COMMITTEE ON CANCER

Staging for Breast Carcinoma

T = Primary Tumor   **N** = Regional Lymph Nodes   **M** = Distant Metastasis

PRIMARY TUMOR (T)
T0	No evidence of primary tumor
Tis	Carcinoma in situ: Intraductal carcinoma, lobular carcinoma in situ, or Paget's disease of the nipple with no tumor
T2	Tumor more than 2 cm but not more than 5 cm in greatest dimension
T3	Tumor more than 5 cm in greatest dimension
T4†	Tumor of any size with direct extension to chest wall or skin

†NOTE: Chest wall includes ribs, intercostal muscles, and serratus anterior muscle but not pectoral muscle.

REGIONAL LYMPH NODES (N) (CLINICAL)
N0	No regional lymph node metastasis
N1	Metastasis to movable ipsilateral axillary lymph node(s)
N2	Metastasis to ipsilateral axillary lymph node(s) fixed to one another or to other structures
N3	Metastasis to ipsilateral internal mammary lymph node(s)

DISTANT METASTASIS (M)
MX	Presence of distant metastasis cannot be assessed
M0	No distant metastasis
M1	Distant metastasis (includes metastasis to ipsilateral supraclavicular lymph node[s])

© 1989, American Cancer Society, Inc.

STAGE GROUPING

Stage 0	Tis	N0	M0
Stage I	T1	N0	M0
Stage IIA	T0	N1	M0
	T1	N1*	M0
	T2	N0	M0
Stage IIB	T2	N1	M0
	T3	N0	M0
Stage IIIA	T0	N2	M0
	T1	N2	M0
	T2	N2	M0
	T3	N1, N2	M0
Stage IIIB	T4	Any N	M0
	Any T	N3	M0
Stage IV	Any T	Any N	M1

*NOTE: The prognosis of patients with pN1a is similar to that of patients with pN0.

2
HOW CANCER IS DIAGNOSED

Malin Dollinger, MD, and Ernest H. Rosenbaum, MD

───────◇───────

Cancer can be treated. But if it is going to be treated with any degree of success, it has to be detected in its early stages and a diagnosis quickly made. This isn't always easy because of the silent period of tumor growth—the months or years when the malignant cells are quietly doubling again and again. There may be absolutely no indication that this process is going on.

So how do we discover that the tumor is there? Your own complaint may be the tip-off. Or your doctor might pick up on some clue that appears during a physical. Whatever sets off the search for cancer, the investigative process that leads to a definitive diagnosis follows a standard pattern. Suspicions are aroused. Questions are asked. Doctors try to find answers through examinations, tests, images of body organs and analysis of tissues under a microscope.

SYMPTOMS
When a lump has grown to a certain size, its presence is signaled in a number of ways.
♦ It presses on nearby tissue, which sometimes produces pain.
♦ It grows into nearby blood vessels, which may produce bleeding.
♦ It gets so large that it can be seen or felt.
♦ It causes a change in the way some organ works. Trouble swallowing (dysphagia), for example, might be the sign of a tumor involving the esophagus, the passage between the throat and stomach. Hoarseness or change of voice might indicate a tumor in the larynx, or voice box.

These symptoms—pressure, bleeding, a mass or interference with function—are reflected in the American Cancer Society's list of *Seven Early Warning Signals*:

1. **C**hange in bowel or bladder habits.
2. **A** sore that does not heal.
3. **U**nusual bleeding or discharge.
4. **T**hickening or lump in breast or elsewhere.
5. **I**ndigestion or difficulty in swallowing.
6. **O**bvious change in wart or mole.
7. **N**agging cough or hoarseness.

Recognizing a symptom is the first critical step in the search for cancer. Unfortunately, many people don't pay any attention to these warning signals. They wait and wait, sometimes for months, before getting the medical attention that could save their lives.

The best chance of diagnosing cancer early depends on someone's thoughtful and perceptive awareness that something new has happened to his or her body—especially the appearance of one of these symptoms.

THE PHYSICAL EXAMINATION
The suspicion that a cancer is growing is often aroused during a routine physical examination, the major part of what should be a yearly checkup of your general health. The physical examination is a thorough, systematic and progressive search throughout your body for signs of

disease or abnormal function. To make sure that no significant area is missed, each physician generally develops his or her own standard pattern or sequence. Some start with the head and work down the body, others examine each organ system as a unit.

Whatever the pattern, a good physical examination with a view to detecting cancer involves a search of the entire body with a special emphasis on the parts that are most prone to malignancy.

♦ The nose and throat are examined. There is a quick and painless mirror examination of the larynx.

♦ The lymph node–bearing areas—such as the neck above the collarbone, under the arms and in the groin—are checked.

♦ Specific attention is paid to the breasts in women and the prostate gland in men.

♦ The abdomen is carefully pushed and probed to detect enlargement of any of the abdominal organs, especially the liver and spleen.

♦ Examination of the pelvic area in women, including a Pap smear, is essential to detect cancers of the cervix, uterus and ovaries.

♦ A probing of the rectum with a gloved finger is an essential part of the physical for both men and women.

During the examination, your doctor will ask you a lot of questions about various body functions. There will be specific questions about hoarseness, signs of gastrointestinal bleeding, constipation, swallowing problems, coughing up blood and so on. A "yes" answer to any of these questions leads to more detailed questions, more specific physical examinations and possibly to blood tests, x-rays or other studies.

You might also be asked questions about any family history of cancer, particularly among close relatives—parents, grandparents, aunts, uncles, brothers and sisters. Detailed answers to these questions will help in the search for any cancers with a genetic basis, such as some breast and colon cancers.

Suspicious findings in any part of the physical examination will lead to further tests. An enlarged lymph node in the neck, for example, might indicate a cancer that has spread from somewhere else. This will set off a vigorous search for the primary site. Persistent coughing, especially with blood, might lead the doctor to look directly inside your lungs with a special instrument (a bronchoscope) to detect tumors.

BLOOD TESTS

The next level of the diagnostic process involves a laboratory analysis of blood samples. Two categories of blood tests are used to help in the diagnosis of cancer.

Non-Specific Tests Most blood tests are non-specific. This means they can reveal an abnormality in the blood that indicates some illness, but not which one.

A blood count, for example, may show anemia. Why would you be anemic? Lots of reasons, including cancer. But the anemia may not be related to a tumor unless you have a history of bleeding in the bowel and x-rays show a cancer of the colon. Similarly, there are tests for liver function that indicate abnormalities in that organ. But the problem might be caused by gallstones, hepatitis, tumors or drug toxicity. Certain patterns in the test results will suggest tumors or some other cause of bile obstruction. Other patterns suggest hepatitis. But essentially these patterns are only important clues. They are not solutions to diagnostic questions.

There are so many tests used to detect abnormalities in different organ systems that physicians usually obtain a whole panel of them—blood counts, tests of metabolism (including levels of minerals such as calcium) and tests for the liver, kidneys or thyroid. The test results may suggest certain types of tumors, but no specific diagnosis can be made on the basis of these tests alone.

Specific Tests Other blood tests are fairly specific for particular kinds of cancer, often several kinds. These tests will be ordered if your doctor strongly suspects one of these cancers.

Tumor Markers The most important are tests for chemicals called tumor markers. These are produced by various types of tumors. Breast, lung and bowel tumors, for example, produce a protein called the carcinoembryonic antigen (CEA). Some inflammatory diseases may produce low levels of this chemical, but some tumors in these areas produce very high levels. If a very high CEA level is found, then a tumor is assumed to be present until proved otherwise. Similarly, prostate cancers and many cancers of the testicles and ovaries produce known chemicals.

Some very exciting research is now being done to find more and more accurate markers for different types of cancer. We can now envision the day in the not-too-distant future when specific blood tests will identify most human cancers. But at the moment, the few tests we do have are invaluable. They not only help make the diagnosis but are especially useful for keeping track of the cancer after treatment. If the marker is elevated at the time of diagnosis, then successful treatment should result in the level falling or disappearing altogether. The reappearance of the marker often signals a relapse. If that happens, even if no other sign or symptom appears, there would be a search for a new tumor and consideration would be given to retreatment.

Other Blood Tests When a cancer is in the blood cells themselves, tests of the blood and the blood-forming organs may be all that's needed to make the diagnosis. Cancer of the white blood cells—leukemia—can often be diagnosed by looking at a sample of blood taken from the finger or arm. The diagnosis can be confirmed by examining cells from the bone marrow, where these cells are made. Bone marrow analysis will also diagnose multiple myeloma, which is basically a malignancy of plasma cells in the marrow.

Table 1: Blood Tests Useful in Cancer Diagnosis

Non-Specific Tests

Alkaline phosphatase	elevated in bone and liver disease
SGOT and SGPT	elevated if there is liver damage
Bilirubin	elevated in liver disease, especially with bile obstruction
LDH	elevated in many diseases, including cancer
Uric acid	elevated in gout, cancers of the blood and lymph nodes, and after cancer treatment
Creatinine and BUN	elevated in kidney disease
Calcium	elevated in cancer that has spread to the bone, with tumors that produce parathyroid hormone-like protein and in multiple myeloma, as well as in some non-malignant diseases

Electrolytes (sodium, potassium, carbon dioxide, chloride)	these levels are useful in metabolic and endocrine disease, and for monitoring both nutritional status and the effects of treatment
Amylase	used to assess pancreatic disease

Specific Tests and Markers

Not all cancers produce these markers

CEA (carcinoembryonic antigen)	elevated in cancers of the colon, rectum, lung, breast and pancreas
CA-125	elevated in cancers of the ovary and uterus
CA 19-9	elevated in cancers of the colon, pancreas, stomach and liver
CA 15-3	elevated in breast cancer
Alpha fetoprotein (AFP)	elevated in primary liver cancer and some cancers of the testis
HCG (human chorionic gonadotropin)	elevated in some cancers of the testis and ovary and some lung cancers. Also elevated in pregnancy
Prostatic acid phosphatase (PAP)	markedly elevated in some cases of prostate cancer
Prostate specific antigen (PSA)	helpful in diagnosing prostate cancer, especially in detecting recurrent disease
Serum protein electrophoresis	abnormal gamma globulin (monoclonal "spike") is found in multiple myeloma
Serum protein immunoelectrophoresis (IgG, IgA, IgM)	similar to above, but can classify the type of abnormal gamma globulin present

TESTS OF FLUIDS AND STOOLS

Our bodies produce wastes—urine and stools—that can reveal clues about disease. But there are also other fluids that can be analyzed to detect cancer cells.

♦ The most familiar test of body fluids is the urinalysis that is part of a regular checkup. Analyzing the urine's composition can reveal all kinds of abnormalities. The presence of protein might indicate kidney disease. The level of sugar might indicate diabetes. Too many white blood cells can indicate an infection. Too many red blood cells could indicate bleeding, maybe because of a tumor, maybe from some other cause. If tumor cells are found, other tests will be done.

♦ A physical or x-ray examination may reveal the presence of fluid in the chest cavity, abdomen or joints. A needle can be inserted into these areas and the fluid drawn out for examination.

♦ A lumbar puncture, also known as a spinal tap, is a special procedure to remove fluid from the spinal canal. It involves the insertion of a needle between the vertebrae, after you've been given a local anesthetic. Tests can identify any infection, inflammation or cancer.

The Hidden Blood Stool Test Blood in the stools is always a sign of something going wrong in the digestive tract. Sometimes this blood can be easily seen in a bowel movement; most of the time it's all but invisible. One simple procedure to find out whether there is blood in the stools is called the occult (hidden) blood test. A small amount of stool is smeared on specially treated paper, then chemicals that will reveal blood are added. If blood is found, the upper and/or lower bowel will be examined with scopes or barium x-rays.

Blood in the stools is often caused by hemorrhoids, but a benign or premalignant tumor (a polyp) or a hidden cancer is always a possibility.

IMAGING TECHNIQUES

Any suspicious findings in the physical exam or the lab test results will make your doctor want to find out what is going on inside your body. He or she could just look inside directly, either with special instruments or by opening up some area. But the first step usually involves the use of one or more devices that produce images of suspicious areas.

These "imaging studies" may show a tumor in a specific organ and the image will help your doctor assess its size and whether it has involved surrounding tissues.

If you complain of indigestion, for example, your doctor may suspect stomach cancer. This would lead to an x-ray or endoscopy of the upper gastrointestinal tract. Lower digestive tract complaints such as constipation or bleeding might lead to an x-ray or endoscopy to diagnose a possible carcinoma of the colon. Blood in the urine may lead to an x-ray of the kidneys to confirm a suspected tumor in the

kidneys or bladder. And complaints of severe headaches, together with other symptoms of increased pressure in the head, may result in a CT scan of the head in search of a brain tumor.

Until fairly recently, radiography (x-ray) was the only imaging technique available. If x-rays couldn't answer critical questions in the diagnostic investigation, then a surgeon would have to open up the body to take a direct look. But new techniques have revolutionized the art and science of diagnosis. Some of the new techniques involve the use of x-rays, others do not.

X-rays This familiar imaging technique involves passing a small dose of electromagnetic radiation through a specific area of the body and onto a film. This produces a two-dimensional picture of the structures inside.

Bones and some other dense substances absorb more x-rays than other tissues, so they show up on the film as shadows that your doctor can interpret. But soft tissues can't be seen very well on x-rays. It is impossible to see the inside of a stomach, for example, without adding a substance that will prevent the x-rays from penetrating.

If your stomach is going to be x-rayed, you will have to swallow a barium "meal." The barium will improve the contrast and so produce a better picture. If your bowel is going to be seen, you will be given a barium enema. If your kidneys are going to be examined, another type of "contrast agent" may be injected into a vein to fill the kidneys, which will allow them to be seen.

A fluoroscope might also be used. This lets the doctor see a continuous, moving image. In this procedure, the x-ray beam strikes a small fluorescent screen and the image is amplified through a video system.

Nuclear Scans Radioactive isotopes that emit gamma rays can produce an image on photographic film or on a scintillation detector. Some of these isotopes, generally given by injection, are organ-specific, which means that they concentrate in that part of the body suspected of harboring cancer.

Different organs react to the isotopes in different ways. The isotopes used for liver scanning concentrate in normal tissues but are not taken up by cancer cells. So the image shows "cold spots" that may be cancerous areas. The isotopes used for bone scans, however, work in the opposite way. Cancer cells make the bone react to the isotope to a greater degree than normal bone, so "hot spots" light up the image of the skeleton. Hot spots can be produced by diseases other than cancer, however, such as bone injury or arthritis.

Angiography This is a very useful way to study the blood vessels in a specific area of the body. Angiography is sometimes used to diagnose and precisely locate tumors in the pancreas, liver and brain, especially when surgery is being considered.

Angiography is also used in some chemotherapy treatments, when a plastic tube (catheter) is placed in an artery to deliver anticancer drugs to the tumor. It is especially important in those cases to know the exact size of the tumor to make sure all of it is treated. It makes no sense to insert the catheters and then miss a portion of the tumor not supplied by the blood

vessel being used. Angiograms safeguard against this problem by defining the blood vessels within the tumor, which have a different quality and appearance than the arteries next to the tumor.

CT Scans For the past several years, computerized tomography (CT) scans have made it possible to see parts of the body that are difficult or impossible to view any other way. The images produced are far superior to those obtained by traditional x-rays. And the images are even clearer if you drink a contrast agent or get an injection before the scan is done.

The CT machine scans the area being investigated—chest, brain, abdomen or any other part of the body—by taking x-rays of one thin layer of tissue after another. A computer puts the images together to create a cross-section of the area. Total-body scans are also done.

Although there is higher x-ray exposure with CT scans than with conventional x-rays, *not* undergoing the procedure is much riskier if cancer is strongly suspected. The information from the scan is not only useful for diagnosis but is very helpful in planning treatment.

Magnetic Resonance Imaging (MRI) The MRI scan can complement or even supplant the CT scan in some cases. The images look similar to CT scan images,

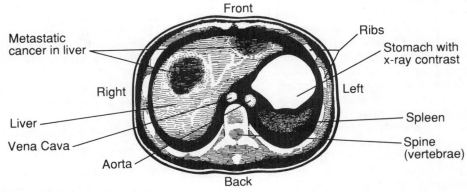

CT image of the upper abdomen, showing metastatic cancer in the liver.

but there are no x-rays involved. The MRI scanner uses a powerful magnetic field to make certain particles in the body vibrate. Extremely sophisticated computer equipment measures the reaction and produces the images.

MRI has a few important advantages apart from no risk of x-ray exposure. Cross-sections can be obtained not only across the body, as in CT scanning, but also from front to back and from left to right. This lets your doctor see your body from all three directions. In some cases, the images provide more information and are superior to those obtained by CT scans. This is especially true for images of the central nervous system and the spine.

MRI is not suitable under some conditions, however. Implanted devices such as a pacemaker, clip or pump can be affected by the strong magnetic field.

Ultrasound This is a harmless and painless imaging technique. It is "non-invasive," meaning that nothing enters your body except sound waves.

The technique involves spreading a thin coating of jelly over a particular area of the skin, then bouncing high-frequency sound waves through the skin onto internal organs. It works basically on the same principle as the sonar used by the navy to detect submarines, where sound waves are sent through the water and the "ping" of the sound bouncing back is analyzed. In a similar way, the complex ultrasound scanning apparatus draws a picture of whatever organ the sound waves are bouncing off. This picture can reveal a lot of information.

Many people are aware of ultrasound as a safe way to examine a fetus to search for abnormalities. But it is also useful for detecting possibly malignant masses or lumps without the need for x-rays.

Ultrasound is used to examine the neck for tumors of the thyroid gland or of the parathyroids. It is the standard method to diagnose gallstones, since the sound

waves bounce quite nicely off the stones. And it is often used in the pelvis to study possible enlargement of the prostate or an ovary. Benign ovarian cysts are common, and other ways of examining this part of the body are not very precise. It has also recently been adapted to help stage rectal and esophageal cancers.

ENDOSCOPY

Sometimes images are not enough. The use of direct visualization has become more and more important in recent years, not only for diagnosing malignancies but in some cases as an aid in treatment (*see* Chapter 9).

Rigid, thin telescopes have been used for years to look inside body cavities with natural openings. A bronchoscope inserted into the mouth or nose and through the windpipe (trachea) can be used to look inside the lungs. A cystoscope inserted into the urethra can be used to examine the bladder. Sometimes mirrors are used with these rigid scopes to examine, for example, the nasal passage and the back of the mouth (nasopharyngoscope) and the larynx (laryngoscope).

Flexible Scopes Lately, flexible fiber-optic "telescopes" have come into widespread use. These scopes use bundles of glass fibers that can bend around corners and form perfect pictures of the tissues at their far ends. Doctors looking through one end of the scope can look into many areas of the body safely, often with a minimum of sedation or local anesthetic. Not only can your doctor see exactly what's going on in these areas but he or she can also take photographs or remove cell samples.

The inside of the lung passages can be examined easily and quickly with the fiber-optic bronchoscope. A diagnosis of lung cancer can often be made by this method alone, without resorting to the surgical procedures that used to be necessary.

Similar instruments have revolutionized the diagnosis of tumors in the stom-

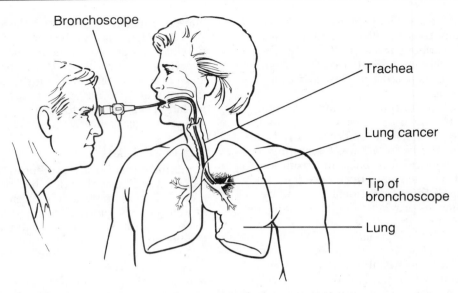

Bronchoscope

Trachea

Lung cancer

Tip of bronchoscope

Lung

Lung cancer can often be diagnosed and biopsied through a bronchoscope.

ach and bowel. With a flexible gastroscope or colonoscope, the entire stomach or colon can be clearly seen and pieces of tissue can be collected. Similar specialized instruments for other body cavities have made diagnostic procedures much safer. And the procedures can be repeated after treatment to see how effective the treatment has been.

ERCP Clever adaptations of these endoscopic methods and tools are sometimes used for specialized diagnosis and therapy. In a procedure called endoscopic retrograde cholangiopancreatography (ERCP), for example, a doctor can pass a flexible fiber-optic telescope into your stomach, visualize the opening of the ducts releasing bile from the liver, insert a tube into these ducts from inside the stomach and take pictures showing the exact location of tumors in the bile ducts and exactly how involved the ducts are.

A new technique is used when lung cancers partially or completely block air passages or when a tumor blocks the esophagus or colon. A beam of laser light can be passed through a flexible scope to create or enlarge an opening in the center of the tumor (*see* Chapter 9).

CYTOLOGICAL STUDIES

Cytology is simply the study of cells. In cancer diagnosis, the term cytological studies means the examination of cellular material removed from the body. The cells might be removed by natural means, such as coughing up sputum (phlegm). They might also be removed by washing a body cavity with a salt solution—the inside of the abdomen after abdominal surgery, for example—or by scraping the surface of an organ or a suspected cancer.

The best-known cytological test is the one developed by George Papanicolaou—the Pap smear. The cervix is scraped and brushed to remove for analysis cells that could be abnormal or cancerous. In the same way, the tongue, esophagus, stomach or the lung's air passages can be easily scraped using a small brush through a scope.

The removed cells are put on slides, stained with dyes and examined under a microscope. The cytologist will look for the characteristic appearance of malignant or pre-malignant cells. A pathologist will also examine the slides and either diagnose cancer or report a strong suspicion of cancer. In many cases, a conventional surgical biopsy will usually be done to confirm the diagnosis.

BONE MARROW ANALYSIS

Bone marrow is analyzed to diagnose blood or bone marrow cancers and to find out if a malignancy from somewhere else has spread to the bone marrow.

The procedure is simple and brief. It can be done in a doctor's office using a local anesthetic similar to the one used by your dentist. In much the same way as blood is taken from your arm, a needle is inserted into either the breast bone or the pelvic bone, both of which are just under the skin and are easily entered. A small amount of liquid bone marrow is drawn into a syringe, placed on slides and examined under a microscope for evidence of leukemia, lymphoma or any other cancer cells.

Sometimes a bone marrow biopsy may be done. A special cutting needle can be put into an anesthetized area of the pelvic bone and tiny bone chips can be removed. This procedure may be necessary for several reasons—to diagnose certain types of blood and bone marrow malignancies, to see if other cancers involve the marrow or as part of the staging process.

Bone marrow examinations are also sometimes done to check for infections, follow up the effectiveness of treatment or discover how well the bone marrow could produce blood cells if really aggressive chemotherapy were to be given.

BIOPSIES

Ultimately the diagnosis of cancer depends on examining a small bit of tissue to see if it has the characteristic patterns and cell types defined as cancer. In fact, the definitive way to diagnose a suspicious area is to go right to a biopsy even before doing other tests.

This microscopic examination is carried out by a pathologist who is expert in the very exact criteria that separate malignant cells from normal or benign ones. It is essential to obtain a specimen of tissue to do this examination. The biopsy is the procedure for obtaining the tissue.

There are two types:
♦ an incisional biopsy involves cutting into a portion of the tumor, then stitching the area closed;
♦ an excisional biopsy involves removing the entire tumor.

The excisional biopsy is often done with tumors that are easily accessible, such as those involving the skin, the mouth or nasal cavity, lymph nodes or a woman's reproductive system.

Biopsies are often done during the surgery that may be needed to expose the tumor. In such cases, it's customary to take tissue samples not only from the apparent site of the tumor but also from the lymph nodes or other tissues in the neighborhood. This will help measure the tumor's potential or actual spread. This defines the stage of the cancer, so the staging process may be carried out at the same time as the diagnostic process. Of course, the surgeon may also try to carry out the most appropriate therapy at the same time by removing all the visible tumor.

Needle Biopsies For easily accessible tumors and also for some tumors inside the body—in the kidney or pancreas, for example—needle biopsies have become quite common. In this procedure, an anesthetic is placed both in the skin and in the soft tissues under the skin. A very thin needle is then directed into the tumor, and a small bit of tissue is withdrawn for examination. This is called fine needle aspiration (FNA).

It's very important to be sure the needle is actually in the tumor, so needle biopsies of internal areas are often done in the x-ray department, where an x-ray machine or CT scanner can show the needle's position accurately.

Tumors in the lung and the liver can be diagnosed by a needle biopsy. Even a tumor involving a deep organ like the pancreas can be diagnosed in this way about 80 percent of the time. But the amount of tissue obtained through a needle is not usually enough to diagnose can-

cers of the lymph glands accurately.

A needle biopsy is not always advisable. When there are vital structures in the area—over the collarbone, for example—there is a risk of complications such as bleeding or nerve damage.

The Next Step Once the biopsy is performed and the diagnosis confirmed, the medical evaluation should be rapidly completed. At this point, treatment planning can begin.

Types of biopsy for cancer diagnosis

| Excisional biopsy
Complete removal of tumor | Incisional biopsy
Remove part of tumor | **A**
Fine needle
aspiration | **B**
Cutting needle
(core) biopsy |

3
WORKING WITH
THE HEALTH CARE TEAM

Ernest H. Rosenbaum, MD, Malin Dollinger, MD, Lenore Dollinger, RN, PhD,
and Isadora Rosenbaum, MA

After you've been diagnosed with cancer, you enter a world that is probably unfamiliar to you. The cancer treatment system is large and complex. Many different kinds of health care facilities and institutions are involved, and the system is populated by a bewildering array of professionals.

You may feel like you are being processed, sent from one place to another for tests or other procedures for reasons you don't quite understand. And at every turn, you meet new people who seem to speak a different language. It's easy to feel lost and disoriented in such a large system.

But it doesn't have to be that way. You simply have to remember that *you* are the one fighting for your life. And all the people and facilities are there to help you in your battle. Fighting cancer is fighting a war, and the more highly trained forces you can gather to attack the invader the more successful you are likely to be.

WHO DOES WHAT IN THE CANCER TREATMENT SYSTEM

Cancer treatment today is very much a team effort that emphasizes total care. A wide range of medical specialists, therapists, technicians, counselors, social workers and others become involved in your treatment and your rehabilitation.

Diagnosis If you have been diagnosed as having cancer, you have already come in contact with several members of the health care team, even if you haven't met them all personally.

♦ Your cancer symptom may have been detected by your internist or primary physician—whoever it is you call when you have a fever, a pain you think should be looked at or when you're just feeling generally sick. If you are a woman, the primary physician may have been a gynecologist. If your child has the cancer, the primary physician may have been a pediatrician. Or it may have been a specialist in family practice, still fondly remembered by some as a GP, or general practitioner.

♦ A laboratory technician may have drawn your blood for tests.

♦ The tissue for a biopsy may have been taken by your primary physician, by a general surgeon or possibly by a radiologist or medical oncologist doing a fine needle aspiration.

♦ Your tissue sample was then examined under the microscope by a pathologist, an expert in the analysis of tissue to identify disease.

Treatment Planning Once the diagnosis is made, the treatment team is assembled. Depending on the most appropriate kind of treatment for your particular tumor, you may deal with internists, surgeons or medical or radiation oncologists.

♦ Internists are specialists in many fields

of internal medicine. They may specialize, for example, in the blood (hematologists), cancer (oncologists), the endocrine system (endocrinologists), the gastrointestinal or GI tract (gastroenterologists), kidneys (nephrologists) or the brain and nervous system (neurologists).

♦ Medical oncologists—internists with additional training in the treatment of cancer—prescribe chemotherapy drugs as well as hormones and other biological agents.

♦ Surgeons—who cut out as much cancerous tissue as possible, ideally before it has a chance to spread—also often specialize, operating only on specific areas of the body. But you should be aware that medical practices aren't always the same in all communities. Most general surgeons, for example, will operate on organs in the abdomen. Most will operate on the colon and rectum, although in larger cities there are usually surgeons who specialize in this area of the body (proctologists). Some general surgeons do chest surgery, others don't. Some back operations will be done by neurosurgeons in some communities but by bone and joint (orthopedic) surgeons in others.

♦ Radiation oncologists are specialists in the use of high-energy x-rays to cause tumors to shrink. Within the radiation department, the radiation oncologist is supported by diagnostic radiologists, who interpret x-ray studies, and radiotherapy technologists and radiation physicists, who check the radiation dosage to make it as safe as possible.

Support Many other health care professionals work as a united team to help you through your cancer treatment and recovery.

♦ Oncology nurses play an essential role on the health care team. They have specialized knowledge and skill in giving chemotherapy and in meeting the special needs of cancer patients. They may specialize even further, as radiation oncology nurses, for example (*see* Chapter 15).

♦ Nutritionists evaluate any deficiencies in your diet and prepare individualized plans that take your condition into account and make sure you get enough nutrients.

♦ Physical therapists can make sure you maintain proper muscle tone and adapt to any changes to your body that result from treatment.

♦ Occupational therapists help teach activities of daily living—how to eat, swallow and use your body efficiently.

♦ Enterostomal therapists specialize in the care of ostomies.

♦ Respiratory therapists help you keep your lungs and breathing passages clear.

♦ Speech therapists work with people who have lost their voice box (larynx) and have to learn to speak in a new way.

♦ Psychologists, psychotherapists and other emotional counselors such as clergy and social workers help you through depression, fear or other emotional problems you may have because of your cancer or its treatment.

♦ Dentists evaluate the state of your mouth before treatment and help you deal with treatment side effects such as mouth sores.

♦ Cosmeticians ensure proper skin care during treatment and help you cope with physical changes.

♦ Laboratory technologists perform specialized blood tests.

♦ Pharmacists prepare complicated medications and ensure correct dosages.

♦ Technologists make sure that breathing machines, chemotherapy pumps, home oxygen equipment and other mechanical devices work properly at all times.

Direction As with any effective team, one person usually takes charge of the overall direction of the team's efforts. He or she is essentially the commander of the forces brought to bear on your cancer. He or she decides what "intelligence" information is needed, delegates specific tasks to the people best able to perform them, analyzes all the options and makes the key decisions.

Most important, he or she is the one who reports to you on your situation. How do things look? What can be done? What are the risks? What are the odds? What are the alternatives?

In some cases, the overall direction will be the responsibility of your primary physician. But since cancer treatment is so complex and so many specialists may be called in at various times, direction is now more often in the hands of an oncologist. And because medical oncologists are also specialists in internal medicine, they often assume overall responsibility.

There are many advantages to this chain of command. Medical oncologists see many cancer patients and are knowledgeable about the effects and likely results of the most up-to-date treatments. Oncologists also tend to do a lot of talking with you because cancer is serious business. Drugs are serious, radiation and surgery are serious, side effects are serious and so is the prognosis. Nothing is trivial.

CHOOSING AN ONCOLOGIST

There are several straightforward ways that an oncologist can become involved in your care. The most common is through a referral from your primary physician, who may recommend a specialist he or she has worked with before, has confidence in and is an expert in the specific kind of cancer care you need. Sometimes you may know a specialist yourself, either because of your own experience or the experience of a family member or friend.

It is unusual these days that you have to choose a specialist without any help from family, friends or general physicians. But if you do have to start from scratch, the American Cancer Society or other medical societies in your area can supply you with names of several qualified physicians.

When you are choosing an oncologist, you can look into his or her credentials in a number of ways, the easiest being to check the *American Medical Directory* or the *Directory of American Specialists* at your local library. The latter lists doctors who have had special training and have demonstrated their competence to a recognized medical certification board (such as the American Board of Surgery or the American Board of Internal Medicine). You can also call PDQ (Physicians Data Query) or, from within the U.S., 1-800-4-CANCER, a National Cancer Institute resource, for a list of specialists. There are excellent oncology specialists who have had full training and are competent and up to date yet are not board-certified. But if you are starting from scratch, the board certification may give you a little extra reassurance that you are in good hands.

UNDERSTANDING WHAT YOUR DOCTOR IS SAYING

Right from the time you hear the cancer diagnosis, the medical team has to get a lot of new information across to you and your family. This isn't always an easy process, either for you or for your doctor. Each stage of cancer care involves a tremendous amount of information that is generally unknown to the lay public. And all too often doctors use technical terms that any non-medical person has trouble understanding. Yet open and clear communication has become an essential part of a good medical relationship.

Cancer is a family affair. One member gets the disease, but the whole family goes through the experience. So it is very important that both you and your family know and understand all aspects of your disease. You should know how it is treated, what side effects there might be and how you best can cope. Trying to learn how to deal with your new life situation may improve how you cope with your treatment program.

The Initial Visit Exactly where and how you find out about the diagnosis isn't always up to you. Yet this first confrontation with the fact that you have cancer can affect your relationship with the disease, your doctor and the medical system.

Most doctors realize that difficult problems come up when someone is told he or she has cancer right in the recovery room after biopsy surgery. No one can fully appreciate what's going on in those circumstances. Most doctors also dislike telling someone he or she has cancer over the phone. It's very traumatic and it doesn't help the relationship. So doctors often try to make sure you are in a proper emotional state and have time to ask questions and discuss various aspects of treatment.

The proper emotional state is hard to achieve, though. Your initial visit to an oncologist's office can be a very trying experience. Fear and anxiety about cancer, no matter how controllable or curable it might be, often limit the effectiveness of the visit. And the diagnosis, once made, often makes you unable to concentrate on the information being given. Faced with a serious, life-threatening illness, it is often difficult to express feelings, ask questions or assimilate all the new information.

When you are under such emotional stress you often cannot think clearly. In our experience, one woman—a medical social worker—walked out of the office and her sister asked, "What did the doctor say?" She said, "I forgot." She hadn't even made it to the reception area.

Sharing the Information For this reason, many doctors encourage family members or close friends to come to the consultation. For this reason too, some doctors record the initial consultation and dictate the letter to the referring physician in front of the patient during the office visit. A separate tape to "translate" the technical letter and to explain the disease, treatment and side effects, along with pertinent questions and answers, can also be very helpful. In a study at Minnesota's renowned Mayo Clinic, it was found that patients had to listen to a taped explanation at least three times before understanding the whole message.

If your doctor tapes your initial consultation, you will find it very beneficial to take the tape home, listen to it as often as you need to, review it with your family and friends in a calm, relaxed atmosphere or even send copies to family members in other cities who wish to be informed.

Ignorance, confusion and unspoken fears can isolate people from one another. In a situation filled with anxiety, the isolation can be especially severe and painful. When family and friends share information about treatment plans, medications and side effects, cancer becomes more understandable and bearable for everyone concerned.

Besides reducing misunderstandings and improving communication, the use of audiotapes has the advantage of making the doctor's explanations more organized and concise. For the doctor, it will also mean fewer unanswered questions and fewer calls from family members trying to find out what's going on.

Getting More Information Besides the discussion and the audiotapes, your doctor may provide you with information in the form of handouts, pamphlets or recommended reading. These are available free from the National Cancer Institute, the American Cancer Society and many support organizations.

Pamphlets and books have their place in giving you both general and detailed information about your cancer and its treatment, but videotapes can accelerate the learning process. Videotapes may be especially important in the period just after your diagnosis because the emotional adjustment you have to make to having cancer can interfere with the concentration necessary for reading. A decrease in attention span and comprehension—a kind of emotional or mental paralysis, really—is not unusual. So videotapes to explain CT scans, radiation therapy, good nutrition, exercise or any other aspects of cancer and cancer therapy can be very helpful.

Videotapes also bring the family together to watch and learn and talk about the procedures shown. Videotapes can present helpful ideas on how to cope and how to solve simple problems such as how to set up a bedroom or tackle more serious problems. This can become a "quickie course" for family members to learn their role in supportive and home care.

The Doctor's Responsibility Doctors are well aware of the problems you and your family go through when you get the diagnosis of cancer. And your doctor does have a responsibility to reduce fears and confusion and to make it as easy as possible for you to understand what he or she is saying.

But not all doctors have learned to communicate effectively. If your doctor doesn't use techniques such as audio- and videotapes, ask about them. With your doctor's permission, perhaps you could take your own tape recorder into your consultations. Experience has shown that this technique promotes active discussion and doesn't intimidate physicians, patients or families.

COMMUNICATING WITH YOUR DOCTOR

When you have cancer, the worry, fears and concerns never stop, even after treatment. If your cancer is cured or permanently controlled, you always have that nagging fear that it might come back with a vengeance sometime in the years ahead. If it is not completely controlled, you worry that the treatment won't work, that you'll be a burden to your family or friends or that you'll suffer pain and disability. No matter how hard you try to put these fears to rest, they reawaken and rise

back up with each visit to the doctor.

You don't know whether you should be reassured by having extra tests or reassured by not having extra tests. You are always waiting for clear, definite answers to all the questions bombarding your brain. Am I really in remission? Is the cancer really gone? Will the pain go away? Can I go back to work? Will I ever feel safe? How long will I live?

While you are trying to understand everything your doctor is telling you, you may feel at a loss about how to get your concerns across. After all, you've had no training in how to deal effectively with specialists or even deal with that nagging voice in your head that keeps whispering all the questions and fears.

What Helps and What Blocks Communication Two main factors affect the way you communicate with your doctor. Both can either help the process along or block effective communication.
♦ Your attitudes and feelings about yourself and about your illness.
♦ Your need to be realistic, to understand your expectations and to express your needs clearly.

The attitudes and feelings that help communication are easy to list—openness, honesty, respect, clarity, responsibility, accountability and a willingness to listen and to learn.

What blocks effective communication are anger, resentment, dishonesty, intimidation and holding back information. And unless you do something to remove these blocks, you won't be receiving the best care your doctor can offer you.

Anger It isn't the anger you might feel about having cancer or anger over a test result that can hinder communication. It is a generalized anger that some people feel toward doctors, an anger that says "they charge too much, they never listen, they're insensitive, they don't really care, they think they're God."

25

You may have good reason to feel angry. Your doctor may keep you waiting for an hour and then spend only five minutes with you. It may take forever for your calls to be returned. Whether your anger is justified or not, communicate how you feel. If you don't say it openly, the anger will be communicated anyway and will always be a barrier to openness and honesty.

You can express your anger and still be respectful. Write down how you feel clearly and concisely. If you write it down it will be easier to speak without resentment. Then respect your doctor's time. Let the appointment desk know you want extra time during the next visit to talk about things that are bothering you and interfering with your ability to have a good working relationship.

When you tell your doctor how you feel, give him or her reasonable suggestions for resolving the problems, such as getting the first appointment of the day so you won't have to wait. Ask him or her what time calls are usually returned and say that you will call only at those times unless there's an emergency. Then stick to it.

Doctors know that anger is a secondary feeling, rising up in response to fear, anxiety or frustration. But doctors are also human and under a lot of pressure. So it might be difficult for your doctor to respond to you in a supportive way if you confront him or her only with anger. Ask yourself what lies beneath the anger—fear? rejection? disappointment?—and express those feelings. If it's emotional support you want and your doctor doesn't seem to have the time or compassion to meet your needs, ask if there is someone else who can. You have to be willing to accept your doctor's limitations but be unwilling to accept less than *you* need.

Intimidation This is a two-way street. Many patients feel intimidated by their doctors. Patients can be afraid that doctors will think they're stupid if they ask too many questions or not like them for taking up so much time. This is fear, pure

and simple. Make it work for you. Simply say, "I'm afraid to take up your time but I'm more afraid for myself." You'll be amazed how that kind of honesty can work for you.

The other side to intimidation is when the patient intimidates the doctor. If you think to yourself—or say right out (in a joking way, of course)—"I know as much as you do, so don't try to talk down to me," again recognize the fear at the source of this need to intimidate. Express this fear openly and honestly. If you really think your doctor is doing less than he or she should, talk about it and listen to how the doctor responds. Only then can you make a rational decision about what action you should take.

Withholding Information Holding back or not being completely honest and clear about how you feel not only blocks good communication, it puts your doctor at a terrible disadvantage and doesn't serve your best interests at all.

If you have a lot of new symptoms, you may be afraid of sounding like a hypochondriac or appearing to be too emotional. So when the doctor asks you how you are, you reply, "Just fine." When you say that, you lose a golden opportunity to communicate your needs. These new symptoms may be causing you all kinds of worry and distress, but by your two little words you've made sure that your doctor will not be able to put your mind at ease. You can only hope your doctor doesn't believe you.

And when your doctor explains a procedure, treatment or test result and asks if you understand, don't just automatically say, "Sure. Got it." If you don't really understand, say so. All pretending can do is add to your confusion and increase your anxiety.

Dealing with Fear It should be clear by now that the feeling of fear can block communication. If fear stops you from asking perfectly reasonable questions or accepting needed treatment or if it comes out as anger, it can badly damage your relationship with someone who is doing his or her best to make you well again.

But fear can also work for you in communicating with your doctor. Fear can make you stop and think for yourself. It can make you think seriously about all the alternatives before you and ask for explanations and support. Only then can you realistically evaluate the risks you have to take.

Talking About "What If. . .?" There is one subject that many cancer patients don't want to talk about. Sometimes this is called the "what if. . .?" scenario. What if the treatment doesn't help? What if everything that might help has already been done? What if the only goal now is to try to stay comfortable, physically and mentally?

It is hard to talk about all the aggressive treatments that might be used, the side effects and your critical need to always have hope, and at the same time discuss "what if?" You may not want to talk about it at all. You don't always need to. And your doctor will respect your wishes. But if you do want to discuss it, let your doctor know.

There is one aspect of "what if . . .?" that really should be discussed. If your situation does become grave, your doctor will need some guidance on how you want things handled. How heroic do you want your doctor to be, especially if the end seems near? If the situation does reach that stage, you may not be in any condition to discuss the question rationally. Your doctor may be able to talk it over with your family, but it is *your* wishes that are most important (*see* Chapter 28).

HOW YOU CAN HELP YOURSELF GET AN EFFECTIVE REVIEW

Fifteen minutes may not seem like a lot of time to cover critical information that may be important to your very survival. But a lot can happen during a fifteen-minute office visit. Unfortunately, a lot of time can also be used up by relatively trivial matters.

From the doctor's point of view, it sometimes may take about three minutes to cover the strictly medical procedures. A schedule for a chemotherapy program, the dosage and the side effects can be covered quickly. But a doctor has to deal with what happened last week, how you felt about things, what your hopes and fears are—all the secret things going on beneath the surface that might be important. So the other 12 minutes are often given to psychological evaluation and counseling, rather than purely technical matters.

All questions and problems are in some way important, but some are more important than others. And if you want to help yourself get the best chance of an effective review, there are certain rules or guidelines you should be aware of.

♦ *Focus on the matter at hand* Doctors try to take care of the most pertinent issues first. The doctor's most important questions will be about what's happening with you right now. Do you have a sore mouth? Are you losing weight? Do you have any major complaints? Do you have diarrhea? What's new since your last visit? The doctor then has to try to analyze and make sense of what's changing. Doctors are always trying to anticipate changes so they don't have to play "catch-up." Until you have a problem, your doctor can't solve it. So give the clearest, most detailed answers you can without holding anything back. It might help if you keep notes of significant symptoms or events that you noticed between visits.

♦ *Be cooperative* Every doctor has seen

patients who, because of anxieties—the fear of illness or death—simply aren't cooperative. They object to having extra blood tests or doing things that are sometimes necessary but that they simply don't want to do. When they come into the office, they should undress for an examination, yet some say, "I don't want to get undressed today." That's not the best way to get help. You have to follow certain patterns and be cooperative if you expect results.

♦ *Avoid raising irrelevant problems* Your doctor is always ready to deal with important problems like weight loss or nausea or a swollen arm or leg. When all that has to be covered during the office visit, it's hard to deal with a stubbed toe or whether the pimple on your backside has to be removed. Talking about a half-dozen minor problems can use up half the appointment. Of course, the doctor realizes that what you are really saying is, "I'm scared. I'm frightened for my life." But still, discussing extraneous problems is not the most effective use of office time.

♦ *Ask the pertinent questions* Unless you try to limit your questions to the most essential problems, you lose both focus and the chance for better explanations. All questions are relevant, but if you take a long list of questions you're going to defeat yourself before you begin. As a patient, you have an obligation to be practical and to do your best to work with your physician rather than frustrate each other.

4
DECIDING ON THE APPROPRIATE TREATMENT

Malin Dollinger, MD, and Ernest H. Rosenbaum, MD

"Cancer is one of the most curable chronic diseases in this country today."
—*Vincent T. DeVita, Jr, MD*

Medicine has now reached the stage where almost half of all diagnosed cancers are cured. Of course, this statistic is an average. The cure rate for some cancers is much higher than for others. And some cancers can come back even after the "five years cancer-free" that is used to define "cure."

But even with cancers still considered incurable, proper therapy often yields tremendous benefits. Treatment can add months or years to a reasonably normal life. It can also greatly improve the quality of your life by relieving pain or ensuring the relatively normal functioning of your body processes. Many people live a normal life span with chronic cancer before succumbing to some other disease.

Unfortunately, far too many people still think a cancer diagnosis is a death sentence. Far too many take the attitude that if it can't be cured there's no point in undergoing treatment. What is even more unfortunate is that this attitude is found not only among people with cancer and the lay public but within the medical community.

In many cases, cancer truly is an incurable disease. But it's not the only one. Diabetes and heart disease can't be cured, but they can be treated on an ongoing basis. They're treated all the time. Few people take the "why bother?" attitude with either of them. Why? Because they know both can be managed day by day

and that people with either disease can lead long, active and productive lives. The same can be true for cancer patients.

The key to getting the chance for cure or successful management is getting the best treatment as soon as possible after your diagnosis. What that treatment is, you will have to help decide. Yes, you should rely on experts with training and experience in fighting cancer. But it's your life on the line, and ultimately, the decisions must be yours. And you will have to base those decisions on a detailed analysis of your disease and the recommendations of your primary physician or cancer specialist.

WHAT ARE THE OPTIONS? A TREATMENT OVERVIEW

The three mainstays of cancer therapy over the years have been surgery, radiation and chemotherapy. These have now been joined by biological therapy, which uses the body's immune system to combat growing cancer cells. The goals, procedures, risks and side effects of each of these four kinds of therapy (sometimes referred to as modalities) are detailed in the next four chapters. Here, the treatment options are briefly reviewed.

 Surgery This is the oldest and most successful approach to cancer treatment. If it is possible to "cut it out" safely and there is no residual disease, you may be cured. Two key questions have to be answered when deciding if surgery is the right thing to do.

♦ Is the tumor just in one place (localized)? Once the cancer has spread, surgery may or may not be appropriate.

♦ Can the tumor be removed without damaging vital organs or causing major functional problems? A cancerous lung or a kidney can be removed because everyone has a spare. But a surgeon can't cut out the whole liver or vital parts of the brain.

There are two surgical approaches. In the one-stage approach, the diagnostic biopsy might be followed immediately by the removal of the tumor while you are still under anesthesia. After the operation, you can discuss whether you need additional therapy and what the most effective method or sequence would be, particularly if several therapies might be realistic alternatives.

In the two-stage approach, only the biopsy is done. You then discuss the results with your doctor. If the biopsy shows cancer, you and your doctor plan the definitive cancer treatment. If surgery is an option, the operation to remove the tumor will then be carried out.

 Radiation Therapy The purpose of radiation is to make tumors shrink or disappear. Radiation does this by damaging the genetic structure (DNA) of the tumor cells so they can't grow or divide. The damage is done by a beam of x-rays, gamma rays or electrons aimed directly at the tumor from a high-energy x-ray machine set up at a specific distance from your body or by radioactive materials placed inside or close to the tumor.

There is no pain or discomfort during radiation therapy. Undergoing treatment is much the same as having a chest x-ray, except the machine is left on for several minutes instead of a second or two. Radiation may be the only treatment need-ed for some localized cancers, or it might be used along with other kinds of therapy.

 Chemotherapy This term is often misunderstood. What it means is treating some medical condition with chemicals (drugs). Treating cancer with 5-fluorouracil is chemotherapy. So is treating an infection with penicillin or a headache with two aspirins.

Yet when chemotherapy is mentioned in connection with cancer, the term generates a lot of fear. Almost everyone has heard horror stories about serious side effects. These side effects can be unpleasant, but they are in general greatly exaggerated. It's true that a few people cannot tolerate chemical therapy at all. But most can tolerate it reasonably well. Others have moderate to significant reactions. When approaching the subject, also keep in mind that many drugs are used in chemotherapy and not all of them have serious side effects. The side effects themselves can often be reduced or controlled by antinausea drugs or other medications.

While surgery and radiation treat cancers that are growing in one particular place, chemotherapy is generally used for cancers that have traveled through the blood and lymph systems to many parts of the body. In the past, chemotherapy was used only when surgery and radiation were no longer effective. But now it is the treatment of choice for some kinds of cancer and is often used in combination with surgery and radiation, especially for localized cancers.

 Biological Therapy This is a relatively new way to treat cancer. It takes advantage of recent research that shows that the immune system may play a key role in protecting the body against cancer. The immune system might even play a part in combating cancer that has already developed.

The immune system consists of white blood cells called lymphocytes that act as a defense system against foreign organisms such as bacteria and viruses. One type of lymphocyte—the T cell—is formed in the thymus gland and is a natural killer of foreign cells, including cancer cells. Another lymphocyte—the B cell—is produced in the bone marrow and lymph nodes and makes antibodies in response to stimulation by a foreign protein. B lymphocytes can also kill cancer cells. Another white cell—the monocyte—interacts with T and B cells.

Biological therapy consists mainly of using highly purified proteins—interferon and interleukin-2 are the best known—to activate the immune system. In many different ways, they boost the lymphocytes' cancer-killing properties.

COMBINATION AND ADJUVANT THERAPIES

Five or 10 years ago it was common to think about treating cancer only by surgery *or* radiation *or* chemotherapy, depending on the stage of the disease. Two or all three therapies might be used, but usually only one at a time and in the sequence mentioned—surgery if the tumor was localized, then radiation if there was an actual or potential recurrence, then chemotherapy if the cancer involved vital organs or had spread so far that surgery or radiation had to be ruled out.

Recently there has been great interest in using what is called combination or multimodality treatment. Many aggressive forms of cancer therapy incorporate two or three of the standard treatment methods. There is no universal agreement yet on what the best combination or best sequence is for most malignancies. But broad principles have emerged.

♦ When tumors are large, locally aggressive and touch adjacent structures, radiation or chemotherapy might be given before surgery. This will shrink the tumor

and make the surgical procedure much simpler. In hospitals with special radiotherapy equipment, radiation will sometimes be given during surgery to kill invisible or microscopic tumor cells that might cause the cancer to come back in the future.

♦ Both radiation and chemotherapy may be given after surgery. Radiation will usually be used if the surgeon finds during the operation that the tumor is invading nearby tissues that couldn't be removed.

♦ Radiation and chemotherapy have also been combined in an attempt to produce a more powerful antitumor effect than either treatment can produce alone. Radiation, for example, has a more powerful killing action against smaller tumors, so chemotherapy is sometimes used to shrink the tumors before radiotherapy.

A number of procedures (clinical protocols) use both methods—together or in sequence—to take advantage of the increased sensitivity a tumor may have when both treatments are used. The combined therapy does not usually produce more toxic effects, side effects or complications than each treatment produces on its own. But the dosages of both may sometimes have to be reduced to prevent really major side effects.

♦ The new biological therapies—interferon alpha, beta and gamma, interleukin and other investigational programs—are being blended with standard radiotherapy and chemotherapy. But research on these combinations is still in a fairly early stage. It will probably be several years before it is known what sequence, dosage or combination is the most helpful or even whether adding biological therapies to the others is more effective than today's standard treatments.

Adjuvant Chemotherapy The purpose of giving chemotherapy after surgery—called adjuvant therapy—is to wipe out tumor cells that may be invisible to the surgeon's eye but that might cause a recurrence later on. There has been a great deal of interest in using chemotherapy after surgery because studies of experimental tumors in animals have shown that chemotherapy can cure very small tumors. In fact, chemotherapy is most effective when tumors are so small that they are invisible. Adjuvant radiation therapy is also given after surgery to kill remaining cancer cells.

The interest in adjuvant therapy has been especially high in the treatment of breast cancer. Women whose breast cancer has spread to the lymph glands under the armpit (axilla) have a high probability of cancer showing up in other parts of the body within 10 years after surgery. Studies have now shown that almost half the premenopausal women who otherwise would have a recurrence can be cured by adjuvant therapy.

HOW YOUR PHYSICIAN DECIDES ON THE BEST TREATMENT

Making the decision on which treatment to use is a stepwise process. It really begins with the suspicion of cancer aroused by signs or symptoms, then proceeds through the diagnostic process outlined in Chapter 2. Once the diagnosis is confirmed by a positive biopsy, several factors have to be considered.

The Stage How far along the tumor is in its development is the most critical factor. Sometimes the stage isn't known until a surgeon actually has a look at the tumor. But there are other ways to find out what stage the malignancy has reached.

During the staging process many parts of the body will be searched for evidence of cancer. Tests will discover the extent of the spread and the involvement with other tissues at the primary site. This will involve blood tests to see how organs such as the kidneys and liver are functioning. Imaging techniques such as chest x-

rays and CT scans will be used to see if there is any involvement of the lungs either directly or by spread.

Other specialized tests will be ordered according to the primary site and the type of tumor being investigated. Each type of cancer has a typical pattern of spread, so different specific areas of the body will be investigated in each case.

Prostate cancer, for example, usually spreads to bone, so bone scans, bone x-rays and blood tests will be quite important. Lung cancers can spread to the center of the chest (mediastinum), an area that can be mapped with a CT scan and looked at directly through a scope (mediastinoscopy). Cancers of the stomach and bowel commonly spread to the liver, so liver scans and blood tests will be needed to be sure about those areas.

It is important to understand that *when a cancer spreads, it remains the same cancer*. A breast cancer that spreads to the bone does not become bone cancer. If it spreads to the lung, it does not become lung cancer. Wherever it lands, it grows as breast cancer. It's like blowing the seeds off a dandelion—whether the seed lands in a field, a forest or a crack in a sidewalk, what grows is still a dandelion.

This is important because cancer treatment depends mainly on where the tumor starts, *not* where it lands.

The Biology of the Disease An analysis of the disease—its cell type, biology and expected behavior—is an important factor to consider. The tumor's biology strongly affects the likelihood of a particular therapy slowing down or stopping the disease process.

State-of-the-Art Alternatives Once the staging process is completed, your doctor has to consider all the treatments that might be appropriate considering the type of tumor, the site of origin and the stage of spread. In some cases, only one specific therapy may be generally accepted as appropriate. But in many cases, a variety of approaches might be used.

Cancer treatment is always evolving. Every year new discoveries are made and old methods are modified or discarded. It's hard even for specialists to keep up with all the developments in the field. But there are several ways your primary physician can find out about the most current treatment methods that are considered state-of-the-art.

♦ Tumor specialists (medical oncologists) are often consulted at this stage. So are surgeons or specialists in radiotherapy.

♦ The most recent medical literature can be reviewed, perhaps along with a computer search of your disease via a database like PDQ (*see* Chapter 31).

♦ Physicians and specialists attend many of the hundreds of cancer meetings that take place every year where important research findings and other cancer information are presented.

Tumor Boards Another way to get information and discuss the best treatment, especially with unusual types of cancers, is to attend a meeting called a Tumor Board. These boards are held frequently in all hospitals where cancer treatment is offered. They allow a group of doctors specializing in cancer to meet, discuss particular cases and give their opinions about the advantages and disadvantages of treatment alternatives. It is very common at this meeting for biopsy results to be presented and explained by the pathologist and for the radiologist and nuclear medical specialists to present all the x-rays and scans.

Your primary physician or oncologist will present your case (anonymously) so that each physician there has the same information your doctor has in making his or her decision.

In many larger hospitals there are specialty Tumor Boards that review cases in one particular field—breast cancer, urologic cancer, gynecologic cancers or head and neck cancers, for example.

When it comes to recommending treatment then, your doctor has had the benefit of input and ideas from a wide range of professionals.

Personal Factors: Benefits and Risks
Which treatment is finally recomended will also depend on such personal factors as your age, other medical problems (which might make surgery risky) and especially the possibility of significant side effects with one or another treatment.

Age comes into the decision because the patient who is forty years old may be able to tolerate the aggressive chemotherapy drugs that bring about a substantial rate of remission. The same drugs given to an eighty-year-old could be risky. At that age the kidneys don't function as well as they do earlier in life and the risk of therapy could outweigh the potential benefit. But each case has to be decided on its own merits.

Both you and your doctor have to consider the relative advantages and disadvantages of each therapy. You have to weigh the chances of achieving remission or cure with the risks and side effects of treatment. You and your family are partners with your physician in this decision-making process.

Your Decision In making the final decision on treatment, nothing replaces a good discussion between you and your doctor. He or she should be able to explain to you the staging process, the tests that were done, their results and all the available methods of treatment.

He or she may present the information from any Tumor Board that was held. Or he or she can sometimes pass on the consensus of the informal consultations with other doctors that often take place in medical groups having several physicians involved in the cancer field. Your doctor should also have alternative forms of therapy in mind and should outline what could be done if your tumor doesn't respond to treatment or if some other problem comes up.

Informed Consent There may be legal principles regarding "informed disclosure" that come into play during these discussions. In the State of California, for example, patients with breast cancer must be given a pamphlet published by the State describing the various methods of primary treatment and the advantages and disadvantages of each. Although this document appears to be comprehensive, its coverage of many important areas is incomplete and outdated.

A brochure certainly cannot replace the important and key discussion between physician, patient and family. Nothing can. This initial comprehensive discussion about deciding on therapy is *the most important single meeting* that you have with your physician. It forms the basis for all of the decision-making that follows.

WHEN AND HOW TO ASK FOR A SECOND OPINION

As noted, by the time your doctor explains the recommended treatment to you, he or she has probably already reviewed the literature, consulted other doctors, met with pathologists and radiologists, drawn on his or her own experience and perhaps met with a Tumor Board.

Nevertheless, you may still feel insecure about the treatment options you've been given. You might want to discuss them with another physician. This is a perfectly acceptable, rational and appropriate thing to do.

There should be no hesitation on your part in asking your doctor if he or she would have another specialist review all the material relating to your case. Second opinions are not unusual. They are actually required by some insurance companies.

In view of your need for a continuing relationship with your primary physician or specialist, it would be helpful to express your satisfaction with his or her decision and care. You can simply say that you wish to have someone else review the case to assure yourself that your decision to accept treatment will be made on the most thoroughly informed basis possible.

Who to Consult You may have a certain consultant in mind or you might ask your doctor to select a senior specialist in your city or at a major medical center, depending on your diagnosis. Many times your oncologist may recommend a second opinion and refer you to a local specialist or a specific cancer center where researchers with a special interest in your disease are working. Your doctor should have no hesitation in making your case material, including slides and x-rays, available to the second opinion consultant. This consultation is generally done fairly quickly so it does not delay treatment.

It is not a good idea to get a second opinion "in secret." Ultimately, it is not in your best interest. Second opinion consultations are done by physicians for physicians. They are done to review and help improve your medical care. Consultants cannot really evaluate your case properly unless they have at least the same information your primary doctor has, including the slides, x-rays and results of laboratory tests and other procedures.

Don't think your doctor will take offense or feel hurt. Your doctor should welcome the opportunity to satisfy your need for a second opinion.

CONSIDERING A CLINICAL TRIAL

Depending on the type and stage of your cancer, your doctor might recommend a new kind of treatment. The word investigational might come up. Or experimental might be the term used. If the standard treatment options available to you aren't likely to be effective, your doctor might simply suggest that you take part in a "clinical trial."

All these terms might make you feel more than a little anxious. They shouldn't. Investigational treatments that are being given a clinical trial are used only under very stringent conditions. They wouldn't be used at all if there wasn't some hope they would be more effective than other treatments.

What a Clinical Trial Is Advances in cancer treatment are rarely made by one scientist or physician working with a single or even a few patients. Advances usually come about because of some clever idea or concept for a new therapy proposed by a cancer research physician. This idea is eventually tested in a large number of patients to find out two things: Is it effective? And is it as good as or better than conventional treatments?

It takes several hundred and sometimes several thousand patients to prove quickly and reliably whether a new treatment will work and is worthwhile. It is almost impossible to conduct a trial in any single hospital or cancer center. The concept of cooperative clinical trials was developed for just this reason. The rules and procedures for clinical trials are standardized and quite specific.

The Clinical Protocol A clinical trial consists of an exact written description of a treatment program that is called the clinical protocol. This is formulated and written with great care. Not only do the researchers need to be sure that the trial will answer the two main questions about effectiveness, but the rights of the patients being treated have to be safeguarded too. The risks involved have to be minimized and disclosed.

The clinical protocol outlines the criteria for patients who might participate in the trial. It also describes what tests will be done and how the researchers will determine if a tumor is responding. Systems for monitoring the patient and checking for any adverse effects will be detailed. And there will be provisions for "informed consent."

Who Approves the Trial The entire project has to be approved by a Human Use Committee made up of physicians and non-physicians who have no relationship with the study. The members of this committee certify that the patient's rights are protected, that the trial is reasonable and logical and that the study will answer the question it is supposed to answer. These same committees review the studies again during and after completion of the trial as originally proposed. The Cancer Therapy Branch of the National Cancer Institute also keeps watch on these investigational studies.

The Importance of Clinical Trials Almost every advance in cancer treatment over the past 20 years has come about because of clinical trials. In fact, just about every chemotherapy drug and radiation treatment now considered standard therapy was first given in a clinical Phase I trial. These treatments were given to patients who were willing to be in the forefront of advances in medical knowledge.

The willingness of thousands of women to participate in clinical trials by the National Surgical Adjuvant Breast Project (NSABP), for example, has resulted in answers being given to extremely important treatment questions. These trials have formed the basis for adjuvant chemotherapy in breast cancer patients with a high risk for recurrence even though no apparent tumor is left after surgery. This has saved many lives. All because of the usefulness of these clinical trials.

The Three Phases of Clinical Trials Whether for surgery, chemotherapy, radiotherapy or biological therapy, clinical trials are always conducted in three phases.

A chemotherapy clinical trial, for example, proceeds this way:
♦ *Preliminary* After a new anticancer drug has been found to be effective against one

or more experimental tumor systems in the lab, it is tested in rats or other small animals to find out which dosage might be both effective and reasonably safe.

♦ *Phase I* About 20 human patients are treated with the same drug. There is no assurance or certainty that a significant tumor response will occur, although, again, every single anticancer drug now useful in therapy was initially a Phase I agent.

Patients selected for these trials are almost always in cancer research centers and have already received all known effective anticancer therapy. After the proposed treatment is explained to them, they may volunteer to receive the new treatment. There is, therefore, no moral objection to giving this new treatment. Since there is "nothing to lose," it is hoped that a specific new agent may in fact prove effective.

This phase is completed when no unusual problems or toxic effects have been found and the dose necessary to produce a biologic effect has been determined. The study can then move to the next phase.

♦ *Phase II* Ten to 20 patients are treated, each with various types of tumors known to be responsive to chemotherapy. These might include lymphomas, breast cancer or colon cancer. Since these tumor types are known to be responsive, the patients will be those who have already received all standard forms of therapy that seem reasonable. The use of a Phase II trial does not deprive anyone of any therapy known to be effective. If a significant number of patients with each type of tumor respond to the therapy, the trial moves to the next level.

♦ *Phase III* In this phase the new therapy is compared with standard treatment to see if there is an improvement in the response or if the same response rate is achieved but with less-toxic side effects.

A therapy tested in a clinical trial does not necessarily involve a drug not already in clinical use. A new treatment often con-

sists of standard drugs used in a new combination or a new sequence, in new dosages or even simply given in a new way. But if a new drug is involved and the Phase III trial is successful, the National Cancer Institute will approve the drug for general use. Eventually, the new therapy might become the standard therapy.

Clinical Trials and the "Approved" Uses of Drugs When using anticancer chemicals, it is important for both you and your doctor to be aware of how the pharmaceutical industry works. Once drug companies have fulfilled the lengthy and complex testing— and the drawn-out legal procedures— required to market a new drug, they tend *not* to devote a lot of effort to discovering new uses for that drug. They more or less delegate this responsibility to the cancer physicians conducting clinical trials.

But every drug comes with an official "package insert" detailing what dose to use for what illness. This information is also listed in the *Physician's Desk Reference*. These summaries usually contain only the information "passed" by the government's approval agencies. Why this is important is that many drug programs in standard use are not listed as "approved." They are used because experience with patients has shown they are effective. About *half* of all the current uses of anticancer drugs in the United States and Canada are for indications and schedules *not* given in the official inserts.

Since the inserts do not necessarily reflect the most up-to-date cancer research, the current standard use of these drugs, nor even their optimum use, your doctor should not be restricted to printed drug-listing materials.

This is another reason why an oncologist can be a useful member of your health care team. Cancer physicians are up to date on the most recent research findings and important advances in treatment even though that information may not appear in the drug-related literature.

5
WHAT HAPPENS IN SURGERY

Carlos A. Pellegrini, MD

◇

If you have cancer, there is a very good chance that you will see a surgeon during the course of your treatment. Surgery plays a crucial role in treating the disease. It is the oldest form of treatment and also the most effective. More cures are achieved by surgery than by any other form of therapy.

Surgery's role in cancer treatment has expanded considerably over the past few years. Better understanding of the natural history of many tumors, safer anesthetic techniques and improved pre-operative and post-operative care have led to better immediate and long-term survival rates. Surgeons can now also plan operations more effectively because a tumor's size and location can be determined more precisely with modern imaging techniques.

Surgery can support other treatment methods too. For example, the development of pumps and similar devices that allow precise, continuous and comfortable delivery of drugs has added a new dimension to cancer treatment. So has the implanting of radioactive seeds to deliver measured doses of radiation to internal tumors. Surgery is critical to the effective use of these techniques.

WHY SURGERY MIGHT BE RECOMMENDED

Since surgery is used in the diagnostic, treatment and post-treatment phases of cancer management, your primary physician or oncologist might suggest surgery in a variety of circumstances. The many different types of surgery each have their own

goals. In general, there are eight reasons why surgery might be recommended.

♦ *To prevent or lower the risk of developing cancer* Some benign diseases associated with a high risk of developing cancer are commonly referred to as pre-cancerous conditions. To avoid the risk of cancer, therefore, it may be beneficial to remove an organ affected by one of these diseases.

Ulcerative colitis, for example, is a benign inflammatory condition of the large bowel. Colon cancer develops in about 40 percent of people whose large bowel has been affected by the disease for over 20 years. If a younger person has ulcerative colitis affecting the entire colon, then it *may* be appropriate to remove the colon before cancer appears.

Any operation performed to prevent cancer—commonly called prophylactic surgery—must be discussed in detail by both you and your doctor. The risks of developing cancer have to be weighed carefully against the risk of surgery itself and the permanent changes that surgery will cause. The situation may not always be clear and options may be possible. In such cases, you, the surgeon and your oncologist have to study all the facts and decide on a course of action that takes your preferences into account.

As an example, consider that several risk factors significantly increase the chance that some women will develop breast cancer. A prophylactic mastectomy would prevent the breast cancer but would also result in the loss of the breast.

Whether to perform the surgery is up to the woman. Some women may feel more comfortable avoiding surgery at an early stage and living with the risk. Others may feel otherwise.

♦ *To diagnose or stage the disease* Although many non-surgical techniques can diagnose cancer accurately, in most cases it is still necessary for an oncologist planning therapy to have a sample of tissue to analyze. A surgeon can remove a small amount of tissue by inserting a very fine needle into the area of the tumor and drawing out a few cells to be examined under a microscope. This needle aspiration—or aspiration cytology—is the easiest and most comfortable technique used to obtain sample cells, but the very small amount of tissue involved may not be enough for an accurate diagnosis.

When more tissue is needed, a larger needle can obtain a "core" of tissue for microscopic examination. If that sample is still not enough, a small operation—an incisional biopsy—may be performed to remove a portion of the tumor. When the tumor is small, the surgeon might do an excisional biopsy, meaning that the entire lesion is removed rather than just a sample of it. This is very common with skin lesions, where the doctor has to know whether the lesion is a benign condition, malignant melanoma or some other skin cancer.

To stage the disease properly a more formal operation may be needed to obtain tissue from several areas of the body. This is common with lymphomas, where a staging laparotomy—opening and examining the abdomen—may be required to remove sample tissues from the liver and lymph nodes and to remove the spleen.

It is important to remember that diagnostic surgery is just that—an operation designed merely to obtain tissue to confirm a diagnosis or to help plan adequate treatment. The goal is not to cure the cancer.

♦ *To remove the primary tumor* For many cancer patients, removal of the tumor may be the best form of treatment. In some cases, surgery might lead to a cure. This form of surgery is referred to as surgery for the primary lesion. For this to be possible, the tumor has to be localized in an organ or area of the body that can be safely removed.

This type of surgery generally involves a major operation requiring admission to the hospital, general anesthesia and several days for recovery. The surgeon will try to remove the affected organ or area along with an adjacent area—called the margin—of normal-looking tissue. This is done because cells and small parts of the tumor may extend beyond what the surgeon can see as obvious cancer.

The lymph glands connected to the organ with the tumor might also be removed, since most tumors spread to lymphatic glands quite early. Removing the nodes along with the tumor improves the chance of removing all the cancer and, therefore, the chance of cure.

The removal of the tumor, lymphatic tissue and a rim of normal-looking tissue is referred to as a radical operation, and is the most common operation performed when attempting to cure the cancer.

After the operation, the surgeon passes the entire specimen—the "gross" (visible) cancer, the margin and the lymphatic glands—to a pathologist for examination under a microscope. The pathologist will be able to find out the exact kind of tumor involved and how far it extends into normal tissues and glands. As always, the extent of the tumor determines the prognosis and the need for additional forms of therapy. It usually takes two or three days for a specimen to be processed and examined, so the surgeon will not usually be able to discuss the final diagnosis or prognosis with you or your family for a few days after surgery.

♦ *To remove other tumors* Besides removing the primary tumor, surgery may also be performed for residual, metastatic or recurrent lesions. Surgery for "residual" tumors means that the operation has been preceded by radiation therapy or chemotherapy. The idea is that certain tumors shrink or even disappear with radiation or chemotherapy and that the surgeon can then remove the rest of the affected organ.

In other cases, after the original tumor is removed the surgeon may remove the metastases, those small cancer cells that have broken off the tumor and spread to other organs. Patients with colon cancer, for example, who develop a single metastasis to the liver and in whom there is no other evidence of disease can benefit from the removal of the metastatic tumor.

Finally, if the tumor has returned at the original site—"recurrent" disease—the surgeon may attempt a second removal of the tumor. This operation may be performed with some melanomas or breast cancer, for example.

♦ *To relieve symptoms* Some tumors produce mechanical problems in the body. If the tumor becomes large enough to block some part of the gastrointestinal tract, food cannot move properly through the system. A large tumor could also block the biliary tract so that bile could not get into the intestine. Or a tumor could press on a nerve and cause pain. When the tumor cannot be removed safely, surgery can still be useful to bypass an obstruction or relieve the compression on a nerve. This kind of surgery is referred to as palliative.

Other symptoms caused by tumors can also be palliated. A cancer of the stomach may bleed a lot, for example. If the tumor is extensive and the presence of metastases makes surgery for cure impossible, the tumor may still be removed solely to stop the bleeding. In that case the operation would be considered a palliative one.

♦ *To reconstruct or rehabilitate* Removing an organ or tumor can sometimes produce some deformity or functional problem. When that happens, surgery can often improve appearance, function and the quality of life. Excellent techniques provide reconstruction for women who have had a radical mastectomy. There are also ways to restore appearance and function after head and neck surgery.

It is not unusual for both doctor and patient to focus so sharply on treatment that they simply accept some of the crippling results of major surgery and overlook alternatives that can improve the quality of life. So be aware of this form of

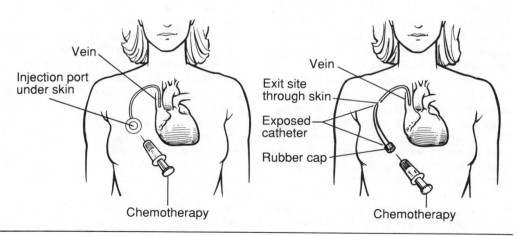

Implanted port for intravenous infusion.

Implanted external catheter for intravenous infusion.

Liver

Arpatic artery

Infusaid pump

Skin

Chemotherapy

Side view

Artery to liver

Infusaid pump for prolonged internal infusion.

surgery and discuss the alternatives for reconstruction with your oncologist, surgeon or other doctor involved in your treatment.

♦ *To support chemotherapy and radiation therapy* Surgery is often used to support other forms of cancer therapy. If you need to have drugs administered intravenously, for example, you may have a port, catheter or pump surgically implanted. Ports and catheters are implanted under local anesthetic in an operating room, although general anesthetic can be given to people who prefer less discomfort.

A port is essentially a small chamber placed under the skin, usually near the shoulder. The chamber connects to a small tube inserted in a vein and threaded through it into larger veins. Access to the port is easy for the person injecting the drug and avoids the pain and discomfort often associated with intravenous injections.

Catheters may sometimes need to be placed into large veins through the skin. The catheter differs from the port in that its end is left outside the skin; the tube enters the body through a small puncture. Catheters usually have up to three inner

lines so that different solutions—medication or nourishment, for example—can be given.

Pumps are more sophisticated devices. They have a large chamber that is filled with a drug, usually 1 to 1 1/2 ounces (30 to 50 mL). The pump has a mechanism, driven by the body's heat, that allows the drug to be delivered constantly through a small catheter inserted into a vein or artery without the need for a stay in the hospital. It is sometimes possible to target a specific organ such as the liver and deliver large amounts of chemotherapy drugs directly to it through an artery.

To support radiation therapy, an operation can be performed to implant catheters that are subsequently loaded with a radioemitter. Surgery is also used to expose a tumor so that a large dose of radiation can be given directly to the tumor or the tumor bed (*see* "Intraoperative Radiation" in Chapter 6).

♦ *To treat complications* Tumors or their treatments often suppress the immune system. This can lead to infections, bowel perforations or obstructions that may require surgical treatment.

PREPARING FOR SURGERY

Before you have surgery, your doctors will study the kind and extent of the tumor involved, then discuss what kind of surgery you need. The intensity of preparation for the surgery will depend on the kind of operation planned. If the surgery is for diagnosis and will involve a needle biopsy, there may only be a need to make sure your blood will clot so that bleeding from the needle puncture will stop quickly.

Preparation is much more elaborate for a major operation. Assuming that the tumor has already been studied thoroughly, two areas will be given special attention—the identification of any abnormalities or associated diseases and their correction before the operation. Patients are examined less or more comprehensively depending on the type of operation planned and their age. As people get older they tend to develop diseases of the heart, lungs and other organs that can jeopardize their recovery from an operation.

Diagnosis of Associated Diseases It is important for a surgeon to know if you have diabetes, if you are being treated for some other disease, what medications you are taking, how many white and red blood cells are in circulation, how well your blood clots and so on. Much of this information can be obtained through blood tests. Blood-clotting abnormalities can be discovered with tests, but the best indicator of an increased risk of bleeding during surgery is a history of bleeding problems.

Similarly, a chest x-ray will give the surgeon an idea of the state of your lungs and an electrocardiogram (ECG) will help evaluate the state of your heart. Tests of lung (pulmonary) and heart function may also be performed. These will not only help evaluate the overall risk of surgery but also help determine the kind of anesthetic and other drugs you may need.

Correction of Associated Diseases Once problems have been identified, as many abnormalities as possible should be corrected. High blood pressure (hypertension), for example, should be treated before the operation. Infections can be treated with antibiotics, blood can be replenished if the blood counts are not high enough, and there may be ways of improving pulmonary function.

One of the most common problems people with cancer have is malnutrition. It is very important to correct this before the operation, since good nutrition gives your body the strength to get through the trauma of the operation and to heal properly. If necessary, additional feedings through a small tube in the stomach or an intravenous line can provide your body with an extra 2,500 to 3,000 calories a day.

WHAT YOU CAN DO TO PREPARE

While your doctor will look after most of the abnormalities noted above, there is a lot you as a patient can do to improve the outcome of the operation.

First, if you smoke, stop. Whether or not you intend to stop forever (which is always beneficial), you should stop as soon as the decision to operate is made. Lung and breathing problems are the most common type of complication after surgery and they can be minimized if the pulmonary system is working well. Clearing the lungs for as many days as possible before surgery will significantly improve your chances of not developing these problems.

Second, become as physically fit as possible. This will make both the operation and your recovery a lot easier. Eating appropriately and losing weight if you are overweight will also help. And any form of exercise, including walking, will be beneficial because it improves both circulation and pulmonary function.

Third, make sure to discuss with the

surgeon the details of the operation and what you can expect afterward. Knowledge of the hospital, the intensive care unit, the staff and the procedures to be followed will help you prepare for the operation emotionally.

Fourth, discuss the use of blood. Most major surgery requires administering blood and there is some risk involved, albeit a small one. That risk can be completely abolished if you use your own blood. If your blood count is high enough and the state of your tumor permits, it may be appropriate to store your own blood two weeks before surgery so it can be returned to you if needed (*see* Chapter 14).

ANESTHETICS

Modern anesthetic techniques have greatly increased the safety of major cancer surgery and the ability of surgeons to combat cancer. Anesthesia is safe and comfortable. Each form of surgery requires a different form of anesthetic, the major kinds being local, regional and general.

♦ *Local anesthesia* is used for procedures that are short and superficial, in other words, near the skin. A biopsy or catheter placement, for example, can be performed under local anesthetic. The surgeon injects a drug such as lidocaine that numbs the site. You will remain awake and will usually feel some pressure as well as minor pulling of tissues in the area. If you do feel any pain, tell the surgeon so you can get additional anesthetic.

♦ *Regional anesthesia* involves giving the anesthetic agent near the spinal cord. The drug may be given by a single injection (called an epidural) or continuously through a small catheter tube placed directly into or near the spinal canal (peridural).

This form of anesthesia is excellent for operations in the lower part of the body, especially the lower extremities and the pelvis. The main advantage of regional anesthesia is that it gives you complete pain relief for many hours and that it wears off slowly, allowing you to take other forms of pain relief as needed after the operation. Another advantage, especially if you have lung problems, is that you stay awake throughout the operation, eliminating the interference with breathing that takes place with general anesthetic. Remaining awake, however, may be considered a disadvantage by some people.

♦ *General anesthesia* is normal in most major operations for cancer. Anesthetic agents are given by intravenous injection, through a breathing mask or both. They act directly on the brain to produce a temporary loss of consciousness. In most cases, the anesthesiologist will also use muscle relaxants to produce a profound relaxation of the body. This will make the surgery easier to perform and will mean less pain afterward. Because your muscles will not be functioning, you won't be able to breathe spontaneously. But a tube will be placed in your windpipe (trachea) and connected to a machine (ventilator) that will deliver air to your lungs every few seconds.

The anesthesiologist monitors breathing by periodically checking the concentration of oxygen in the blood. The anesthesiologist is also in charge of administering fluids intravenously, including blood when needed. The amount and the quality of the fluids are regulated carefully to maintain adequate blood pressure, an adequate amount of circulating blood and adequate blood flow to the body's organs.

AFTER THE OPERATION

Contrary to popular belief, waking up from general anesthesia is not always unpleasant. In fact, it is not too different from waking up from any deep sleep. You will usually wake up in a recovery room, although you may not remember the experience.

Depending on the operation, you may find upon awakening that one or more intravenous lines are running into your body. You may also find drains in some body cavities. You may feel some discomfort and not be able to eat for a few days. The surgeon will have covered all these points with you before the operation.

Pain Control Most patients worry about pain after the operation, but there are several relatively easy ways to control it. If low-level pain relievers (analgesics) like aspirin and codeine won't do the job, pain can be controlled by the injection of stronger analgesics, the most potent being narcotics like morphine. These drugs provide relief from pain for three to four hours and should be readministered by the clock or as soon as the pain reappears.

Traditionally, patients have had to call a nurse each time they felt the need for an injection, but patients themselves can now activate devices that deliver the analgesic. The "patient controlled analgesia" (PCA) device has a compartment for the morphine, a trigger button to press and a small computer that delivers a fixed dose of the drug. There is also a lock-out period set by the doctor and nurse—usually at 20 minutes—to make sure the drug isn't administered too often. The main advantage of this form of pain control is that the pain can be relieved as soon as it felt, which usually means that smaller amounts of medication are needed.

Another way to control pain is with morphine or a local anesthetic administered into the spinal canal, just like the epidural given during the operation. This will control the pain completely, but usually causes bladder malfunction. A catheter, therefore, will be needed to drain the bladder of urine.

These options should be discussed and a basic plan devised before the operation. The main point to remember is that pain can be controlled and that there is no need to suffer. It's also useful to note that taking liberal doses of morphine or other analgesics in the post-operative period *does not* lead to drug addiction.

WHAT ARE THE RISKS?

It is important for you to discuss with the surgeon before the operation the risk of anesthesia, the risk of the surgical procedure itself and any potential complications. You should also discuss the operative mortality—usually defined as a death that occurs within 30 days of an operation—that can result either from the underlying disease or from complications that develop during the operation.

♦ *The risk of anesthesia* is related to your age, the magnitude of the operation and the presence of associated diseases. The American Society of Anesthesiology has devised a formula to classify the status of patients, divided into five classes. As the age or the associated diseases increase, the number of the class increases to indicate a greater risk. Class 1, for example, is a middle-aged patient with no significant associated disease who has a localized process requiring a limited operation. Class 3 patients have severe systemic disturbance from other diseases, such as low pulmonary function, vascular complications or heart disease. The overall risk of anesthesia, however, is very small.

♦ *The operative risks* vary greatly with the kind of operation performed. They are usually divided into immediate risks (occurring within a few days or weeks of surgery) and late risks (occurring months or years after the operation). Just as in the case of anesthesia, the immediate risks are increased by the presence of other diseases.

Bleeding is usually quoted as a common risk of surgery, but very few patients suffer much from it. The most common immediate complications are pulmonary and usually result from earlier lung disease, a history of smoking or the fact that postoperative pain and being in bed prevent the lungs from expanding. These complications can be prevented or minimized by vigorous coughing, as a nurse may request, and by getting up and walking around as soon as possible.

Another complication that may occur after a prolonged period in bed is the development of a clot in the legs brought on by poor circulation. The major risk is that part of the clot might break loose and lodge in the lungs. This is called a pulmonary embolism and is a potentially serious complication that can be prevented by walking or by moving your legs, particularly the calf muscles, while in bed.

Other common complications in the postoperative period have to do with the operative wound. Infection can set in around the incision, but infections can be easily treated and shouldn't cause you much physical or emotional discomfort.

Late complications of surgery have to do with the scarring that is an inevitable part of the healing process. Scarring in the abdomen can occasionally lead to a bowel obstruction or some other form of mechanical blockage.

CHOOSING A SURGEON AND A MEDICAL FACILITY

This is not usually an overwhelming problem. In most cases, your oncologist or the general physician who diagnosed your cancer will recommend someone whom he or she knows and has worked with before. In other cases, you may know of a surgeon personally or by reputation and can either use him or her directly as the surgeon or as a source of information.

If you want to make the choice yourself, it is a good idea to get information from the local medical society about doctors who are Board-certified in surgery. While certification by the American Board of Surgery does not necessarily mean outstanding performance, it does have implications about a surgeon's level of knowledge and adherence to certain standards.

Most reputable surgeons are also Fellows of the American College of Surgeons, which can also help you with names of surgeons practicing in your community. Write to American College of Surgeons, 55 E. Erie Street, Chicago, Illinois 60611 or telephone (312) 644-4050.

When the procedure you are facing is minor or has to do with one of the more common forms of cancer, chances are that the operation can be performed successfully by most surgeons. But if your oncologist says your disease is out of the ordinary or if the operation you need is a major or complex one, it is usually best to seek out the services of an experienced surgeon working in a sizable hospital or other medical institution. His or her experience is an important asset, but more important is that the specialists, sophisticated equipment and advanced techniques that may be needed to react to problems during and after an operation are available only at large medical centers.

Once you have made a preliminary decision about a surgeon, it is a good idea to arrange a meeting. Decide for yourself whether he or she is the kind of person you want to entrust your life to. If you feel positive about it, follow through. If not, it is easy enough to find another surgeon who can perform the operation just as well.

At this point you might also want to get a second opinion. Another opinion can be very useful, especially with a case that is difficult, complex or uncommon. You will be able to compare the two approaches to the disease, and that may give you more confidence as you face your operation.

When all this has been done, you are ready for surgery.

6
WHAT HAPPENS IN RADIATION THERAPY

Lawrence W. Margolis, MD, and T. Stanley Meyler, MD

About half of all people with cancer need radiation therapy as part of their overall treatment plan at some point in their illness. It is often recommended as the primary treatment, but can also be used along with chemotherapy or surgery. When used with surgery, it might be given before, during or after the operation. When used with chemotherapy, it may be given before or after the program begins or at the same time as chemotherapy.

There are two main goals in radiation therapy:

♦Cure the cancer. This usually requires a long and complex course of treatment.

♦Relieve symptoms (palliation). Treatment to achieve this goal is usually less complex and takes less time.

HOW IT WORKS

Radiation therapy—which is also called radiotherapy—uses high-energy x-rays, electron beams or radioactive isotopes to kill cancer cells without exceeding safe doses to normal tissue.

Radiation accomplishes its purpose by killing cancer cells through a process called ionization. Some cells die immediately after radiation because of the direct effect, though most die because the radiation damages the chromosomes and DNA so much that they can no longer divide.

The key to successful treatment is getting the appropriate amount of radiation to the tumor in the most effective way. There are several technical ways of doing this. The most common way is by external radiation in which a radiation beam is directed at the tumor from a machine. Internal or systemic radiotherapy delivers radiation by giving a radioactive source intravenously or by injection—intravenous radioactive iodine or radioactive gold into the abdominal cavity, for example. With intracavity radiotherapy, an applicator containing radiation seeds is placed into an organ such as the uterus. In interstitial radiotherapy, the sources are placed directly into the tumor. These methods are usually used in combination with external radiation.

PLANNING THE THERAPY

All radiation treatment is supervised by physicians who are generally Board-certified specialists trained to evaluate and treat cancer patients using radiation. Your specialist may be called a radiation oncologist, radiotherapist, radiation therapist or therapeutic radiologist.

Whatever the term used in your particular hospital, this specialist is an important member of your cancer team. He or she may be consulted at any time during your treatment, from immediately after the diagnosis to well along in your therapy. At whatever stage the radiation oncologist joins your team, the treatment planning process follows several standard steps.

The Goal The first thing the radiation oncologist has to do is thoroughly evaluate your case. He or she will give you a physical examination, review all scans, diagnostic x-rays, pathology slides and operative reports, then will discuss your case with your primary physician, medical oncologist or possibly a surgeon. After the evaluation has been completed, a decision will be made on what role radiation therapy will play—will the goal of treatment be curative or palliative? At this point, the radiation oncologist will also decide on the method of radiation to be used—external, the various internal methods or a combination. Then the detailed planning starts.

The Simulation If external radiation is going to be used, the first step in the detailed planning stage is called a simulation, performed on a special x-ray machine built to resemble the machine that ultimately will be used. Certain "contrast agents" or probes may be used to aid in the simulation. The point of the exercise is to make all the necessary measurements to fix the precise location of the tumor. Marks will be made on your skin with a colored ink to outline the target the radiation oncologist will be aiming for—the "radiation port"—which has to be the same every day.

While the simulation is being done, the radiation oncologist may use the services of a clinical physicist and dosimetrist. The physicist is specially trained in the clinical application of radiation therapy and will give advice on technical matters that the radiation oncologist will incorporate into the plan. A dosimetrist is a person who, with the use of computers, helps design the specialized treatment plan developed for each individual.

Following the simulation, you will be ready to start treatment either that day or possibly several days later if your case is complex. The reason for the delay is that all the data from the simulation will be fed into a computer. The treatment team will need time to study the various plans and tailor-make any shielding or blocking devices that may be needed to keep radiation away from your healthy tissues.

The Dosage The amount of radiation you receive is measured in units that used to be called rads. The term used now is centigray (cGy), but since one gray equals 100 rads the two terms are interchangeable.

Deciding what dosage of radiation to give is a critical part of the treatment plan. Careful planning allows the radiation oncologist to deliver the maximum effective dose to the visible tumor and any invisible tumor cells that might be nearby while protecting the surrounding normal tissues as much as possible.

Calculating a dosage figure that balances these two goals can be complex, since the size and stage of the tumor have to be taken into account and since different tissues tolerate different levels of radiation. The liver, for example, will tolerate 3,000 cGy, the lungs 2,000 and the kidneys 1,800. Higher doses can be delivered to small parts of one of these organs, but if the entire organ is given higher doses than these, normal tissues will be harmed.

The radiation oncologist prescribes the total dose necessary to destroy the tumor, then calculates the daily dose over a specific period. This is called the fractionation schedule. Throughout, the radiation oncologist works with a figure called the therapeutic ratio, defined as a comparison of the damage to the tumor cells compared with normal cells. The therapeutic ratio can be enhanced in a number of ways—by using altered time fractionation schedules, careful treatment planning, selection of the optimum radiation energy for the specific problem and by the use of experimental techniques such as high LET radiation or chemical modifiers that either make the tumor cells more sensitive to radiation or better protect normal tissues.

The Number of Treatments Radiation is

usually given daily five days a week. That schedule can continue for two to eight weeks depending on the tumor, the kind of treatment being used and the dosage required. The point of using multiple treatments instead of a single treatment is to give normal cells a chance to recover and repair themselves.

TYPES OF EXTERNAL RADIATION

Radiation oncologists now have a variety of ways to deliver the most effective amount of radiation to specific tumor cells. Which method to use is based on many factors, including the biology of the tumor involved, the possibility of side effects or complications, the physical characteristics of the various sources of radiation and how these different sources affect the body's many different cells, tissues and organ systems. The methods can be broadly divided into external and internal radiation, with several options available within each category.

External radiation—the delivery of the dosage from a source outside the body—can vary according to the photon energy of the machines involved, the type of beams produced (electrons, x-rays, gamma rays), when the treatment is given and the number of beams involved in the treatment procedure.

High and Low Energy Radiation External beam treatment uses special equipment that uses either low energy (orthovoltage machines) or high energy (megavoltage machines). All the machines used today are quite precise about where they deliver the radiation dose.

Orthovoltage Equipment Orthovoltage x-rays are produced in a tube in which a filament is heated to a high temperature. Electrons are emitted and strike a tungsten target, producing x-rays with energies up to 300 kilovolts. This type of machine delivers its maximum dose on the surface of the skin and has a very limited range of penetration. These days, orthovoltage machines are used only for surface tumors such as skin cancers.

Megavoltage Equipment These are high energy machines with energies greater than 1,000 kilovolts. Megavoltage machines let the radiation oncologist treat internal tumors without giving an excessive dosage to the skin. Commonly used megavoltage machines include Cobalt 60 and Linear Accelerators that produce the maximum dose at an internal depth determined by the energy of the machine. A 25-megavolt Betatron, for example, delivers its maximum dose almost 2 in. (4.5 cm) beneath the skin.

♦ Cobalt 60 became available in the 1950s and is still used. This machine contains a radioactive source housed in a specially designed lead container. As the cobalt isotope decays over time, it produces a beam in the megavoltage range.

♦ The Linear Accelerator, one of the most popular machines now being used, is available in energies ranging from 4 to 35 megavolts. Many of these machines can treat patients with x-rays or electrons or a combination of both. The combination is called a mixed beam and allows the radiation oncologist to tailor the treatment to a specific tumor and reduce the dose to surrounding tissues.

The machine works by producing electrons that are accelerated along a wave guide to a high velocity. These electrons can be directly used for treatment in the electron mode or they can be directed at a target within the machine to produce the x-rays that are then used for treatment. The high energy electrons used in the electron mode have a specific range of penetration into tissue, determined by the energy of the beam selected. The higher the megavoltage, the greater the penetration. Because an electron therapy beam produces a high skin dose, the whole course of treatment will seldom be given with only the electron beam unless you are being treated for skin cancer.

Intra-Operative Radiation Therapy (IORT) People with localized tumors that can't be completely removed or have a high risk for a local recurrence—carcinoma of the pancreas, for example—may be candidates for IORT, a treatment carried out during surgery. The surgeon localizes the organ containing your tumor and removes as much of the tumor as possible. He or she then moves the normal tissue out of the path of the radiation beam. Radiation equipment may then be brought into the operating room or you may be wheeled to a radiation department. A treatment cone connected to a Linear Accelerator is placed directly over the tumor, which is then treated with a single high dose. Normal tissues are spared since they are outside of the beam.

Stereotactic (Stereotaxic) Radiosurgery
This was introduced in the 1950s by Dr. Lars Leksell of Sweden who found that he could treat deep-seated blood vessel malformations within the brain by using a number of cobalt sources.

If you are receiving this treatment, your head will be placed in a special frame that helps to maintain alignment and localize the treatment volume. With the frame in place, you will have a CT or MRI scan or an angiogram study. Technical information from the scan is then fed into a treatment-planning computer and a dose distribution is calculated for the Linear Accelerator. You will then be transported to the Linear Accelerator, which will direct high doses of radiation from specific angles outside your head so that they converge on the target area. Surrounding tissues are for the most part spared.

The computer revolution and the availability of Linear Accelerators has made this form of treatment especially useful for vascular malformations, meningiomas, acoustic neuromas and some malignant brain tumors.

TYPES OF INTERNAL RADIATION

Modern radiation treatment makes extensive use of methods that deliver radiation to cancer cells not from a distance but by being inserted directly into or around the tumor. Radioactive sources can be injected, housed in special applicators or implanted in the form of needles or seeds.

Internal (Systemic) Radiation Therapy
With this type of treatment, radioactive isotopes are given intravenously or placed in an organ such as the bladder or abdomen.

♦ One of the most common forms of systemic treatment involves the use of radioactive iodine (I-131), which is sometimes used for carcinoma of the thyroid. Its use in thyroid cancer is limited because many thyroid cancers fail to take up iodine. But if a thyroid cancer does show iodine uptake in preliminary tests, then by giving I-131 the isotope will be concentrated in the gland, thereby administering a high dosage of radiation to the organ while sparing other tissues.

♦ At one time, radioactive phosphorus isotopes were placed within an abdominal cavity to treat malignant fluid (ascites) or to prevent reaccumulation of that fluid. But its use today is quite limited.

♦ An agent called strontium 89 is currently under investigation for treatment of bone metastases from prostate and breast cancer. Given intravenously, this isotope shows promising preliminary results.

Interstitial Radiation Therapy This method, also called brachytherapy, places the sources of radiation directly into the tumor and surrounding structures. It's most commonly used in tumors of the head and neck, the prostate and the breast. It is also usually used in combination with external radiation.

There are two types of implants:
♦ A permanent implant involves small radioactive seeds such as gold or iodine

placed directly into the affected organ. I-125 seeds, for example, are used for prostate cancer. Over several weeks or months, the seeds slowly deliver a specific dose of radiation to the tumor.

♦ A removable implant is the most common method of interstitial radiation therapy. The operation, usually carried out under general anesthesia, involves placing narrow, hollow stainless steel needles through the tumor. Once the placement seems satisfactory, Teflon tubes are inserted through the needles and the needles are then removed, leaving the tubes in place. The operation is then terminated and you return to your room, where a small ribbon of radioactive seeds will be inserted into the tubes in a procedure called afterloading.

With computerized treatment planning, the specific strength of each seed can be selected, thereby providing the desired dose to the tumor volume over a specific period. Once the dose is reached, the tubes and the seeds are removed. This type of implant is commonly used for tumors of the head and neck or as a boost after external beam radiation of breast cancer after a lumpectomy.

Intracavitary Radiation The most common use of this method is in gynecologic tumors, such as carcinoma of the uterus. Specially designed hollow applicators are placed into the uterus under general or spinal anesthesia. X-rays are taken in the operating room to determine correct positioning, and once the placement is satisfactory the operation is ended. After you return to your room, a small plastic tube containing the required number of sources of radioactive isotope of a specific strength are inserted into the hollow applicators. The sources and applicators are left in place for 48 to 72 hours, during which time you have to stay in bed. The seeds deliver the dose over the specified time, and once the dose is reached, the applicator and the sources are removed.

The advantage of this method is that a very high dose of radiation can be delivered to the tumor while the rapid fall-off in the dose gives maximum protection to the surrounding structures.

Intraluminal Radiation Therapy This method has limited use with some tumors in hollow organs like the esophagus and biliary tract. In esophageal carcinoma, for example, a specially designed tube is placed into the opening (lumen) of the esophagus. Then under x-ray visualization—fluoroscopy—several small radioactive sources are placed into the tube opposite the tumor. The tumor receives a high dose of radiation while the dose to the surrounding structures is minimized. Intraluminal therapy is often used in combination with external radiation.

NEW TECHNIQUES TO IMPROVE RADIOTHERAPY

Today's researchers are exploring several ways to make radiation therapy more effective, building on important advances in biology, physics and engineering. Some have already produced significant results.

Hyperthermia The effect of heat on some types of cancer has been observed for more than 100 years. In 1893, W. B. Cooley reported that high temperatures had an effect on 38 patients, 12 of whom had a complete regression of their cancers. Many malignant cells show a therapeutic response to high temperatures. And even moderate hyperthermia (108° F/42° C) can cause destruction of malignant cells.

The problem has always been how to heat the tumors properly. Recent advances in the engineering and physics of hyperthermia have led to various devices that can safely and reliably produce the specific temperatures needed. It is now possible to heat all of the body, specific regions of the body or just the tumor itself. Compared to radiotherapy alone, the combination of heat plus radiation has increased the response rate of certain tumors such as melanoma, and there are also promising preliminary results from treating brain tumors using interstitial implants plus heat.

Researchers are now studying the use of a new "multimodality" treatment—the combination of radiation therapy, chemotherapy and heat—which may increase the response rate for some tumors (*see* Chapter 10).

Clinical Modifiers Research continues in the hope of finding chemical compounds that will modify radiation effects. Since radiation is more effective in cells with a good oxygen supply, one of the first approaches to modifying radiation sensitivity was through the use of hyperbaric oxygen chambers. Patients were placed in a closed chamber so they could breathe air with a higher than normal concentration of oxygen.

More recently, radiation sensitizing agents that have an effect similar to oxygen have been developed. Other compounds now being investigated are "radioprotectors" that may decrease damage to normal tissues.

High Linear Energy Transfer (LET) Radiation Radiation with accelerators that use heavy particles or subatomic particles rather than electrons, x-rays or gamma rays is now being studied in many centers. Several types of heavy particles are under investigation, including protons, helium ions and neutrons. Two features seem to make this type of radiation—called High Linear Energy Transfer (LET) heavy particle radiation—more effective. First, it can kill poorly oxygenated cells better than standard radiation can. Second, tumor cells are less able to repair sublethal damage from high LET radiation.

Several tumors have been identified that may benefit from high LET particle radiation—including sarcomas of bone and soft tissue, salivary gland tumors, some head and neck tumors and melanomas of the eye—and the search is on to find others. In the past few years, high LET radiation has been used with patients with advanced malignant disease. But it is still an investigational treatment and is available only in a few facilities in the United States.

DEALING WITH SIDE EFFECTS

The common side effects of radiation therapy can be divided into generalized (systemic) and localized effects. What the effects are and how severe they become generally depend on the area treated, the size of the radiation port, the daily dose rate and the total dosage delivered.

Not everyone who has radiation therapy suffers side effects. Many people go through treatment experiencing only minimal effects or none at all. But for some people, the side effects can be significant and uncomfortable.

Systemic Effects One of the most common systemic side effects is fatigue or malaise. This is especially common among patients receiving treatments to large areas, such as the whole abdomen or total lymph node radiation.

A lot of people associate nausea and vomiting with x-ray treatments, but both these symptoms are unusual in radiotherapy patients. Again, it depends on the area being treated. Nausea and vomiting may occur in patients receiving radiation to the upper abdomen, but it is rare in patients getting radiation to the head and neck, chest or pelvis. Even when you are receiving treatment to the abdomen, nausea and vomiting can usually be controlled by adjusting the dosage, changing the diet or using antinausea medications.

Localized Side Effects As certain parts of your body are treated, you may experience several common localized side effects. Your radiation oncologist will go over these with you before treatment and will give them individualized attention if they occur.

♦ *Skin* All radiation has to pass through the skin, but with today's high energy machines and daily treatment techniques using multiple ports, the side effects on the skin are seldom a problem unless the treated area actually involves the skin.

Most skin reactions appear as a redness called erythema. This is similar to sunburn and goes through the same stages—redness, gradual tanning, then peeling. Once the condition is treated, the reaction will usually go away within a week or 10 days. If the dose has been high, late skin changes may appear in the form of increased pigmentation, which may be more noticeable in people of dark complexion.

If you develop any of these symptoms, it is important not to put any creams or lotions on your skin without your radiation oncologist's approval.

♦ *Head and neck* One of the most significant side effects is irritation of the membranes lining the body cavities, such as the lining—or mucosa—of the mouth. If you are being treated for a cancer of the head and neck, the mucosa surrounding the tumor may become red. And as treatment progresses, quite a few small superficial ulcers may develop. This can cause a lot of discomfort and will probably interfere with swallowing and nutrition. Fortunately, the effect is temporary and will disappear as soon as the treatment is finished.

Radiation to the head and neck may also interfere with taste if your tongue is in the primary radiation beam. And the amount of saliva produced can be significantly reduced if the salivary glands happen to be in the treatment beam (*see* "Special Problems of Radiation Patients" in Chapter 18).

♦ *Chest* Most patients receiving chest radiation will not have any local symptoms. But the esophagus, which carries food from the mouth to the stomach, pass-es through the chest and may develop a mucosal reaction similar to that described for the mouth. If this happens, you may develop heartburn-type symptoms, which can be relieved by taking liquid antacids such as Amphogel, Gelusil, Maalox, Mylanta or Riopan.

♦ *Abdomen* The most significant side effects of radiation are associated with treatment to the abdomen. The larger the radiation port and the higher the dosage, the more likely you are to experience these effects.

Radiation to the upper abdomen can cause nausea and vomiting, usually during the first few days of treatment. As the treatment progresses the symptoms often diminish.

Treatment to the pelvis can be associated with cramps, perhaps followed by diarrhea during the second and third weeks of treatment. A low residue diet or antidiarrhea medications such as Lomotil, Imodium or Kaopectate will usually control the problem.

Most patients getting radiation treatment to the pelvis do not develop any significant bladder problems. But it is not unusual to have to urinate often, to feel an urgency to urinate or to feel some pain when urinating. Fortunately, these symptoms are usually temporary and will go away soon after the treatment course is completed. In the meantime, medications such as Pyridium or Urispas will usually ease the problem.

♦ *Hair loss* Only hair within the radiation port will be affected by treatment. So you will lose scalp hair only if you are receiving radiation to your head, usually for tumors involving the brain. If the entire brain needs to be treated, the radiation can affect the entire scalp. But only a part of the scalp might be affected if a smaller portion of the brain is radiated. Whether the hair loss is temporary or permanent depends on the dosage (*see* "Hair Loss" in Chapter 17).

7
WHAT HAPPENS IN CHEMOTHERAPY

Malin Dollinger, MD, and Ernest H. Rosenbaum, MD

◇

The idea of treating cancer with chemical agents or medications has been around since the days of the ancient Greeks. Yet the practice of cancer chemotherapy as it's known today really only began in the 1940s. Near the end of that decade, nitrogen mustard became the first drug approved to fight tumor cells. Over the next 20 years, chemotherapy was essentially an investigational treatment.

But in the last 30 years, more effective antitumor drugs have been developed, and other new drugs and supportive techniques have come along to reduce the side effects of the cancer-killing agents. Now, with greater understanding of the nature of cancer and of how chemicals interact, chemotherapy has become a standard therapy. Either alone or in combination with other treatments, chemotherapy can now cure some common forms of cancer—testis cancer, leukemia, choriocarcinoma, many cases of Hodgkin's disease and non-Hodgkin's lymphomas and some cases of ovarian cancer.

The Range of Drugs For many years, researchers looked hard for one single drug—a "magic bullet"—that would cure cancer. This has yet to be found, if it exists at all. Today, about 50 anticancer drugs are available on the market. About a dozen others have not yet been approved for general distribution but have proved to be useful in some forms of cancer. These experimental or investigational drugs are supplied to clinical trial investigators under a special government license.

To make drugs available earlier for therapy, some drugs with an established role in treatment are also made available to practicing oncologists, even though they are not yet on the retail market. In 1989, for example, a year before it was released to the general market, the National Cancer Institute made the drug levamisole available to be used in combination with 5-fluorouracil for treatment of Dukes Stage C carcinoma of the colon. This new policy may mean earlier release of new drugs in the future.

THE GOALS AND POSSIBLE RESULTS OF THERAPY

Your doctor might recommend chemotherapy for several reasons. The goal might be:
♦ to cure a specific cancer;
♦ to control tumor growth when a cure isn't possible;
♦ to relieve symptoms such as pain;
♦ to shrink tumors before surgery or radiation therapy; or
♦ to destroy microscopic metastases after tumors are removed surgically.

While surgery and radiation therapy are used to treat localized tumors, chemotherapy treats the whole body. It destroys malignancies of the blood, bone marrow and the lymphatic system (leukemias and lymphomas). It destroys cancer cells that have broken off from solid tumors and spread through the blood or lymph systems to various parts of the body.

Adjuvant Therapy When chemotherapy is

used to eliminate small invisible metastases after surgery or radiation therapy, it is known as adjuvant therapy. This is given when there is a high risk of a cancer recurring because small cells that couldn't be detected during surgery or any other way many remain and later grow back.

Adjuvant chemotherapy usually involves combinations of drugs known to be effective against particular tumors. They are given in the highest dosages the patient can tolerate. And they will usually be given as soon as possible after surgery or radiotherapy since the longer the delay, the less chance of cure.

What Chemotherapy Can Achieve There are four possible results of chemotherapy given for visible or known areas of cancer.

♦ *Complete remission* The tumor may seem to disappear completely, meaning that there is a complete response to the drugs. This clearly indicates the treatment is working, though it has to continue for a while so any "hidden" cancer cells will be destroyed. Current detection methods can miss an internal tumor smaller than half an inch (about 1 cm) and if treatment is stopped too soon there is a high chance for a relapse.

Some remissions, especially for very responsive tumors, may be permanent. Others are temporary, lasting for months or even years. But then the tumor reappears or begins to grow again. Complete remission, therefore, is not necessarily the same as a cure. "Cure" usually means the lack of any sign of cancer for at least five years, but how it's defined really depends on the kind of cancer being treated and on the individual patient.

♦ *Partial remission* The tumor may shrink by more than half its size but not disappear. This is obviously a good result, but therapy has to be continued until the tumor either completely disappears or stops shrinking. If it simply stops shrinking, the drug program may be changed or surgery or radiotherapy may be used to try to wipe out the remaining tumor cells.

♦ *Stabilization* The tumor may neither shrink nor grow. This can be looked on as a favorable result of therapy, but doctors tend to be nervous when this happens. They basically worry that the effect may be brief and the tumor will start growing again. The period of stabilization can sometimes last months or years.

♦ *Progression* The tumor may keep growing despite therapy. The doctor's task is to discover this as soon as possible after the therapy has had a fair trial. Then a different treatment program can be worked out.

HOW ANTICANCER DRUGS WORK

Like normal, healthy cells, cancer cells go through a continuous process of change. Each cell divides into two daughter cells. These cells grow, rest and then divide again. The drugs used in chemotherapy are powerful chemicals designed to interrupt this cycle and stop the cells from growing.

Several different types of drugs are used in chemotherapy. Each type kills cells at a different stage of the cell's life cycle. Each does its job in a different way.

Antimetabolites attack the cells during the process of division, when they are more easily killed. The antimetabolites imitate normal cell nutrients. The "anti-vitamin" methotrexate, for example, resembles the normal B vitamin, folic acid. The cancer cell consumes the drug— "thinking" it's getting a good meal—and starves to death.

Alkylating agents attack all the cells in a tumor whether they are resting or dividing. These drugs bind with the cells' DNA in various ways to prevent reproduction.

Antitumor antibiotics insert themselves into strands of DNA. They either break up the chromosomes or inhibit the DNA-directed synthesis of RNA that the cell needs to grow.

Alkaloids prevent the formation of chromosome spindles necessary for cell duplication.

Hormones such as estrogen and progesterone inhibit the growth of some cancers, although how they do it is not clearly understood.

Drug Combinations It used to be that anticancer drugs were given one at a time. But now combinations of drugs are usually given, all according to a plan designed to inhibit or kill as many cancer cells as possible.

Drugs that attack tumor cells at every stage of their life cycle—called non-cell-cycle-specific drugs—may be given first to reduce the size of the tumor. This may activate the remaining cells to divide. When they do, cell-cycle-specific drugs that attack dividing cells will be given. Other sequences of other drugs can also be devised to maximize the therapeutic effect.

This is much like fighting a war, making sure you use all your forces on several fronts with repeated attacks. Your chances of winning the battle are greatly improved.

Drug Resistance There's another good reason for giving drug combinations: it reduces the chance that you'll develop a resistance to any one drug.

Resistance is one very common reason why these agents fail to do what they're supposed to. A course of chemotherapy is often quite successful at first. The cancer responds, leading to a remission. But then, even though the drugs are still being given, there is a relapse and the cancer starts to grow again. A resistance to therapy has developed just like the resistance to penicillin or other antibiotics that can develop when treating an infection.

When this happens, the drugs in the treatment program have to be changed. Unfortunately, if you develop resistance to one drug or group of drugs there may be less chance that your body will respond to another drug program.

Why Resistance Develops One of the mysteries of cancer therapy is why some people respond really well to a treatment while others have problems. About 10 years ago, research on drug resistance led to speculation that multiple resistance developed during therapy and that this was responsible for progressive and uncontrollable metastatic disease.

More recent research has begun to explain how cancer cells become resistant to drugs. There is a protein called P-glycoprotein on the surface of a cancer cell. This protein acts like a pump, regulating the passage of drugs into and out of the cancer cell. Tumor cells with larger amounts of P-glycoprotein may not allow any drugs to enter. This, of course, makes chemotherapy ineffective.

There are now ways to measure the amount of this protein, so it can often be predicted whether a cancer will be resistant to chemotherapy. P-glycoprotein genes have also been discovered, which may explain why some cells in a tumor are resistant to drugs while others are not. This in turn may explain why some drugs are not effective when administered even when a drug sensitivity test indicates that the tumor *should* be sensitive to a certain drug. Researchers are now trying to overcome drug resistance related to P-glycoprotein.

HOW THE DRUGS ARE GIVEN

The drugs used in chemotherapy are very powerful. The line between a therapeutic and a toxic dose is so fine and the consequences of the wrong dose so severe that general physicians without special training don't prescribe them. So chemotherapeutic agents are usually given only by oncologists, usually medical or pediatric oncologists (specialists in the medical treatment of cancer) and hematologists (specialists in diseases of the blood), although some surgical and gynecological oncologists also give chemotherapy.

Delivery Routes and Methods The drugs can be delivered to your circulatory system by many different routes. They can be taken orally in capsule, pill or liquid form. They can be injected through a syringe into a vein, artery or muscle. Or they can be given intravenously through an IV drip device.

Single or multiple drugs can be injected directly into organs such as the liver, using a small pump to ensure a constant flow. An external pump might be used, although internal pumps can now be surgically implanted and remain in the body for several weeks or months or permanently (*see* Chapter 5 for illustrations of catheters, ports and pumps).

Each delivery route has its advantages and disadvantages.

♦ *Intravenous* For intravenous delivery, you have to have a vein that can be entered easily and without causing a lot of discomfort. This isn't always easy. Some people naturally have small veins. Sometimes the veins get "used up" after several chemotherapy sessions.

If a vein isn't easily accessible, a temporary plastic tube can be implanted under the skin in the chest or in an arm or leg. These catheters, as they are called, extend into larger veins. They provide an access point either for injections or for the slow drip (continuous infusions) of therapy over hours or even days. All kinds of fluids can enter the vein through the catheter—chemotherapy drugs, nutritional formulas, antibiotics, blood or platelet transfusions, antinausea drugs or morphine or other pain-killing narcotics.

The catheters avoid any discomfort from vein "sticking" and also any worry about having shots of irritating drugs that might leak out into the tissues. They can't be pulled out with an average pull or jerk, so they are quite safe. And they are simple to care for. They just need occasional cleaning and changing of the injection cap and periodic injections of heparin, a drug that prevents blood clotting in the catheter.

♦ *Implanted infusion ports* Another type of catheter is completely under the skin. It is called a port, and it's filled by placing a special needle through the skin into the chamber. The chamber contains a rubber or Silastic cover that can be punctured thousands of times with a special needle to deliver therapy, antibiotics or nutrients directly into a large vein.

The advantage of the implanted system is that since it is completely under the skin, no dressings or cleaning are needed and care is much simpler. Heparin injections won't be needed so often either. The disadvantage is that there is a slight risk of the drug leaking out. Also, a port can occasionally get out of position and become more difficult to enter.

♦ *Ambulatory pumps* Small portable pumps that deliver chemotherapy while you go about your normal activities are called ambulatory pumps. ("Ambulatory" just means you can walk around.)

These devices are often about the size of a deck of cards. They hold the drug supply, a mechanism for injecting it slowly and smoothly into an attached catheter, a battery to power the mechanism and controls for regulating the rate of drug delivery. Many of the pumps have become very sophisticated. Some have alarms. One of the newer systems can deliver four separate drugs in a preset time sequence.

Several types are available. The balloon pump (Travenol infuser) is the cheapest and simplest, consisting basically of a large plastic reservoir. The pump is filled, then attached to a port or catheter. The pump empties automatically when it's connected.

♦ *Central nervous system delivery* Some patients, such as those with acute leukemia, need chemotherapy drugs injected into the spinal fluid. This can be done by repeated lumbar punctures (spinal taps), but the preferred method is to use an Ommaya reservoir. This is a rubber bulb usually placed under the scalp. A tiny tube connects the reservoir to the spinal fluid compartment. This requires a minor operation for placement of the reservoir and tube. Drugs are injected through the skin into the reservoir. Infection in the reservoir area is a possibility, so patients are usually monitored for side effects such as tenderness, inflammation, fever, stiff neck and headaches.

♦ *Intraperitoneal* This technique which involves delivering drugs directly into the abdominal cavity is sometimes used for ovarian or abdominal metastatic cancer. A catheter is connected to a chamber, usually on the chest or abdominal wall. The drugs are injected into the chamber, which releases them into the abdominal cavity. This eliminates the need to put a new tube into the abdomen every time drugs have to be given. High doses can be given this way, higher than would be possible with any other method of delivery.

♦ *Intra-arterial* Drugs are often given to specific areas such as the liver, head and neck, or pelvis through the artery supplying that area. This is usually done in the hospital, where the delivery system can continuously infuse chemotherapy over a specific time. The drugs are given through a pump that can overcome arterial pressure.

♦ *Infusaid pumps* This special pump was developed to be surgically implanted within the abdomen. The pump is shaped like a hockey puck and has two chambers—one for the drug, the other for a fluid that forces the drug into the catheter. It also has a side port for chemotherapy injections. The pump can deliver a drug for as long as two weeks, then the chemotherapy solution can be replaced with salt water to give your system a rest.

Which Route to Use This decision depends on several factors, mainly the type of tumor and the drug being used. There are many questions to answer. Can the drug be absorbed in the stomach? How big a dose is required? What are the side effects? Are they tolerable?

Ultimately, the decision will be made on the basis of what is the most effective way to get the highest dosage of the right drug to the right place. Whichever route is chosen, your doctor will give you and your family or friends complete information on the usual effects of the drug, its side effects, any safety precautions to take and what reactions to report.

Where the Drugs Are Given Intravenous administration of some drugs requires a stay in the hospital for a few days. Injections are usually given in a hospital or in the doctor's office, although oncology nurses can give the drugs as part of a home care service.

If pills, liquids or capsules have been prescribed, you can take them at home or at work. Even if you are taking the chemotherapy orally, however, you will still have to visit your doctor's office every so often so the tumor's response can be monitored and your blood counts analyzed. Some drug programs require more frequent office visits because the schedule can be fairly complex.

HOW LONG TREATMENT LASTS

Cancer therapy is a fast-changing field with new treatment schedules always being tested in clinical trials. While new chemotherapeutic drugs are being developed, it is often the same drugs in new combinations or given on different schedules that make the difference between success and failure in destroying cancer cells.

So there are few hard and fast rules on how often drugs are given or how long treatment lasts. Apart from the ever-changing recommended treatments, every person is different, every tumor is different, and every chemotherapy program is tailored to fit the situation.

Just as an example, a cycle of therapy may consist of one drug being given every day for two weeks with other drugs being given on particular days in the two-week period. After a rest period to allow normal tissues to recover, the entire cycle might be repeated every few weeks for six months or longer.

The length of treatment varies with different treatment programs.

♦ For programs that may be able to cure certain forms of cancer, even if widespread, the therapy is typically given for no more than about six months or up to a year in a few cases. This is true of Hodgkin's disease, some lymphomas, cancer of the testis and adjuvant therapy for breast and colon cancer.

♦ Where a remission has been achieved in various forms of metastatic cancer, treatment will be given until the maximum effect has been observed and then for a little while longer in an attempt to destroy hidden tumor cells. If therapy is stopped—unmaintained remission—it may be a long time before the tumor begins to grow again and more therapy is needed. But sometimes chemotherapy is continued indefinitely—maintained remission—until a relapse occurs, at which time the drug program will be changed.

♦ For programs in which chemotherapy is combined with radiotherapy, specific rules and formulas apply to each treatment protocol—prescribed doses, schedules and drug combinations—which are generally followed exactly.

♦ There are similar standards for adjuvant chemotherapy programs for patients who have a high risk for recurrence. The therapy to wipe out small nests of cancer cells that cannot be detected is generally given for six months to one year.

SELECTING THE RIGHT DRUGS

Which drugs to use, alone or in combination, is decided on the basis of many factors, including the extensive guidelines for treatment in the cancer literature. Yet each treatment program is, in a sense, an experiment, since the results cannot be predicted. There are no guarantees. It is not possible to state ahead of time whether a certain drug or combination of drugs will stop or slow down tumor growth in a particular individual.

Doctors are able to estimate, for example, that perhaps 30 or 55 or 73 percent of patients can be expected to respond to a particular drug program for a particular tumor. But they cannot know until they conduct the treatment trial whether any one individual will respond with the hoped-for tumor shrinkage.

What "Response Rate" Means A misconception often arises when a doctor says that a drug has, say, a 60 percent response rate. Patients sometimes think this means that the drug will be at least partly effective against tumors in all treated patients. But to say a drug has that response rate is like saying that a diaphragm or condom is a 95 percent effective way of preventing conception. That figure doesn't mean that all women will become 5 percent pregnant. It means that those contraceptives work 100 percent of the time in 95 percent of the people who use them and don't work at all for the other 5 percent.

Similarly, a drug with an average response rate of 60 percent means that 60 percent of the patients receiving it will respond. But 40 percent will not, although tumor growth might be delayed in some of them.

Devising the Plan As with any plan for cancer treatment, the chemotherapy program your doctor recommends will be tailored to the precise stage of your particular kind of tumor, your age, physical condition and any other medical problems. He or she will be generally guided by some specific information.

♦ *What's worked in the past* Oncologists rely primarily on experience from clinical trials involving many patients with similar tumors. They will usually consult reports in medical journals and the research findings presented at cancer meetings. Since more and more literature on drug treatment is being produced every month, the updated cancer information provided by the Physicians Data Query (PDQ) system of the National Cancer Institute should also be consulted. Such computer databases are now essential for physicians who want to keep track of the rapid changes in the field.

♦ *Drug sensitivity* A lot of research over the past 15 years has been devoted to finding ways of predicting which drugs would kill which tumor cells most successfully. This research has involved growing an individual patient's cancer cells in the laboratory and testing a whole battery of anticancer agents on them.

This drug sensitivity test program—called a clonigenic assay—may give a doctor some guidance on which drugs to use. But it's especially useful for indicating which drugs *not* to use. If a drug doesn't kill single cancer cells in the lab, then it probably won't be effective in the body. So any drugs that are inactive in a laboratory test of a patient's tumor cells would not usually be used with that patient.

The latest research in this area (1990) showed that useful information was obtained from more than two-thirds of the patients whose tumors were grown and tested under this system. The tests are not the final solution to the problem of drug selection, however, since their usefulness is limited by a number of factors:

♦ The tumor may not grow in the laboratory, or only certain drug-sensitive cells may grow.

♦ There may be differences between the way the drug works in the body and the way it works in a test tube. In the body, the drug can be bound and inactivated, eliminated by the kidneys or not be allowed to get through the P-glycoprotein "gate" on the cell surface.

♦ These test procedures apply only to one or, at most, two drugs tested one at a time. But chemotherapy cures are generally produced only by combinations of many drugs.

♦ *The possibility of using other therapies* There is no one absolutely right choice in cancer therapy, and the treatments recommended can change over the course of the illness. One reasonable choice at a particular time may not be appropriate at a later time.

A woman whose breast cancer recurs in a non-vital place, for example, may have several options. Her doctor may recommend: surgery, radiation treatment to the region to possibly control the cancer for years, hormone treatments, simple chemotherapy, complex chemotherapy or even doing nothing until the cancer grows and starts to bother her in six months' or a year's time.

Each treatment option has advantages and disadvantages, and there may be more than one option that is sensible.

SELECTING THE RIGHT DOSAGE

Larger doses of chemotherapy drugs do result in more cancer cells being killed. But a balance has to be struck between improved therapeutic effects and unacceptable toxic effects.

It may *not* be a kind act for your doctor to limit the dosage to avoid toxic effects. For those tumors that can potentially be cured with chemotherapy or have a good chance of going into remission, reducing the dosage to minimize toxicity will also reduce the possibility of cure or remission. The kindest act is to provide the maximum safe dose for cure, even at the cost of some toxicity. When the risks are weighed against the benefits, it doesn't make sense to take all the risks yet fail to get the benefits because the dosage was too low.

When Therapy May Be Stopped Because of Side Effects There is no reason to stop therapy when the drugs produce few problems and the control of the tumor is very satisfactory or even barely satisfactory. But major or objectionable side effects or complications can only be justified by a very significant and pronounced antitumor response.

The decision to stop therapy really depends on how you and your doctor define "objectionable" and what you are willing to put up with. Most men with metastatic testis cancer, for example, can be cured with less than six months of chemotherapy. Naturally, both doctors and patients are usually willing to put up with more discomforting side effects in that case because of the improved chance of cure. The alternative would be fatal.

What is important is for the doctor to give an adequate dosage of drugs—one that would be expected to produce results if that particular tumor in that particular patient happens to be sensitive. Then, after waiting an appropriate time—often about two or three months—tests will show if the tumor is shrinking.

MEASURING THE RESPONSE

There are several ways to tell if a tumor is responding to treatment. They are pretty much the same methods used to diagnose the tumor in the first place—physical examination, x-rays, blood tests and scans. These same tests will have been done before treatment to establish a baseline for future comparisons.

♦ A lump or a tumor involving lymph nodes can be felt and measured directly. The size of the liver, spleen and other organs can also often be determined by physical examination. Your doctor will record these direct measurements in your chart and compare them from time to time to see if the size of the tumor is decreasing.

♦ Some tumors, such as those involving the lungs, show up on x-rays. If new x-rays are taken at one-, two- or three-month intervals, the size of the tumors on the x-ray film can be measured directly with a ruler.

♦ Internal tumors, such as those involving the liver or other organs, are more difficult to measure. So special techniques have to be used—scanning using radioactive tracer isotopes, CT or MRI. Again, the size of the tumor as shown on the image can be measured directly at various intervals.

♦ Sometimes blood tests provide a clue to tumor response. Both non-specific tests, such as liver function tests, and tests for specific tumor markers may be used.

MONITORING BLOOD COUNTS

The drugs used in chemotherapy are growth inhibitors. They are especially good at turning off cells that are growing very quickly. Unfortunately, the drugs are not selective in their action. They turn off every fast-growing cell. There's no way the drug can tell an abnormal cell from a normal one.

The most important rapidly growing normal cells affected by the drugs are the blood cells. The red cells that carry oxygen are not usually affected very much. But the levels of the white cells that fight infection and the platelets that stop bleeding usually fall during chemotherapy.

There are no signs or symptoms of a minor decrease in blood counts. A slight decrease isn't harmful anyway. In fact, blood counts are expected to fall. This ensures that the drugs are being given in the maximum possible safe dose. The lowered counts also show your doctor that the drugs are doing what they are supposed to do—stop fast-growing tissues from growing. If there is enough drug in your system to stop white blood cells, then there is enough to have a potential effect on other rapidly growing cells, namely the cancer cells.

Still, it is very important that your doctor keep a close watch on the blood cells. The blood counts have to be measured regularly, usually before each chemotherapy treatment. If the counts are normal, it may be safe to give the standard dose or even increase the drug dosage. If one of the counts is too low, a drug dose can be modified or even put off for a while. When a therapy session is skipped because of low counts, this does not mean that the cancer cells will get out of control. The rest period is a normal part of the therapy, done for safety reasons.

The Danger of Infection A very low white blood cell count could lead to serious infections, and a very low platelet count could lead to bleeding. If the white blood count or platelet count falls lower than is safe, a rest period will allow the blood counts to recover. If you have fever, chills or any other sign of infection, like a cough or sore throat, during chemotherapy, call your doctor so therapy can be stopped until the infection has been treated effectively. Chemotherapy may suppress your immune system, making it harder for you to fight off infections. Any infection might spread and could become serious.

DEALING WITH SIDE EFFECTS

The prospect of chemotherapy can be frightening. This is not surprising, seeing as how the side effects have been portrayed so horrifically in the popular press. Word of mouth hasn't helped either. Everyone seems to know an uncle of a friend of someone at work who had just a terrible time. But the side effects are usually not nearly as bad or troublesome as your friends may have told you or as you may have read about or seen on TV.

Many people tolerate chemotherapy very well and have few negative reactions. The person who visits the doctor's office, gets a shot for colon or breast cancer, then goes home or back to work and functions fairly well rarely appears on television or gets written up in the papers (*see* Chapter 17).

Taking the Right Approach You should bear in mind that more than 50 drugs are used in cancer chemotherapy. Some produce very few side effects and are easy to take. Others have major problems that have to be combated with appropriate medications. It is also important to remember that some of the most active drugs against cancer are also the ones that provoke the most side effects.

You should try hard to put any fears behind you. Fear of treatment and fear of side effects is a major problem, for anxiety can make the reaction worse. Supportive care, counseling and anti-anxiety drugs may became vital to making sure therapy continues. A more relaxed attitude toward chemotherapy may well lead to fewer bad experiences.

You should approach chemotherapy with the knowledge that it is impossible to attack cancer cells with drugs without also affecting normal tissues. As mentioned earlier, the drugs are most effective against rapidly growing cells. Tumor cells grow rapidly. So do hair follicles, the bone marrow and the cells in the lining of the gastrointestinal tract—mouth, stomach and bowels.

There are basically two kinds of side effects of chemotherapy, immediate and chronic.

Immediate Side Effects These are mainly nausea and vomiting. Both can occur soon after treatment, but both usually go away fairly quickly. Fortunately, a number of very effective antinausea medications have been developed over the past few years. They are often given two, three or four at a time, sometimes intravenously, and can usually prevent major problems with both nausea and vomiting. Very often your doctor will have to try different combinations of antinausea medications if the first combination isn't working as well as you both would like.

Sometimes these nausea medications produce their own side effects, mainly sleepiness or general fatigue. But these minor effects are well worth the trade-off if you can avoid feeling sick. Treatment schedules can also be arranged so that the medication does not disrupt your life too severely. Chemotherapy may be given on a Friday, for example, so that any tiredness will wear off enough by the following Monday that you can return to work.

Chronic Side Effects Since fast-growing cells are affected most, there may be some hair loss, sore mouth, nausea and diarrhea or depressed blood counts.

Hair Loss The amount of hair loss can vary from a slight thinning to baldness. The loss may be gradual or sudden. Sometimes all body hair—head, eyebrows, legs, armpits and pubic areas—may be lost. Depending on the drug used (and on the individual), hair loss on the head can be reduced by using a tourniquet or an ice cap. These narrow the blood vessels in the scalp so that less drug reaches the hair follicles.

The hair loss will be less upsetting if you plan ahead. Before treatment, get a short haircut so the loss won't be so noticeable. Get fitted for a scarf, turban or wig. And keep in mind that hair loss is temporary. Many people find that their hair starts growing back while they are still getting chemotherapy.

Sore Mouth Sores in your mouth or a sore mouth are common side effects but last only a few days. Your doctor can prescribe medication to relieve any pain. Choosing soft, bland foods, rinsing frequently with mild mouthwashes and using a soft toothbrush will help.

Low Blood Counts Depressed blood counts can have several effects, depending on which blood component is low.

♦ Low red cell counts may lead to a general feeling of weakness. You can offset this effect by making sure you get enough rest and not overtaxing yourself in your daily activities.

♦ Low white cell counts leave you vulnerable to infection, so it will be important to avoid people with colds or the flu and to take other preventive measures (*see* Chapter 20).

♦ Low platelet counts may lead to easy bruising and bleeding, so you'll have to take care to avoid cuts, burns or injuries and to avoid aspirin and alcohol. If the platelet count is very low, you can get a transfusion. The bone marrow will usually return to normal in two or three weeks.

Some drugs have very specific side effects. Your doctor can spell these out for you, indicate your chance of having them and outline special measures you can take to minimize or prevent them (*see* Chapter 17).

If you need additional information, several excellent books can be consulted, including *Coping with Chemotherapy*, by Nancy Bruning, *Nutrition for the Cancer Patient*, by Janet Ramstack and Ernest H. Rosenbaum, and *A Comprehensive Guide for Cancer Patients and Their Families*, by Ernest H. Rosenbaum and Isadora Rosenbaum.

8
WHAT HAPPENS IN BIOLOGICAL THERAPY

Raphael Catane, MD, and Malcolm S. Mitchell, MD

◇

Biological therapy is a relatively new way to treat cancer. It is based on the idea that the human immune system, which is designed to eliminate and destroy any foreign substance found inside the body, can play a role in destroying cancer cells.

There are several problems with this approach. One of the biggest is that the immune system doesn't always treat cancer cells as "foreign." It is easy for the system to recognize bacteria or viruses, since they are completely different from normal human cells. But the difference between a tumor cell and a normal cell is small.

Great strides have been made, however, and biological therapy is now an accepted treatment for some cancers. The therapy consists mainly of treating the immune system with highly purified proteins that help activate the system or help it do its job more effectively. Interferon and interleukin-2 are the best known of these proteins. Many others are being evaluated.

HOW YOUR IMMUNE SYSTEM WORKS

To understand the role biological agents play in cancer treatment, you have to know how the normal immune system works.

When something foreign, such as a bacteria or virus, gets into your body, several kinds of cells go into action in what is called the immune response.

♦ *Monocytes or macrophages* These large cells are the body's front line of defense. They are the first cells to recognize and engulf foreign substances. The reason for the two names is that they are called monocytes when found in the bloodstream and macrophages when found in tissues.

♦ *Lymphocytes* These smaller round cells are the most important immune cells. They are divided mainly into B and T cells.

B lymphocytes produce antibodies—proteins (gamma globulins) that recognize foreign substances and attach themselves to them. This process is referred to as humoral immunity.

T lymphocytes make direct contact with foreign materials. When contact is made, the T lymphocytes produce a wide variety of proteins (lymphokines) that either destroy the foreign organisms or send signals to other immune cells. This process is referred to as cellular immunity.

♦ *Polymorphonuclear leukocytes (PMNs)* This is a general name for a group of white blood cells consisting of neutrophils, basophils and eosinophils.

Neutrophils are the most common immune cells in the body. If you have an infection, their number increases rapidly. They are the major constituents of pus and are found around most common inflammations. Their job is to "eat" (ingest) and destroy foreign material.

Basophils and eosinophils are PMNs that contain large granules—storage sacs—inside the cell. They interact with certain foreign materials. Their increased activity may lead to an allergic reaction.

How the Cells Interact The immune response is a coordinated effort. All these immune cells have to work together, so they have to communicate with each other. They do this by secreting a large number of special protein molecules called cytokines that act on other cells.

Interleukins and interferons are cytokines, and there are others such as tumor-necrosis factors and colony-stimulating factors. If you are given any of these cytokines, your immune system may become more active. And the judicious use of the right doses and combinations of them may have an effect on tumor cells.

TYPES OF IMMUNOTHERAPY

There are really five ways to improve the workings of an immune system. They are analogous to ways you could make an army more effective if it was fighting a battle in the field. You could increase the number of your troops, both foot soldiers and more specialized units. You could help the troops focus their efforts more effectively by helping them communicate with each other. You could quickly replace any troops already lost in the fight. You could give them more precise weapons. Or you could make sure their efforts aren't wasted in a scattershot way by clearly identifying or highlighting the targets they're shooting at.

In a similar way, cancer immunotherapy can be conveniently characterized by five broad strategies.

♦ *Active stimulation* This is based on the idea that everyone has some intrinsic anti-tumor immunity and that if the defensive cells can just be aroused in some way they may have an effect against cancer cells.

There are both non-specific and specific strategies involved.

The non-specific strategy uses bacterial or chemical booster substances (adjuvants) to "turn on" a whole range of immune cells—macrophages, natural killer cells and other non-specific killer cells. One effect of stimulating macrophages is that T cells are activated too.

The specific strategy uses the tumor cells themselves or tumor-associated antigens to trigger specific "effector" cells such as killer T cells.

♦ *Adoptive* This strategy involves transferring immunological cells or molecules that carry information (especially lymphokines, the cytokine secreted by lymphocytes) that will help the immune system do its work in a more coordinated way.

♦ *Restorative* Cancer itself and treatments like radiation and chemotherapy can decrease the number of immunological cells available to take part in the immune response. The restorative strategy involves replacing these cells or accomplishing the same goal indirectly by inhibiting the action of suppressive influences on the immune system, such as suppressor T cells.

♦ *Passive* This strategy involves giving the immune system specific "weapons" such as antibodies or short-lived antitumor "factors," that can attack specific cells. Special kinds of antibodies can also be programmed to deliver killer molecules such as radioactive isotopes or toxins to tumor cells.

♦ *Tumor cell modulation* This category isn't generally recognized yet, but "tumor cell-modulating immunotherapy" is really the most appropriate term when talking about biological agents such as the interferons. All types of immunotherapy depend on the immune cells recognizing the tumor cells. The only way they can do this is by spotting certain antigens on the surface of these cells, which is not always an easy thing to do. "Cell modulation" means that the tumor-associated antigens are highlighted, giving the immune cells a kind of flashing billboard to aim for. This strategy may also be useful to modify the metabolism of chemotherapy drugs.

BIOLOGICAL AGENTS

Over the past few years, many biological agents and many approaches to biological therapy have been investigated. Most clinical trials originally concentrated on one or another of the strategies outlined above, trying to understand and exploit individual approaches to improving the immune response of cancer patients.

With the data from these trials in hand, it is now becoming possible to design useful combinations of strategies and agents. At the moment, a range of biological agents is being researched. These include biological response modifiers that have no direct antitumor effect but are able to trigger or stimulate the immune system and so indirectly affect tumors.

The Interferons (IFN) There are several interferons. One of them—interferon-alpha—was the first of the cytokines shown to have an antitumor effect, both a direct effect and indirect effects through a more active immune system.

So far, studies have shown that interferon-alpha causes tumors to shrink 15 to 20 percent of the time in patients with kidney cancer (renal cell carcinoma) and melanoma. Other studies have shown it to have a major effect in 90 percent of patients with the rare hairy cell leukemia and with the more common chronic myelocytic (myelogenous) leukemia. Interferon-alpha is also occasionally effective in people with indolent non-Hodgkin's lymphoma and in some people with AIDS who develop Kaposi's sarcoma.

Researchers are now investigating interferon-beta and interferon-gamma, both of which have some similar antitumor effects. And all the interferons are being evaluated in combination with other cytokines or in combination with chemotherapy. What isn't understood very well yet is the exact mechanism that makes the interferons effective. They may make the tumor cells seem more foreign (increase the antigenicity), which makes them more vulnerable to attack by antibodies or by the various immune cells.

Interleukins There are also several interleukins (IL-1 through IL-9). The one being most intensively investigated by the National Institutes of Health and many universities is interleukin-2, which increases the activity of lymphocytes. The lymphocytes that have been non-specifically activated by IL-2 are called LAK cells (lymphokine-activated killer cells), and these do a much better job of identifying and destroying tumor cells than ordinary lymphocytes. All the other interleukins are still in an early investigational stage, but several will soon be studied in cancer patients.

Some researchers believe that IL-2 treatment can be even more effective if lymphocytes are collected from a patient's blood through a special machine, activated with IL-2 in the laboratory, then returned to the patient as LAK cells along with even more IL-2. An alternative is to activate lymphocytes from a patient's tumor, producing what are called tumor infiltrating lymphocytes (TIL cells).

Studies of treatment with IL-2 show a response rate of 20 to 25 percent in patients with kidney cancer. IL-2—with or without the addition of LAK or TIL cells—also produces a response rate of about 20 to 25 percent in cases of advanced malignant melanoma. These responses are usually partial; complete responses are rare.

Colony-Stimulating Factors (CSFs) The CSFs are not directly effective against tumors, but they do play a major role in increasing the number and the activity of neutrophils and/or macrophages.

What makes research with CSFs particularly exciting is that high-dose chemotherapy dramatically reduces the number of white blood cells (including neutrophils) that fight infection, making chemotherapy patients vulnerable to various infectious diseases. It is for this reason that the dosage of chemotherapy often has to be kept low, thwarting any attempts to give higher and potentially more effective doses. But if the number of neutrophils can be increased by using colony-stimulating factors (such as G-CSF, GM-CSF and possibly IL-3 and IL-5), both the severity and the duration of low white blood counts can be reduced. Infections should therefore be less common and less severe. This should allow greater doses of chemotherapy to be given, which in turn should lead to more complete remissions.

T Cells Some investigators are studying the use of T cells rather than less specific cells in the fight against cancer. The T lymphocyte is a very important component of the immune response. It recognizes tumor cells and either makes helper factors that stimulate the rest of the immune system or makes killer factors that destroy tumor cells.

Tumor vaccines depend on stimulating T cells in the body. But another approach is to take T cells *out* of a patient's body—either from the bloodstream or from within the tumor itself—make more of them and at the same time stimulate them with IL-2, then return them in greater numbers than the patient could generate by himself or herself.

Although this approach is in its early stages, there have been some promising results in animals and in early studies with humans. Once again, melanoma and kidney cancer seem to be the most readily affected. As additional T cell growth factors are produced by genetic engineering, it should be possible to do a better job of growing T cells outside the body and causing them to be more highly activated than is now possible with IL-2 alone.

Tumor Vaccines One type of immunotherapy that has been studied for years and is only now coming of age is "active specific immunotherapy," more commonly known as the use of tumor vaccines. These would in theory work the same way as vaccines for measles, smallpox or other diseases.

Studies have shown responses in some people with some widespread tumors, particularly melanoma in about 25 percent of patients and in kidney cancer in about the same proportion. It has also been possible to prolong the survival of people with melanoma by treating them with vaccinia-treated, or Newcastle disease virus-killed, melanoma cells.

In another study involving colon cancer, patients with large primary tumors who had surgery were compared with similar patients who had surgery and then were injected with their own irradiated tumor cells and the booster substance BCG. The vaccinated patients survived longer than the group having surgery alone.

Many universities are now studying active immunization for other cancers including pancreatic cancer and lymphomas. There is no reason why this approach shouldn't be useful for a wide variety of tumors. It is probable that under the right circumstances the human body has the potential for developing immunity against all of them.

Tumor Necrosis Factors (TNFs) TNFs are a group of proteins that can destroy tumor cells. They occur naturally in the body in small numbers and can be produced in a laboratory by stimulating macrophages and lymphocytes. They have been found to be effective against certain tumors in animals (mainly mice), and clinical trials are now trying to find out if they are also effective in humans, either alone or in combination with other biological therapies.

ANTIBODY THERAPY

Antibodies are proteins (gamma globulins) that are produced by B lymphocytes. Every B lymphocyte produces one kind of antibody that recognizes a "foreign" protein structure, or antigen. The foreign structures are usually part of bacteria, viruses or other antigenic proteins. If the antibody can make contact with the antigen, it will become attached to it. This is important because a tumor cell surrounded by antibodies is more vulnerable to destruction by the cells of the immune system.

Vulnerability is increased because the antibodies have two parts—a variable part and a constant part.
♦ The variable part recognizes the antigen, or the specific structure of the "foreign" invader.
♦ The constant part, or the "tail," is recognized by the effector cells of the immune system such as monocytes, macrophages, T lymphocytes, neutrophils and LAK cells. So this constant part attracts the working immune cells, which then attack and destroy the structure to which the whole antibody is attached.

Monoclonal Antibodies A very modern and sophisticated way to use antibodies is to produce them in the laboratory as monoclonal antibodies (MAbs).

What makes MAbs different is that the antibodies produced naturally in the body by the many different B lymphocytes are always a mixture of different antibodies. But antibodies produced in a lab by a colony of B lymphocytes are all derived from the same parent cell (from the same "clone"). These antibodies won't be a mixture, but a pure accumulation of the specific antibody of the parent cell. The goal of this procedure is to produce a large culture of antibody-producing cells and then to select from the culture only the clones of those cells that make the specific antibodies against the antigens found on the surface of the cancer cell being treated.

How the Clones Are Made Live human cancer cells carry the antigens that are going to be the targets for the antibodies. So the cancer cells (or their tumor-specific antigens alone) are injected into mice. The immune systems of the mice are activated, and the mice produce lymphocyte colonies in their spleens. Each of these lymphocytes has reacted to an antigen from the cancer cell. These activated B lymphocytes are then removed from the spleens and "immortalized" by fusion with a special B cell. This produces a "hybridoma"—basically, a factory that can indefinitely manufacture antibodies against a specific antigen of the original cancer cell.

Normal antibody-producing B cells do not survive for more than a few days in a lab culture. Only the advent of cell fusion methods has made it possible to cultivate large colonies of B lymphocytes and so produce enough antibodies to use in cancer treatment.

The Effect on Normal Cells One problem with monoclonal antibodies is that while many MAbs can be produced to recognize tumor-associated antigens, most tumor antigens are not specific for the tumors. This means that these antigens may also be found on normal cells. This could create problems. But what saves MAbs as a treatment is that many antigens are found in large quantities on tumor cells and only in very limited amounts on normal cells. So an antibody designed to react against such an antigen will be able to destroy quite a few tumor cells without causing too much harm to normal cells.

Programming MAbs The ability to make antibodies in the lab has raised all sorts of possibilities. Clones can, in effect, be designed or programmed to serve several purposes besides reacting against specific cancer cells.

♦ MAbs can be programmed to be specific against cell growth factors, for example. This will interfere with the growth of cancer cells, which are frequently dependent on such factors.

♦ MAbs can be very helpful in some cases of bone marrow transplantation. Often, a cancer patient will donate his or her own marrow before heavy radiotherapy or chemotherapy, with the idea that it will be returned after treatment. But one problem with this kind of procedure (called an autologous transplant) is that cancer cells might be in the bone marrow. If the marrow is removed, stored and reintroduced, the cancer cells would be put right back and the cancer would recur. MAbs can be effective in purging the bone marrow cells of any cancer cells if the marrow is treated while it is outside the body.

♦ MAbs against a specific cancer cell can also be programmed to carry a radioisotope source to the tumor. This "radioactive-labeled" antibody will find the cancer cell and attach to it; the radioactive particles then destroy the tumor cells.

One problem is that the therapy requires an isotope strong enough to kill cells in the area of the target cancer cell. With radioactive iodine (I-131)-labeled antibodies, this treatment has been used successfully in cases of lymphomas, which are very radiosensitive tumors. But it is hard to deliver enough radiation to kill cells when treating many other kinds of tumors. Cancers of the colon, pancreas, stomach and esophagus, for example, are not very sensitive to radiation. With more research it is hoped that this technique may soon have better success.

♦ In the same way, MAbs that are specific against a certain cancer can be programmed to deliver other anticancer agents such as chemotherapy drugs or cell toxins like ricin to the tumor. As with the radioactive-labeled therapy, this is really antibody-guided treatment. The monoclonal antibody homes in on the cancer cell, latches on to it and lets the payload of drugs or toxins do their work.

Problems and Promise Antibodies—plain or bound to radioactive materials or other toxic substances—are being evaluated as therapy for cancer in clinical trials. The verdict on their usefulness isn't in yet, though theoretically they have a potential for specifically targeting and destroying many tumor cells.

What is clear so far is that the success of antibody therapy depends on how specific the monoclonal antibody is against the target antigen on the surface of the tumor cell, on the blood supply to the cancer and on how any one person's system handles the antibody. Unfortunately, there are still many problems to be overcome.

♦ It is difficult to precisely match the antibody with the antigen. Cancers are not pure. They have many different types of cell proteins, and only a specific cell line is affected by a specific MAb. This is much like direct-dialing from New York to Hong Kong. Get one number wrong and you could end up talking to Zaire.

♦ After receiving repeated courses of mouse MAbs, the human body develops antibodies against mouse immunoglobulins.

♦ Repeated courses of MAbs can also cause allergic reactions, with symptoms including fever, chills, itching, skin rashes, nausea, vomiting and flushing. A severe form of hypersensitivity known as serum sickness has also been reported.

SIDE EFFECTS

All cytokines are proteins, which means they can be destroyed by stomach enzymes. So they cannot be taken orally. They have to be given by injections into a vein, into a muscle or under the skin. Antitumor antibodies—polyclonal or monoclonal—are also given by injection.

There can be side effects at the site of the injection, just like the reaction you get with a smallpox "scratch" on your arm. But since biological agents are getting into your system, the side effects can also be generalized, or systemic.

◆ Most of the cytokines cause fever, fatigue and occasionally chills and a skin rash. They may cause changes in blood pressure, usually decreasing it.

◆ Interferons and TNFs cause general malaise, sometimes called flu-like syndrome.

◆ IL-2 can give rise to extremely severe and life-threatening side effects. IL-2 causes the peculiar capillary leak syndrome. If this develops, you may rapidly gain weight, experience a drop in your blood pressure and find it difficult to breathe. Tissues become swollen as fluid accumulates and there are sometimes toxic effects on the heart. Unless treatment is discontinued at this stage, IL-2 may cause kidney shutdown or respiratory arrest and death.

For these reasons, IL-2 is usually given in an intensive care unit, where blood pressure, urine output and breathing can be closely monitored and side effects treated promptly to avoid failure of a vital organ.

◆ Antitumor antibodies—polyclonal or monoclonal—can cause an allergic reaction varying from a mild skin rash, coughing and wheezing to an acute and severe reaction called anaphylaxis. With a full-blown anaphylactic reaction, blood pressure drops, various parts of the body swell, a severe skin rash breaks out and breathing can become difficult. This reaction can be fatal unless it is treated promptly with epinephrine and corticosteroids.

The possibility of allergic reactions to antibodies (or to any foreign substance) increases markedly with every additional injection, because eventually you become immunized against the foreign molecules. Your immune system will rapidly destroy these molecules, with the allergic reaction being a sign of your immune cells'

increased activity.

◆ The side effects of antibodies vary with their target. An antibody aimed at a colon antigen may cause diarrhea. One directed against white blood cells will cause low white blood cell counts.

WHEN BIOLOGICAL THERAPY IS APPROPRIATE

Researchers are investigating the possible role of biological therapy in the treatment of several tumors, especially kidney cancer, chronic myelogenous leukemia and melanoma. But all the agents included in biological therapy are still considered experimental, with one exception—interferon-alpha for hairy cell leukemia and Kaposi's sarcoma.

As an investigational treatment, biological therapy will usually be offered only after a trial of conventional treatment. But when there is no effective standard therapy and biological therapy offers some promise—with kidney cancer or advanced melanoma, for example—it may be recommended as a first-line treatment.

Patient Beware Many promoters of unproven and useless anticancer treatments claim that their product or therapy improves the immune system and so will probably cure cancer. As an educated consumer of health care services, you should beware of any such false claims about new agents that augment the immune system.

Except for some rare tumors such as Kaposi's sarcoma and some lymphomas that often result from immune suppression, there is as yet *no definite proof* that cancer is caused by failure of the immune system. The initial limited success of IL-2 and interferon may lead many people to jump to the conclusion that any improvement in the immune system will have a beneficial effect on malignant disease. But the truth is that how IL-2 and interferon actually work is not completely understood yet. And any unbalanced change in the immune system may be more harmful than beneficial.

Many agents with proved immuno-augmenting activity have failed to pro-duce a long-lasting antitumor effect. Although there is considerable promise, there is still a long way to go until we can reliably use the immune system to fight cancer.

9
LASER THERAPY

Carlos Pellegrini, MD, Ernest H. Rosenbaum, MD, and Malin Dollinger, MD

◇

Laser therapy involves the use of high-intensity light to destroy tumor cells. Lasers are fairly new weapons in the anti-cancer arsenal, and their role is still limited. In a few select cases laser therapy can cure a cancer. But the technique is now used mainly to relieve serious symptoms such as bleeding or obstruction, especially when the cancer can't be cured by surgery, radiation or chemotherapy or when standard treatment can't be used because of advanced age, malnutrition or heart or pulmonary disease.

The verdict isn't in yet on whether laser treatment can truly be a curative procedure or if it is useful only for palliation. The final answer will have to await results from more studies.

HOW LASERS WORK

The word *laser* is an acronym for "light amplification by stimulated emission of radiation." The light is produced by devices that can "excite" substances such as carbon dioxide, argon and neodynium:yttrium-aluminum-garnet (Nd:YAG) to a higher energy state. As these substances return to their "resting" state, they release their extra energy in the form of a powerful light with a special "energy" that is capable of vaporizing human tissue, including tumor cells.

What makes this type of energy so useful in cancer treatment is that it can be aimed so precisely. Lasers focus on very small areas with extreme accuracy.

Endoscopic Laser Therapy Laser therapy is usually given by activating the special light beam through a flexible tube called an endoscope, the same instrument used to diagnose many cancers. The scope can be passed through any opening in the body—the mouth, nose, anus or vagina.

A laser operator looking through the scope can see the tumor directly and aim the light beam precisely into the target tissue. The operator then activates the device and the energy is produced. On contact with the tissue, the laser beam produces an intense heat. At 60° C (140° F), this heat can coagulate protein. At 100° C (212° F), it can vaporize tissue. The tissue usually burns for just a few seconds, giving off a bit of smoke and leaving a hole or ulcer.

Removing a tumor with a laser beam is not as effective as removing it with conventional surgery. A surgeon removes all the visible tumor, the tumor below the surface of the organ and a wide margin of tissue on each side. The laser operator removes only the visible tumor on the organ's surface. But tumors are like icebergs. What is visible is simply the tip of a much greater mass below the surface. After laser treatment, the bulk of the tumor is still in place.

Photodynamic Laser Therapy In some cases, laser therapy can be made more effective by the use of photodynamic therapy. This involves injecting a chemical before the laser treatment that can make tissue more sensitive to light. Malignant tissues have a special affinity for light with a specific wavelength. After a tumor is sensitized by hematoporphyrin, for example, the laser is more selective in its cell-destroying action.

WHEN LASER THERAPY MIGHT BE RECOMMENDED

Laser therapy is used primarily to treat cancers of the skin, trachea, lungs, esophagus, stomach, colon, rectum and anus. It can't replace surgery, radiation or chemotherapy as a definitive cancer treatment, but it can complement these therapies in a variety of ways.

Direct laser therapy to the skin or cervix can be very successful. But the usual objective of laser therapy is to help relieve an acute obstruction. This might be done so that surgery, radiotherapy or chemotherapy can be used effectively. Or it may be done to keep some vital body tube open—the esophagus for swallowing, the trachea for breathing or the colon, rectum and anus for eliminating stool.

The benefits are usually short-term, however, and there are technical limitations. The best results are usually obtained in centers where the procedure is performed frequently by highly experienced endoscopists.

Planning the Treatment Before laser therapy is even attempted on the trachea, bronchi or gastrointestinal tract, the first thing to decide is whether an endoscopic biopsy needs to be done to verify the diagnosis.

The next step is a thorough clinical assessment. This may involve specific kinds of x-rays (such as a barium swallow or barium enema), CT or MRI scans and ultrasound. These imaging studies are needed to estimate the risk of bleeding and to map the exact shape and size of the tumor and any sharp angles (as in the colon or esophagus) that will have to be dealt with.

Endoscopic ultrasonography may help, since it allows the tissue beneath the surface to be assessed. It is very important to know how much of the tumor is within the opening, or lumen, of the body tube and how much of it has extended through the wall of the lumen into surrounding tissues. The status of the lymph nodes is important too, and this staging can be done quickly if an emergency arises.

Treating an Obstruction in the Trachea
Tumors in the windpipe (trachea) can't be treated very successfully with standard treatments. Less than 30 percent of patients are candidates for surgical removal of the tumor, and radiotherapy has few long-term survivors. Yet if the goal of treatment is palliation, laser therapy is a reasonable alternative.

Tracheal and endobronchial cancers can be directly seen through an endoscope and can be treated with a YAG laser, with or without the light-sensitizing hematoporphyrins. The tumor usually grows back and another treatment will be needed in four, eight or twelve weeks. With intrabronchial lesions, this interval can be stretched out by "afterloading" iridium-192. This involves placing empty catheters next to the tumor through an endoscope, then inserting the radioactive materials into the catheters to deliver a specific dose of radiation.

TREATING COLORECTAL AND ANAL CANCER

Laser treatment might cure a few cases of colorectal and anal cancer, though surgery along with radiation therapy is considered the primary treatment, with chemotherapy for certain stages. So the goal of laser therapy once again is usually palliation.

Colorectal Cancer If the purpose of laser treatment is to reduce or stop bleeding or to reduce the bulk of a tumor, one or two treatments will usually be enough.

When the obstruction is large, it may be hard to get the endoscope into the tumor.

It may be necessary to pass a guidewire through the tumor mass and use a smaller scope. An alternative is to use a guidewire to insert a balloon to dilate the constricted area, which will also allow a small scope to be passed to accomplish laser treatment.

♦ The most successful treatments occur when the tumor is growing inward, extending into the bowel lumen rather than outward toward the layer of the colon or rectum beneath the inner surface (submucosa).

♦ Short or smaller tumors and straight rather than curved or angulated areas of the colon are more successfully treated.

♦ The treatment is not curative and will require follow-up treatment to keep the lumen open every four, eight or twelve weeks, depending on how fast the tumor is growing.

♦ In rare instances, an obstruction of the bowel from colorectal or anal cancer may be decompressed by endoscopic laser therapy. This may allow surgery or other therapies to be planned on an elective rather than an emergency basis.

Anal Cancer What is often treated is a growing adenoma or an obstructing cancer when surgery, radiotherapy and chemotherapy are not appropriate treatments. Again, the best results from laser treatment are when the tumor is within the lumen rather than extending through the wall to adjacent tissues. A well-differentiated cancer that is small (less than 1 in./2.5-3 cm), non-ulcerating and growing into the lumen may have the best results.

The procedure is the same as for colon cancer and can be repeated after about 48 hours if you are in the hospital or about a week later if you are being treated as an outpatient. Several treatments might be needed to completely remove the obstruction.

♦ Fluid might accumulate in the tissues, which may temporarily intensify the obstruction or require pain-relieving medications.

♦ Retreatment is usually necessary four, six or twelve weeks after the obstruction is first removed.

♦ Many studies have shown that the obstructed lumen can be kept open in approximately 90 percent of cases. Bleeding can be controlled in over 85 percent of cases.

LASER THERAPY AND ESOPHAGEAL CANCER

Theoretically, laser therapy might be the only form of treatment needed for a very small tumor in the esophagus that could be completely vaporized.

Still, if the tumor can be cured with surgery, laser therapy isn't recommended for esophageal cancer. For one thing, tumors that small are very, very rare. For another, your doctor could never be sure the tumor hadn't invaded the wall of the esophagus beyond the laser's reach.

But if the cancer can't be cured by surgery (and esophageal cancer can seldom be cured), lasers can still help relieve the symptoms. When the tumor becomes so large that the opening of the esophagus—the lumen—gets blocked, you can't swallow food or even saliva. About 50 percent of patients can maintain their ability to swallow throughout their illness when a laser restores the lumen by vaporizing the tissue blocking it.

Laser vs Prosthetic Placement There are alternatives to laser therapy to treat swallowing problems. A tube, or prosthesis, placed in the esophagus can achieve an esophageal opening for swallowing in 95 percent of patients. But the procedure has a 13 percent complication rate and a 4.3 percent mortality.

Prostheses have a number of problems. They tend to get out of position and may block the esophagus on their own. They also don't propel food down to the stomach, so you may be limited to fluids or semi-solids. In general, they are not good for palliation of swallowing problems.

Laser therapy, on the other hand, offers 100 percent chance for success, with a 3.6 percent complication rate and approximately 1 percent mortality when performed by experienced practitioners. Laser is also considered better for high esophageal obstruction, where plastic prostheses such as Celestin's tubes cannot be fitted.

Endoscopic Laser Treatment Pretreatment evaluation will again involve mapping the exact geometry of the tumor and staging the disease. The size, depth of penetration of tumor invasion and lymph node status will determine whether the tumor is operable.

In the procedure itself (YAG laser with or without hematoporphyrin), the endoscope will be passed through your mouth and down the esophagus to the tumor site. Only the top layers of the treated area will be affected and only small pieces of tissue will evaporate. Three or more sessions might be needed to achieve an opening. These sessions are often spaced at 48-hour intervals to allow tissue breakdown to be more complete and to give the patient a rest. The technique varies and is decided upon by the operator. He or she will usually treat the lowest part of the tumor first, then come higher with each treatment session.

♦ Lasers are most useful in the middle and lower esophagus, which is straight, and least valuable for tumors outside the esophageal wall.

♦ It is difficult to know how deep to go into the submucosa since there are no good landmarks.

♦ There may be very narrow spaces (strictures) involved, which makes laser treatment more difficult. Dilating the esophagus first may help.

♦ There is acute angulation—a corner—at the junction of the esophagus with the stomach that makes laser therapy in this area very difficult.

♦ Since only the tumor within the lumen is removed, tumors usually come back quickly. The therapy will have to be repeated every two to eight weeks to keep the passage open.

♦ Laser therapy can help control bleeding as well as open a passageway to allow foods to be swallowed.

Combining Lasers and Other Treatments Different degrees of swallowing difficulty merit different approaches. Dilation of the esophagus before using chemotherapy or radiotherapy to help shrink the tumor may be the best way to get a functional esophageal opening that will improve the quality of life.

♦ Obstruction may occur with squamous cell esophageal cancer or with an adenocarcinoma of the stomach that grows upward to obstruct the esophagus. Lasers might be used in combination with standard treatments for these cancers.

♦ There may be a longer survival for squamous cell carcinoma with laser and radiation therapy. Squamous and adenocarcinoma have the same results for laser treatment, with tumors on the surface (Stage I) being easier to treat than tumors under the surface (Stage II).

♦ Results are better if the lesions are less than 2 in. (5 cm) in diameter. In one study, lasers gave almost all the patients (97 percent) an open passageway, but only 70 percent could eat satisfactorily.

♦ After the obstruction is removed, radiotherapy with afterloaded iridium-192 seeds can help prolong the swallowing interval.

10
HYPERTHERMIA

Penny K. Sneed, MD

◇

The idea of using heat to help destroy tumors has been around for a long time. In the early 1800s, there were medical reports that some people with cancer showed signs of tumor shrinkage after they developed high fevers. By the end of the last century, there were reports of some complete remissions because of high body temperatures.

But hyperthermia—the word means elevated temperature and refers to the use of heat in the treatment of cancer—has only recently been added to the arsenal of anticancer weapons. It is a specialized weapon, since hyperthermia techniques are still not applicable to all types of tumors. But in certain cases, when heat is applied for about an hour once or twice a week in conjunction with radiotherapy or sometimes chemotherapy, the results have been very promising.

HOW IT WORKS

When temperatures rise above 106° F (41° C), the heat starts to damage cells. How much damage is done depends on the temperature and how long the exposure lasts. The temperatures now used range from about 106 to 113° F (41 to 45° C).

Combining Hyperthermia with Other Therapies Heat is particularly effective when combined with radiation, for heat is especially destructive to two types of cells that tend to be resistant to radiation:
♦ cells making DNA in preparation for division; and

♦ cells that are acidic and starved for oxygen (poorly oxygenated). Unlike normal tissue, many tumors are likely to have poorly oxygenated cells that are particularly susceptible to hyperthermia, and tumors can often be heated to higher temperatures than surrounding normal tissues.

Heat also makes cells more sensitive to radiation by preventing them from repairing radiation damage. Heat and radiation work best together when the two treatments are given simultaneously or within perhaps an hour of each other. Hyperthermia treatments are usually given only once or twice weekly, because after cells are exposed to heat, they become resistant to subsequent exposures for about three to five days.

Heat also seems to improve the effect of some of the drugs used in chemotherapy, such as bleomycin, cisplatin, cyclophosphamide, melphalan, mitomycin C and the nitrosoureas.

Heating Techniques During the past 15 years devices have become available to heat tumors directly and safely.

Hyperthermia treatment techniques can be divided into three broad categories—localized, regional and whole body heating.
♦ Localized heating of tumors in or near the skin is often performed using an external applicator. This square or round box is placed on the outside of the body over the tumor. The applicator is connected to equipment that supplies different types of energy—microwave, radiofrequency or ultrasound—that will heat the tumor cells.

Localized heating can also be accomplished internally in a process called interstitial (inside the tumor) hyperthermia. Under anesthesia, needles or plastic tubes are placed into the tumor. Heat sources are then inserted directly into the plastic tubes or radiofrequency current is passed through the needles. Interstitial techniques often raise the tumor temperatures much higher than could be done with external techniques and without doing much damage to surrounding normal tissues.

♦ Regional hyperthermia involves using microwave or radiofrequency applicators to heat large volumes of tissue deep inside the body.

♦ Whole body heating can be accomplished by using hot water blankets, specialized oven-like devices or other methods. This procedure is safe, using temperatures up to about 107° F (41.8° C). This temperature may not be high enough to be effective in combination with radiation therapy alone, but may become useful with chemotherapy. Whole body and/or regional hyperthermia can also be combined with localized hyperthermia to improve results.

Although the hyperthermia treatment may be given externally, the temperatures inside the tumor usually have to be carefully monitored to control the treatment properly. This often means that tiny thermometers have to be placed into the tumor region, usually inside one or more small needles or tubes that are gently inserted through the skin under a local anesthetic.

Side Effects Hyperthermia does not cause any marked increase in radiation side effects or complications. Superficial hyperthermia by itself, however, can cause discomfort or even significant local pain in about half the patients treated. It can also cause blisters, which generally heal rapidly. Less commonly, it can cause burns, which tend to heal very slowly and occasionally need surgical repair.

How often blisters and burns occur depends on whether the tumor involves the skin and on the degree of skin cooling used during the treatment. In one study, heat blisters occurred in 10 percent of the superficial areas treated, but normal tissue ulceration occurred in less than 1 percent of cases. This indicates that burns can normally be avoided with careful monitoring and control of surface temperatures.

WHEN HYPERTHERMIA IS APPROPRIATE

As a form of treatment, hyperthermia has had very limited success when used by itself. In one study, only 13 percent of superficial tumors treated with hyperthermia alone had a "complete response"—in other words, disappeared completely. But many studies in patients with superficial malignancies have shown benefits when hyperthermia is added to radiation therapy. A review of 15 studies revealed a complete response rate of 37 percent for tumors treated with radiation alone, and 63 percent for tumors treated with radiation and hyperthermia.

The tumor response was often evaluated by comparing the results with different tumors in the same patients. In these same-patient comparisons, the complete response rate was 31 percent for tumors treated with radiation alone versus 71 percent for tumors treated with radiation and hyperthermia.

Superficial hyperthermia has been used successfully in combination with radiation therapy to treat:

♦ advanced primary breast cancer

♦ chest wall recurrences of breast cancer after a mastectomy and/or radiation therapy

♦ advanced or recurrent tumors involving lymph nodes containing metastatic cancer

♦ recurrent primary or metastatic melanoma in the skin or in tissues just under the skin

♦ melanomas in the eye
♦ primary cervix cancer
♦ soft tissue sarcomas

Interstitial hyperthermia—applying heat with probes inserted into the tumor—has been used for some tumors in the head and neck, breast, pelvis and skin or soft tissues. There is also now a lot of interest in using interstitial hyperthermia and radiation for brain tumors.

New Directions Many exciting areas of investigation could make clinical hyperthermia much more useful in the near future. Studies are in progress to find out just how much hyperthermia is needed to improve the results of radiation treatment. Several methods may soon be available to help predict a tumor's response to hyperthermia based on small samples of the cancerous cells.

It may also soon be possible to improve results by manipulating the flow of blood to the tumor or by manipulating its sensitivity to heat. Computer-based treatment planning, incorporating knowledge of blood flow in tumors and normal tissue, could be used for more effective hyperthermia treatment planning.

Although many tumors are unfortunately still difficult to heat with available devices, great improvements are being made in technology and treatment techniques that will allow hyperthermia to be applied to many more tumors.

11
HYPERTHERMIC PERFUSION THERAPY

Robert E. Allen, Jr, MD

Regional perfusion is a way to deliver chemotherapy drugs to tumors in parts of the body that can be isolated from the circulatory system—that is, the arms and legs.

The first reported use of this technique was in 1950, when nitrogen mustard was infused into the arteries supplying blood to tumors while the veins returning the blood were blocked. This maximized the exposure of the tumor to the chemotherapeutic drug.

The technique was refined in 1957 by using a tourniquet to isolate an extremity and adding a heart-lung machine to the process. The machine supplied oxygen and circulated the mixture of blood, drug and mineral solution (the perfusate) throughout the isolated limb. This method allowed an increase of 6 to 10 times the normal dosage of drug that could have been given locally to the cancer. The drug's toxic effects to the entire body were reduced and the rate of response was increased. The first report of a large number of patients treated with isolated limb perfusion at normal body temperature showed they had a survival rate 20 to 25 percent better than those treated in the conventional way.

A later development added heat to the perfusion system. Heat will kill tumor cells more often than normal ones at certain critical temperatures. The tumor-killing effect depends on the amount of heat used and the length of time it is applied. Using a heated perfusate improved the response rate in a 1967 study and heat has played a role in the procedure ever since.

What makes isolated limb perfusion particularly effective is that it delivers high-dose chemotherapy not only to the tumor but to the entire limb below the tourniquet, including potential sites of metastases. All that limits the dosage of the chemotherapy drug to be given is local tissue toxicity.

WHEN THE PROCEDURE IS APPROPRIATE

Perfusion can be used to treat a variety of cancers in the arms and legs. Melanomas, sarcomas and some localized cutaneous lymphomas have been treated with this method, but it has been most widely and effectively used to treat cutaneous malignant melanoma.

This cancer can be cured surgically if the tumor is discovered at an early stage, but isolated heated limb perfusion is suggested for people with extensive local tumors. And perfusing may be the treatment of choice for those who have melanomas involving the palms of the hands, the soles of the feet and the fingernails and toenails (subungual areas). Melanomas in these locations tend to have a poor prognosis.

People who have locally recurrent melanomas or spreading melanomas that are traveling away from the primary site toward nearby lymph nodes—the prognosis is very grave in both situations—are best treated by perfusion.

Results of Treatment Whether the treatment leads to a beneficial outcome depends on the stage of the cancer. There is some controversy about whether people with high-risk Stage I melanoma should have prophylactic perfusion or just surgery alone. One report has shown increased disease-free survival for Stage I patients treated with perfusion.

The five-year cure rate for acrolentiginous melanomas treated with perfusion ranges from 70 to 78 percent; the cure rate for the same lesions treated without perfusion ranges from 38 to 50 percent. On the average, perfusion offers people with Stage II or III melanomas a 20 to 25 percent increased survival over other treatment methods.

The following survival rates have been reported for the various stages as defined by the staging system developed at the M. D. Anderson Tumor Institute, the system most often used to stage melanomas of the extremities.

STAGE FIVE-YEAR SURVIVAL AFTER PERFUSION

◆ **Stage I**	
Localized primary melanoma	89-94 percent
◆ **Stage II**	
Local recurrence within or adjacent to the scar	74-77 percent
◆ **Stage III**	
Regional metastases	
IIIA In-transit metastases	70-81 percent
IIIB Positive regional lymph nodes	48-54 percent
IIIAB In-transit metastases with regional nodes	30-45 percent
◆ **Stage IV**	
Systemic metastases, positive iliac lymph nodes	20-25 percent

WHICH DRUGS ARE USED

Alkylating agents are the most effective drugs to be perfused. They react with DNA, altering the nucleic acid and eventually killing the cell.

Melphalan (L-phenylalanine mustard) has been the drug most extensively used, either alone or in combination. Other drugs—cisplatin, thiotepa, dactinomycin and dacarbazine—are also used, but melphalan has many of the qualities of the ideal agent for isolated limb perfusion. It is the least toxic single drug, with low toxicity to soft tissues and blood vessel linings. It has a short half life (meaning that it disappears quickly) and its action isn't limited to specific phases of the cancer cell's life cycle.

Whatever anticancer drug is used, its effectiveness is enhanced by two aspects of the perfusion procedure. The use of high oxygen concentrations magnifies the effects of the drugs by sensitizing tumor cells and has a tumor-killing effect of its own. Heat opens the blood vessels so that there is a more even and thorough perfusion.

HOW IT WORKS

There are several steps in the regional hyperthermic perfusion procedure.

Isolating the Limb The technique begins with the process called cannulating, which means that small tubes are inserted into the arteries carrying blood to the limb and the veins carrying blood out. This means placing tubes into the axillary artery and vein when treating an arm and into the external iliac artery and vein when treating a leg. The blood vessels in the thigh (femoral) and behind the knee (popliteal) have also been used when treating a leg.

To make the isolation complete, a rubber tourniquet is placed at the top of the arm or leg and held in place with a mechanical device. The blood vessel tubing is then connected to a heart-lung machine.

Preparing the Circuit The complete perfusion circuit consists of a low flow modular pump, arterial and venous tubing, an oxygenerator with an arterial line filter, a heating and cooling unit and an arterial blood temperature probe.

The circuit is primed with a mixture of your own blood and an electrolyte (mineral) solution, which circulates through the isolated limb with very high concentrations of oxygen. Heparin, a substance that

System used for hyperthermic perfusion therapy.

prevents blood from clotting, is added. Leakage of the perfusate into the general circulation is checked by injecting fluorescein dye into the mixture, and any leakage is monitored and corrected during the operation.

Special thermometers (needle thermistors) are placed in the soft tissues at strategic locations to record the temperature of the limb during the procedure.

Giving the Drug The perfusate temperature is raised to 107.6° F (42° C). The temperature of the extremity is raised to 104° F (40° C) and is not allowed to rise beyond that.

When the average temperature near the tumor is 102.2° F (39° C), the chemotherapy drug is added to the solution and the perfusion continues for one hour (tourniquet time is limited to a maximum of two hours). Flow rates are in the range of 400 to 600 cc/min. for a leg and 250 to 350 cc/min. for an arm, with perfusion pressures never allowed to exceed the average blood pressure in the body.

When the procedure is complete, the drug is drained from the arm or leg and the limb is washed out with a mixture of dextran-40 and a balanced salt solution.

After the Procedure You will have to stay in bed with the extremity elevated for three days after the procedure, during which time you will be given low doses of heparin, the anticoagulating agent.

The oxygen saturation of the perfused limb has to be continuously monitored for four days after the operation. A fall in the saturation usually signals the start of what is called the compartment syndrome, meaning that the limb swells so severely that it may interfere with circulation.

Complications About 30 percent of people who have perfusion will experience complications, but most of them are minor and pass quickly.

◆ Severe bone marrow toxicity occurs in about 5 percent of patients, but this is usually temporary.

◆ The compartment syndrome occurs in 3 to 4 percent of patients. This is an emergency situation and if proper treatment is not given promptly, the limb may have to be amputated.

◆ There is always a buildup of fluid in the tissues (edema), but this does not last long if it is properly treated.

◆ Since anticoagulation is used, there is an increased risk of postoperative bleeding.

◆ Inflamed veins and blood clots in the legs (thrombophlebitis) occur in 10 to 15 percent of patients, but the clots rarely travel to the lungs (pulmonary embolism).

◆ Mortality from the procedure is variously reported from 1 in 2,000 (0.05 percent) to 3 in 200 (1.5 percent).

12
BONE MARROW TRANSPLANTATION

James O. Armitage, MD

Bone marrow contains immature (or stem) cells that are capable of continuously producing new cells. This is what helps make bone marrow the "factory" for normal blood cells—the red cells that carry oxygen, the white cells that fight infections and the platelets that help blood clotting.

Bone marrow can sometimes be defective—for example, not producing enough normal blood cells. Red cells, white cells and platelets are necessary for life, so this is obviously a serious situation. And doctors long ago realized that if defective bone marrow could be replaced with normal marrow from another individual, a critical situation like that could be resolved. But only in the past 20 years has medical knowledge advanced to the point where effective bone marrow transplantation techniques could be developed.

These techniques involve the intravenous administration of immature blood cells capable of reproducing themselves and repopulating an empty bone marrow.

WHY A TRANSPLANT MIGHT BE RECOMMENDED

Replacing the defective bone marrow of an otherwise healthy person is one use of transplantation techniques. But at least 90 percent of all bone marrow transplants are performed to treat cancer.

Direct Benefit Transplanted bone marrow can have a direct effect against a cancer like leukemia. The transplanted marrow— which represents the immune system of another person—can recognize cancer cells as abnormal and destroy them. Unfortunately, this same phenomenon is thought to be related to an unwanted side effect known as graft-versus-host disease. Ideally, it would be possible to have only the effect against the cancer and avoid damage to normal tissue.

To Support Other Therapies A number of cancers are very sensitive to chemotherapy and radiation, but they cannot quite be cured with conventional doses. Unfortunately, the high drug or radiation doses that might cure the cancers can irreversibly damage other tissues.

Bone marrow is the organ generally most sensitive to the toxic action of chemotherapy and radiation. There is a wide difference between the intensity of therapy that leads to lethal toxicity in bone marrow and the higher intensity that leads to lethal toxicity in other organs. So, if the bone marrow could in a sense be written off and replaced after therapy, higher doses of chemotherapy and radiation could be administered without irreversibly damaging other major organs. Assuming the cancer cells are sensitive to treatment, the increased intensity of therapy should lead to higher cure rates.

When a Transplant Is Appropriate Bone marrow transplantation is not a procedure that can be recommended lightly. It is a dangerous treatment and is not appropriate in every case. If a patient can be cured with therapy that does not require bone marrow transplantation, that is obviously the easiest approach. If a patient can be cured only with therapy so intense that other organs as well as the bone marrow are lethally damaged, there is no advantage to having a bone marrow transplant, for survival is unlikely anyway because of the organ damage.

But bone marrow transplantation can be uniquely curative for a patient whose cancer could be cured with high-dose therapy that irreversibly damages bone marrow but does not fatally damage any other organ. Some patients who can almost but not quite be cured with standard therapies could cross the "cure threshold" with increased amounts of therapy. With certain malignancies sensitive to chemotherapy and radiation, it is clear that this "window of opportunity" does exist.

TYPES OF TRANSPLANTS

Transplanting any organ—a heart, a kidney, a lung or bone marrow—from one person to another is a complicated procedure. The immune system is designed to destroy foreign tissues, and "graft rejection" is always a possibility. The risk of rejection can be reduced by matching as much as possible the tissues of the donor and the tissues of the person receiving the transplant.

Depending on the availability of appropriate donors, there are three types of bone marrow transplantation that can be attempted.

Allogeneic This type involves the transfer of marrow from one individual to a completely different individual. The marrow donor is selected through a process known as HLA typing.

Matched vs Unmatched Each individual has genes on one chromosome that code for proteins that appear on cell surfaces and are involved in cell self-recognition. These bits of information, or antigens, can be identified in the laboratory. This makes it possible to tell whether bone marrow from two individuals would be "matched" or "unmatched."

Related vs Unrelated Usually allogeneic transplants are between brothers and sisters. This can be done when all the known antigens are matched or if there is a mismatch at only one site. The treatment will be equally successful in either case. But the better the match, the better the outcome.

Allogeneic transplantation between unrelated people can be done. But given the extraordinary complexity and diversity of HLA antigens—there are more than a billion possible combinations—finding matched but unrelated individuals is very difficult.

The National Unrelated Donor Bank now operates in the United States to try to find unrelated donors. This bank has made it possible to identify donors for most patients with common HLA antigens. Yet it is still hard to find donors for patients with uncommon antigens. Adding to the problem is the uneven distribution of HLA antigens among people with different genetic backgrounds. Because most of the volunteer donors so far are of European ancestry, it is especially hard to find donors for patients with African, Asian or other ancestry. (If you are interested in participating in the National Bone Marrow Donor Program, contact your local Red Cross Blood Center for information about how to volunteer.)

Syngeneic The best donor for any bone marrow transplant is an identical twin. Since identical twins share all the same genes they have exactly the same HLA antigens, so there is no risk of rejection. This is called a syngeneic transplant and, of course, is uncommon.

Autologous A somewhat similar situation

arises if someone receives his or her own bone marrow after high-dose chemotherapy and/or radiotherapy. This can be done by removing marrow before therapy and keeping it in cold storage (cryopreserving) until treatment is complete. This procedure—called an autotransplant or autologous bone marrow transplantation—should avoid the problems associated with introducing cells with different HLA types. There should be no risk of rejection. But it adds the risk of possibly reinfusing cancer cells that were inadvertently stored along with the marrow.

HOW BONE MARROW IS OBTAINED

In newborn children, essentially all bones have active marrow. In adults, active marrow is found mainly in the center of the pelvic bones, ribs, spine and collarbones. When an appropriate donor is identified, active marrow usually is removed from these bones with needles and a syringe. In some circumstances, it is possible to remove stem cells from blood.

Needle Aspiration Most bone marrow transplants involve extracting bone marrow from the bones of the pelvis by repeated needle punctures. The donor is usually under anesthetic during this process, which is a good thing, for it takes 150 or 200 needle punctures to remove enough marrow for a transplant—about 500 to 1,000 cc (one or two pints).

How the bone marrow is handled after it is removed depends upon the type of transplant to be done.
♦ If the transplant is allogeneic and the donor and the recipient have the same ABO red blood cell type, the marrow is immediately given intravenously.
♦ If the red blood cells of the donor and recipient are incompatible, the red cells can be separated out.
♦ If an autotransplant is planned, the cells have to be stored. This requires mixing them

with a substance to prevent ice from forming and then freezing the cells in liquid nitrogen. The cells are sometimes also treated with chemicals or antibodies—in a process called marrow purging—to try to remove potentially contaminating cancer cells. It is not yet known how effective this is.

Getting Cells from the Blood If you are going to have an autologous transplant, immature blood cells can be obtained from your blood by repeated separating (pheresis) procedures. This involves drawing blood into an apparatus that works like a cream separator. The same type of cells obtained by needle aspiration are collected and the remainder returned to you. The procedure has to be repeated several times to get enough cells for transplantation, so the process usually lasts two to four hours. The number of immature cells in the blood might also be increased by the administration of various chemicals.

COMPLICATIONS AND RISKS

The transplant procedure is fraught with risk. The only reason that anyone undertakes this risky venture is that the alternatives are so much worse. Anyone who undergoes a bone marrow transplantation is someone who will certainly die soon without one.

The specific risks are related to the phase of the procedure and can be divided into effects that are delayed or immediate.

Delayed Effects Long-term toxic effects of high-dose therapy can include cataracts in people receiving total body radiotherapy. Delayed effects can also include sterility, although people who've been extensively treated for their cancer before a transplant are often already sterile. But there have been cases lately where women who have had a bone marrow transplant have conceived and borne healthy children.

Immediate Risks Much more threatening are the risks during and soon after the transplant procedure. The high-dose therapy itself, the damage to the immune system and the reaction of the immune system to the transplanted marrow can all cause dangerous complications.

♦ *Toxic reactions from drugs and irradiation* High-dose therapy occasionally has an acute toxic effect on the heart that can be lethal, although this is quite rare.

♦ *Infections* After the transplant, there will be a period of two to six weeks during which the new bone marrow cannot manufacture red cells, white cells or platelets. Though it is fairly easy to transfuse red cells and platelets, it is nearly impossible to transfuse white cells. Going without them for any time is dangerous because the risk of infection is high when blood counts are very low. So anyone getting a transplant will usually be given liberal amounts of antibiotics. Sometimes these are given before any signs of infection appear and are usually not discontinued until the blood counts have returned to a more normal level. They are always given at the first sign of a fever. Most of the time infections can be controlled until normal white cells return. But certain infections—such as fungal infections—can still prove fatal.

It may soon be possible to reduce the period of low white blood cell counts by using agents called hematopoietic growth factors (such as G-CSF or GM-CSF). These normally occurring products can now be isolated and administered in doses that seem to accelerate the return of white blood cells after a transplant. These agents have not yet been released for general use in the United States, but it is hoped they will be soon.

♦ *Bleeding* Platelets can usually be transfused easily, but for a few patients it is difficult to transfuse enough of them. For these patients, serious bleeding is a possibility.

♦ *Graft rejection* This is a major risk, particularly for people having an allogeneic bone marrow transplantation. And the risk seems greater for those who have unrelated or less well matched allogeneic transplants. What usually happens is that the marrow function starts to come back, but then it disappears. This is a serious complication, but it can sometimes be overcome by a second transplant.

♦ *Pneumonia* The lung seems to be the organ most sensitive to the adverse effects of transplantation. It has been suggested that the lung is to bone marrow transplantation what the quarterback's knee is to a football game. A lot can go wrong. The lung can be injured because of infection, because of the toxic effect of high-dose chemotherapy and radiation or because of some unknown cause.

When severe pneumonia develops after a bone marrow transplant, death often—but not always—results. The most common pneumonia in these cases is caused by cytomegalovirus, a particularly severe pneumonia that can develop several months after the transplant. If it does develop, it is often in association with another serious complication, graft-versus-host disease.

♦ *Graft-versus-host disease* After an allogeneic bone marrow transplant, the immunologically active cells in the new marrow can recognize the "host" organism—the patient receiving the transplant—as foreign and go on the attack. The most commonly damaged organs are the skin, liver and intestines.

Medicines can be given after the transplant to reduce the possibility of graft-versus-host disease. If the condition nevertheless develops, it can occur soon after the return of white cells (acute graft-versus-host disease) or much later (chronic graft-versus-host disease).

The two types are similar in some ways, though each has distinctive features. The acute form often doesn't last long but can be quite severe. If it is severe, the prognosis for survival is very poor.

Chronic graft-versus-host disease almost always requires therapy, and most patients recover. One positive note is that when patients develop chronic graft-versus-host disease after an allogeneic transplant for leukemia, they are less likely to have recurrent leukemia.

CHOOSING A TRANSPLANT CENTER

If you are told that you might be referred for a bone marrow transplant, it is usually at a time when things aren't going too well. If there were a simpler way to cure your cancer, there would certainly be no call for bone marrow transplantation.

Having the procedure will sometimes involve traveling a considerable distance to a marrow transplant center. Which center to choose is often a difficult decision, with such factors as convenience, the center's experience with the disease and insurance issues all affecting the decision.

♦ *Experience* When facing a treatment as dangerous as bone marrow transplantation, most people want to be sure they are treated at a highly experienced center so the risk can be minimized. With certain cancers, it might be appropriate to choose a transplant center that has a special interest and extensive experience with your particular type of tumor.

You and your doctor may want to consult the American Society of Clinical Oncology and the American Society of Hematology, which have made joint recommendations for the *minimal* criteria for a center to perform the procedure.

♦ *Costs* Bone marrow transplantation is expensive and, in the United States, all transplant centers, before they will allow admission, will want some guarantee that the cost of the treatment will be reimbursed. Most health insurance companies in the United States now reimburse the cost for transplantation for leukemia and lymphoma, but how willing they are to reimburse for other diseases varies widely.

It's unfortunate, but some patients will be denied this treatment because their insurance company will refuse to pay for it.

Securing a Bed If you are referred to a particular transplant center, you will usually have to go to the facility for a "transplant interview." The center has to decide whether you are a good candidate for the treatment. You have to decide whether you feel comfortable undergoing treatment at that center.

Once this decision has been jointly made, there will be other decisions such as whether more "traditional" therapy might be done to improve the chance for success. An allogeneic donor may have to be found or stem cells will have to be taken and stored for an autotransplant. Then it will be necessary to secure a bed in the transplant unit. Keep in mind that some centers have long waiting lists. Once a bed has been secured, you enter the hospital and begin therapy.

A SUMMARY OF THE STEPS TO A SUCCESSFUL TRANSPLANT

For a successful bone marrow transplant to be performed, your medical team will have to complete a number of steps in sequence. Each step involves critical decisions and potential risks.

1. Determine that the cancer is sensitive to high-dose therapy and cannot be cured with simpler treatment.
For both doctor and patient this is the hardest part of the procedure. The candidate for a transplant has to have a disease serious enough that a treatment as risky as bone marrow transplantation is a reasonable option.

What makes the decision particularly difficult is that transplants are much more useful when patients are referred for treatment early in the course of their disease. Then they are still healthy. There is less cancer and it hasn't become highly resistant to therapy after repeated treatments. But transplant-related deaths are least acceptable in these early stages. The easiest course would be to refer a patient for transplantation when he or she is almost dead from cancer and all other therapies have failed. Unfortunately, at that point we know bone marrow transplantation is not likely to be beneficial.

The best approach, then, is to identify those who might benefit from the procedure and refer them for the treatment as soon as it seems clear that they cannot be cured with a simpler therapy.

2. Identify a source of marrow stem cells.
Once the decision to have a transplant is made, the possibility of your being able to use your own marrow cells or blood stem cells has to be evaluated. If your cells are contaminated by tumor, an allogeneic or syngeneic transplant will be the only choice and a bone marrow donor will have to be found—an HLA-matched brother or sister or a partially matched relative for an allogeneic transplant, a matched but unrelated donor for an allogeneic transplant or an identical twin for a syngeneic transplant.

Allogeneic transplantation is more effective in younger people. The incidence of graft-versus-host disease rises rapidly in those over 30, and most transplant centers will not do allogeneic transplants on people older than 40 to 55.

3. Administer high-dose chemotherapy—with or without radiotherapy—to kill the cancer and, in an allogeneic transplant, destroy your own immune system.
The purpose of the high-dose therapy is to destroy the cancer, suppress the immune system if necessary and empty the marrow to provide space for the new bone marrow cells to grow. If an allogeneic transplant is being performed, your own immune system must be destroyed. If it isn't, your immune cells will reject the

donor's bone marrow cells and leave you without a functioning bone marrow.

4. Infuse the stem cells intravenously.
In a typical bone marrow transplant unit, the day on which the marrow is given is referred to as Day 0. The other days you spend in the hospital are numbered as either a plus or minus, counting from the day the marrow is infused.

5. Manage the complications until the marrow produces enough normal blood cells and, in an allogeneic transplant, until graft-versus-host disease is controlled.
While the high-dose therapy is often uncomfortable, the period after the marrow infusion is the most dangerous. This is when the bone marrow cells begin to proliferate, ideally to the point where the marrow will produce enough red cells, white cells and platelets. This is when you run the risk of infections and bleeding problems. Most patients who don't survive long after a bone marrow transplant die from infections or the effects of graft-versus-host disease after the new marrow starts to grow.

Until you recover adequate white blood cell and platelet counts, you will be kept under close medical observation, usually in a special hospital room. After the marrow starts to grow, you will stay under close medical supervision until it is clear that the new marrow is functioning properly, that there has been no serious graft-versus-host disease and that your cancer has been controlled.

EFFECTIVENESS WITH DIFFERENT CANCERS
The following table summarizes the results of allogeneic and autologous bone marrow transplantation as a treatment for a variety of cancers. These results are only summaries and certainly vary with specific clinical situations.

It is also important to recognize that bone marrow transplantation as a treatment for cancer is a fast-changing field. New high dose therapies or improved transplant techniques might change the results with a particular disease in a very short time.

CURE RATES WITH BONE MARROW TRANSPLANTATION

Type	Late in the Disease	Early in the Disease
Leukemias		
◆ Acute Lymphoblastic and Acute Myeloblastic	10 percent	50 percent
◆ Chronic Granulocytic	10 percent	50 percent
Lymphomas		
◆ Hodgkin's Disease	10 percent	50 percent
◆ Large Cell Non-Hodgkin's Lymphoma	10 percent	40 percent
Neuroblastoma	less than 10 percent	30 percent
Breast Cancer	occasional prolonged remissions	studies too early to determine cure rate

Leukemias The first common cancer to be treated with bone marrow transplantation was acute leukemia. Even patients with "end stage leukemia" could sometimes be cured when they had allogeneic bone marrow transplantation, although there were better results when it was used early in the treatment.

Acute Leukemia The results for allogeneic transplantation in acute leukemia seem to depend very much on age. Patients who have a transplant as part of their initial therapy have a cure rate of more than 50 percent if they're under 20. But as age increases, the cure rate decreases. Results in patients over 40 are much poorer, although successful transplants can still be performed. But the fact that regular-dose chemotherapy also has better results in younger patients—and can sometimes cure them—makes the use of marrow transplantation in the initial control of the disease (first remission) very controversial.

In patients who are initially treated with other therapies for acute leukemia and then relapse, bone marrow transplantation is the only treatment with any real chance for cure. Though the cure rate is less than 50 percent, it has become the generally accepted form of therapy.

The transplantation can be either allogeneic or autologous in acute leukemia. But if autologous transplantation is the choice, there has to be a source of uncontaminated bone marrow cells for reinfusion after high-dose therapy. This is usually accomplished by trying to eliminate—purging—contaminating leukemia cells from bone marrow collected during a period of remission.

Chronic Leukemias Bone marrow transplantation has only recently been used in cases of chronic granulocytic leukemia, a disease that occurs in young adults and is always fatal with standard therapy. During the late 1970s and 1980s, quite a few patients with this cancer underwent allogeneic bone marrow transplantation and a promising number of them were cured. Allogeneic transplantation has now become the treatment of choice for patients of an appropriate age with chronic granulocytic leukemia and who have an HLA-matched brother or sister. Cure rates of over 50 percent have been reported.

Non-Hodgkin's Lymphomas and Hodgkin's Disease Lymphomas are among the tumors most responsive to chemotherapy and radiation. Hodgkin's disease was the first commonly occurring solid tumor shown to be curable with combination chemotherapy, and all types of lymphomas can be cured with radiation when they haven't spread. So it is not surprising that these tumors are among those most likely to respond to very high-dose therapy accompanied by a bone marrow transplant.

Aggressive Non-Hodgkin's Lymphomas
These can be cured between one-third and one-half of the time with primary therapy. But if there is a relapse after initial therapy, bone marrow transplantation can cure a significant percentage of patients.
♦ It apparently can cure about a third of patients who are treated early when their disease is still sensitive to chemotherapy at lower doses (they have at least a partial response to chemotherapy at lower doses but cannot be cured by it).
♦ It can cure 10 to 15 percent of patients who have relapsed after primary chemotherapy but whose tumors are no longer sensitive to lower-dose chemotherapy.
♦ It only very occasionally cures patients whose tumors have never responded to chemotherapy.

There is now considerable enthusiasm for testing the use of bone marrow transplantation even earlier in the course of aggressive lymphomas, perhaps incorporating it into the initial therapy for patients who aren't likely to be cured with standard treatments. As we become better at identifying patients with a poor outlook with primary therapy, this might become an important use of bone marrow transplantation.

Low-grade Non-Hodgkin's Lymphomas
These malignancies are rarely cured with standard therapies, although they are associated with a long average survival. But an average survival of even 10 years is not good enough for people who are 30 or 40 years old at the time of diagnosis. For this reason, several centers have recently begun to treat low-grade lymphoma patients with high-dose therapy and bone marrow transplantation early in the course of their disease. The results so far show that these patients tolerate the transplant process well and a large proportion of them stay in remission for extended periods. It is still too early to know if this treatment can actually cure the disease.

Hodgkin's Disease Patients with this cancer do so well with standard treatment approaches that physicians have been reluctant to refer them for transplantation early enough in their disease for a transplant to be beneficial. But it has become apparent that patients who relapse after high-quality combination chemotherapy have a poor outlook with more standard therapy. And when these patients are referred for high-dose therapy and bone marrow transplantation soon after their relapse, 50 percent or more seem to be long-term, disease-free survivors—in other words, probably cured. The cure rate is much less (10 to 20 percent) when they have the transplant after failing many chemotherapy regimens.

Other Blood Cancers A number of other hematologic malignancies have occasionally been treated with bone marrow transplantation, and some patients with hairy cell leukemia and chronic lymphocytic leukemia have been cured.

More recently, bone marrow transplantation has been used to treat patients with multiple myeloma. Although most patients with this disease are past the age at which bone marrow transplantation is usually attempted, there are still many who might benefit from the treatment. The results aren't conclusive, but it appears that both allogeneic and autologous bone marrow transplantation can bring about complete remissions in some multiple myeloma patients.

Solid Tumors in Adults Bone marrow transplantation has been used in a wide variety of so-called solid tumors—carcinomas and sarcomas—in adults. It can cure some men with advanced testicular cancer, for example, a predictable result given the extraordinary responsiveness of testicular cancer to chemotherapy. A small number of patients with soft tissue sarcomas have also had long remissions after high-dose therapy and a bone marrow transplant.

Unfortunately, many common solid tumors such as lung cancers and gastrointestinal cancers aren't sensitive enough to high-dose chemotherapy and radiation to make the bone marrow procedure beneficial.

One of the most common carcinomas in the United States—breast cancer—*is* reasonably sensitive to chemotherapy and radiotherapy. Recent clinical trials with high-dose therapy and autologous bone marrow transplantation suggest that increased doses of drugs active against breast cancer can dramatically increase the response rate. Some women have had complete remissions and some of these remissions have lasted several years. It will be a while before long-term results on large numbers of patients are available. Yet most investigators are encouraged that bone marrow transplantation might be able to cure some breast cancer patients who have a poor prognosis with standard therapy.

Solid Tumors in Children Most pediatric solid tumors are sensitive to chemotherapy and can sometimes be cured by chemotherapy without bone marrow transplantation. But, as might be expected, high-dose therapy and autologous or allogeneic transplantation can cure some children who can't be cured with standard therapy.

Neuroblastoma is the disease in which the procedure has been most carefully studied. It appears that some children can have long-lasting remissions—in other words, can probably be cured—with high-dose therapy and bone marrow transplantation. But, as with many other diseases, the optimal timing and treatment procedures haven't been identified yet.

Another common group of solid tumors in children—brain tumors—are also undergoing clinical trials with bone marrow transplantation. How useful the technique is in these cases will have to await further studies.

THE FUTURE OF TRANSPLANTATION

Bone marrow transplantation is a rapidly evolving field that is likely to become more and more important in cancer treatment. The advances over the past 20 years have been remarkable.

The first attempt at allogeneic bone marrow transplantation was reported in the 1930s. It didn't work because the scientific advances that led to HLA typing had not yet been made. Autologous bone marrow transplantation was first tested in the 1950s. Once again, the attempt failed, this time because the techniques for cryopreservation of bone marrow cells had not been perfected.

The development of HLA typing in the 1960s made allogeneic transplantation a reasonable possibility, and the first successful transplants were performed at the end of that decade. Through the 1970s, allogeneic bone marrow transplantation gradually became an accepted form of therapy. The successful cryopreservation of bone marrow cells was perfected in the late 1970s, making autologous bone marrow transplantation a widely available therapy in the 1980s.

Now the future for the use of bone marrow transplantation in cancer treatment is optimistic. It is likely to be used for some time to treat leukemia and lymphoma. It also appears that more patients with carcinomas or sarcomas—solid tumors—will be identified who can benefit from, and possibly be cured by, the procedure. And the increased use of hematopoietic growth factors to accelerate marrow regrowth after transplantation will likely make the technique safer and more widely available.

Perhaps most exciting is that the ability to use peripheral blood stem cells has increased the number of patients who might benefit from autologous transplants, while the National Donor Program for identifying unrelated donors has greatly increased the number of patients who might benefit from allogeneic transplants.

13
QUESTIONABLE AND UNPROVEN CANCER THERAPIES

Barrie R. Cassileth, PhD

Surgery, radiation therapy and chemotherapy have been "accepted" cancer treatments for a long time. They are accepted because they were developed after years of study with animals and then humans. The studies were based on logical, scientific principles, and the treatments were then shown to be effective against the growth of tumors in thousands of people.

These conventional cancer treatments are responsible for dramatic improvements in survival over the past few decades. Where few people used to survive for long after a cancer diagnosis, about half of all diagnosed patients are now cured.

Every few years or so, the media present a startling report on some new way to treat cancer. The treatment is typically described as resulting in "miraculous cures" or as being able to prolong lives in some extraordinary fashion. The exact formula or chemical content is usually unknown or is kept secret by the practitioner promoting this new method. Knowledge of the treatment often spreads only by word of mouth or by being publicized in certain types of popular magazines and tabloid papers.

These "cures" are not reported in the scientific literature, however, nor are they backed by the extensive data and research information that accompany reports of new medical tests and therapies. There are two reasons why reports on these cures never show up in scientific journals:

♦ The most common reason is that the practitioners promoting the unorthodox method never actually studied it and so never prepared any report to send to scientific publications. Typically, these practitioners say they are too busy treating patients to spend time on evaluation or research, even though it is only through rigorous evaluation and research that the worth of a treatment can be known.

♦ The other reason is that a report may have been sent to a journal's editorial board but that publication in a medical journal was simply not warranted because the quality of its data was so poor, it lacked accurate information or there was no evidence of benefit.

Most unproven methods have never been studied at all. The only "proof" their developers usually offer is the display of people who—the practitioners say—have been cured by their therapy. The "beneficiaries" of the miracle treatment may be displayed live during some publicity event. Or they may testify to the worth of the treatment in writing, often in a brochure. Of course, it is not possible to know from these kinds of displays whether the person was cured by the unproven method, whether he or she received conventional treatment before or at the same time as receiving the unproven treatment or if, in fact, he or she had ever been diagnosed as having cancer at all.

Stories told by or about a patient are called anecdotal reports, and they can sound very impressive and persuasive. Even assuming they are true, however, no faith can be placed in anecdotal reports about one or even a few patients. Careful study of many clinically similar patients is required before a legitimate conclusion can be drawn about any new therapy.

The Appeal of New Methods To people with cancer and their families, unproven treatments can look very appealing, especially when no conventional treatment is left to be tried. They may be drawn to some unorthodox remedy even if there is no solid evidence that a product or procedure is beneficial. Patients and families may be ready to try anything, feeling that they have nothing to lose.

But there *is* something to lose. The financial losses can be considerable for anyone who pursues a useless treatment, usually at an expensive private clinic. For those who are terminally ill and beyond the help of conventional treatment, false hope can also rob them of the good use of what time they have left. When patients can still benefit from conventional treatment and there is a possibility of a long remission or even cure, what can be lost is a life.

It is understandable that you or your family may be attracted to some unproven therapy. To protect yourselves physically and financially, however, you must become educated health care consumers. You have to understand all medical procedures and services, including unproven methods.

THE ROOTS OF UNPROVEN METHODS

Unproven remedies for cancer and other serious illnesses have been with us for centuries. They have taken many forms, including:
♦ liquefied grasses to drink
♦ small wooden objects with magical properties to hold in the hand
♦ pastes to rub on the skin
♦ radio waves and magnetic forces to direct at various parts of the body
♦ potions made from many different nat-

ural and unnatural items to take

And many others. None has survived very long. These remedies usually enjoyed a brief popularity, then faded from view. But they were soon replaced by some other questionable cure. Understanding the roots and sources for these questionable remedies will help you understand the role questionable remedies play today.

Parallel Medicine in the Nineteenth Century Unproven cancer treatments have typically mimicked or paralleled developments in scientific medicine. The promotion of unproven methods in the nineteenth century arose in response to the development of modern clinical methods and the emphasis on local pathology. In the early 1800s, medical efforts began to be devoted to finding and treating a specific source or cause of illness. At the same time, advocates of questionable remedies began working to make "every man his own doctor" and to develop a "holistic" self-care alternative to a medical system oriented toward disease.
♦ In the early 1880s, the hot/cold theory of diseases—Thomsonianism—gained a wide following. This theory promoted hot baths and emetics (to induce vomiting) while opposing "mineral" drugs and the "tyranny of doctors."
♦ Around 1850, homeopathy became popular. This was based on its Law of Similia, which stated that disease results from suppressed itch ("psora"). Over 3,000 drugs, each a highly distilled organic or inorganic substance, were used for cures.
♦ Naturopathy, a belief system that gained popularity about 1890, was another alternative. In opposition to scientific medicine, it held that disease results not from external bacteria but from violation of the "natural laws" of living. Its cures involved diets, massages and irrigation of the colon.

Twentieth Century Alternatives After these holistic approaches were tried and failed to demonstrate any benefit, there was a shift in the early 1900s to quasi-medicines in pill or liquid form. All kinds of these nostrums appeared, including Radol and Chamlee's Cancer-Specific Purifies-the-Blood Cure.

During the 1920s, in the exciting early days of the electronic age of radio, telephone and other miracles produced by energy, "energy" cancer cures appeared. "Cosmic energy treatment" and "light therapy" became the rage.

Koch's glyoxilide (distilled water) cure of the 1940s was followed in the 1950s by the Hoxsey Treatment in pill and extract form. Injectable krebiozen—which turned out to be essentially mineral oil—was popular in the 1960s and was followed in the 1970s by Laetrile, a substance prepared from apricot pits and often referred to as vitamin B_{17} even though it is not a vitamin. Like all the others, Laetrile was shown upon investigation to have no effect against cancer.

The long history of unproven methods and the fact that none survived for more than a few months or years indicate their lack of usefulness. Still, there is a natural human tendency to respond to claims for new cures, especially ones promoted as more effective or less difficult than existing scientific treatments. This is a major reason why unproven therapies persist.

Today, the concerns of the medical counterculture mirror the nineteenth-century perspective. Just as the "natural" whole-body treatments arose then in response to modern clinical methods, so the currently popular unproven methods stem partly from a reaction to today's technological, heroic medicine. The very specialization and sophistication that offers clinically optimal care also creates dissatisfaction and unease among some patients. Many people are uncomfortable seeing a series of specialists rather than being cared for by a single physician. Many find the marvels of current diagnostic and treatment equipment too technical, cold and mechanical.

It is not surprising that contemporary unproven treatments represent a throwback to nineteenth-century beliefs in disease as a systemic, total-body phenomenon, in demystification and simplification of illness, in self-care and in "natural" cures. Now, as 150 years ago, the medical counterculture is firmly rooted in a political anti-authority context. Now, as then, ambivalence or hostility toward the medical profession is clearly evident.

The cycle of popular unproven approaches has now gone full-circle—from the natural, holistic alternatives of the 1800s, through the quasi-medicines of the early and mid-twentieth century, back to the natural, holistic, dietary regimens of today.

TODAY'S POPULAR ALTERNATIVES

The questionable cancer remedies now getting the most attention range from those that are based on misinterpretations of scientific data to those that are downright fraudulent. All are good examples of why cancer patients and their families must become *educated* health care consumers. You have to review *critically* the principles or concepts on which unproven methods are based so that their logic and accuracy can be evaluated.

Adjunctive Therapies Promoted as Cures

The standard treatments—surgery, chemotherapy, radiation therapy and biological therapy—are all designed to remove or kill tumor cells. But cancer specialists and other doctors may also recommend other types of treatment that are not designed to kill tumor cells. Instead, these treatments aim to bring about some overall improvement in general health and well-being. They are often called complementary or adjunctive treatments because they are used along with the standard therapies.

Nutritional therapy, relaxation therapy, a focus on emotional well-being, the provision of effective support systems, yoga and so on all fit into this category. When used in conjunction with standard therapies, these are legitimate therapeutic approaches. They are helpful in recovery or rehabilitation.

But sometimes these adjunctive or complementary therapies are advertised as having the power to cure cancer on their own. Nutritional programs are promoted as dietary "cures." Relaxation therapy or imagery are promoted as essential to developing the right attitude that will make cancer go away.

Many people are drawn to these "cures" because they are free of the sometimes unpleasant side effects of conventional treatments. But this is a very destructive and unfortunate misuse of otherwise helpful activities. When cancer patients look on these complementary therapies as cures, they may decide—or even be encouraged—to stop their conventional treatments. Some may assume that they no longer have to see their oncologist or receive chemotherapy. If they do so, they lose their only chance for remission or cure.

Immune-Enhancing Therapies After a long period of intense and well-publicized scientific study of the immune system, a number of unorthodox practitioners developed therapies aimed at improving cancer patients' immune systems. Several unorthodox approaches work toward this goal. One aims to stimulate immune function through injected vaccines. Another aims to enhance the immune system through mental imagery and attitude.

These therapies sound legitimate because they address an issue—the immune system—that is a subject of legitimate scientific investigation. Because the terminology sounds scientific and the rationale appears to be a great deal more accurate than it really is, it is important to understand some background information before evaluating these therapies.

There is some scientific experimental evidence showing that the immune system plays a role in the body's defense against cancer. There is very little evidence indicating that the system is helpful against metastatic disease once cancer has developed. But there is no scientific proof that mental imagery or adopting a new emotional attitude influences the immune system in a way that affects the growth of tumors.

Many immune-stimulating agents have been studied in clinical trials. These include the tuberculosis vaccine, BCG, as well as a variety of chemicals that have been shown to stimulate immunity in animals. One immune stimulant—Levamisole—was approved by the National Cancer Institute in late 1989 for use in combination with standard chemotherapy for one stage of colon cancer because this combination produced better results than chemotherapy alone. BCG has also been approved for the treatment of early bladder cancer. Yet very few immune-enhancing substances are known to improve disease in humans. Ongoing studies with other cancers have not yet shown much benefit from immune-enhancing techniques.

Metabolic Treatments These are offered by many practitioners and clinics in the United States and in Tijuana, Mexico. Metabolic procedures vary according to the practitioner, but they generally include at least two of:

♦ "detoxification," typically through cleansing of the colon
♦ special diets
♦ vitamins
♦ minerals
♦ enzymes

Metabolic treatments sound appealing. They emphasize "natural" therapy with treatment directed at "cellular detoxification and restoration." But these treatments are neither natural nor safe. Many people have been harmed by them. Like most unproven treatments, metabolic therapy is based on an invented principle: that toxins and waste materials in the body interfere with metabolism and healing. Cancer and other chronic illnesses are seen as the result of degeneration of the liver and pancreas or of the degeneration of the immune and "oxygenation" systems.

The educated consumer will know that there is no such thing as an oxygenation system. Nor is there any such thing as cellular detoxification and restoration.

Special Diets The "miracle diet" that cures cancer is a staple of the tabloid press. You can read about these diets at the checkout counter of any supermarket, but not in many other places.

Such diets are a good example of the faulty logic that often accompanies a misunderstanding of scientific information. People read or hear that following certain dietary measures can help prevent cancer, as indeed they can. Eating a low-fat, high-fiber diet, for example, can lower your risk of developing some kinds of cancer. But some people then make an illogical leap from prevention to cure and assume that these same dietary measures can cure a cancer once it has started to grow.

Following a special diet or eating certain foods will not make cancer go away. Yet many dietary "cures" are promoted in North America today and they are often accepted at face value. Little attention is paid to how they may rob the body of necessary nutrients or that they may be based on false, illogical concepts. The popular macrobiotic diet, for example, is based on a fanciful and completely faulty concept of how the human body works.

The special diets are usually "practitioner-specific." This means that each promoter offers a different approach to cancer therapy through a different type of diet. Among the diets now attracting attention are the grape cure, the wheatgrass cure,

the vegetarian diet, the raw food diet, the diet based on liquefied carrots and various diets based on Oriental herbal remedies.

None is known to be helpful. Many result in nutritional deficiencies, a situation cancer patients should avoid at all costs. Moderation is still the best approach to diet for all medical problems. Taking excessive amounts of vitamins, minerals or "health food" substitutes may do more harm than good.

HOW TO TELL WHEN A THERAPY IS QUESTIONABLE

If you are going to make an educated decision about a treatment, you have to go beyond testimonials and promises. You have to understand what the unproven method is all about. You have to know what concepts it's based on and what its track record is.

A legitimate treatment method meets each of the following standards. A dubious or questionable treatment does not meet any of them.

♦ The method was studied scientifically and shown to be more effective than no treatment at all.

♦ The benefits of the method clearly exceed any harm it might do.

♦ Studies of the method have been properly conducted. That is, an appropriate research design has been used, the studies have been subject to review by others knowledgeable in the field and a human studies committee has given the study its approval.

If you have any doubt about a therapy, examine it critically against these three standards. Check the brochure or any other available literature to see if the method was studied and found to be better than nothing. The brochure will certainly note the "benefits" of the method, but you will have to look for or ask about any problems.

The third point is the easiest to determine. Legitimate treatment methods are *always* evaluated with the participation of other scientists. They are *always* reviewed and approved by a human subjects committee in an established, reputable medical institution.

"Secret" cures or treatments that are said to work only in the hands of one practitioner are questionable by definition. New scientific therapies are always made available through meetings, talks and publications to the entire community of scientists and researchers. The worth of the treatment can be confirmed only when the results of research can be reproduced by others.

An in-depth, critical evaluation of an unproven program can tell you whether the "cured patients" offered as proof of its worth actually had a diagnosis of cancer confirmed by a tissue biopsy. It can tell you whether the "cured patients" received conventional treatment along with the questionable therapy, even if all credit is given to the unproven method. It will indicate what the problems and toxicities associated with the unproven treatment might be.

Your oncologist can help supply this information and should be your major source for information and assistance. He or she best understands your illness and knows which treatments are useful against it. You can also contact your local offices of the American or Canadian Cancer Society or the American or Canadian Medical Association.

Other sources of information include:
National Council Against Health Fraud
PO Box 1276
Loma Linda, California 92354
(714) 824-4690

Consumer Reports Health Letter
PO Box 52145
Boulder, Colorado 80321-2148

The Skeptical Inquirer
Committee for Scientific Investigation of Claims of the Paranormal
PO Box 229
Buffalo, New York 14215-0229

By using the available resources to become educated health care consumers, you and your family can avoid the many difficulties that await those who pursue treatments that have no benefit. You will certainly save financially. You will spare yourself much anguish. You may gain yourselves precious moments together. And, if there is still a chance for remission or cure, you may also prevent a tragedy of the highest order.

14
BLOOD TRANSFUSIONS AND CANCER TREATMENT

Herbert A. Perkins, MD

◇

Blood is a complex living tissue. It is made up of three kinds of cells that are manufactured in the blood cell "factory"—the marrow cavity of our bones. All these cells are suspended in a liquid called plasma, and each cell plays a critical role in keeping us alive.

♦ Red blood cells carry oxygen to our tissues.

♦ White blood cells—leukocytes—help us fight off infections.

♦ Platelets are necessary to form the blood clots that stop bleeding.

Blood transfusions play a crucial role in cancer treatment. The disease can reduce the marrow's ability to produce blood cells, sometimes so severely that the cells have to be replaced by transfusion. Some forms of cancer—leukemia and multiple myeloma—grow in the marrow cavity, leaving no space for the development of normal blood cells. These normal cells will then have to be provided by transfusion.

But most of the people with cancer who need blood transfusions need them because of the aggressive approaches used to treat the disease. If blood transfusions weren't available, most of the remarkably effective cancer treatments available today could never have been introduced—the chemotherapy used to kill cancer cells, for example, which may also kill developing blood cells in the marrow. Many cancers can also be cured or at least helped by surgery and that surgery may result in loss of blood by hemorrhage to the point where it has to be replaced. No other form of medical treatment can make such a difference between life and death as blood transfusions can.

WEIGHING THE RISKS

Just like other powerful forms of treatment, transfusions can bring about serious complications, although these are uncommon. Some can be fatal, although this is very rare.

Infection Unless you donate blood to yourself, there is always a very slight risk that you could be infected by some organism.

AIDS The risk foremost in everyone's mind lately is the possibility of being infected with the HIV virus that can lead to Acquired Immune Deficiency Syndrome (AIDS). But the risk of getting AIDS from a transfusion is now so low—one in 40,000, and possibly lower—that it should have almost no effect on the decision to have a transfusion that is medically indicated.

Hepatitis The number-one infectious risk associated with transfusion is, and always has been, the serious infection of the liver called hepatitis. The risk has been markedly reduced in the past 10 years, however, and should be reduced another 70 to 80 percent in 1991, since a new test has become available. This test will detect blood donors who are healthy but nevertheless carry the newly discovered hepatitis C virus.

Other Infections Blood banks test for

syphilis and HTLV I and II (HTLV I is a virus that may occasionally cause leukemia). Other infections are rarely transmitted.

Reactions to Differences in Donor Blood
Unless you are transfused with your own blood or have an identical twin who donated blood for you to use, the blood you receive will contain many things that are foreign to you. This is true even when the blood is correctly cross-matched.

The donor's blood—the red and white blood cells, platelets and even plasma proteins—will all have antigens (proteins) your body will have never come in contact with before. What usually happens when you are exposed to foreign antigens is that your immune system reacts. After all, the system is designed to recognize and try to destroy anything foreign that gets into our bodies, especially invading germs such as bacteria or viruses. Fortunately, the immune system rarely recognizes most of the differences between a donor's blood and your own.

Differences in Red Blood Cells These are the most critical. While there are more than 400 recognized differences, only three are of practical importance. These have to do with certain antigens, namely the A, B and D antigens that determine your ABO and Rh blood types.

Antibodies are part of the immune response to foreign antigens. If you have type B blood, you have anti-A antibodies, so if you are transfused with Type A red cells, those cells will be destroyed. Not only will the transfusion not accomplish its purpose but you may experience chills, fever, aches and pains and in rare cases shock, bleeding, even death. Blood banks and hospital transfusion services do repeated tests and checks to be sure patients don't receive blood with the wrong ABO type.

Red blood cells are also either Rh positive or Rh negative, depending whether you have one of the Rh antigens called D. The D antigen is easily recognized as foreign by an Rh-negative patient whose system then makes an antibody against it.

Blood banks always test red blood cells from donors and transfusion patients to see if they contain A, B and D. They also test the serum (a form of plasma) to see if it contains antibodies to these antigens. The hospital transfusion service also checks the serum of each patient who will be transfused to see if it contains antibodies to other red cell antigens. If it does, the blood bank must provide donor blood lacking these antigens. As a final check, the transfusion service does a cross-match, a test to see if the serum of the patient recognizes anything in the donor blood cells as foreign.

Differences in White Blood Cells The white cells have an entirely different set of foreign antigens than the red cells do. The most important are called HLA antigens. These are the same antigens that a laboratory looks for when tissue typing to select an organ donor for a transplant.

Antibodies to white blood cells develop fairly easily through transfusion or pregnancy. They rarely cause serious harm, but they do explain the chills and fevers experienced by about 3 percent of patients receiving transfusions. If you have such reactions to an uncomfortable degree, your doctor can prevent or minimize them in future transfusions by ordering red blood cells from which most of the white cells have been removed (leukocyte-poor red blood cells).

Differences in Platelets Donor platelets have the same HLA antigens as the white blood cells, plus they have antigens unique to platelets. If you have to have repeated platelet transfusions over a long time, your immune system may form antibodies that will attack and destroy the donor platelets, making the platelet transfusions useless. These antibodies can also cause chills and fever when they react with donor platelets.

Differences in the Plasma Reactions to donor plasma in the form of hives happen in up to 5 percent of patients. Hives can sometimes be severe to the point of generalized swelling and, in rare cases, the reaction can result in a life-threatening obstruction to breathing. Allergic reactions to plasma can usually be simply treated or prevented with antihistamines. And if you do have a severe reaction, future transfusions can be given without causing a reaction by washing the blood cells with salt solution to remove the plasma.

WHAT GETS TRANS-FUSED AND WHEN

When someone donates blood, about a pint of blood is usually drawn into a plastic bag. The bag contains a solution that keeps the blood from clotting and helps preserve the red cells. Each bag, with its attached tubing and the needle that goes into the donor's arm, comes as a sterile unit in a sealed pouch and is used only once.

The blood is stored in a refrigerator under carefully controlled conditions until it's used. If it isn't used within five or six weeks, the blood has to be discarded because changes in the red blood cells during storage make it less effective and possibly dangerous, although in special circumstances, red blood cells can be frozen and stored for years. What part of this stored blood is transfused depends on your condition and your needs.

Whole Blood This is used only when a patient is hemorrhaging large amounts of blood in a short time. Almost always, the blood bank separates each unit of blood into red cells, platelets and plasma.

Red Cells Because of your cancer or your treatment, you may become anemic to the point where breathing becomes difficult,

your heart pounds or you become very weak. If that happens, red blood cells will be transfused. If your marrow is not doing its job, it may be necessary to transfuse red blood cells every three to four weeks. Red blood cells will also be transfused when there is a lot of bleeding, as there may be during surgery.

Platelets When your marrow can't produce enough platelets on its own, a platelet transfusion might be necessary to prevent bleeding. Moderate drops in the platelet count do not need treatment. But very low counts—less than 10,000 or 20,000 without bleeding, a little higher with—will require platelet transfusions, often every two to three days. During each transfusion, it is customary to give between six and ten units of platelets.

At least 70 percent of patients who get repeated platelet transfusions will make antibodies to foreign platelet antigens, making the transfusions less and less effective. Blood banks can solve this problem by providing platelets that have the correct HLA type and by doing many cross-matches with donor platelets.

The Apheresis Technique Modern cancer treatment has led to such a voracious need for platelets that the need cannot be met just by making a platelet component from each whole blood donation. So blood banks have turned to a procedure known as apheresis. In this process, a donor's blood is taken from a vein, passed through an apheresis (or separating) device and returned to the donor through another vein. The device skims off and saves the blood platelets while the red blood cells and plasma are returned. When patients no longer respond to the platelets of random donors, family members are often asked to donate platelets by apheresis, since they are much more likely than a random donor to have the same platelet antigens as the patient.

Plasma The plasma component of whole blood is used in a variety of ways.

♦ It may be immediately frozen (fresh frozen plasma) and then used to transfuse missing plasma proteins into patients with unusual deficiencies of clotting factors.

♦ It can be processed into cryoprecipitate, a special product used to treat hemophilia.

♦ It can be made into albumin to treat shock, gamma globulin to prevent hepatitis, and clotting factors.

DONATING BLOOD TO YOURSELF

Since any blood bank component can transmit infections or cause reactions, the safest blood donor is yourself. Getting your own blood is called an autologous transfusion. It is not always possible for people with cancer to donate blood, since it is certainly not appropriate if you are likely to have cancer cells in your blood. But it is worth asking your surgeon whether any of the following approaches are possible or advisable.

Pre-Deposit Donation Many cancer patients can provide their own blood before surgery if time permits and a few basic conditions are met. In this "pre-deposit autologous donation," your blood is taken exactly as it is from a standard blood donor. The usual age limits for donors don't apply, but you can't be too anemic or have certain types of serious heart disease. It is usually possible to collect two, three or four units of blood in the five-to-six-week period that blood can be stored. Since you will be giving blood much more often than is permitted for the usual blood donor, your doctor will usually prescribe iron so that red cell production is not slowed down by iron deficiency.

Hemodilution This is another approach to autologous transfusion. Instead of blood being gradually donated before the operation, several pints are taken in the operating room just as surgery is about to begin. A saline (salt) solution is transfused at the same time so that your total blood volume doesn't change. Your blood is then transfused during the surgical procedure or after the operation as the salt solution escapes from your circulation.

Cell Salvage This approach is possible when fairly large amounts of blood escape into a body cavity during surgery. The blood can be removed, washed with a saline solution, and later returned to you. Cell salvage may not be possible, however, if there is a risk that cancer cells will be returned to your system.

BLOOD FROM OTHER DONORS

If you can't donate blood for your own use, you will have to rely on blood supplied by volunteer blood banks or on blood donated from a relative or friend.

Directed or Designated Donations Directed donors may be selected by a patient or a patient's family in the belief that their blood will be safer than that from the usual blood bank volunteer. Usually, this belief is not correct. Although positive tests for AIDS are rare among both directed and routine donors, directed donations have a *higher* frequency of positive hepatitis tests. In some areas, directed donors also have a higher frequency of positive AIDS tests.

Why Direct Donors Are Riskier There are logical reasons why directed donors are less safe on the average.

♦ People asked to donate for a relative or friend may, because of embarrassment or for reasons they wish to keep confidential, not want to confess that they are ineligible.

♦ Directed donors are usually first-time donors, while more than two-thirds of routine donors have given in the past, most on many occasions. With each donation there was a chance that the medical history or laboratory tests would uncover some reason for ineligibility or that an investigation of an infection in a transfused patient would identify the donor as a possible source.

Despite the arguments against the use of directed donors, most patients and families are convinced that *their* relatives and friends are safer than routine donors. For the peace of mind of the patients and families, most blood banks accept requests for directed donations. In some states they are required by law to do so.

Community Blood Bank Donors These donors are volunteers who have no reason to donate their blood other than the pleasure it gives them to help their fellow humans.

Each blood donor (and this applies to directed donors as well) must read an information sheet that details reasons why a person should *not* donate blood. If the donor concludes that he or she is eligible, a medical history is then obtained using a series of very detailed questions, a number of which are specific about sexual practices.

The donor is then usually given the opportunity to indicate confidentially that the blood he or she donates should not be transfused. This procedure takes care of situations in which the donor knows he or she is not eligible but does not wish this to become apparent to relatives, friends or

co-workers. Finally, the blood donated is tested for a whole series of infectious agents—AIDS, hepatitis B, hepatitis C, HTLV and syphilis, as well as CMV in special circumstances. The result is the safest blood supply by far that this country has ever known.

The Need for More Donors Eighty to 90 percent of transfusions use blood from volunteer donors in the community. The rest are autologous or directed. If blood isn't available when a patient needs it, that patient could die. Yet serious blood shortages, which require rationing of the available supply, are frequent in many communities.

There are many reasons for the shortage of blood donors. Most people who do not give blood fail to do so because they just ignore the need or assume someone else will do it. A quarter of the population has the completely mistaken notion that it is dangerous to donate blood, that one might become infected with AIDS. And a very large number of people are not eligible to be blood donors anymore, based on the strict criteria used and tests performed.

People with cancer cannot donate blood for others. Yet cancer patients should have an unusual awareness of the need for an adequate blood supply. Carry the message to your relatives and friends to become regular blood donors. Then, if you need a transfusion in an emergency, the blood will be there waiting for you.

15
THE ONCOLOGY NURSE

Josefa Azcueta, RN, OCN, and Deborah Hamolsky, RN, MS, OCN

◇

Margaret was a 42-year-old mother of two. She discovered a lump in her breast a few months after she had learned Breast Self-Examination techniques from Nancy, a nurse at the local Breast Examination Training (BET) center. After mammography and fine needle aspiration of the lump, she saw her doctor, who confirmed the diagnosis of cancer. After a Tumor Board presentation, her oncologist reviewed and explained all the options to Margaret and her husband. The decision was made to go ahead with surgery, chemotherapy and radiation.

After her mastectomy, Margaret met nurses like Maria who changed her dressings, gave her medications and sat on the bed and held her hand when she cried in the middle of the night.

After Margaret was discharged, Louise and Joe came to her home for follow-up visits. And when chemotherapy was started in the oncologist's office, nurses like Helen, Irene and Beth taught her about the effects of different chemotherapy drugs. They gave her both the chemotherapy injections and emotional support.

After four months of chemotherapy, Margaret started on radiation. Mary helped explain the treatments to her, drew blood for tests and was always ready with a much-needed hug.

Then, to help them both cope with cancer, Margaret and her husband attended weekly cancer support group meetings, led by Kate, at the local hospital. There they could share their feelings and fears with others who really knew what they were going through.

This story is just one illustration of how many different oncology nurses touch the lives of so many people with cancer.

From before the diagnosis, through the course of treatment and beyond to supportive care, you will continually meet these specially trained nurses. They will share their knowledge and expertise with you. They will help you with their support and understanding when you need it most.

PROFESSIONAL TRAINING

Many nursing studies have shown that people with cancer want and expect many things from nurses. Competency is the most important expectation. People care that the nurse can start the IV and give chemotherapy, change a dressing, insert a catheter and know how to respond to an emergency.

When you are getting treatment for your cancer, you obviously want to know without any doubt that you are in the hands of someone who is an expert, aware of the most up-to-date treatment methods.

Professional Organization In the United States, the national organization of oncology nurses is the Oncology Nursing Society (ONS). Founded in 1975, it is now a large national organization with many local chapters. ONS is dedicated to professional development, promotion of excellence in clinical practice, research, education and political influence. Many oncology nurses belong to local chapters and attend yearly meetings where they learn about medical or other advances that can improve the care they give you and your family. There is also an organization of cancer nurses who specialize in the care and treatment of children, the Association of Pediatric Oncology Nurses (APON).

Specialized Education Oncology nurses have special training in the care of cancer patients within the hospital, the doctor's office, at home or in special facilities such as radiation therapy units. Oncology nurses build on their basic medical knowledge with additional training in:

♦ Giving chemotherapy and managing side effects such as nausea, vomiting and hair loss.
♦ Controlling cancer pain.
♦ Managing cancer emergencies.
♦ Providing emotional support to patients and their loved ones.
♦ Postoperative care.
♦ Care and teaching of long-term intravenous (IV) devices such as Hickman catheters, Groshong catheters and ports.
♦ Participation in clinical research teams or independent nursing research.
♦ Managing new technology and treatments—such as bone marrow transplants or biological therapies—as they evolve.

Nurses can also develop their knowledge in several subspecialties such as radiation oncology, surgical oncology, medical oncology, palliative (comfort) care, cancer prevention and early detection, in-patient nursing, hospice, home care, patient education, research, and ambulatory and office nursing. Some nurses, particularly in large regional cancer centers, may develop an even more specific area of interest such as breast cancer, immunotherapy or pain control.

Radiation Therapy As one example of further education, nurses who specialize in radiation oncology work primarily in radiation therapy departments, either in hospitals or with independent practices. Their specialized knowledge of radiation treatment for cancer includes

♦ how the machines work
♦ what can be expected from the treatment planning, treatment and follow-up care, which treatment courses are expected to cause side effects
♦ managing side effects—fatigue, skin changes, diarrhea, sore mouth—when they do occur
♦ radiation safety
♦ emotional support and education
♦ nutrition.

The nurses work in collaboration with radiation oncologists, radiation physicists, radiology technicians, social workers and dietitians to carry out the treatment plan prescribed by the radiation oncologist for each individual patient.

If you need a radiation implant, you would be hospitalized, usually in an oncology unit, for as long as the implant is in place. But other types of radiation can be given on either an in-patient or out-patient basis. In either case, oncology nurses can help you and your family with information and coping strategies during the course of your treatment.

HOW NURSES WORK WITH YOUR DOCTOR

Treating cancer is very much a team effort these days. And, working closely with other members of the team, oncology nurses are becoming more and more closely involved with the care of people with cancer.

Although your primary physician or oncologist is responsible for the diagnosis and planning of effective treatment, there is now more of a professional collaboration between oncology physicians and nurses than there used to be. The oncology nurse will make decisions about your care within her or his scope of practice. The physician encourages and values the nurses' recommendations and contributions.

♦ In the hospital, it is the nurses who will be with you 24 hours a day, seven days a week. So your doctor will often ask the nursing team for updates on your condition. Nurses may make "walking rounds" with the doctor to find out how you are doing and to make plans for the upcoming day. It is the oncology nurse at the hospital who monitors your vital signs, assesses lab work and physical findings, evaluates your needs and calls the physician when necessary.

♦ On an out-patient basis or in the office, the nurse will work with you at a more independent level. Your doctor still maps out the treatment plan, but the oncology nurse is an invaluable colleague in carrying it out. Nurses may help the doctor plan and decide the most effective way to deliver chemotherapy drugs. And the nurse's opinion will be especially valuable in, for example, choosing the antinausea medications most likely to be effective for your particular chemotherapy treatment.

♦ Nurses and doctors will usually hold patient care conferences to discuss your treatment. Nurses can often point out subtle changes in your condition that your doctors might not be aware of, some of which could possibly change the treatment plan.

♦ In the research field, oncology nurses may work independently or collaborate with physicians, but most of the time, physician and nurse work very closely together. The nurse is a member of the research team that conducts clinical trials of new therapies, collecting data and assessing responses and side effects. When the data are all collected and the analysis done, the nurse's name appears on the published work alongside the physician's.

♦ Because you usually spend many more hours with a nurse than you do with your doctor, a special relationship often develops. Sometimes you can become so overwhelmed with new terms and complex treatment schedules that the nurse may take extra time to explain the information your doctor gives you. Often the nurse will follow up the next day in the hospital or by telephone to make sure you understand and feel comfortable about your treatment.

Your care and treatment is truly a team effort by your oncologist and the oncology nurse. And it is you who benefits most from this collaboration.

NURSING IN THE HOSPITAL, CLINIC AND OFFICE

While there are many nursing roles in the office, hospital, home and hospice, the majority of cancer nurses work in hospitals. Most cancer centers and many community hospitals have wards devoted to cancer treatment—oncology units— staffed by oncology nurses.

Hospital staff nurses provide direct care to patients over eight-, ten- or twelve-hour shifts. During your hospital stay you will probably come in contact with a great variety of nurses with different levels of training and responsibilities.

♦ Nurse's aides or hospital attendants complete a training program and may have many years of experience. They can give you direct hands-on care, but do not give medications.

♦ Licensed Vocational Nurses (LVNs) or Licensed Practitioner Nurses (LPNs) complete an educational program and can give medications and direct care. They work collaboratively with Registered Nurses (RNs).

♦ RNs receive their education from an associate degree program, a hospital training program or a Bachelor's degree program at a college or university. Many hospitals have different clinical levels of expertise and authority where RNs progress over time, based on merit and continuing education. An RN with cancer nursing experience can become an

Oncology Certified Nurse (OCN) by passing an exam that will certify her or his competency.

♦ Some nurses receive Master's degrees in cancer nursing. They practice as nurse practitioners, clinical nurse specialists, managers or researchers. Or they choose to continue to work as staff nurses at the bedside. In advanced clinical practice, these nurses teach and act as role models for other nurses, take part in advanced problem-solving, participate in clinical research trials and provide leadership.

The Ambulatory Care/Office Nurse You may not always receive your cancer treatment in a hospital. The preferred place of treatment in many places recently has shifted away from hospitals. You might, therefore, find yourself in a comprehensive cancer center, an out-patient clinic, an ambulatory care center or a private office.

One major reason for this shift is the tremendous costs of health care today. There is a great push to shorten hospital stays because out-patient care is more cost-effective for patients, insurance companies and health care plans. But more important, you benefit by going to an office or clinic, getting your treatment and then going home to recover in your own home and sleep in your own bed.

Antinausea treatments have become so sophisticated that many of the negative side effects that used to mean a long stay in the hospital for treatment have been eliminated. Of course, specialized or research cancer treatments still usually have to be given in the hospital so your condition can be closely supervised and monitored. But even then, you can spend more time outside the hospital than used to be the case.

Out-patient nursing includes giving all types of chemotherapy treatments ranging from a rapid injection to a five- to seven-hour infusion. Out-patient nurses learn the latest treatment protocols and investigational studies and can give you and

your family important information about your disease, treatment, possible side effects and how to manage your medications. These nurses are experts at starting IVs or any of the surgically implanted catheters such as the Hickman, the Port-a-Cath and the Infusaid pump, to name a few. Their job may include mixing and preparing the chemotherapy drugs, syringes, IV bags or bottles.

NURSING IN THE HOME AND HOSPICE

For the same reasons that out-patient treatment has become more widespread, home care is becoming an important part of oncology care. There are now a variety of home care agencies that are staffed by oncology nurses. Many people choose this type of treatment simply because they prefer to get their chemotherapy in the privacy of their own homes with family and friends close by.

Care in the Home Nurses can spend anywhere from a few hours to 24 hours in your home. Chemotherapy is not the only treatment you can get at home. Under the direction of the oncologist, the oncology nurse can provide you with wound care, central venous (CV) line care and teaching, intravenous (IV) hydration, IV antibiotics and total IV nutrition.

Hospice Care Hospice can be an important alternative if your cancer becomes very advanced. In the terminal stage of cancer, hospice care gives you the choice of spending the final days not at a hospital but at home with loved ones by your side.

As with other oncology specialties, hospice nurses are closely involved with both you and your family. Under your doctor's guidance, the hospice nurse provides pain medication, including narcotics by many different routes.

They teach family and friends how to care for their loved ones and decrease their distress. The hospice nurse, together with social workers and clergy, also helps the family deal with the impending death and handle the bereavement period that follows. During that time, the hospice nurse spends many hours with the family and is available at all hours of the day or night.

SUPPORT FOR YOU AND YOUR FAMILY

The role of the oncology nurse varies depending on where and what kind of care is needed at any particular moment. But improving the quality of life for people with cancer is a primary goal of cancer nursing practice. To reach that goal, the oncology nurse is devoted to reducing your physical discomfort and providing emotional support to you and your family.

Managing Symptoms Cancer and the side effects of treatment may have symptoms that are distressing or affect your day-to-day life. Your health care team has to work together to identify and relieve these symptoms. There is now a great deal of nursing knowledge that lets the oncology nurse evaluate, advise and effectively take the edge off symptoms like nausea and vomiting, pain, constipation, diarrhea, mouth sores, shortness of breath, loss of appetite and emotional distress.

Support Groups and Other Resources It is important that whatever needs you have for emotional support be matched with the resources available in your community. These needs often change over the course of an illness and may depend on individual differences and the availability of family, friends and community support.

There are nurses, social workers, psy-

chologists and psychiatrists in private practice who have a special interest in and experience with people who have cancer. Most oncology nurses and social workers will be able to give you information about support resources. Nurses are especially active in referrals for support services, particularly the cancer support groups that are widely available. These groups can be led or facilitated by social workers, psychologists or psychiatrists. Many are co-facilitated by nurses. There are many groups led by professionals who have themselves been diagnosed with cancer.

Not everyone with cancer wants or needs to take part in a structured support group. Many patients successfully use friends and family members as a source of strength. Some people choose individual psychotherapy, either along with or instead of a support group. Yet you should be aware that many people with cancer have credited their support groups with fostering hope and supporting their recovery.

A Special Relationship Many cancer nurses choose to specialize in oncology because they want to make a difference. They want to establish ongoing and meaningful relationships with people who have cancer and their loved ones. The oncology nurse truly touches many lives in many different ways. The nurses who specialize in oncology develop the technical skills needed for cancer care. They will support and inform you and your family throughout your illness. They will always be your advocate.

Simply stated, oncology nurses strive to treat you with kindness and caring, expertise and competence, warmth and good humor and, above all, dignity.

PART II:
SUPPORTIVE CARE

16
LIVING WITH CANCER

Ernest H. Rosenbaum, MD, Malin Dollinger, MD, Isadora Rosenbaum, MA,
and Lenore Dollinger, RN, PhD

⟡

Cancer used to be thought of as a virtual death sentence. Yet more and more people have learned to view this disease in a very different light. Many now recognize that living with cancer means learning to live with a chronic disease. It means learning how to manage symptoms and treatments while returning to as many of the normal activities of daily living as possible.

It's important to have life go on as usual or at least as close to usual as you can make it. Maybe you won't be able to take a planned vacation. Maybe you won't be exercising or playing sports or making love as vigorously or as often as you used to. Then again, maybe you will. The point is that a cancer diagnosis doesn't have to be absolutely devastating—although it can be if you let it.

The key is to not feel as though you are a helpless victim of blind fate. Do that and you may easily lose the will to live. If you're going to be cured, go into remission or even just improve the quality of your life, *you have to take an aggressive stance.*

Fighting cancer is a joint effort, a shared responsibility between you and your medical team. This partnership is based on honesty, communication, education and a willingness to do your part. The medical team assumes responsibility for planning the most effective treatment and giving therapy and support. You have to assume responsibility for working on proper nutrition, proper physical exercise and the proper mental attitude.

Do your part and the result will be a much greater ability to cope, a strengthened will to live and a much more enjoyable life. Sometimes it may seem like a struggle, but you—just like many people before you—can learn to live with cancer.

TALKING TO FAMILY AND FRIENDS

Not too many decades ago, some illnesses were never discussed openly, even among family and friends. Tuberculosis was rarely mentioned in front of other people, for example. And any mention of cancer was made in hushed tones more suitable to talking about bubonic plague. *Cancer* gradually became the most feared word in the English language. It still is. Today, many people remain reluctant to talk about it, even though it is now a rather common disease and often a curable one.

How open you should be about the fact that you have cancer or about how your treatment is going is entirely up to you. There is no single "right" way to talk about it. There are no "right" words to use. Like everyone else, you will have to find your own comfort area and the words you're most comfortable using. If you would rather talk about your "malignancy" or "tumor" or "growth" or "lump" or "problem" than keep using the word "cancer" all the time, so be it.

Deciding Who to Tell Some people prefer to keep their cancer a very private matter, not telling anyone outside the family. One person in our experience has had cancer for 19 years and no one knows but her husband and her daughter, now age 21. The cancer started in 1971 with breast cancer metastatic to her liver and bones. Yet she works, she runs track and is active in the community. One of the reasons she has survived is because she is living with her cancer. For her, this approach is a very positive one. She wants to forget about it and get on with her life.

Others who need outside help pick one or two close friends who have indicated that they would be available emotionally to provide comfort and support when it is needed.

Deciding What to Say Although it can be hard, it makes sense to be open and direct with your family and close friends if you feel comfortable doing that.

Without candor and openness, concerned relatives and friends are left with their own darkest imaginings. They have their own fears and frustrations that will only grow into terrifying phantoms if they are left behind a veil of secrecy and ignorance of what you are really experiencing. The mutual confrontation of fears is a good way of keeping your own fears and the fears of others under control.

Being open doesn't mean that you have to start every conversation with the story of your latest aches and pains. Nor, if someone asks how you feel, do you necessarily have to answer with a long, detailed description. The litany of the person who wants sympathy or empathy—"I've got it bad. It hurts here and here. I've got to get this treatment"—makes a lot of people want to avoid you. People with cancer are often avoided because, by their own conversation, only bad things seem to happen to them.

Another person in our experience—a military man and pharmacist who had lymphocytic leukemia and, concurrently, colon cancer—was a very open, extroverted person. But if someone said to him, "How do you feel?" he always said, "I never had it better in my life." For him, this was a great opener, ending any conversation about his cancer that he could have found depressing, demoralizing or inappropriate. It also made the association with others far less uncomfortable and much warmer because no one was made uneasy.

Short-circuiting painful conversations like this is one way of coping and getting on with your life. But, again, it is not the only way. What is right for you is your own decision. For you, it might not be helpful to just say "fine" if someone asks how you are doing. Such an automatic social response might be appropriate for friends, relatives or co-workers you are not particularly close with, but not if the person asking is someone close who is trying to be supportive.

The same caution applies the other way. When you are feeling low physically or mentally, many people will try to buck you up by telling you, "Don't worry, everything will be fine." This is a common, socially acceptable statement we are all taught to make to show support. But the true message seems to be, "Don't tell me that you don't feel good, so tell me you're okay."

When you really aren't feeling so good, this kind of support obviously contradicts what you know to be true. At such times it is especially nice to have a close friend or relative who can say, "I'm sorry you're feeling down and I'm glad I'm here for you." For that special someone to be there for you, you have to be able to communicate truthfully how you really feel.

COPING WITH SPECIAL FAMILY PROBLEMS

Cancer is a personal disease, but everyone close to you suffers in some way. Cancer is especially hard on family members, particularly when you are in the hospital for an extended time. The period of separation can be traumatic.

Family caregivers are often very stressed. Everyone in the family wonders where you will be in a month or two months down the road—in the hospital, a nursing home, at home and needing nursing care? They are afraid you will have great discomfort or pain.

Very often, the family struggles with questions about how needs can be met and care arranged in such a way that insurance companies will pay for it. They wonder how other caregivers can become involved so they can get back to work. Relatives who live some distance away may have to make plans for taking care of their children so they can come and provide help for a few weeks or a month. Schedules may have to be rearranged, but people are often uncertain about when they should come.

And all members of the family have fears of losing someone who is an important part of the family's life, with meaning and value for love and companionship.

The Needs of Children When you are away in the hospital or when you are back home but feeling tired from treatment, it is not unusual for children to feel lost or neglected. You and other family members have to reassure them often that they are still loved. With younger children you may also have to quickly eliminate any notion that they somehow caused this illness.

Teenagers are especially vulnerable to stress. They have all the same worries that other members of the family have. They have the same needs for reassurance as younger children. And at the same time they may be burdened by having to take on adult responsibilities around the house. If all this becomes too much to bear, they can rebel by cutting the number of visits to the hospital, not doing their new chores at home or even taking alcohol or drugs.

Strained Relationships Not all families are supportive all the time. Realistically,

not everyone is able to be open, loving and intelligently supportive in a crisis. Families sometimes feel death before it even happens. Oncologists have seen patients take a turn for the worse, then have seen family members decide emotionally and psychologically that all is over and stop coming around to the hospital for visits. The family goes into mourning while the patient is still trying to get better and have hope. It's sad to say, but oncologists sometimes see family members fighting at the bedside over wills and codicils.

But even close families and stable relationships can be threatened by the pressures of a long-term illness. Emotional and physical exhaustion, frustration and constant worry and care can all take their toll. Anger and guilt can surface in sudden attacks, recriminations or indifferent or oversolicitous behavior. Other problems that may have been latent in a relationship for years can suddenly emerge.

All these possible strains just emphasize the need for everyone to look after his or her own needs. You have to do all that you can to look after yourself. Your family members have to be reminded that they need time for themselves. They need moments of rest and relief to keep themselves on an even keel emotionally and psychologically.

Both you and your family may be suffering from the same feelings of inadequacy, the same burdens of guilt, the same quiet anguish, the same sheer tedium of prolonged illness. Any or all of these can break the spirits of the most loving and courageous people.

No one can or should be blamed or criticized for the ways he or she responds to the crisis of cancer or the threat of change or loss. Some people and some relationships grow stronger. Some waver but hold fast. Some collapse. Some experience new heights of love, respect and understanding.

DEALING WITH NEGATIVE EMOTIONS

Nothing can undermine your will to live and your "battle-ready" posture so much as the negative emotions that are so often the response to a cancer diagnosis—anger, fear, loss of self-esteem and feelings of isolation. These emotions have to be resolved. If they aren't, helplessness, futility and resignation can easily take over.

Resolving Your Anger How you react to the cancer diagnosis depends on your personality and how you usually adapt to life's problems. If you are the sort of person who looks on adversity as one more problem to be attacked with determination or as simply something you have to make the best of, then your normal positive attitude will probably carry you through the initial shock of the diagnosis and the tough times ahead. But if you usually react to adversity by asking "why me?" you may spend most or all of your emotional energy being angry at the disease, the "gods" or other people for bringing this catastrophe down on your head.

Anger is a normal reaction. In some ways it can help you through the period of grieving that comes after the diagnosis. In fact, if you don't feel some anger and find some way of expressing it, you may be setting yourself up for a period of depression. But there is a time for anger and a time to put anger aside.

If anger stays unresolved, it takes away the energy that could be channeled into coping with the disease and living life as fruitfully as possible. The first step in resolving it is to recognize why you are angry. If you don't, you may find yourself taking out your anger on others, finding fault with friends or family, making a big deal about trivial matters or flying off the handle at the slightest provocation. The result may well be that you drive needed people away just when you need them most. But if you recognize your anger for what it is, you will be getting your mental attitude set to cope with it.

It's important to let your anger out. Talk about it. Scream. Punch a pillow or throw things around—anything to help release anger's hold on you. Then work to apply that energy in a positive and useful direction. Tell the world you just ain't ready to go, and put your anger to work to make sure you don't have to.

Coming to Terms with Fear Most people hear the word *cancer* and immediately think of suffering, prolonged disability or the phrase "nothing can be done." These responses may be okay for the movies, but except in unusual circumstances they don't have a lot to do with the reality of cancer treatment today. Something can almost always be done. Pain and other side effects of treatment can be controlled. Disability is not inevitable. Most people are surprised to learn that their ideas about cancer are much more pessimistic than the facts warrant.

But no one with cancer has any experience or training in how to deal with the sometimes scary events that happen day to day, week to week or month to month. Even if the surgeon "got it all out" or the radiation or chemotherapy seems to be working, there is always a fear that the cancer will come back.

Fear is a terrible master if you let it get a grip on your life. You can be literally "frightened to death." It is a documented phenomenon in modern medical practice that people who accept a cancer diagnosis as a death sentence can die quite quickly, long before the disease has progressed far enough to cause death by itself.

A diagnosis of cancer is not a death sentence. The first question people usually ask when they get the diagnosis is, "How long have I got?" Unfortunately, some doctors still answer with an unqualified "six months" or "a year" or "two years." Specific predictions like these are simply not valid. Such figures may be published averages for people with a specific type of cancer, but they are only averages. Obviously, some people did not live as long as the estimate, some lived longer.

No estimate of *individual* survival can be made until therapy has begun and the response to it has been established. Until then, predictions are, at best, guesswork and uncertainty that can only stifle hope and the will to live.

Knowledge and understanding are the keys to freeing yourself from unreasonable fear. If you want to know the truth about cancer, talk to oncologists and other members of your health care team. Don't listen to what friends, relatives or acquaintances tell you or take reports in the press as gospel. Fears can be resolved if you understand clearly the problems you face, if you understand the treatments and supportive measures that might be taken and if you have a reasonable and realistic estimate of the discomfort or inconvenience you can expect.

Dealing with the Fears of Others Even if your own fear is under control, well-meaning friends or family members can communicate their fears to you. Unless you are prepared for this, you might find your reserves of emotional energy drained and a depression coming on.

The only way out of this situation is to either hide the fact of your cancer or make sure your family and friends understand your disease and treatment. You may even want to include some of them in your consultations with your doctor so they can become part of your "informed" support team. This may also help your doctor, for, from the doctor's point of view, many of the problems in communication come from the family— the husband or wife, the sister or brother, the cousin or friend who has heard about a cure somewhere or about someone who's had better treatment. By making sure that all interested parties are kept informed, everyone can focus their ener-

gies and efforts in the most constructive channels.

Overcoming a Loss of Self-Esteem Your self-esteem can be threatened by the very idea of having cancer. Unfortunately, it's not unusual to feel that if you were somehow a better or more complete person you wouldn't have been stricken in the first place or that the cancer is some sort of divine punishment.

These are all superstitious beliefs that, sad to say, still cling to the word *cancer*. But having cancer doesn't mean that you are unworthy in any way or that you are guilty of some terrible wrongdoing. Cancer can happen to anyone. It will happen to one out of every four Americans.

Even if you don't fall victim to these superstitions, however, cancer can take away or change some of the things that have always given you a sense of self-esteem.

Your Body Image Changes to your body as a result of surgery, radiotherapy or chemotherapy can have a devastating effect on your self-esteem, especially if the changes are visible to other people. If you lose some part of your body, if you have scars or skin changes or if you lose your hair or a lot of weight, everyone can't help but notice. And you're bound to feel uncomfortable when they do, at least at first. If you have to have an ostomy you may feel humiliated by having to collect your body wastes in a bag. If you have surgery to your genitals, you may feel that you are no longer a "real man" or a "real woman."

But your body is not your self. Your true self is your spirit and your soul. It may be hard for you to accept this truth, but you can come to accept it with help and encouragement. Become involved with a support group and get to know other people who have had similar body changes. Just as you will be able to relate to them, other people will be able to relate to you just as you are. The volunteers who work with groups or other social agencies can help you adjust emotionally. You, in turn, may eventually be of value to others going through the same changes.

Loss of Independence and Control To some extent, these are inevitable for anyone with cancer. In the beginning, you will have to depend on the medical system for your very life. When you are in the hospital, other people may well determine when you eat, sleep, bathe, walk or even go to the bathroom. You may feel uncomfortable or humiliated by having to use a bedpan or having your body exposed to doctors, nurses and medical staff.

When you get home, you may have to depend on family, friends or social service agencies for help around the house, personal body care or meeting your financial obligations. You may start to feel "useless" or feel guilty about being a burden to people you care about.

You may have to simply accept your loss of independence for a while, but your sense of self-esteem can be improved if you take as much responsibility as you possibly can in the areas you *can* handle.
♦ Look after as many self-care tasks as you can.
♦ Be methodical and dedicated about eating the right foods and doing regular exercises to increase your strength and mobility.
♦ Keep charts of your progress to help you feel a sense of accomplishment.
♦ Carefully choose some little jobs you can do around the house, whether it's tending plants or caring for a pet or finding some other outlet for your ability to nurture.

Your self-esteem can also be improved if you get involved in a range of supportive programs such as special group counseling or patient support organizations. If there are no support groups in your area, talk to your local medical staff, social workers, clergy and other people with cancer and start one yourself.

Avoiding Isolation Our society likes to think that it is compassionate and willing to rehabilitate people who are disabled or suffering from chronic diseases. The reality is that disabled people are often shunted aside or even shunned. Employers and co-workers can keep their distance. Family and friends, attentive and sympathetic at first, can drift away over time as they deal with their own problems and live their own lives. Everyone can feel uncomfortable talking to someone who is seriously ill, not knowing quite how to relate or what to say. At times like these, it is easy to feel abandoned and lonely.

Even when you are surrounded by caring friends and family, you may feel cut off. Any life-threatening disease can put you in touch with the essential aloneness humans feel when contemplating their own mortality. Some people turn their attention and energies inward to such a degree that they lose contact with life and the rest of humanity.

Isolation and loneliness can often be self-inflicted. If you focus on grieving or feeling sorry for yourself or if you accept the diagnosis as a death sentence, you may snip your ties to the world and live as though you already belong to the dead. When that happens—just as when isolation comes from the outside and old connections are broken by others—you have to make new connections, building new bridges to people and activities that can renew your energy and zest for living.

You may be frightened or pessimistic about taking the first steps toward making a new life. But you *can* change direction. The benefits of doing so make the effort more than worthwhile.

SUPPORT GROUPS

Some people need special help to cope with their cancer, and their doctors can't always provide it. Doctors are as interested in their patients' emotional well-being as they are in their physical well-being, yet medical appointments are usually taken up with talks about treatment problems, side effects, precautions and complications.

Doctors do recognize the importance of dealing with emotional concerns and can often refer you to the many external support groups and systems available to you. These groups give all cancer patients the kind of help that only interested and dedicated people, often sufferers of the same disease, can provide.

At the Hospital Many local hospitals, especially those with cancer treatment centers, have support groups that are run by health professionals and often meet every week. These are groups designed just for individuals with cancer and for family members.

Some of these groups are specialized, dealing only with the common physical and emotional problems of people who have been treated for specific tumors. For example:

♦ People who have had ostomies—artificial openings created in the colon, intestine or bladder—have to learn what they can do to live as normal a life as possible.

♦ People who have had their larynx, or voice box, removed have to learn how to speak all over again.

♦ Women who have had a mastectomy have specific emotional problems. So do men with testicular cancer.

OUTSIDE THE HOSPITAL

The American Cancer Society and other professional organizations have programs that help deal with physical, emotional and mental problems associated with having cancer. The Reach to Recovery program for women with breast cancer and the I Can Cope program of weekly seminars are two examples. Both include a comprehensive educational process for cancer patients and their families.

The Wellness Community is another example of an organization devoted to improving the quality of life of people with cancer. It features educational programs, seminars, discussion groups and the opportunity for everyone with cancer to relate to others with the same fears and worries. Many people find the approach of this rapidly expanding organization—which encourages you to become an active participant in your fight for recovery—extremely helpful (*see* Chapter 26).

Depending where you live, there also may be organizations designed to meet the needs of young adults who do not always feel comfortable in other support organizations. An organization called Vital Options, for example, meets these needs. This organization started in Los Angeles and is rapidly expanding nationally.

How the Groups Work There are great advantages to taking part in a group when you feel well enough to participate. A group of people in circumstances similar to yours can offer companionship and the chance to discuss many concerns and feelings.

How the support groups are designed and structured and what they cover vary. But they all have in common the gathering together of people with similar experiences. In these groups:

♦ You can tell your story, sharing your experience of cancer and its effect on your life.

♦ You can hear the stories of others, support their similar experiences and decrease their sense of isolation, fear and loneliness.

♦ You can share information and resources that will help you cope with specific problems.

Each group functions for better or worse, depending on the members and the leadership. *Not everyone is suited for a group.* Some people prefer and would do better not participating in a group. But many people with cancer have given credit to their support groups for helping them maintain hope and setting them on the road to recovery.

Where to Find the Right Group Local chapters of the American Cancer Society usually have a current listing of which groups are offered. Many cancer newsletters contain this information, and most oncology nurses and social workers can help you find support resources.

GETTING BACK TO WORK

Many people don't realize how much their feelings of self-worth depend on their being active, productive and capable of taking care of themselves and others. Then an illness strikes and it soon sinks in just how important all that is. Of course, a job is pretty much essential for financial well-being. But it can also be essential for psychological well-being.

This is especially true when you have cancer. The loss of self-esteem that often follows a cancer diagnosis or treatment can be magnified by sitting around doing nothing while you depend on family and friends for personal care, financial assistance and help around the house. So it is vital to your peace of mind to find ways of returning to productive work in some capacity. It might mean getting back to your old job. It might mean learning a new skill, studying or even simply doing work around the house.

Keeping a Positive Attitude Admittedly, getting back to work can sometimes be a problem. You may be disabled in such a way that you can no longer do the same job you had before treatment. And, you may have to confront some discrimination in the job market or prejudice in the workplace.

It's unfortunate, but there is still some stigma attached to having cancer. Employers and co-workers may react out of a vague fear or uneasiness about cancer in the abstract. Co-workers can stay at arm's length either because they just don't know what to say or because they have the irrational and completely mistaken notion that they'll catch something terrible if they go near you. Employers might be afraid of decreased production or financial losses because of the time you might need to take off for treatment.

A study by the American Cancer Society in the 1970s showed that cancer patients did face some discrimination in hiring, firing, job assignments, benefits and attitudes.

♦ Almost a quarter of the people who took part in the study reported either being rejected for jobs because of cancer treatment or being the target of negative attitudes.

♦ Slightly more than half described at least one illness-related problem.

But the good news was that 46 percent said they had *never* had problems at work because of their cancer. And over three-quarters said that after treatment they had earned salary increases because of promotions or increased responsibilities. Since that study was done many American states have passed legislation to outlaw discrimination because of medical conditions, including cancer.

What is absolutely essential is that you keep a positive attitude despite some rejection. Medical social workers, physical and occupational therapists and vocational counselors can all help ease the transition back into the workforce. They can help you match your skills with available jobs or help you get retraining if that is necessary. But learning to live with cancer is the key. Your positive attitude will strengthen your resolve and also just might rub off on employers and co-workers.

YOUR NEED FOR RECREATION

Recreation is an important part of living. We all need a break from the routine and stress of daily life to keep us steady even in the best of circumstances. Although it is sometimes hard to summon up the energy or the will, recreation is even more important when we are sick. Engaging in some kind of recreational activity helps relieve tensions and bring on a feeling of relaxation. It also contributes to feelings of self-worth and well-being.

When you are being treated for cancer, you may forget about recreation. Or you may think it's not important, inappropriate or just too hard to pursue. It is none of these. No matter what your limitations, you can start many activities while you are in the hospital and continue when you go home.

Being with a Group Working with a group or simply working on your own among other people engaged in the same activity has a lot of advantages. The companionship can give you the opportunity to talk about any problems or concerns you have. Better yet, it gives you the chance to talk about all kinds of things that have absolutely nothing to do with cancer. Either way, being with others can lift your spirits and calm your anxieties.

If you are up to it, you can arrange outings with one or more companions. You might want to do something as simple as take a walk in the park with an old friend or take in something entertaining like a movie or a play. If you are involved with craft work, go on an outing to a museum or library to pick up new information or broaden your appreciation of craft activities.

There are many outside resources you can contact, both for learning opportunities and companionship—the YMCA/YWCA, local clubs, schools, colleges and universities, community centers, religious organizations. And keep looking in local newspapers and magazines for recreational activities that change from week to week.

Things to Do on Your Own If you feel more comfortable with solitary pursuits, check out the library in your neighborhood or at the hospital for suggestions. There are many games, crafts and other activities that you can become involved in no matter what your limitations in strength and energy. The list of possibilities is almost limitless, but you might:

♦ Start a scrapbook. Put all your loose photos and mementos into some pleasing arrangement. Divide them by subject or theme and write captions or amusing comments. Maybe you could devote part of the layout to tracing your family tree.

♦ Take up sketching, painting or some other artistic activity. If you have no experience with art, start with line drawings of still life. Once you've got the basic contours of the object on paper, fill in details and shadings and add color. Experiment with various materials. You might find you have talents you never dreamed you had.

♦ Listen to music. It not only "soothes the savage breast," it can raise your spirits, help you sleep, relieve pain and make mealtimes more pleasant and satisfying. Listening to music is not only enjoyable, it's downright therapeutic.

♦ Rent funny movies. If you have a VCR, watch as many comedies as you can. Whether your taste for humor is satisfied by Charlie Chaplin, the Marx Brothers, the Three Stooges or Monty Python, many comedies are available at your local videotape outlets.

♦ Watch comedians. Let Johnny Carson, Jay Leno, George Carlin or anyone else you like tickle your funny bone. Laughter can change your whole outlook on life.

♦ Crochet or knit. Both activities can be very entertaining. And you can see the results of your labors quickly. Even if you've never done either before, you can easily learn to make simple afghans, scarves, shawls or hats for yourself or as gifts for others.

♦ Collect stamps, coins, figurines, recipes, sports cards or anything else that catches your interest. Collecting gets your mind working on organizing, classifying and physically arranging your collection, as well as on what you need to make the collection more complete.

♦ Set up a golf putting course in your home or yard. A very simple arrangement is all that's needed. It will give you an opportunity to stay active and give you a challenge every day.

What kind of recreational activity you pursue is entirely up to you. But whatever you choose as a diversion should be just that—something enjoyable and fun that diverts your mind away from your illness. The relief from stress and the positive attitude fostered by enjoyment can be critically important to your recovery.

THE GOAL OF TOTAL REHABILITATION

Overcoming your anger and fears, developing the right attitude, getting your support system in place and arranging for productive work and recreation are just the start of your rehabilitation and recovery. All these "set the table" for all you have to do during the tough times ahead.

Once you have made the critical decision that you want to get well, you have to be willing to make sacrifices and believe that achieving the goal is worth the effort. You will have to pay attention to all kinds of things that are detailed in the next few chapters—coping with side effects, maintaining good nutrition, getting enough exercise, learning how to relax, becoming secure enough to express yourself sexually, and many more.

You will have to know your strengths and limitations and be able to set realistic goals. And you will have to be willing to compromise, to accept what cannot be changed and move on from there. Having cancer means that your life has to be restructured if you are going to get as full a rehabilitation as possible. This doesn't mean that you have to change the habits of a lifetime, even if you could. But it does mean you will have to make adjustments in your daily living patterns so that your time can be used in the most efficient and constructive ways.

If you pay attention to your mind and body and spirit, you will be well on your way not only to living with cancer but to achieving the highest level of success possible in the circumstances.

17
COPING WITH TREATMENT SIDE EFFECTS

Ernest H. Rosenbaum, MD, Malin Dollinger, MD,
Barbara F. Piper, RN, MS, and Isadora Rosenbaum, MA

When you are ill, your overriding goal is to get well and return to an active life. If you are going to reach that goal, every part of your rehabilitation program is important—the psychological and social dimensions, nutrition, pain control and all the others. But unless the side effects of treatment are looked after, you might not have the energy nor even the desire to get back to a normal life. Side effects can be debilitating. They can sap your strength, weaken your resolve and generally just make life unpleasant.

With support from the medical team, family and friends, you can manage these side effects and eventually overcome them. It may take quite an effort on your part. But the benefits will be well worth that effort.

FATIGUE

No one knows exactly why people with cancer become so fatigued. The tumor itself may make the body function in an overactive (hypermetabolic) state or compete for nutrients at the expense of the energy needs of normal cells. Or there can be a whole range of contributing factors that are related to cancer treatment.

♦ Many people feel very tired during and sometimes after radiotherapy or chemotherapy. These treatments may cause fatigue because of unknown metabolic changes or because of the buildup of toxic substances that are released by cancer cells as they die.

♦ Certain chemotherapy drugs, such as the Vinca alkaloids (vincristine, Velban), appear to cause fatigue as a result of neurotoxicity. Antiemetics and sedatives compound the problem.

♦ If you are receiving radiation therapy, you will need more energy for repair of damaged tissues. You may have a 20 percent increased need for calories and protein during treatment and you will feel tired if you can't satisfy that need.

♦ Complications or side effects of the disease and/or the therapies—anemia, infection and fever, for example—can create energy needs your food intake can't supply.

♦ Fatigue also can be made worse by other side effects or symptoms such as loss of appetite, nausea, vomiting, pain, depression, lack of sleep and loss of muscle tone and strength because of inactivity. Muscle exhaustion can lead to an excess of lactic acid that reduces muscle power, worsening the fatigue even more.

Whatever the cause, fatigue sometimes can become so severe that it affects your ability to function in any useful way. Sometimes it can affect treatment too, making it necessary to limit dosages of chemotherapy or biological therapy. The goal for both you and your medical team should be to prevent fatigue from becoming chronic and unrelenting.

Fighting Fatigue The best way to fight fatigue is to reduce the problems that cause it. Unfortunately, it is not always easy to know what the cause is. Your doctor will have to assess all the possibilities thoroughly. If your fatigue is related to anemia, blood transfusions can help your body carry enough oxygen for its metabolic needs. Other causes can be managed on an individual basis, with a special emphasis on maintaining good nutrition (*see* Chapter 18).

HINTS ON HOW TO COMBAT FATIGUE

ASSESSMENT

♦ Keep a diary for one week to identify the time of day when you are most fatigued or have the most energy.
♦ Identify which activities make the fatigue worse and which make it better.
♦ Develop a plan to pace yourself, scheduling activities according to your fatigue-energy pattern.

MANAGEMENT

Nutrition

♦ If you are losing weight, have lost your appetite or experienced any taste changes, ask for a nutritional consultation to help you correct any deficiencies in your diet.
♦ Drink 8 to 10 glasses of fluid a day to help your body eliminate toxic metabolic substances.
♦ Eat highly complex carbohydrates like grains and vegetables that provide energy over a long period rather than sweets, which give you a quick burst of energy but then leave you more tired than before.

Activity and Exercise

♦ Space activities out over the week and plan adequate rest periods between activities.
♦ Be selective in the type of activities you choose to do when your energy is at a low point.
♦ Do range-of-motion exercises or bed exercises to maintain your muscle tone and strength.
♦ Once cleared by your doctor, walk or do other exercises to increase your aerobic endurance.

Symptoms

♦ Control other symptoms you may have—fever, infection, nausea or vomiting—as best you can. Use medications if necessary.
♦ If you can't sleep, try to figure out why. Take a sleeping pill as prescribed, if you need to.

Psychological

♦ If you are depressed or feeling anxious about things, talk with someone who is a helpful listener—a friend, spiritual counselor or psychiatrist.
♦ Ask your doctor about prescribing mood-elevating drugs.
♦ Ask your doctor or nurse to describe some of the relaxation and distraction techniques that many people have found helpful.
♦ While you are healing, delegate non-essential tasks to other people.

NAUSEA AND VOMITING

Nausea is a feeling of stomach distress or wooziness accompanied by a strong urge to throw up. Nausea and vomiting are temporary side effects of both chemotherapy and radiotherapy. They can also be brought on by an obstruction in the intestine, irritation of the gastrointestinal tract (gastritis) or brain tumors.

Constant vomiting naturally makes it impossible for you to eat or take fluids, so whatever can be done to reduce nausea should be done *before* vomiting starts. Paying attention to nausea's psychological causes and using antinausea drugs will help control what can be disturbing events.
Nausea and Chemotherapy Drugs The goal of chemotherapy is to deliver a thera-peutic amount of drugs with the least side effects. But each chemotherapy agent and each drug combination has a potential for causing nausea and vomiting. Getting three or four drugs at a time, which is often the case, can make the reaction even more severe. The dosage and the number of cycles to be given can also contribute to the reaction.

You, your family and even your friends should talk with your doctor about the type of chemotherapy you'll be getting. For each drug, a program should be established so that you feel you have some control over the situation. With psychological factors playing such a big part, it is very important that you be a participant in preventing nausea and vomiting.

CHEMOTHERAPY DRUGS AND THEIR POTENTIAL TO CAUSE NAUSEA

Highest Potential	Intermediate Potential	Least Potential
◆ cisplatin	◆ Adriamycin/doxorubicin	◆ bleomycin
◆ dacarbazine	◆ nitrosoureas (lomustine, BCNU)	◆ 5-fluorouracil (5-FU)
◆ nitrogen mustard (Mustargen)	◆ procarbazine (Matulane)	◆ etoposide (VP-16)
◆ dactinomycin	◆ Cytosar (cytosine arabinoside ARA-C)	◆ methotrexate
◆ Cytoxan	◆ mitomycin C	◆ chlorambucil
◆ streptozotocin	◆ ifosfamide	◆ vincristine/vinblastine
	◆ carboplatin	◆ mercaptopurine
		◆ melphalan (Alkeran)

Nausea Before and During Treatment It is estimated that up to half of all people receiving chemotherapy experience some nausea or vomiting not after they receive the drugs but *before* their treatment. This is known as anticipatory nausea and vomiting (ANV) and it usually makes the nausea and vomiting even more severe when the chemotherapy is actually given. This can eventually become such a set psychological pattern that it affects the amount of chemotherapy that can be given. And once the psychological pattern of ANV is established, it is much harder to control nausea and vomiting before and after treatment.

Anticipatory nausea is the result of a conditioned reflex. This means that if chemotherapy made you throw up once or twice, then you will will feel nauseated whenever you take the treatment or even when something triggers the very idea of treatment. This conditioned aversion often takes hold after two to four chemotherapy sessions and can last a long time. A standard joke among doctors is the one about the patient who passed her oncologist on the street three years after therapy and threw up on the spot.

Your anxiety state, how you feel about yourself and your cancer and how you respond to stress and disease are all important factors in setting up this psychological pattern. And once the pattern is established, all kinds of stimuli can trigger feelings of nausea—the colors or odors in the room where the chemotherapy is given, the smell of alcohol used to prepare you for the IV needle, the sight of the nurse entering the room.

To deal with this problem, you will have to take steps both to relax before your chemotherapy and to not inadvertently set up situations that become associated with nausea.

♦ Try to relax in a quiet, darkened room before your treatment sessions.

♦ Use behavioral techniques to help you relax and control any triggering stimuli—hypnosis, relaxation therapy, imagery or listening to a tape of your favorite music or a relaxation tape (*see* Chapter 25).

♦ Perhaps try acupuncture or acupressure, which have been effective in controlling nausea or vomiting in some cases.

♦ The time of day when you get treatment can sometimes make a difference. If you have a problem with either the morning or the afternoon, try to change your appointment schedule.

♦ Avoid eating hot, spicy foods or other dishes that might upset your stomach or gastrointestinal tract.

♦ Eat slowly so you don't develop gas or heartburn.

♦ Try to avoid cooking odors that may bring on nausea by having friends or family prepare meals at their own homes and bring them over to you.

♦ Always avoid your favorite foods when you are getting chemotherapy. You might start to associate these foods with treatment, nausea and vomiting and develop a strong aversion to them.

Nausea After Treatment Nausea and vomiting are common side effects after chemotherapy (or after radiation therapy). They may begin one to three hours later or even as long as two to four days after treatment.

Like anticipatory nausea, post-therapy nausea and vomiting can have significant therapeutic implications. You may start to fear therapy, a fear that can gnaw at you and make you want to avoid treatment. It may also make problems such as pain control and maintaining an overall good quality of life much harder to deal with.

Fortunately, a wide variety of antinausea drugs has been developed and some combination tailored to your specific needs will usually do the trick to minimize or prevent the problem.

Antinausea Medications Two areas in the brain have been identified as being responsible for nausea and vomiting, and certain drugs and other methods can selectively block these areas. Your doctor can work out a program to combat your nausea, although if one drug or drug combination doesn't work as well as you would both like, you may have to experiment with different programs.

Generally, antivomiting drugs (antiemetics) should be taken 30 minutes before chemotherapy so that they have time to take effect.

♦ If vomiting has already started and you can't keep a pill down, suppositories such as Compazine or Tigan may help.

♦ Long-acting spansules such as Compazine can be very helpful, since they work for 12 hours.

♦ Ativan and Decadron may help block the brain's vomiting center. It is also a very powerful combination to block anticipatory nausea and vomiting. Ativan can be taken under the tongue for rapid absorption during severe nausea.

♦ Ativan is also an antidepressant and sleeping tablet that can cause amnesia, which might take the edge off any memory of vomiting once the episode is over.

♦ Some forms of marijuana—the natural

delta-9-tetrahydrocannabinol (THC) and the synthetic Marinol—may successfully control nausea and vomiting by working on the higher brain centers. But they can also cause drowsiness, dry mouth, dizziness, a rapid heartbeat and sweating.

♦ A new antiserotonin drug is the 5-HT3 receptor blocker Ondandsetron (Zofran).

It is the most significant new drug used to control nausea and vomiting caused by intensive chemotherapy and radiotherapy and has just been released on the market. It suppresses vomiting in 60 to 80 percent of patients and is even more effective in combination with other antinausea drugs.

COMMON ANTINAUSEA DRUGS

	Oral	IM	IV	Suppository
♦ Compazine (prochlorperazine)	X	X	X	X
♦ Ativan (lorazepam)	X	X	X	
♦ Reglan (metaclopramide)	X		X	
♦ Haldol (haloperidol)	X	X		
♦ Inapsine (droperidol)			X	
♦ Decadron (dexamethasone)	X	X	X	
♦ Benadryl (diphenhydramine)	X	X	X	
♦ Tigan (trimethobenzamide)	X	X		X
♦ THC (marijuana tablets)	X			
♦ Torecan (thiethylperazine)	X	X	X	X

SORE MOUTH

The lining, or mucosa, of the gastrointestinal tract—which includes the inside of the mouth and throat—is one of the most sensitive areas of the body. Many chemotherapy drugs can inflame the lining, a condition called mucositis. Many drugs can also cause small ulcerations or sores to develop. Radiation delivered to the head and neck can irritate the lining and cause sores, too, and so can mouth or throat infections, especially fungus infections like monilia (thrush). All these can be very painful or at least uncomfortable.

If you are going to get over your mucositis, mouth care is very important. You will have to make sure your mouth stays clean and moist and that you eat the proper foods and get medication for any infections that develop.

Oral Hygiene A good oral hygienic program includes dental cleaning and scaling, followed by daily brushing and flossing to reduce plaque.

Any scaling, cleaning, tooth extractions or repair of cavities should be done before your cancer therapy begins. Extractions especially should be completed at least two weeks before therapy to give your mouth a chance to heal. Ill-fitting dentures should be fixed or replaced.

Before any dental work is to be performed, your blood counts should be checked to be sure that counts are adequate to take care of any possibility of infection or bleeding (low white cell counts can lead to infections and a low platelet count may lead to bleeding). So any periodontal or dental work has to be coordinated with your oncologist. If you have any mouth injury because of a dental procedure, antibiotics are certainly recommended.

The following daily steps will help your mouth stay in good shape:

♦ Use a soft-bristle toothbrush and soften it more by soaking it in warm water. You may also find that brushing with a paste of baking soda and water may be less irritating than commercial toothpaste.

♦ If brushing your teeth is painful, use either a cotton swab or commercial Toothettes, a sponge-tip stick impregnated with a dentifrice.

♦ Avoid commercial mouthwashes. Some of these have ingredients (especially alcohol) that can irritate your mouth even more. Lemon glycerin swabs may make your mouth feel clean but they are not recommended, because glycerin will make your mouth drier.

♦ A Water-Pik to cleanse your mouth is helpful.

♦ Peridex (oral rinse) will help gum inflammation and bleeding.

Dry Mouth Chemotherapy and radiation to the salivary glands can make your mouth very dry. This can make your mucositis or mouth sores more painful, so you should do everything you can to keep your mouth moist.

♦ Commercial preparations such as Moistir or MouthKot—an oral natural saliva substitute—may help.

♦ You can make your own mouthwash with liquid Xylocaine, baking soda and salt dissolved in 1 quart (1 L) of water.

♦ Sucking sour lemon hard candies or Tic Tacs can help. You can also suck on popsicles or flavored or plain ice cubes.

♦ Use lip balms or lipstick if your lips are dry.

Mouth Sores If the soreness in your mouth becomes severe, there are quite a few anesthetic agents you can use on a short-term basis. If your symptoms persist, you should have a complete dental hygienic evaluation.

♦ Benadryl elixir, lozenges and analgesics may help reduce mouth pain.

♦ Swishing and swallowing the anesthetic

jelly viscous Xylocaine or Hurricane can also help you eat if you have pain in your mouth, pharynx or esophagus (a spray is also available).

♦ It may help to swish diluted milk of magnesia, Carafate slurry or Mylanta around your mouth.

♦ Orabase—with or without Kenalog—is a dental salve that covers mouth sores while they are healing. You may have to apply it several times a day.

Infections Mouth infections can be dangerous and have to be cared for. You should examine your mouth every day for any irritation or early fungus growth (white spots inside your mouth that don't wash off). Look under your tongue and at the sides of your mouth and report any changes to your doctor. If you do get an infection, it should be treated promptly.

♦ If you have a herpes virus—acute or recurrent—your doctor may prescribe oral Acyclovir.

♦ Monilia requires antifungal agents, including mycostatin oral suspension Nizoral tablets, Mycelex Troches or Mycostat Pastilles.

♦ You can freeze Nystatin Liquid in medicine cups in the refrigerator and let it melt in your mouth.

Nutrition A normal high-protein, high-calorie diet—with supplements as needed—will help your sore mouth or tongue heal faster. Drinking lots of fluids will also help the healing process as well as help make your mouth sores more comfortable.

A high-calorie, high-protein diet would include scrambled eggs, custards, milk-shakes, malts, gelatins, creamy hot cereals, macaroni and cheese and blenderized or pureed foods. Commercial supplements such as Ensure, Sustacal or Carnation Breakfast Drink can also be helpful.

Until your mouth sores heal you should avoid:

♦ Very hot or very cold foods.

♦ Tomatoes and citrus fruits such as grapefruit, lemons and oranges, which can burn your mouth.

♦ Salty foods, which can cause a burning sensation.

♦ Hot, spicy, coarse or rough foods, including toast, dry crackers and chips.

♦ Alcoholic beverages and tobacco, both of which irritate the lining of the mouth.

♦ Any medications such as mouthwashes or cough syrups that contain alcohol.

LOSS OF APPETITE

Loss of appetite, called anorexia, is one of the most common side effects of chemotherapy. It can also result from radiation therapy, stress and anxiety, depression and the cancer itself.

For the sake of your health, your strength and your ability to fight cancer, you have to get enough nutrition. But it's hard to keep your appetite when your mouth and tongue are sore or you have trouble swallowing. Fortunately, these side effects are usually short-term, lasting only three to eight days. But even after they go away, you still might have trouble getting your normal appetite back.

You can talk to a dietitian, nurse or your doctor about ways to improve your appetite. If you don't seem to be making too much progress, you might also ask your doctor about medications that can stimulate your appetite, such as:

♦ Prednisone, a corticosteroid hormone, when given in small doses of 10 to 20 mg a day (there are side effects to consider).

♦ Megace (a progestin), 40 mg two to four times a day.

♦ Marinol, a legally available synthetic form of marijuana in capsule form. It is usually used as an antinausea drug, but stimulation of appetite is a positive side effect.

Tips to Reduce Loss of Appetite

♦ Plan your meals in advance and arrange for help in preparing them. You might also better tolerate meals prepared by friends or family, since cooking at home might produce offensive odors that will put you off food.

♦ Make your mealtimes a pleasant experience.

♦ Stimulate your appetite by exercising for 5 or 10 minutes about a half-hour before meals.

♦ Have an aperitif such as a small glass of wine before meals. It will help you relax and stimulate your taste buds.

♦ Relax for a few minutes before meals, using relaxation exercises.

♦ Eat frequent, small meals and have snacks between meals that appeal to your senses.

♦ Add extra protein to your diet. Fortify milk by adding 1 cup (250 mL) of non-fat dry milk to each quart (liter) of whole milk or milk recipe. Be creative with desserts. And use nutritional supplements.

TASTE BLINDNESS

Many chemotherapy drugs can change your sense of taste and smell. What these changes are depends on the individual, but they are most common with foods that are either very sweet or very bitter. Oddly enough, sweet foods might taste sour and sour foods taste sweet. Chewed meat may have a bitter taste because of the release of proteins in your mouth. Sometimes there is a continuous metallic taste in your mouth after chemotherapy, which naturally enough can affect what you eat and how you eat.

Taste changes may not last long. But while you are experiencing them, you can do several things to lessen their effect.
♦ Brush your teeth several times a day and use mouth rinses such as diluted bicarbonate of soda.
♦ If foods and beverages taste bitter, add sweet fruits, honey or NutraSweet.
♦ If meat tastes bitter, substitute bland chicken or fish, eggs and mild cheeses or tofu. All of these might taste better if you use them in casseroles or stews.
♦ It will also help if you marinate meats, chicken or fish in pineapple juice, wine, Italian dressing, lemon juice, soy sauce or sweet-and-sour sauces.
♦ Add whatever flavorings you enjoy, but avoid spicy, highly seasoned foods.
♦ You might find that starchy foods such as bread, potatoes and rice have a more acceptable taste if you eat them without butter or margarine.

CONSTIPATION AND IMPACTION

Constipation means infrequent bowel movements. It also means a collection of dry, hard stools that get "stuck" in your rectum or colon. When you are constipated, you will often feel bloated and not have much of an appetite. If constipation persists, it may cause a stool "impaction"—a very large hard stool that you will have great difficulty passing.

It is important to try to prevent constipation and stool impaction, for both can cause great distress and pain. Patients with heart, respiratory or gastrointestinal diseases can be especially aggravated by the discomfort and pressure of an impaction.

Causes All kinds of things can make you constipated—lack of exercise, emotional stress, various drugs or simply a lack of high-fiber or bulk-forming foods in your diet.

Chemotherapy drugs such as vincristine and vinblastine are often constipating. So are narcotics such as morphine and codeine, gastrointestinal antispasmodics, antidepressants, diuretics, tranquilizers, sleeping pills and calcium- and aluminum-based antacids.

When prescribing these drugs, your doctor should anticipate the need for a stool softener and/or a mild laxative. Enemas or suppositories might also be needed.

Laxatives and Stool Softeners If you become constipated, talk to your doctor about a laxative program. It is essential that you take laxatives—and suppositories and enemas as well—only under your doctor's supervision. Don't try to diagnose and treat yourself since there may be more to the situation than you may realize. For example, diarrhea can occasionally develop at the same time as a stool impaction, with the liquid stools moving around the impaction. If you decide to take antidiarrheal drugs, you can make the situation much worse.

There are many different ways to treat a wide variety of conditions, and your doctor may recommend several kinds of medications depending on your condition and other personal factors.
♦ *Stool softeners* help the stool retain water and so keep it soft. Stool softeners—Colace (docusate sodium 50 to 240 mg per day with a full glass of water) and Surfak,

for example—should be used early, before the stools become hard, especially as it can be days before any effect is noticeable.

♦ *Mild laxatives* help promote bowel activity. Examples are milk of magnesia, Doxidan, cascara sagrada and mineral oil (a lubricant).

♦ *Stronger laxatives* include Phospha-soda(Fleet's), magnesium citrate and senna (Senokot).

♦ *Contact laxatives* such as castor oil or Dulcolax suppositories or tablets cause increased bowel activity.

♦ *Bulk laxatives* include dietary fiber, bran, methyl cellulose (Cellothyl) and psyllium (Metamucil).

♦ Laxatives with magnesium should be avoided if you have kidney disease. Laxatives with sodium should be avoided if you have a heart problem. (Laxatives that contain magnesium can also cause diarrhea.)

♦ If you are taking narcotics you should use stool softeners and mild laxatives rather than bulk-forming laxatives, because the combination can cause high colon constipation.

♦ Non-stimulating bulk softeners such as docusate (Colace) help to soften the stool and mineral oil or olive oil can be used to loosen the stool.

♦ Glycerin suppositories or Dulcolax suppositories may be used to stimulate bowel action as a contact laxative. (Dulcolax may cause cramping.)

♦ Bowel stimulants such as Reglan may be useful.

♦ Lactulose (chronulac) is an acidifyer that softens the stool and increases the number of bowel movements.

All laxatives should be used with care. If you use them continually, you might develop a gastrointestinal irritation that can make it difficult to regain your normal bowel habits once you stop taking them. Increasing doses can also make your colon and rectum insensitive to the normal reflexes that stimulate a bowel movement.

Hints to Prevent and Relieve Constipation

♦Eat foods that are high in fiber and bulk. These include fresh fruits and vegetables (raw or cooked with skins and peels on), dried fruit, whole-grain breads and cereals and bran. Avoid raw fruits and vegetables, including lettuce, when your white blood cell count is lower than 1,800.

Note: You should start a high-fiber diet before taking a chemotherapy drug that causes constipation.

♦Drink plenty of fluids—8 to 10 glasses a day. *Avoid dehydration.* Try to drink highly nutritional fluids (milkshakes, eggnogs and juices) rather than water, since liquids can be filling and may decrease your appetite.

♦Add bran to your diet gradually. Start with 2 tsp. (10mL) per day and gradually work up to 4 to 6 tsp. (20 to 30 mL) per day. Sprinkle bran on cereal or add it to meatloaf, stews, pancakes, baked goods and other dishes. Dietary bran is helpful.

♦Avoid refined foods such as white bread, starchy desserts and candy. Also avoid chocolates, cheese and eggs, since these can be constipating.

♦To make your bowel movements more regular, take prunes or a glass of prune juice in the morning or at night before bed. Prunes contain a natural laxative as well as fiber. Warmed prune juice and stewed prunes will be the most effective.

♦ Eat a large breakfast with some type of hot beverage, such as tea, hot lemon water or decaffeinated coffee.

♦ Get enough rest and eat at regular times in a relaxed atmosphere.

♦ Get some exercise to stimulate your intestinal reflexes and help restore normal elimination.

Treating Stool Impaction A stool impaction develops when all of a stool doesn't pass through the colon or rectum. The stool gradually gets harder and harder as water is absorbed by the bowel. Then the stool gets larger and larger. If you can't pass it, it may partially obstruct the bowel or cause irritation of the rectum or anus. If you do pass it, it may cause small tears or fissures in the anus.

The primary treatment is to get fluids into the bowel to soften the stool so it can be passed or removed. Using enemas—either oil-retention, tap water or phosphate (Fleet's)—may help accomplish this goal. Sometimes it might be necessary for a health professional to use a gloved finger in the rectum to break up a large bulky mass or to extract the stool.

DIARRHEA

Diarrhea is a condition marked by abnormally frequent bowel movements that are more fluid than usual. It is sometimes accompanied by cramps.

You may get diarrhea because of chemotherapy, radiation therapy to the lower abdomen, malabsorption because of surgery to the bowel or sometimes a bowel inflammation or infection. Some antibiotics, especially "broad spectrum" antibiotics, can cause diarrhea, and it might develop because of an intolerance to milk.

Treating Diarrhea Effective treatment depends on finding the cause. A good general approach is to limit your diet solely to fluids to allow the bowel to rest. Drink plenty of mild liquids, such as fruit drinks (Kool-Aid and Gatorade), ginger ale, peach or apricot nectar, water and weak tea. Hot and cold liquids and foods tend to increase intestinal muscle contractions and make the diarrhea worse, so they should be warm or at room temperature. Allow carbonated beverages to lose their fizz—stir with a spoon—before you drink them.

When you are feeling better, gradually add foods low in roughage and bulk—steamed rice, cream of rice, bananas, applesauce, mashed potatoes, dry toast and crackers—eaten warm or at room temperature.

As your diarrhea decreases, you may move on to a low-residue diet. Frequent small meals will be easier on your digestive tract. Low-residue nutritional supplements such as Precision Low Residue, Vivonex, Flexocal or Citoein can also help.

Foods to Avoid Many types of foods are likely to aggravate your diarrhea and should be avoided. These include:
♦ fatty, greasy and spicy foods;
♦ coffee, regular (non-herbal) teas and carbonated beverages containing caffeine;
♦ citrus fruits such as oranges and grapefruit;
♦ foods high in bulk and fiber, such as bran, whole-grain cereals and breads, popcorn, nuts and raw vegetables and fruits (except apples); and
♦ beverages and foods generally that are served too hot or too cold.

Replacing What Is Lost Diarrhea can cause dehydration, so you will have to drink plenty of fluids. To replace the fluid, sugar and salt you will lose, a good general formula is: 1 quart (1 L) boiled water, 1 tsp. (5 mL) salt, 1 tsp. (5 mL) baking soda, 4 tsp. (20 mL) sugar and flavor to your taste. As with any specially prepared concoction, however, you should check with your dietitian or doctor to make sure you can tolerate the particular ingredients.

Potassium is also lost in diarrhea. It is a necessary mineral, and it must be replaced. Foods high in potassium include bananas, apricot and peach nectars, tomatoes, potatoes, broccoli, halibut, asparagus, citrus juices and milk. Supplementary potassium tablets sometimes have to be taken.

Milk Intolerance Some people are born with lactose intolerance and some develop it as they grow older. The intolerance results from a deficiency of lactase, an enzyme that digests milk sugar (lactose) in the intestine, and is marked by cramping and diarrhea.

A lactase deficiency can sometimes develop after intestinal surgery, radiation therapy to the lower abdomen or chemotherapy. Because you can no longer digest milk sugar properly, you feel bloated and experience cramping and diarrhea.

♦ If your diarrhea is caused by milk intolerance, you should avoid milk and milk products such as ice cream, cottage cheese and cheese. Depending on how sensitive you are to milk, you may also have to avoid butter, cream and sour cream.

♦ If you are very sensitive, look for lactose-free, non-fat milk solids. You can even make your own lactose-free milk by adding Lactaid—a tablet containing lactase—to your milk and keeping it in the refrigerator for 24 hours before using it.

♦ You can use buttermilk or yogurt because the lactose in them has already been processed and is digested. You might also tolerate some processed cheeses.

♦ You might try Mocha-mix, Dairy Rich and other soy products, or some lactose substitutes like Imo (an imitation sour cream), Cool Whip or Party Whip.

Diarrhea Medications

♦**Kaopectate**. Take 2 to 4 tablespoons (25 to 50 mL) after each loose bowel movement.

♦**Lomotil**. One to two tablets every four hours as needed. You can take Lomotil with Kaopectate or Imodium. Maximum eight Lomotil tablets per day.

♦**Imodium.** Two capsules initially, then one to two capsules every two to four hours. Maximum 16 capsules per day.

♦**Paregoric**. Take 1 tsp. (5 mL) four times a day. It may be used with Lomotil.

♦**Cholestryamine**. A bile-salt sequestering agent. One packet after each meal and at bedtime.

♦**Donnatal or Robinul**. Anticholinergic, antispasmodic agents for bowel cramping. One to two tablets every four hours as needed.

♦When all else fails, try Metamucil plus Kaopectate.

SWOLLEN LIMBS (LYMPHEDEMA)

Lymphedema—the medical term for swelling caused by the buildup of fluid (lymph) in the soft tissues—develops because of some blockage of the lymphatic system. Most lymphedema in cancer patients results from scarring after the surgical removal of lymph nodes or after radiation therapy. It usually involves areas next to large collections of lymph nodes in the armpit (axilla), pelvic region and inguinal (groin) areas. The lymphatics are obstructed and swelling in the arms or legs is the result.

In its early phase, the swelling of the limb will "pit" with finger pressure. Elevating the arm or leg or using an elastic support arm glove or stocking will help reduce the swelling and improve the lymphatic flow.

Acute and Chronic Lymphedema Acute lymphedema may be a temporary condition. It can happen after a radical surgical procedure with lymph node dissection or after an acute inflammation such as an infection in the limb. More often seen in cancer patients is chronic lymphedema. Sometimes it results in only minor swelling and discomfort. But occasionally it can lead to grave disability and disfigurement.

Chronic lymphedema is more difficult to reverse than the acute variety because the more the limb swells the harder it is to drain the fluid adequately. People with chronic lymphedema are also more susceptible to infections or local injuries, which results in more scarring and additional lymphedema. Infections of the limb—known as cellulitis—often develop after even minor cuts or abrasions and they can often only be controlled with long-term antibiotics.

Occasionally lymphedema becomes prolonged and severe. It can be aggravated by poor protein intake that may result from loss of appetite or nausea and vomiting from chemotherapy. It can also be aggravated by a decrease of the protein in the blood called albumin. The decrease results in leakage of water into the tissues, which leads to additional arm or leg swelling.

Who Gets It A small number of people with cancer develop lymphedema. It is not unusual after treatment for several common cancers.

♦ Breast cancer. Primary radiotherapy to the breast is rarely associated with lymphedema. It is more common if you are treated with radiotherapy after surgery to the regional lymph node areas.

♦ Malignant melanomas with lymph node dissection and/or radiation involving an extremity.

♦ Prostate cancer or gynecologic cancers after surgery, with or without radiation.

♦ Testicular cancer with lymph node dissection, with or without radiation.

♦ Patients who have had several courses of radiotherapy to the axilla, shoulder or groin, especially if surgery has also been performed there to treat recurrent cancer.

Preventing Lymphedema If you have had any of the above procedures, you will have to take extra special care of the limb that might be affected. You should treat your arm or leg with the same care and attention you give to your face.

You can do a lot to prevent lymphedema—good nutrition with a high-protein diet, active physical exercise to help your muscles pump the lymphatic fluid, control of obesity. You should also try hard to avoid infections from small cuts you might get working around the house or by doing physical work that might damage or injure the skin on the affected arm or leg.

Even if you follow a prevention program faithfully, lymphedema can occasionally develop years after surgery. This often happens after a local infection, although sometimes it happens for no apparent reason at all. If you develop any evidence of inflammation or infection (cellulitis) with redness or increased swelling, report it to your doctor. He or she can evaluate your condition and prescribe any necessary antibiotics. You may have to stay on antibiotics for several weeks or even months.

Milking Your Muscles Exercising your muscles is vital if you want to prevent lymphedema. It is just as vital if you want to control it. The compression of your muscles helps to milk the fluid in the lymphatics back toward your heart.

Physical therapists can recommend the most appropriate exercises for you. Many people are often encouraged to walk or ride a bicycle to help improve the lymphatic flow. Breast cancer patients are usually instructed to go through a series of hand and arm exercises after surgery. A similar program is used by patients with melanomas involving the limbs. Therapists can instruct you in the use of lymphedema milking pumps that can reduce your swelling, which can be an effective approach for chronic lymphedema.

Hints for Preventing and Controlling Lymphedema

1. Whenever possible, keep the swollen arm or leg elevated, preferably above the level of the heart. When you are sitting, put your leg on a chair or stool.

2. Clean and lubricate your skin every day with oil or skin cream.

3. Do everything you can to avoid injuries and infection in the affected limb:
♦ use an electric razor to shave the limb to avoid skin cuts
♦ wear gloves when gardening or doing housework and wear thimbles when sewing
♦ suntan gradually, if at all, and use a sunscreen
♦ wear foot coverings when on the beach or wading in water
♦ use insect repellants and wear protective clothing to avoid insect bites
♦ clean any breaks in your skin with mild soap and water, then apply an antibacterial ointment
♦ use gauze wrapping instead of adhesive tape on any skin wounds
♦ if you develop a rash, consult your doctor
♦ try to minimize all the "invasive" procedures for drawing blood and giving medications—injections, finger pricks and IVs—on the affected arm or leg
♦ take good care of your nails and don't cut the cuticles
♦ cut your toenails straight across
♦ see a podiatrist for any foot care problems
♦ keep your feet clean and dry and wear cotton socks
♦ avoid extreme hot or cold—ice packs and heating pads, for example—on the swollen limb.

4. Avoid constrictive pressure on your arm or leg:
♦ don't cross your legs while sitting
♦ wear loose jewelry and clothes with no constricting bands
♦ carry handbags on the non-swollen arm
♦ don't use blood pressure cuffs on the swollen limb
♦ wear only elastic bandages or stockings without constrictive bands
♦ don't sit longer than 30 minutes without changing position.

5. Check the limb daily for signs of change. Especially watch for signs of infection—redness, pain, heat, swelling or fever—and call your doctor immediately if any signs appear. Be sure to report any sensation of swelling or sudden increase in fluid.

6. Practice your drainage-promoting exercises faithfully.

7. After the limb has healed, *gradually* return to your normal activity. But always practice protective procedures—edema can come back if you get an injury.

HAIR LOSS

Losing your hair (alopecia) can be quite an emotional experience. As the most visible side effect of cancer treatment, it is often the most upsetting. In fact, you may find it helpful to have your mate or a close friend or relative with you when you talk to your doctor about the potential for hair loss.

Why You Might Lose Your Hair Chemotherapy drugs circulate throughout your body and they aren't selective about which cells they affect. They change normal as well as malignant cells and have an especially destructive effect on rapidly growing cells like your hair and the cells lining your mouth and gastrointestinal tract. So hair loss is a common side effect of chemotherapy, especially with drugs such as Cytoxan, Adriamycin and vincristine. Your chances of losing your hair are increased if you are getting combination therapy.

When You Lose Your Hair You may not lose all your hair. It may just become thin or patchy. The loss might also be sudden or gradual. It usually happens within the first cycle (usually around Week 3), but it may not happen until the second cycle. And, whether the loss is partial or complete, you may develop some scalp irritation, dermatitis or scaling that will need medical attention.

The hair almost always comes back. It may take three to six months or it might come back while you are still on chemotherapy. When it does come back it might have a slightly different texture or color or curl.

Hair Loss and Radiation You might lose some hair after radiation therapy to the skull or brain. This may be total and permanent, but if lower doses are used the hair sometimes comes back within two to three months.

Preparing for Hair Loss This is one side effect you can plan for well in advance. There are several things you can do before you begin treatment that will make losing your hair not quite as upsetting.
♦ Get a short haircut so that the hair loss won't be as noticeable either to others or to you when you look in the mirror.
♦ Treat your hair and your scalp gently by avoiding hairsprays, perms and dyes.
♦ Select hair covers that you'll need during the period of hair loss—turbans, scarves, hats, wigs and scarves with hair fringes that look like your own hair. Many insurance companies will pay for a hair piece or wig since they are a "part" of treatment, so ask your doctor for a prescription. To get the best possible match, buy a wig before you lose your hair.

Tourniquets and Ice Caps Scalp tourniquets and ice caps can be used to prevent or reduce hair loss. But they are not very useful when the chemotherapy drugs tend to stay in the bloodstream for several hours or if the drugs are taken orally, which leads to the same time effect. Even so, using caps and tourniquets during therapy might make you feel better by reducing anxiety.

Tourniquets and ice caps are *not* recommended if you are being treated for cancers that are likely to have hidden scalp metastases—melanoma, kidney cancer, leukemia, lymphomas and tumors that spread in the bloodstream.

18
MAINTAINING GOOD NUTRITION

Ernest H. Rosenbaum, MD, Malin Dollinger, MD, and Lawrence Margolis, MD

◇

Good nutrition is vital to all of us all the time. It is impossible to stay in good health without consuming the right foods in the right amounts. Good nutrition gives us the energy and the building blocks our bodies need to function properly and stay in good repair.

Good nutrition is even more necessary when you have cancer. Your body is fighting disease and food is a critical weapon in the fight. You will need even more nutrients than usual—a metabolic need about 20 percent higher than a healthy person who engages in moderate activity. The extra nutrients will help your body fend off weakness, repair damaged tissues, help boost your immune system and create a feeling of general well-being.

COMMON PROBLEMS

Many people with cancer have a hard time maintaining good nutrition since the cancer itself and the therapies that fight it can make it hard to eat enough food. There are several major common problems.

♦ *Loss of appetite* This is the most serious problem. Pain, nausea, vomiting, diarrhea or a sore or dry mouth can easily make you lose interest in food. You may also tend to eat less because of fear, anxiety or depression about having cancer.

♦ *Malabsorption* For a number of reasons, nutrients may not be absorbed normally into the bloodstream from the intestines. Cancer of the pancreas can cause a decrease in the digestive juices that regulate absorption. Abnormal connections between surgically created loops in the intestine may divert food past the parts of the intestine where nutrients are usually absorbed. The intestines may become less able to absorb nutrients if your normal food intake is reduced for a lengthy time.

♦ *Physical problems* Tumors in the mouth and neck area, as well as radiation therapy directed to those areas, can make it hard to swallow or cause pain in the mouth or throat. Radiation directed to the abdomen or the removal of part of the stomach or intestinal tract can cause diarrhea, cramps or decreased absorption.

♦ *Changes in smell and taste* Chemotherapy or radiation to the neck and mouth can distort the perception of smell and taste, and the loss of taste tends to be greater if the tumor is more advanced. Some foods can start to taste bitter or rancid, especially meat, which might taste bitter and metallic. It is common to develop strong aversions to foods such as meat, eggs, fried foods or tomatoes. All these changes make your appetite worse, making it even more difficult for you to avoid weight loss.

♦ *Early filling* The feeling of being full after taking only a few bites of food is a common problem and will lead to weight loss if you try to stick to the usual three meals a day.

Because of all these problems, many people with cancer become malnourished almost to the point of starvation. And malnutrition can have very serious effects.

THE DANGERS OF WEIGHT LOSS AND MALNUTRITION

Malnutrition affects your whole body, making you steadily weaker. It can also decrease your immunity and make you more susceptible to infections. It can promote tissue breakdown that can lead to "fistulas"—leakage from the natural gastrointestinal tract—and poor healing of any surgical wounds. Malnutrition can also worsen any problem of malabsorption of food you may have as a side effect of treatment, resulting in cramping, bloating and diarrhea.

But the worst effect of malnutrition is the excessive weight loss so often seen in cancer patients. Losing a great deal of weight unfortunately sets up a vicious cycle. A decreased appetite and weight loss lead to fatigue and depression. Depression and progressive weakness lead to reduced activity and an even smaller appetite. More weight loss and weakness lead to a lower resistance to disease and a decrease in immunity. Lower resistance may limit the amount of chemotherapy, radiation therapy or surgery that can be delivered, leading to a poorer prognosis.

Anyone with cancer who is potentially curable may fail to be cured because of poor nutritional management.

Planning for Improved Nutrition The key to keeping this cycle at bay is to do everything in your power to prevent malnutrition from occurring in the first place. Once weight loss begins, it is hard to reverse. The time to start thinking and planning for proper nutrition is not when you have already lost a lot of weight but when the diagnosis is made or your treatment gets under way.

If you lose more than 5 percent of your usual weight, you and your doctor should consider the loss significant. Losing 10 percent of your normal weight is a danger signal. A 15 percent weight loss may result in a further decrease in your appetite, depression, fatigue and progressive weakness that will limit your chance of recovery.

HOW MANY CALORIES AND HOW MUCH PROTEIN DO YOU NEED?

Your normal weight _____pounds

Your desirable weight _____pounds

♦ Your *minimum* daily protein requirement = _____grams
desirable weight (pounds) x 0.5

♦ Your *minimum* daily calorie requirement = _____calories
desirable weight (pounds) x 18 (men)
desirable weight (pounds) x 16 (women)

♦ Keep a daily record of your weight
(and your protein and calorie intake).

If you are losing weight, increase your protein and calorie intake to:

protein grams = desirable weight x 0.7 = _____grams

calories: desirable weight x 20 (men) = _____calories

calories: desirable weight x 18 (women) = _____calories

THE BEST APPROACH TO EATING

What you will need is a totally different approach to eating. Forget the signals that have always told you when to start eating and when to stop. They will no longer be a reliable guide. You will have to approach eating as a necessary part of your therapy and learn to eat even if you don't feel like it.

Nutritional support is usually best directed by your physician, preferably at the start of therapy. But the hospital nutritionist can plan an individualized program for you after two or three days of observation and analysis of any deficits in your intake of calories, protein or fat. You and your family can be instructed in basic nutritional requirements, such as the four basic food groups—protein, milk, vegetable-fruit and bread-cereal.

The nutritionist can also explain how you can deal with the special dietary problems associated with cancer and cancer therapy, such as anorexia, bloating, heartburn, constipation, diarrhea, nausea, vomiting, sore or dry mouth, indigestion and taste blindness.

Special Diets Your nutritional needs may change during therapy. After surgery, for example, you may need to go on a liquid diet and work your way up through a soft diet before getting back to your regular foods. You may need a lactose-restricted diet, a high-fiber diet and/or a high-protein diet. You might also need special food supplements, either with or between meals, to increase your daily intake of nutrients.

There are diets to prevent kidney stones from forming and diets to prevent diarrhea, constipation, nausea and vomiting. There are diets to help improve taste and appetite. All of these preventive and palliative techniques, including occupational therapy to improve your ability to swallow, can be used along with other supportive programs to control depression, relieve any pain and promote physical activity.

A Team Effort With guidance from your doctor, the nutritionist and a few good pamphlets and brochures, you and your family should be able to handle most nutritional problems at home.

And remember that good nutrition is a team effort. It requires not only the expertise of nutritionists and the medical team but the tact and concerned attention of family and friends. Your support team should know that you will be more likely to respond to enjoyable company and gentle encouragement than to harassment and manipulation. The preparation, serving and sharing of food expresses the concern of care givers, family and friends. And that concern can have a direct effect on your sense of well-being.

Also remember that planning for good nutrition early in your disease not only may result in your being able to take more intensive therapy but can also make the difference between survival and death.

So eat often and well. You will feel better mentally and physically. You will heal faster after surgery and have fewer unpleasant side effects from radiation or chemotherapy. You may be able to tolerate more chemotherapy. Your radiotherapy will not have to be interrupted as often. Your immune system will be better able to resist infection. And, not least, you will be able to lead a more active and enjoyable life.

Guidelines for Overcoming Weight Loss

♦ Help ease the problem of early filling by eating smaller portions of food more frequently throughout the day and by drinking fluids between meals instead of with food.

♦ Snack between meals with high-protein diet supplements, milkshakes, eggnogs and puddings.

♦ Add extra calories to your diet by adding cream or butter to soups, cooked cereals and vegetables and by using gravies and sauces with vegetables, meat, poultry and fish.

♦ Add extra protein to your diet by using fortified milk, peanut butter, cheese and chopped hard-boiled eggs.

♦ Taste blindness makes it critical that you do everything you can to enhance the smell, appearance and texture of food. So cook dishes that appeal to your sense of smell and be especially creative with desserts.

♦ Choose foods that you like, within any dietary restrictions your doctor or nutritionist tell you about.

♦ Exercise about half an hour before meals to stimulate your appetite.

♦ Make mealtimes pleasant by doing relaxation exercises beforehand to reduce stress, by setting an attractive and colorful table and by eating with family or friends.

♦ Plan daily menus in advance. If possible, prepare many portions of food and have them frozen and ready to heat and serve.

TUBE AND INTRA-VENOUS FEEDINGS

The *ideal* way to get enough food is by eating normally—put the food in your mouth, chew it well and swallow. The food is absorbed naturally, using a functional gastrointestinal tract to meet nutritional needs. This is also the least expensive method of nutritional support.

But there are times when normal eating just isn't practical. You may not be able to swallow. You might be suffering through a bout of nausea, vomiting or diarrhea. Your mouth, throat, esophagus or stomach might be so inflamed that you can neither chew nor swallow. You might also have some obstruction or irritation in the gastrointestinal tract.

These kinds of problems are not unusual after surgery, chemotherapy or radiotherapy. And it is when you have these kinds of problems that the possibility of malnutrition becomes a critical concern. Your body must somehow get enough nutrients.

Enteral Nutrition As long as your stomach and bowel are still working properly, enteral—or tube—feedings can be a practical and low-cost way of providing good nutrition.

Feeding tubes can be placed:
♦ through your mouth (orogastric);
♦ through your nose (nasogastric); or
♦ directly into your stomach through the abdominal wall (gastrostomy) or the small bowel (jejunostomy). This can be done during or after surgery, when the need for high-calorie and high-protein nutrition is most critical. There is also a

new technique called percutaneous gastrostomy that allows a stomach tube to be placed without the need for surgery.

Enteral Formulas Obviously, solid food can't be delivered to your stomach through a tube. So you will need enteral feeding formulas. These can be prepared by pureeing food, or you can buy any of the nutritionally complete formulas your physician or nutritionist might prescribe. Which formula to use depends on your individual situation. There are special formulas for lactose intolerance (lactose-free) and for high-calorie, high-protein intake. Or you may need a low residue and/or chemically defined liquid diet.

♦ Sustacal and Meritene are soy-based lactose-free high residue formulas and are very palatable.

♦ Ensure, Resource, Isocal and Osmolite are lactose-free low residue diets for lactose-intolerant patients.

♦ Vital-HN and Vivonex-TEN are low-residue, lactose-free chemically defined diets with hydrolized protein and crystalline amino acids. These are useful when you have malabsorption problems or an inflammatory disease like gastroenteritis.

Side Effects of Enteral Feeding Though effective in delivering enough nutrition, feedings through nasogastric tubes can produce some side effects.

♦ You may suffer some throat irritation, nausea or vomiting.

♦ Some formulas, including cold or concentrated formulas, may cause diarrhea. The formula may have to be changed to either lactose-free hyperosmotic concentrated solutions or warmer feedings.

♦ Impaction and constipation can occasionally develop, possibly leading to an obstruction in the intestine.

Parenteral Nutrition When neither oral nor enteral nutrition methods are practical, you can still get all the nutrients you need through a process called hyperalimentation. This is also called total parenteral nutrition (TPN). What it means is that you get all the proteins, vitamins, minerals and/or fat you need intravenously through the familiar IV drip. High-calorie (fat) and high-protein fluids can be used simultaneously.

SPECIAL NUTRITIONAL PROBLEMS OF RADIATION PATIENTS

Radiation oncologists try to select the most effective dose of radiation to destroy a tumor while still protecting normal tissues. Nonetheless, there are often acute effects during treatment, mainly on rapidly growing tissues such as the skin, the mucous membranes (mucosa) in the esophagus, the bladder, small intestine and rectum. These tissues usually heal within a few weeks after radiation. There may also be late chronic effects that can result in the formation of scar tissue, ulcerations or damage to an organ.

Depending on which part of the body is irradiated, you may develop special problems that will affect your ability to get enough nutrition. But many of these problems can be prevented or eased by careful planning and treatment. Your close cooperation with your radiation oncologist and dietitian will let you complete your treatment with as few side effects as possible.

Mouth Problems Radiation to the mouth and throat may result in painful sores on membranes (mucositis), dry mouth, dental problems and taste changes or the loss of taste.

♦ *Dental problems* If you are getting radiation to the oral cavity or pharynx, a complete dental evaluation is essential before treatment. Your teeth should be x-rayed and any decayed teeth either repaired or removed. If you have to have a tooth extracted, the site must be completely healed before treatment to avoid late and irreversible bone damage. Radiation treatment should generally not start until about 14 days after any extraction. Your other teeth should be treated daily with a topical fluoride to help prevent cavities.

♦ *Mucositis* Radiation mucositis frequently occurs after radiation to the head and neck. If the membranes lining your mouth and throat are inflamed, you will need a nourishing soft diet. Sharp-edged or salty foods, such as pretzels and potato chips, should be avoided. So should extremely hot or cold foods that may irritate the membranes even more. You should also stop drinking alcoholic beverages and smoking or chewing all forms of tobacco immediately, since they can irritate the mouth and throat.

When you have mucositis, good oral hygiene is crucial. Frequent use of a gentle mouthwash can help reduce discomfort or pain, especially if you use a solution of baking soda and salt dissolved in warm water instead of commercial mouthwashes that might irritate the mucosa.

If the mucositis is severe and interferes with eating or drinking, you can use a topical anesthetic such as viscous Xylocaine, gargling 1 tsp. (5 mL) before meals. A slurry of sucralfate (Carafate)—prepared by dissolving sucralfate in water and sorbitol, which is available at most drug stores—can also coat the oral membranes and soothe any discomfort.

Your radiation oncologist will have to check your mucositis carefully and often to rule out monilia (fungus) infection. These infections can be treated locally or systemically with mycostatin (Nystatin) oral suspension or tablets, ketoconazole (Nizoral) or Difulcan.

♦ *Dry mouth* Xerostomia, or dry mouth, isn't unusual after radiation to the mouth or pharynx, since you can't produce as much saliva after irradiation of the salivary glands. This may be a temporary condition, though if the total dose exceeds 4,000 cGy, you may have some degree of permanent mouth dryness. You can minimize symptoms by using an artificial saliva such as Salivart, moisturizing gels such as Oral Balance and a special dry-mouth toothpaste such as Biotene. It will also help if you increase your intake of fluids, particularly with meals, and if you use creams, gravies and sauces to moisten dry, hard food.

♦ *Loss of taste* Irradiation of the taste buds can make you lose your sense of taste. The decrease in, or the thickening of, saliva from irradiation of the salivary glands can contribute to the problem too. Taste will usually come back within two months after radiation treatment is completed.

Problems in the Esophagus Radiation is frequently delivered to the upper chest (thorax) to treat lung cancer, esophageal cancer and lymphoma. And the esophagus usually has to be within the radiation port. If you get doses over 3,000 cGy in three weeks, the lining of your esophagus may react, causing some pain when you swallow. The reaction will go away gradually. But it is possible that the daily dose can be reduced or your treatment interrupted for a short period to allow rapid healing.

In the meantime, a soft, bland diet, antacids and a topical anesthetic such as a viscous Xylocaine (lidocaine) solution will often minimize the symptoms. A slurry of sucralfate will coat the esophagus and soothe the discomfort as it does in the mouth. If symptoms persist, you may have a candida infection, which can be effectively treated with ketoconazole (Nizoral) or mycostatin (Nystatin).

Problems in the Bowel (Radiation Enteritis) With their rapidly dividing cells, the membranes lining the large and small bowel and the rectum are quite sensitive to even low doses of radiation. So any radiation delivered to the upper abdomen or pelvis can cause an irritation of the bowel known as radiation enteritis.

Only 5 to 15 percent of people treated

with radiation to the abdomen will develop chronic problems, and the severity of the symptoms will depend on several factors—how much of the abdomen or pelvis is irradiated, the daily dose, the total dosage required and the possible use of chemotherapy at the same time. People with a history of abdominal surgery, pelvic inflammatory disease, atherosclerosis, diabetes or hypertension are also more likely to suffer radiation injury.

Symptoms If you are getting radiation to the upper abdomen, you may experience bouts of nausea and vomiting. Pelvic irradiation is more likely to cause irritation in the rectum, frequent bowel movements or watery diarrhea. These disturbances to the intestinal mucosa may change the way your gastrointestinal tract absorbs nutrients from the food you eat. It may become much more difficult to absorb fat, bile salts and vitamin B_{12}, for example.

Your doctor will evaluate the extent of the enteritis by assessing how often you have diarrhea, the character of the stools, whether you have any rectal bleeding and whether your abdomen is enlarged (distended). He or she will also watch for possible dehydration or an electrolyte mineral imbalance in your blood resulting from diarrhea and/or malabsorption.

Managing Enteritis The medical management of radiation enteritis includes dietary changes, medication and, in severe cases, an interruption of radiation treatment. If you are getting abdominal or pelvic radiation you should start on a low-fat, low-fiber, low-residue diet right from the beginning of treatment.

Foods to Avoid

- Whole-grain or high-bran breads and cereals.
- Nuts, seeds, coconut and beans.
- Fried, greasy or fatty foods, which may be hard to digest.
- Fresh and dried fruit and some fruit juices (such as prune juice).
- Raw vegetables.
- Rich pastries.
- Popcorn, potato chips and pretzels.
- Strong spices and herbs.
- Chocolate, coffee, tea and soft drinks containing caffeine.
- Alcohol and tobacco.
- Milk and milk products. Exceptions are buttermilk and yogurt, which are often tolerated because lactose is altered in the presence of lactobacillus. You might be able to tolerate processed cheese, because the lactose has been removed. You may use milkshake supplements such as Ensure, which are lactose-free.

Foods to Enjoy

- Fish, poultry and meat (preferably broiled or roasted).
- Bananas, apple juice, peeled apples, apple and grape juices.
- White bread and toast.
- Macaroni and noodles.
- Baked, boiled or mashed potatoes.
- Cooked vegetables that are mild, such as asparagus tips, green and wax beans, carrots, spinach and squash.
- Mild processed cheese, eggs, smooth peanut butter, buttermilk and yogurt.

Helpful Hints

♦ Eat foods at room temperature.

♦ Drink 12 glasses of fluids per day. Let soft drinks and other carbonated beverages go flat before you drink them. You can help the process along by stirring the drink until the bubbles disappear.

♦ Add nutmeg to food. This will help to increase mobility of the gastrointestinal tract.

♦ Start a low residue diet on Day 1 of radiation therapy.

Medications If radiation enteritis persists despite changes in your diet, it may be necessary to reduce the daily dose of radiation to the abdomen and pelvis. You may also have to use medications such as:

♦ Kaopectate (2 to 4 tablespoons/25 to 50 mL after each loose bowel movement).

♦ Lomotil (one to two tablets every four to six hours as needed to a maximum of eight tablets a day). Most patients find they need only two or three tablets per day after the diarrhea has been controlled.

♦ Imodium (two capsules initially, followed by one capsule after each loose stool, the total dosage not to exceed 16 capsules per day). Imodium is also available in a liquid form (half-dose strength) that does not require a prescription.

♦ Donnatal or Robinul (one or two tablets every four hours for abdominal cramping).

♦ Paregoric (1 tsp./5 mL orally every four hours for diarrhea).

♦ Compazine (10 mg every four hours) or Reglan tablets or liquid (10 mg four times daily, 30 minutes before each meal and at bedtime) can usually control nausea.

19
CONTROLLING PAIN

Ernest H. Rosenbaum, MD, Malin Dollinger, MD, and Elliot Krames, MD

"Pain is an even more terrible lord of mankind than death itself."
— *Albert Schweitzer*

◇

Fear of pain is a big part of the fear of cancer. This is a realistic concern. Between 60 and 90 percent of cancer patients have pain severe enough that they need some kind of medication, including narcotics. For most people, pain is not an early symptom of cancer. But it can create an awful lot of problems as the disease progresses.

Pain can have a terrible effect on the way you live. It can lead to depression, loss of appetite, irritability, anger or an inability to sleep or cope. If it's not controlled, pain can destroy the quality of your life and your will to live.

Fortunately, *pain can be controlled*. What is needed to control it is an understanding of what actually is causing your pain, an assessment of the type of pain you are suffering and a well thought out plan of appropriate therapy. Your doctor and/or a pain specialist are well equipped to handle your pain.

SOURCES OF PAIN

Pain is a complex phenomenon. It has physical causes, certainly. But it has emotional and psychological components too. Even your cultural upbringing and beliefs are factors. Certain cultures—American Indians, for example—teach tolerance of pain. And some individuals from many cultural backgrounds have learned to be stoic. They "bear the pain" without complaining or even expressing their needs. Others have a low threshold of pain tolerance and emphasize their feelings.

How each person responds to pain depends partly on prior experience with pain, partly on religious, cultural and racial background, partly on psychological state and, of course, very much on the extent of disease.

Physical Sources There are two kinds of physical pain. Acute pain is sudden and intense. It can come on strong and fade quickly. Chronic pain can sometimes be just as intense, but it's usually just there in the background. The level rises and falls, but it never seems to go away. It just keeps nagging and throbbing.

For people with cancer, acute pain may be a result of surgery, a broken bone or an obstruction in the intestine or urinary tract. Sometimes, the pain is a side effect of treatment—a sore mouth from chemotherapy, postsurgical pain or skin irritation after radiation.

Chronic pain can have many causes. It may be a direct response to a tumor growing and pressing on nerves or to a tumor obstructing or blocking an internal hollow organ such as the gastrointestinal tract. It could be brought on by a blood vessel obstruction, inflammation, infection, swelling of arms and legs or aches in the joints. It may simply be the cumulative effects of a prolonged illness. But chronic pain rarely results from the cancer therapy except as an unusual result of some chemotherapy medications such as cisplatin or vincristine.

Emotional Sources Pain is made worse by worry and fear—fear of death, suffering, deformity, financial disability or isolation. All these fears can be magnified when a kind of pain in the spirit comes on. This might be triggered by surroundings, the level of emotional support or feelings of loneliness and desperation. At such times pain can feel much worse.

How you approach the problems of life makes a big difference to how you perceive pain. And that makes a big difference to how pain is controlled.

THE TREATMENT PLAN

Treating and controlling pain is a major challenge to any medical team. Every pain control program has to be tailored to the individual and the phase of the disease. Depending on the extent of local disease, pain during the initial phase will be very different than pain during the period of metastases. Pain late in the disease also feels different than the pain early on.

Your doctor will assess your pain before administering therapy. He or she will ask you about the nature of the pain, where it is, how long it lasts and what triggers it. The goal of pain therapy is complete pain relief with total comfort. Sometimes, however, complete pain control cannot be obtained and comfort becomes the major goal. You should talk about this concept early on in your treatment and work out a plan to relieve the fear of pain in case your cancer gets worse.

The Pain Control Ladder The tailoring of pain control follows steps in the pain control ladder.
Step 1. *Non-narcotics* Aspirin, Tylenol (acetaminophen) and non-steroidal anti-inflammatory drugs
Step 2. *Stronger pain relievers* Propoxyphene (Darvon)
Step 3. *Weak narcotics* Codeine, oxycodone (Percocet, Percodan), Vicodan (hydrocodone)

Step 4. *Strong narcotics* Morphine, hydromorphone (Dilaudid), dolophine (Methadone), Demerol and levophanol (Levo-Dromeran)

Simple measures such as aspirin, Tylenol with or without codeine, or ibuprofen may do the job well enough. But when pain is severe, the medication has to be increased. Sometimes only increasing the dosage or taking the medications more often may be all that's necessary. If not, you have to step up the ladder—from non-narcotics to weak narcotics to oral morphine or its derivatives such as Dilaudid or Methadone. Strong narcotics may be given along with non-narcotics such as aspirin or Tylenol to decrease the dose needed to control the pain or to make the effect last longer.

When to Take Your Medications Up to a quarter of cancer patients do not get adequate pain control because the most appropriate methods available are not prescribed. In part, this is because pain medications are often prescribed "as needed." Usually, this means that you get pain medication only when pain becomes more intense or when a pain that had gone away comes back. For optimal pain control, pain medication should be given "by the clock." Some medications can be taken every three to four hours and some long-acting preparations can even be taken every 8 to 12 hours, with appropriate dose increases for adequate control. This is far preferable to using medications only after you start feeling pain. It takes at least 30 minutes for any pain medication to work. Taking the medication by the clock rather than when you feel pain will give you much better pain control.

Side Effects Narcotics often have side effects—constipation, nausea, vomiting, dizziness, low blood pressure, mental confusion and urinary urgency or retention. If you are taking strong narcotics such as morphine, you may feel sleepy or drowsier than normal during the first few days, but this effect tends to wear off. Depending on which side effects occur, the dose may have to be adjusted as part of the pain control plan. Remember that side effects can be controlled too.

MYTHS ABOUT MORPHINE AND CANCER PAIN

A lot of cancer patients want to avoid taking narcotics. In today's society the term has an unsavory ring. But it is very poor practice if you experience a high degree of pain and don't use narcotics when they are necessary and indicated. Patients whose pain is relieved by morphine get more rest and better nutrition. They not only do better in general but they can tolerate cancer therapy better than those living in continual pain.

Even some doctors resist giving morphine. But to withhold strong narcotics from moderately to severely ill cancer patients is a tragedy that can sometimes apply even to earlier stages. Tolerance is not an issue. The dose of narcotics can be as high as needed.

The problem is that there are a great number of myths about morphine, other narcotics and cancer pain.

Myth 1. *People given morphine for pain control are always doing worse or are near death.* Just because a person is placed on morphine does *not* mean that he or she is gravely ill. Morphine is a well-known, highly effective medication that can be used and is used at all stages of the disease.

Myth 2. *All patients getting morphine will become addicts.*

Physical dependence *can* happen with prolonged narcotic use, but physical dependence is not necessarily addiction. The biggest concern is the psychologic need for drugs developing in people using morphine for pain control. But psychologic dependence—addiction—*rarely* if ever develops when narcotics are used for can-

cer pain. If the pain stops, the narcotics can be withdrawn safely and easily.

Myth 3. *Patients who take morphine develop tolerance and always need more and more medicine.*

Someone who needs increased amounts of narcotic painkillers is usually a victim of poor pain control through underdosing. Adequate pain relief can be achieved, often through increased doses. But the dose of morphine may rise to meet a physical need then fall when the cause of the pain is controlled or relieved. Morphine tolerance—the need for a higher dose—does not usually develop rapidly and if it does it often means an increase in disease, not tolerance. Increasing the dose also does not mean that the doctor who prescribes morphine has given up on the patient. What you need to know is that there is no such thing as too much morphine. If you are in more pain you need more drug.

Myth 4. *Morphine is dangerous because it can make breathing harder for a terminally ill patient.*

Morphine in patients with cancer and pain is not a dangerous respiratory depressant. It is usually given in specific doses which are gradually increased as needed.

Myth 5. *People taking morphine always have to get shots since morphine is poorly absorbed by mouth.*

Oral morphine, when used early, can be an excellent means of controlling pain. In fact, oral preparations for long-acting morphine have become very popular, because they reduce the number of times a day the medication has to be taken and administration is much simpler. Higher doses are needed because so much of the medication isn't available to the body for pain control and is wasted. But the pain equivalency between oral morphine and parenteral (intravenous or intramuscular) morphine is known to be 3 to 1. So 10 mg of injected morphine is equivalent to 30 mg of oral morphine.

Using Morphine Morphine can be taken in a variety of ways. All methods control pain very effectively.

♦ Intravenous or direct IV morphine can be used when you are in the hospital.

♦ It is available in pills or oral solution—short-acting (3 to 4 hours) and long-acting (8 to 12 hours).

♦ It is available as a rectal suppository.

♦ It can be given by injection under the skin. You can even easily learn how to give your own shots if no one else is available, just as diabetics give themselves shots of insulin.

♦ It can be given through a portable infusion pump with a small butterfly needle inserted under the skin, or as a slow intravenous infusion (morphine drip).

All these ways of getting morphine into your system are easy. Another method is very useful and may reduce the narcotic dose. Intermittent injections of morphine either around the spinal canal (epidural) or within the spinal canal (intrathecal) can be an effective way of getting proper pain control. The injections have to be given through a catheter or by a continuous infusion pump. The pump might be external, though there are also implantable ones.

The advantage of spinal morphine is that very small doses relieve pain for a long time—often 18 hours or more. Morphine has several times the concentration in the spinal canal than morphine given orally or by injection. Because the small dose goes such a long way, side effects are minimal and quality of life generally improves.

WAYS TO IMPROVE PAIN CONTROL

An effective pain control plan isn't limited to painkilling medications. Many other procedures and techniques can be used to help reach the goal of complete pain relief with total comfort.

Heightening the Effects of Analgesics Nerve pathways run between the site of pain and the spinal cord. Other pathways from the spinal cord relay pain information to the brain. Morphine and other narcotics work to control pain at several levels by blocking pain receptor sites in the spinal cord and the lower and higher brain centers.

Several drugs can reinforce these effects. Antidepressant drugs such as Elavil (amitriptyline), for example, enhance the effect on the pathway from the brain down to the painful area.

Other medications can be helpful in other ways. Non-steroidal anti-inflammatory drugs such as Naprosyn (naproxen) and Motrin (ibuprofen) help by blocking the pain at the original site such as a broken bone or a surgical incision.

Cortisone (prednisone, Decadron) can help relieve pain through an anti-inflammatory action. And medications such as tricyclic antidepressants, corticosteroids and non-steroidal anti-inflammatory drugs given with Tylenol, codeine or morphine can double or triple those analgesics' ability to control pain.

Patient Controlled Analgesia (PCA) This is a helpful device if you are taking morphine or other analgesics intravenously. Whenever pain increases, you simply push a button and another intravenous dose of narcotics—preset by your doctor—is pumped into your system. An automatic system prevents overdose. This can make for much better control of both chronic and acute pain.

Nerve Blocks In extreme cases, neurosurgical and anesthetic techniques might have to be used to control pain. In surgical procedures called cordotomy or rhizotomy, nerve fibers are cut to relieve pain. But nerve-cutting procedures are used only when simpler methods of pain control aren't satisfactory. When the cancer is very advanced, simple nerve blocks—

done by injecting local anesthetics or nerve-killing drugs around the nerve—can completely relieve the pain, making narcotics unnecessary.

Supportive Techniques It is important to look after the emotional and psychological components of pain too. Psychological counseling can help in many ways—finding sources of emotional support, reducing any sense of loneliness and isolation, coming to terms with your situation or planning for the future. Talking with clergy or other trusted spiritual advisers might also reduce anxieties and fears that contribute to your pain.

Basically, anything that helps you relax can help your efforts at pain control. Relaxation exercises, massage, nerve stimulation, acupuncture or acupressure may all be of help.

And, perhaps surprisingly, one very effective pain control device may be as close as your stereo. Music has been rated to have an analgesic effect twice that of a plain background sound. So listen to your favorite musical works and artists. Music can help you relax, raise your spirits, give you great joy *and* help you control your pain.

20
GUARDING AGAINST INFECTIONS

Margaret Poscher, MD, Lawrence Mintz, MD, W. Lawrence Drew, MD, PhD,
Ernest H. Rosenbaum, MD, and Malin Dollinger, MD

◇

Everyone with cancer runs a high risk of catching some sort of infection. This is so because the cancer and the methods used to fight it affect the immune system defenses that normally keep infections at bay.

Our first line of defense against infection is the outer and inner linings of the body—the skin and the mucous membranes. Both these barriers are punctured by the invasive procedures necessary to diagnose or treat cancer problems. Chemotherapy and radiation are particularly damaging to mucous membranes. And the needle in the arm to draw blood for testing, the IV lines, the catheters and pumps all create potential ports of entry for infectious organisms.

Once an infection does get into our bodies, one of the most important defenses—the white blood cell—usually goes into action. But the number of these cells is dramatically reduced by chemotherapy, radiation therapy, leukemia and bone marrow transplants. Low white blood cell counts are common in cancer patients, and as the count decreases the risk of infection increases.

Another defense mechanism is known as cellular immunity, in which specialized white blood cells called T lymphocytes attack invading organisms. But some cancers such as Hodgkin's disease can cause defects in cellular immunity, and so can chemotherapy, radiation and drugs that suppress the immune system.

Another part of the immune defense system is known as humoral immunity. Here other specialized white blood cells called B lymphocytes produce proteins—antibodies—to fight infections. This part of the system can be damaged in cases of multiple myeloma and chronic lymphocytic leukemia or when treatment requires the removal of the spleen.

We all have "resident" bacteria (called normal flora) that are usually harmless but can cause serious infection when our defenses are down. We can try to prevent infections, but nevertheless they do occur.

THE DIFFERENT TYPES OF INFECTIONS

Infections are defined by the type of organism involved and the location in the body. The most common organisms fall into three broad categories.

Bacterial Infections These result from organisms that are usually found in the gut (gastrointestinal tract). In a phenomenon known as sepsis, these organisms find their way into the bloodstream and can "seed" various organs.

Bacteria on the skin can can get into the bloodstream if an IV line is in place, resulting in sepsis or a local infection called cellulitis. A urinary catheter to drain the bladder can sometimes lead to a urinary tract infection. You may also catch pneumonia or some other lung infection from other people, infections that you would be able to fight off if your immune system was working normally.

Once any area of your body is infected with bacteria, the opportunity exists for bacteria to get into the bloodstream, spread and cause sepsis.

Viral Infections When your cellular immunity is decreased, new viruses can take up residence in your body and old viral infections can be reactivated. Cold sores, for example, are caused by the herpes simplex virus. This is a virus that stays with you, although it can have long quiescent periods. When your cellular immunity is damaged, the virus can flare up and give you quite severe cold sores. Another herpes virus—the same one that causes chicken pox—can reactivate and cause shingles that can become widespread and quite severe.

Fungal Infections These usually occur when fungi normally present on the skin take advantage of a depressed immune system. Fungal infections are common when white blood cell counts are profoundly low and IV lines are in place.

SIGNS AND SYMPTOMS

There are several common signs and symptoms of infection. Some might be caused by something other than an infection, but you should consult your doctor as soon as any of them appear.

♦ Fever. This is a very reliable sign of infection and has to be attended to immediately, especially if your white blood cell count is low.

♦ Shaking chills.

♦ Severe night sweats.

♦ Nausea and vomiting, especially if accompanied by fever.

♦ Diarrhea, especially with a fever or with blood in the stool.

♦ Burning or pain when urinating, which could indicate a bladder infection.

♦ Coughing, shortness of breath or chest pain, all of which may be the first signs of pneumonia or bronchitis.

♦ Headache or neck stiffness with fever. This could indicate meningitis, a very serious infection of the nervous system that should be treated immediately.

DIAGNOSIS

Once you notice any of these signs and symptoms, your doctor will start searching for the origin of the infection. He or she will follow the usual steps in the diagnostic procedure, first asking you about your medical history, which may provide some clues about where the infection comes from. Shaking chills and fever are clues that sepsis may be present, which will prompt your doctor to order blood cultures. A cough might indicate pneumonia, which can be confirmed by a chest x-ray. Soreness and pains will lead the search to specific areas of your body.

The physical exam can confirm the leads given by the symptoms and may lead to the discovery of abnormalities you may not be aware of. Your abdomen will be examined for signs of enlargement or tenderness in organs that may be involved with infection. Your skin will be checked for signs of redness or tenderness. Even if there are no symptoms, pneumonia might be detected simply by listening to your chest. A careful neurologic exam will be done and sophisticated tests can be ordered if the exam reveals any abnormalities.

Once the history and physical exam are completed, your blood, sputum and urine will be analyzed. Stools, spinal fluid and skin lesions might be tested too. Depending on the results of the complete blood count and serum chemistry panel, you may undergo other diagnostic studies—x-rays, CT or MRI scans or nuclear medicine studies such as gallium or indium scans.

All the information from the history, exams, tests and studies will be used to plan the most appropriate therapy.

TREATMENT

There is a huge array of antibiotic, antifungal, antiviral and immune modulating therapies available to fight infections. Which to use depends on the organism involved and the site of infection. Someone with multiple myeloma, as well as some other patients, might benefit from the boost to the immune system provided by intravenous immune globulin. Someone with a herpes virus might need an antiviral drug like acyclovir. Someone with a serious fungal infection might be give an antifungal drug like amphotericin B.

In an ideal world, the infecting organism would be identified quickly and the most effective drug against it would immediately be given. But cultures and lab test results may take 24 to 48 hours to get. While the offending organism still isn't known, what is called "empirical" therapy will begin, meaning that broad spectrum drugs will be directed against the most likely culprit. Someone with leukemia, for example, with a fever and a low white blood cell count would be given a combination of broad spectrum antibiotics effective in treating the kinds of bacteria known to infect this type of patient.

Once the organism is identified, treatment can be modified, if necessary. The broad spectrum drugs may be replaced by a specific antibiotic most effective against the bacteria or may be continued if tests show they are likely to be effective. If the fever and low white cell count continue after a week or 10 days of antibiotic therapy, an antifungal drug might be added.

Length of Treatment When to stop antibiotic treatment depends on the situation. If you've had fever and a low white cell count but neither the organism nor the site of infection could be identified, then antibiotics will usually be continued until the fever is gone and your white cell count is returning to normal.

If the site of infection is known—as in pneumonia, for example—and your temperature and white blood cell count is normal, antibiotics will be continued for one to two weeks.

If blood tests have isolated the organism, your fever is gone and the white count is back to normal, antibiotics will usually be stopped five to seven days after the fever disappears.

WHAT YOU CAN DO TO AVOID INFECTIONS

There will be certain times during the course of your illness when you will be more susceptible to infections, particularly when your white blood cell count is at its lowest. This point is called the nadir. Infections are most likely when the nadir is down to 1,000 cells per cubic millimeter or less. You should do everything you can to avoid possible sources of infection at all times. But be especially vigilant when your susceptibility is greatest.

The best single preventive measure you can take against infection is to wash your hands often and well. Also keep the following guidelines in mind:

♦ Stay away from people with colds or the flu.

♦ Avoid intimate contact with people who have open sores such as cold sores or other viral infections.

♦ Avoid enclosed public areas where there is little ventilation, such as airplanes, theaters and shopping malls.

♦ Cut your nails carefully to avoid small nicks.

♦ Shave with an electric razor rather than a blade.

♦ Use gloves for protection when doing physical work that might damage the skin.

♦ Avoid dental work or cleaning if you are taking chemotherapy or if your white cell or platelet counts are low (less than 3,000 WBC or less than 100,000 platelets).

♦ Avoid raw vegetables and fruit that can't be peeled.

♦ Avoid lettuce completely when the white cell count is very low.

♦ Don't eat undercooked meat and poultry.

♦ Avoid constipation, using a stool softener if necessary. The act of straining can cause small tears in the anus and the lining of the intestine. This is dangerous when the white blood cell count is low.

♦ Avoid rectal thermometers and any other manipulation of the anus or rectum.

♦ Don't clean cat litter boxes or bird cages. Avoid all contact with animal stool and urine.

♦ Don't garden. It doesn't make sense to "play in the dirt." For this reason, plants (except plastic or silk ones) are usually kept out of patients' hospital rooms when the white cell count is very low.

21
LIVING WITH AN OSTOMY

Kerry Anne McGinn, RN, BSN, MA

◇

Some of my good friends just happen to have ostomies.

Like Virginia. She's the one stretching her four-foot 10-inch self so that her head shows above the podium for the speech she's giving. After 10 years with a colostomy—10 years of energetic work as an organizer, publicity person and grandmother—she says, "My colostomy's just part of me."

Like Joe. "My urostomy is a positive asset. When we go camping and everyone has a little beer, I'm the only one who doesn't have to get up in the middle of the night to trudge to the Porta-toilet."

Like Carol. She may be hard to find, between her trips to Australia and Finland with her husband, her teaching and her writing contracts. She says, "My ostomy is a minor nuisance. I barely remember it most of the time. Actually, I did have to be a little extra-cautious when I ran the marathon in Helsinki."

These three are a few of the hundreds of thousands of people who have had a passageway constructed through the abdominal wall as an exit for feces or urine. This change becomes necessary if their normal outlet cannot be used because of disease, trauma or birth defect.

Without their ostomy surgeries, none of these people would be alive. With their ostomies, each is happily, comfortably, normally alive.

A FEW DEFINITIONS

There are various kinds of ostomy—the surgical creation of an "opening into"

some organ to connect it with the skin. A tracheostomy can be performed to improve breathing, for example. Most ostomies are performed to allow the elimination of body wastes through the abdominal wall.

"Ostomy" is the word for the total change the surgeon makes. "Ostomate" is one common term for a person who undergoes this change in personal plumbing. The new opening that can be seen on the abdomen is called a stoma.

There are three general categories of these abdominal exit ostomies:

♦ *Colostomy* is the rerouting of the colon, or large intestine. This change may be permanent or temporary.
♦ *Ileostomy* is such a detour in the ileum, the last section of the small intestine.
♦ *Urostomy*, or urinary diversion, covers a number of surgical procedures that redirect urine to the outside of the body when the bladder or another part of the urinary tract has to be bypassed or removed.

COLOSTOMIES

A colostomy is the most common ostomy. Surgeons perform colostomies for colorectal cancer, for other cancers of the abdomen or pelvis that press on or invade the large intestine and for conditions that have nothing to do with cancer.

In this surgical procedure, part of the colon is removed or disconnected and all or part of the rectum may be removed too. The end of the remaining colon is brought to the surface through the skin of the

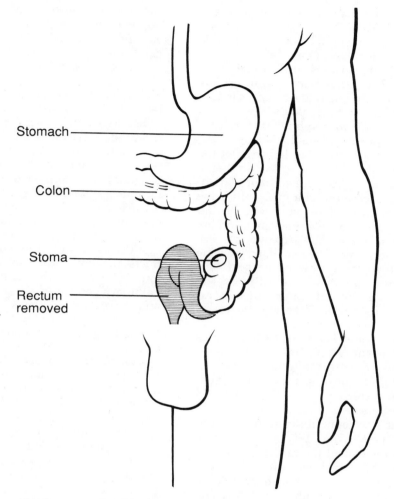

Sigmoid colostomy, after abdominal-perineal resection for rectal cancer.

abdomen, folded back like a turtleneck and stitched in place to form the stoma.

Adjusting to the Ostomy How does your body change when you have a colostomy? What stays the same?

Everything we eat, from apple pie to zucchini, must be broken down into tiny particles and changed to simpler chemical substances that can be absorbed into the bloodstream. The resulting nutrients make their way to cells throughout the body,

providing constant fuel and materials for energy, growth and rebuilding. This complex process of digestion takes place in the long—28 ft. (8 m) or longer in an adult—twisting channel that starts at the mouth and ends at the anus.

By the time food reaches the colon—the last 6 ft. (2 m) of the channel—most of the nourishment has been absorbed. Here the major tasks are absorbing water and some mineral salts in the first portion of the colon, then transporting and storing the

149

indigestible remains of the food in the rest of the colon and the rectum. At the far end is the anus, a ring-like sphincter muscle that opens to release feces.

The body adjusts quite nicely to a shortened digestive tract. If your ostomy occurs near the end of the colon, as it does in many colostomies, you've lost only a storage area and a sphincter to release feces. If your ostomy is higher up in the digestive tract, you may lose part of the ability to absorb water so the discharge will tend to be less formed, more liquid. (This is much more of a problem for the person with an ileostomy, who has no colon and may have a problem absorbing mineral salts also. But ileostomy surgery is rare for cancer.) The remaining intestine eventually takes over some of the water-absorbing function. The kidneys, the major regulators of water and mineral salts, handle the rest of the adjustment.

Temporary and Permanent Colostomies
With new surgical techniques available, surgeons are performing fewer "permanent" colostomies—in which the rectum and anus are removed—than they did several years ago.

But if a cancer occurs near the very end of the digestive tract, this may be the best way to remove all the cancer and save a life. An abdominal-perineal (A-P) resection is the usual surgery, with the surgeon making incisions in both the abdomen and the perineal area around the anus to remove the cancer and construct the colostomy.

Often, a surgeon constructs a "temporary" colostomy, which can sometimes last for years. This operation involves bypassing, but not removing, the rectum and anus. For instance, a surgeon might cut out a colon cancer but want the area to heal without feces passing over it. Or a large tumor that can't be removed causes pain because it's blocking the passage of stool. Using one of several techniques, the surgeon can form a colostomy using the colon

ahead of the affected section, leaving the problem area alone. Stool then can pass out of the body, but through a new exit. Later, the colostomy can be reversed so that stool moves through the anus again.

How the Stoma Functions The stoma that results from a colostomy could be described as a soft valve. Since it is made from the digestive tract that winds from the mouth to the anus, it is the same red-pink color as the mouth, and is lined with essentially the same kind of soft velvety mucous membranes. It stretches to permit waste to be expelled. During inactive periods, the tissue pulls together rather like puckered lips (stoma, in fact, means mouth). Although it expands and contracts, the stoma does not have the firm muscle control of the anal sphincter. So voluntary control of a bowel movement must be replaced by something else.

For many people with colostomies, that "something else" is a pouch (also called an appliance or bag). This is made of thin flexible plastic or rubber, which adheres to the skin over the stoma to hold feces until a convenient time for disposal. These are comfortable, odor-proof and secure.

An alternative for many colostomates with fairly solid stool is "irrigation," a kind of enema through the stoma done every day or two. This permits them to empty the bowel at a convenient regular time. They wear only a tiny pouch or a soft pad over the stoma the rest of the time.

URINARY DIVERSIONS

Urinary diversions or urostomies are often performed for cancer in the urinary tract.

Normally, once the kidneys have filtered wastes out of the blood, they flush excess fluid and wastes as urine through narrow tubes to an expandable storage area—the bladder—and then out of the body. At least some kidney function is essential for life, but any other part of the urinary tract can be removed or bypassed. Because reasons for urostomies vary from birth defects to bladder cancer, the age range of ostomates is wide and many different surgical techniques are used.

Making the Conduit To treat bladder cancer, surgeons may create an ileal conduit (also called an ileal loop or Bricker loop). The surgeon removes the bladder or sometimes just bypasses it. A section a few inches long is cut away from the last part of the small intestine (the ileum), keeping the blood and nerve supply intact. This section is closed at one end, the narrow tubes from the kidney are attached to it and the open end is brought through the abdominal wall to form a stoma.

The remaining ends of the intestine are reconnected and resume their function of moving feces out of the body. If the surgeon prefers to use a section of colon rather than ileum, the ostomy is called a colonic conduit.

The conduit is not an artificial bladder. It doesn't store urine. It is simply a passageway, and urine continues to drip out of the stoma all the time. This means that if you have this kind of urinary ostomy you wear a pouch at all times and drain it into the toilet as needed.

TAKING CARE OF YOUR STOMA

Although the stoma usually shrinks somewhat in diameter as postoperative swelling subsides and you resume your normal diet and exercise, the red-pink color remains.

Unlike an incision, a stoma requires little healing. A urostomy stoma starts to expel urine immediately, even before the new urostomate has left the operating room. Colostomies start discharging feces in a few days, usually with a lot of gas and watery stool until the bowel settles down after surgery.

Stomas come in many shapes and sizes, depending on the kind of ostomy and the person who owns it. Since it is made from

the large intestine, a colostomy will be wider than an ileal conduit urostomy made from the small intestine. Some "temporary" stomas may be quite large and have two openings in one stoma or two stomas near each other. Most stomas should protrude from the skin enough so that feces or urine discharge away from the skin rather than pooling around the stoma.

At first, it's a temptation to feel overprotective about a stoma. You might feel that it is so fragile it might be damaged by a breeze or a bump. While reasonable protection is essential, the stoma is surprisingly tough. It is not harmed by water, by contact during sex or even by gentle bumps against furniture. But it does bleed easily, even from as little cause as an overzealous wipe with a washcloth, because many tiny blood vessels are very close to the surface of the stoma. A pouch or a soft pad will protect it from the friction of clothes.

GETTING SUPPORT

When you have an ostomy you can eat, work and play normally. But there are new skills to learn. Fortunately, there are many resources to help and give you moral support.

♦ An enterostomal therapist (ET nurse) is a registered nurse with special training in the care of ostomies and ostomates. ET nurses work in hospitals or have private practices. With their information and caring, they are a godsend for both new and long-time ostomates.

♦ The United Ostomy Association (UOA) is an organization of more than 50,000 people with ostomies. The association holds local meetings and provides ostomy visitors—volunteers matched for sex, age and type of ostomy—for the new ostomate. Some people come to the meetings for information, some for moral support, some for the social contact. Some people come because they are having problems, others because they have solved problems and are happy to pass on their experience.

Some are desperate, discouraged, depressed. Many of them find answers and all of them find support and a place where they can talk freely about what concerns them. Local chapters of UOA may be listed in the phone book or can be located through the American Cancer Society. The national organization publishes a quarterly journal and holds regional and national conferences.

Keeping a Positive Attitude Hearing that you have cancer and need an ostomy is a double jolt for anyone. It takes time, information and support to adjust. But it's not the end. Definitely not.

I'll never forget Roger. A year before I met him, the doctor in his small town had diagnosed rectal cancer and had recommended colostomy surgery. "No way," stormed Roger. "You're not going to see me with one of those awful bags."

Despite his doctor's urging, Roger refused surgery. He underwent radiation and chemotherapy, but the tumor spread. When Roger came to our big-city hospital and, by some administrative quirk, to my orthopedics floor, he was deathly ill. But he was still adamantly opposed to "those damned bags."

I was scarcely an ostomy expert at the time, but I knew someone with a colostomy—my mother. So I knew people could be happy with a colostomy, bleak as Roger's chances seemed to be. So Roger and I talked. Just quiet talk. I passed on what information I had and my own confidence that ostomy surgery might make him feel much better. Meanwhile, his bowel became totally blocked, his pain became agonizing and his temperature soared. The bowel had burst and infection had set in. Too ill to protest much, Roger agreed to surgery. The doctors did minimal surgery, creating a "temporary" colostomy so that stool would no longer spill into his abdomen.

To our astonishment, Roger survived both the surgery and a very rocky postoperative course. As he grew stronger, we started teaching him about caring for his ostomy, created in haste and none too neat. Remembering my mother's experiences with the United Ostomy Association, I asked the doctor's permission to call UOA for an ostomy visitor to see Roger, a real boost indeed. Eventually, still with his "temporary" colostomy, Roger was well enough to go home to his hometown hundreds of miles away, where we alerted the UOA chapter to expect him.

After he left, I wondered how he was, what had happened to him, whether he was still alive. His chief pleasure at home, besides his family, had been riding his horse, but I rather doubted that he'd ever be able to do that again.

Nine months later he returned to our hospital and was again admitted to our floor.

"Roger! What's the matter?"

"You'll never believe it, Kerry," he said, with a fine combination of sheepishness and pride. "I was at the rodeo."

"Hey, that's great! You've been getting out of the house some. Have you been able to ride at all?"

"Sure, that's what I was doing, roping cattle at the rodeo."

I took a deep breath. "But Roger, what about your colostomy?"

"No problem. The pouches you gave me stick on fine. You know, I just wish I'd known back then how easy a colostomy is. If only I'd known."

"Why are you here?"

"Well. . . I took a tumble from the horse and broke my ankle."

22
THE "LOOK GOOD. . . FEEL BETTER" COSMETIC PROGRAM

The Cosmetic, Toiletry, and Fragrance Association Foundation

Just about anyone's quality of life is seriously diminished during cancer treatment. Fatigue and changes in daily routine, in physical appearance, personal emotions and reactions from family, friends and colleagues can all weigh heavily on cancer patients.

If you are a woman getting cancer treatment, you may find that physical changes are especially hard to bear. Your personal appearance directly affects your self-image and your psychological well-being. And if you are experiencing some of the common side effects of radiation or chemotherapy, you may start to believe that you're in worse medical shape than you really are. The face you see in the mirror each morning is a harsh reminder of your disease. Every day you can't escape your loss of hair, eyelashes and eyebrows or the changes in your skin tone and texture.

Looking in that mirror, you may start thinking that you couldn't possibly lead a "normal" life. But in today's world, leading a normal life—with all the family relationships, work and social demands normal life involves—is essential while you are getting cancer treatments. What you need to get back to a good quality of life is help to overcome the changes in appearance that cancer treatments bring.

Fortunately, a program has recently been developed in the United States to help you do just that. Look Good. . . Feel Better© is the name of a free national public service program designed to teach women with cancer—through practical hands-on experience—the beauty techniques that help restore their appearance during chemotherapy and radiation treatments.

So while your medical treatment helps heal the inside of your body, the Look Good. . . Feel Better program helps you renew your self-esteem by enhancing your "outside" appearance. It encourages you to pay attention to yourself during a time of dramatic physical changes.

HOW THE "LOOK GOOD. . . FEEL BETTER" PROGRAM WORKS

Until recently, the kind of service offered by the program was largely unavailable. Then, three national organizations pooled their resources to develop the service and make it available to women across the country. The program was founded and developed by The Cosmetic, Toiletry, and Fragrance Association (CTFA) Foundation —a charitable organization supported by the members of the cosmetic industry's trade association—in partnership with the American Cancer Society (ACS) and the National Cosmetology Association (NCA). The NCA is a national organization that represents hairstylists, wig experts, estheticians, makeup artists and nail technicians, among others.

These three organizations provide:
♦ Patient education—through group or individual sessions—by volunteer cosmetologists and beauty advisers.

◆Complimentary makeup kits for everyone participating in a group program. (Look Good. . . Feel Better is "product neutral" and does not promote any specific cosmetic product line or manufacturer.)

◆Free program materials such as videos and patient information pamphlets.

The Look Good. . . Feel Better program is administered nationwide by the ACS and is designed to meet the needs of local communities. The NCA organizes volunteer cosmetologists who can evaluate your skin and hair needs and who will teach you the appropriate beauty techniques to deal with the appearance-related side effects of cancer treatments. The CTFA Foundation provides the makeup, materials and financial support for the program.

All volunteers for Look Good. . . Feel Better are trained and certified for participation by the ACS and the NCA at local, statewide and national workshops. The purpose of this training is not only to discuss important hygienic guidelines and helpful cosmetic tips, but also to promote sensitivity and understanding about what a cancer patient goes through during treatment. This is a necessary step for each volunteer.

Group Sessions Each group session usually consists of eight to ten women led through a one-and-a-half to two-hour program by beauty professionals. Through practical hands-on experience, the women learn a 12-step makeup program and are shown beauty tips about hair, wigs, turbans and scarves. To ensure that every participant gets the same working tools, each woman in a group program receives a complimentary bag of makeup containing 12 items, which match the 12-step program.

THE TWELVE-STEP MAKEUP PROGRAM

1. Cleanser	7. Eyeliner
2. Moisturizer	8. Eyeshadow
3. Concealer	9. Eyebrows
4. Foundation	10. Mascara
5. Powder	11. Lipliner
6. Blush	12. Lipstick

Look Good. . . Feel Better group programs are located in comprehensive cancer centers, hospitals, ACS offices, and community centers.

Personal Consultation A free one-time consultation in a participating salon may also be available, depending where you live. A list of all salons willing to provide this service has been compiled by the NCA and has been distributed to all ACS divisions as well as to a toll-free number you can call for information.

Program Materials There are several materials available free of charge from the ACS. These include the patient pamphlet, a 14-minute inspirational video and a 33-minute video, which includes a detailed demonstration of the 12-step program.

HOW AND WHERE TO FIND PROGRAMS IN YOUR COMMUNITY

Many doctors, nurses, social workers and other medical professionals recognize how important outward appearance is to their patients. And with their help, Look Good. . . Feel Better is now reaching out to tens of thousands of women across the United States.

The growth of the program has been remarkably rapid and widespread. Two pilot programs were successfully operated at the Memorial Sloan-Kettering Cancer Center in New York City and the Vincent T. Lombardi Cancer Research Center at Georgetown University Hospital in Washington, DC, in the fall of 1988. By March 1989, the program was off and run-ning. Since then, Look Good. . . Feel Better has been developed in 40 states and con-tinues to expand. In 1990 group programs served more than 20,000 women with can-cer. And plans are being considered to expand the program to include adoles-cents and men.

To find out if your state has programs or participating salons, call your state or local American Cancer Society office.

To learn about Lood Good. . . Feel Better, call the toll-free number 1-800-395-LOOK.

23
BECOMING SEXUALLY ACTIVE AGAIN

*David G. Bullard, PhD, Ernest H. Rosenbaum, MD, Malin Dollinger, MD,
Jean M. Stoklosa, RN, MS, and Isadora R. Rosenbaum, MA*

Cancer affects all aspects of your life. So it's not surprising that it can affect your sexual feelings and the ways you express those feelings. But you and your spouse or partner remain sexual beings. You have much the same needs and desires as you had before the illness struck.

Sexuality can be expressed in many ways—in how we dress and how we move and speak, as well as by kissing, touching, masturbation and intercourse. Changes in body image, tolerance for activity and anxieties about survival, family or finances can strain the expression of sexuality and can create concerns about sexual desirability. But if you were comfortable with and enjoyed your sexuality before your illness, the chances are excellent that you will be able to keep or regain a good sexual self-image despite any changes brought about by cancer.

Many people, healthy or dealing with an illness, find that being sexually active is not important to them. This can be a healthy, normal choice for any individual or couple. But if sexual intimacy has been a comfort to you, you may want to continue being sexually active once your cancer has been diagnosed and treated.

This may require some adaptation of your normal sexual patterns, and it might be a challenge to change them. Support groups with the right orientation can give understanding and encouragement, and open, comfortable communication with your partner is essential. You may also need specific information and guidance from your doctor. But the subject of sexual health for people with chronic illnesses—especially cancer—has been neglected for far too long. Members of your medical team may find it hard to initiate discussions about sexual problems. But don't make the mistake of trying to be a "good" patient by not complaining and simply suffering in silence. Sexuality is a legitimate area of concern. Take the initiative and ask your doctor any questions you have about your sexuality. You can overcome many problems, reduce tensions and get much more sexual satisfaction.

THE PHASES OF SEXUALITY

Understanding the phases of sexuality and how cancer can affect one or more of them can help you increase your satisfaction with sex.

♦ *Desire* This varies from person to person, ranging from an uninterested, indifferent attitude to a very active desire for sex. Desire can often be increased by physical, visual or fantasy stimulation.

♦ *Excitement* The body reacts to stimulation with increased blood flow in the sex organs and increased heart rate and blood pressure. Sexual interest and stimulation are characterized by an erection in men and increased vaginal lubrication in women.

Sexual problems often occur during the excitement phase. This can lead to considerable anxiety and distress. Men may lose the ability to get or keep an erection. Women may not have enough vaginal lubrication for comfortable penetration, making intercourse difficult or painful.

♦ *Orgasm* This is a peak of pleasurable expression followed by a gratifying relaxation. It is both a physical release and an emotional high.

When there are sexual problems, a man might ejaculate only after prolonged stimulation. Sometimes nothing happens despite prolonged effort. Or the ejaculate might be reversed into the bladder (retrograde) rather than going forward and out the penis. Orgasm still occurs, but there is no semen or liquid.

For women, the painful intercourse (dyspareunia) that sometimes follows cancer treatment can affect orgasm by inhibiting nerves and emotions.

♦ *Resolution* Following orgasm there is relaxation and satisfaction. When there are problems in the excitement or orgasm-phases, the satisfying resolution is often replaced by sexual tension, discomfort in the pelvis, pelvic blood congestion or other problems.

THE SEXUAL PROBLEMS OF SPECIFIC CANCERS

Treatment for some cancers may have little effect on sexuality beyond the effects of fatigue, pain, weakness or other temporary side effects. Younger men who receive extensive chemotherapy, however, might consider sperm banking before treatment in case the sperm count does not return to normal. But the treatment of several kinds of cancer may directly affect how well you function sexually.

Bladder Cancer Surgical therapy for bladder cancer can lead to decreased desire, a reduced ability for men to get an erection, retrograde ejaculation and orgasm prob-

lems including a lower intensity. About half the women who have this therapy end up with a shorter and narrower vagina, making penetration more difficult. Communication with her partner will become especially important, as will the use of lubricants such as K-Y jelly or Crème de la Femme.

Breast Cancer Psychological counseling is helpful for all women with of breast cancer given the symbolic sexual significance of the female breast. Even 10 percent of women who have a *benign* biopsy have some sexual problems. And 30 to 40 percent of women who have a modified radical mastectomy experience sexual dysfunction. Fewer sexual problems are reported if a lumpectomy is done, which results in less change to body image.

Colon Cancer There is twice the amount of sexual dysfunction after surgery for colon cancer than there is after surgery for benign causes such as an ilieostomy for ulcerative colitis. People with ostomies may have increased sexual problems because of embarrassment or worry about their partner's reaction.

Gynecological Tumors A woman having gynecological surgery may have a premature loss of estrogen. This in effect is a premature menopause with hot flashes, mood swings, sleeping problems, anxiety and depression. Sexual partners often have a hard time coping with these changes. All this can reduce a couple's ability to have sex or their inclination to even think about it. With the feelings of abandonment and rejection that often follow, the relationship can definitely suffer. But the right kind of help and counseling can help the couple cope with these problems.

Hysterectomies and radiation treatment to the female genitals may lead to problems in the excitement phase. The surgery might also affect orgasms, and painful intercourse can result from radiation. The frequency of intercourse might be reduced. Women who have had hysterectomies for benign disease have similar problems—a decrease in sexual desire especially in the first six months after the operation, with desire usually returning to normal after a year.

Radical surgery to the vagina and vulva can so change the physical aspects of the genitalia that sexual activity can become very difficult both physically and psychologically because of the fear of pain or bleeding during intercourse. Plastic surgery to reconstruct the organs, along with sex counseling, can be very helpful.

Hodgkin's Disease About 20 percent of men and women with this type of cancer lose energy and interest in sex. Hodgkin's disease doesn't usually affect the ability to get an erection, but problems with ovaries may lead to painful intercourse for women. Marital problems are fairly common too, partly because of lengthy treatments and impaired fertility.

Cancer of the Penis and Testicles Men who lose part of their penis may still be capable of getting erections, having orgasms and ejaculating. Removal of the whole penis naturally causes very severe sexual difficulties. But orgasms may still be possible with stimulation of the bones, pubis, perineum and scrotum and ejaculation through a urethrostomy.

With testis cancer, the sexual problems depend on the type of tumor. With non-seminoma, removal of a testicle and the lymph nodes in the area usually result in a decrease in fertility and sexual activity. Some men with seminoma who have had a testicle removed plus radiation therapy report low or no sexual activity, decreased desire, problems with erections and orgasms, and decreased volume of semen.

Prostate The diagnostic biopsy might result in less seminal fluid in the ejacula-

tion. Surgical removal of the prostate can cause similar problems and, with hormonal therapy, the ability to get an erection and ejaculate may be lost altogether.

Radiation produces problems too, but only half as many as the surgical approach. When the pelvic lymph nodes are removed and a radiation implant is used for localized tumors, 15 to 25 percent of men have erection problems and about 30 percent have a retrograde ejaculation. New surgical approaches may help reduce erection and ejaculation problems.

Drugs That Affect Sexual Activity Most cancers occur in people over 50, many of whom are usually already experiencing some decrease in sexual activity. This decrease can be accelerated by the very fact of having cancer and by the drugs that are often taken for other diseases such as high blood pressure, diabetes, alcoholism or psychological problems. A great many drugs can affect sexual activity and can lead to sexual dysfunction:

♦ anticancer drugs and hormones
♦ antihypertensive drugs, including beta blockers
♦ pain medications
♦ antidepressants
♦ sleeping medications
♦ codeine or other narcotics
♦ psychedelic and hallucinogenic drugs

EXPRESSING YOURSELF SEXUALLY AFTER TREATMENT

With all the possible effects of cancer treatment, the prospect of having a normal sex life may seem out of reach. But whatever your cancer, there are steps you can take that will help you increase your sexual enjoyment.

If You've Had an Ostomy People with ostomies and their partners have to learn about ostomy appearance, care and control, paying attention to such seemingly small details as special undergarments for women that cover a pouch while still permitting sexual stimulation. Specially designed and esthetically attractive pouches are available.

If You've Had a Laryngectomy Laryngectomy patients should be acquainted with how to deal with sounds and odors escaping from their stomas. Wearing a stoma shield or T-shirt will muffle the sound of breathing and will minimize your partner's feeling the air that is pushed through the stoma.

If You've Had a Mastectomy After a mastectomy, you may be worried about how you look. Undressing in front of your partner or sleeping in the nude may feel awkward and uncomfortable. That's natural, especially in light of the overemphasis our culture places on the sexual significance of breasts. Grieving over what you have lost is important. But with time and patience, most women overcome their self-consciousness and feel secure and comfortable with their bodies again.

♦ Some women have found it helpful to explore and touch their bodies, including the area of the scar, while nude in front of a mirror. You may want to try this alone at first and then with a spouse, lover or close friend. Share your feelings about your new body.

♦ Be aware that your partner may not know what to say. Your spouse or lover may not know how or when to bring up the topic of sexuality and so wait for you to do it. Your partner may be afraid of hurting or embarrassing you and want to protect your feelings. Sometimes this "protection" may feel like rejection. Although you might feel that it's risky to break the ice and approach the topic yourself, most people feel relieved once they've done it.

♦ You both may also worry about pain. If your incision or muscles are tender, minimize the pressure on your chest area. If you lie on your unaffected side,

you can have more control over your movements and reduce any irritation to the incision.

♦ If you feel any pain, stop. And let your partner know why you are stopping. If he knows that you'll tell him what is painful, he will feel more relaxed and will be less inhibited in exploring and experimenting with you. Taking a rest or changing position may help you relax, and relaxing will usually decrease any pain. With communication and cooperation, you can work together to find positions and activities that give you the most pleasure.

♦ Experimentation and time seem to be the keys to finding satisfactory ways of adapting to the loss of such a symbolically important part of the body as the breast. Talking with other women who have had mastectomies—women from the American Cancer Society's Reach to Recovery program, for example—can provide support and encouragement as well as suggestions about clothes and prostheses.

♦ Some women find breast reconstruction important for their emotional well-being.

If You've Had Treatment to the Genitals or Reproductive Organs Even the prospect of surgery or radiation treatments for these cancers can make you intensely concerned about your body image. But it is usually impossible to predict the effects of treatment for any one person. Treatment can affect some people's ability to get erections, ejaculate or have intercourse. The same treatment for someone else might result in little or no change in sexual functioning.

Anxiety Sexual problems that seem to be the physical results of treatment may actually be due to anxiety. You can reduce your worry by discussing potential problems and possible solutions with your doctor or other members of the health care team *before* treatment. This discussion will

159

also reassure you that if problems do come up there are ways of handling them. Since in most situations there is no completely reliable way to sort out the physical from the emotional causes of sexual problems, your exploration and experimentation about what you can do is very important. Your diagnosis does not dictate what is possible for you sexually.

Painful Intercourse If you find that intercourse is painful after treatment for genital cancer, have a gynecological examination to find the cause. The problem may be related to surgery, radiation or chemotherapy. Then again, it may result from a simple problem like an infection.

♦ If the cause is not enough lubrication, natural lubrication such as saliva or products such as water-soluble lubricants or baby oil can reduce friction. Artificial lubricants such as K-Y jelly, Jergen's Lotion and other creams may make coitus possible where the lack of circulating estrogens has caused dryness. A new way to get adequate lubrication for sexual arousal and intercourse is Replens, a vaginal gel applied three times a week. In some cases, small amounts (one-third to one-half a tube) of a poorly absorbed estrogen like Dienestrol may help restore lubrication and atrophy of the vagina. But if breast cancer has been diagnosed, any use of estrogens is usually unwise.

♦ Surgery or radiation therapy can cause shortening of the vagina or make the vagina less elastic. Either situation may make intercourse difficult. Your doctor may recommend dilators to exercise and stretch the vagina. Getting back to intercourse soon after treatment can also help prevent these problems. Different positions during intercourse, especially sitting or lying on top of your partner, may let you move in pleasurable ways.

Communication Again, the most important thing to remember is to stop when you first feel pain. And tell your partner

ahead of time that you will let him know immediately about any pain. Stopping to rest, slowing your movements, breathing deeply and sharing your feelings will help you relax. By exploring together, you and your partner will eventually discover the kinds of sexual activity that suit you best.

If You Have Trouble Reaching Orgasm
The natural interruption in the ability to experience sexual pleasure after an illness may make having orgasms more difficult for some women. If this is a problem for you, learning to re-explore pleasurable body sensations may be helpful.

It is important to do this when you can be alone and not distracted by having to please or perform for your partner. So find a comfortable place where you can be alone—your bedroom or bathroom—and a time when you won't be interrupted. Undress slowly and gently stroke your whole body. Then focus on the most sensitive areas—your neck, breasts, thighs, genitals or any other area that feels good to you.

Use different kinds of touch, soft and light, firm and strong. Try moistening your hands with oil, lotion or soap. Pay attention to the sensations you feel and discover which ones are most pleasurable. Learning which kinds of touch feel best will help you heighten your sensation and will give you information to share with your partner.

If You're Having Trouble with Erections
Since some drugs can temporarily interfere with the ability to have erections, you may want to ask your physician about possible side effects of your treatment.

Physical and Emotional Causes If you can get an erection by masturbating or you wake up with an erection in the night or morning, it is most likely that anxiety or "trying too hard" is the cause, and it's not a physical problem. If you are not sure of the cause, ask your doctor to refer you to a urologist or sex therapist for evaluation and treatment.

Taking the Pressure Off The more options you have for sexual expression, the less pressure there is on having erections. This in turn makes it more likely that they will happen. Many couples report that they have learned to have very pleasurable sexual experiences without erections or intercourse. Many kinds of sexual expression and stimulation do not require an erect penis. It may be reassuring to know that to have an orgasm many women need or prefer direct stimulation by hand or mouth on or around the clitoris. This is stimulation that even an erect penis in a vagina can't provide.

If you explore other kinds of sexual touching and expression for a while, you may discover that erections will return with time or that the increased variety of sexual options satisfies both you and your partner. Patience, communication and time are critical factors in developing pleasurable sexual experiences.

Counseling If erections don't come back and intercourse is important to you and your partner, ask your doctor to refer you to a sex therapist for counseling. Counseling will help you with relaxation techniques, with planning time for proper stimulation and with methods for using visual stimulation and fantasy. Group counseling with cancer survivors who have had the same problem can also help.

If you are still not getting erections, the counselor may refer you to a urologist. Together with you and your counselor, the urologist can assess whether a penile implant would suit your needs.

GENERAL GUIDELINES FOR RESUMING SEXUAL ACTIVITY

Whenever you are sick, your usual sense of control over your body may be lost.

You may feel inadequate and helpless. An illness can change the way you experience your body or it might actually change the way you look because of surgery, amputation, scarring, or weight loss.

These changes can create painful anxiety. You wonder whether you'll be able to function in your usual social, sexual and career roles. You wonder what people will think of you. This anxiety—and the depression and fatigue that often go along with it—understandably make sexuality seem less important. But once the immediate crisis has passed, sexual feelings and how to express them may become important again.

Feeling anxious about resuming sexual activity is normal and natural. It is easy to "get out of practice." You may have questions about whether sexual activity will hurt you in some way. You may wonder how you will be able to experience sexual pleasure and your partner may share the same worries. He or she may be especially concerned about tiring you out or hurting you somehow.

But once you resume sexual relations, your comfort and confidence should gradually increase. If not, sexual counseling may help you discover ways to deal with whatever problems you are having. For many people, a "new start"—by themselves or through counseling—is refreshing. It might even create opportunities for greater intimacy and sharing than ever before.

What to Do When You Are in the Hospital Your cancer treatment might involve long stays in the hospital and long separations from those you love. Hospitals or convalescent facilities don't usually provide much privacy, so there may be little opportunity for sexual expression unless you speak up.

Although health care facilities are rarely designed to ensure patients' privacy, there is no reason why you and your partner can't have time for intimate physical contact in the hospital. With a little friendly intervention doctors might be able to arrange for a special room where you and a loved one can spend some time alone. Or you can always make a sign reading "Do Not Disturb Until ___ o'clock" or "Please knock" and hang it on the door to your room. The nurses will respect your wishes.

If this sounds important to you, ask your doctor to speak to the hospital staff and help foster a caring and respectful attitude toward your need to express your sexuality with guaranteed privacy. It takes some education and maybe a change in the "way things are always done around here," but it's well worth the effort.

Developing Helpful Attitudes and Practices Whenever you are ready to become sexually active again, there are a few things you should keep in mind.

♦ *You are loved for who you are, not just for your appearance.* If you were considered lovable or sexually desirable before you got cancer, chances are that you will be afterward too. Your partner, your family and your friends will still love you and value you, as long as you let them.

♦ *We are all sexual beings.* Whether we are sexually active or not, sexuality is part of who we are. It is not defined just by what we do or how often we do it.

♦ *Survival overshadows sexuality.* If you've lost your good health, it is normal and natural for stress, depression, worry and fatigue to lower your interest in sex. Just coping with basic everyday decisions can seem like a burden. But take one day at a time and be patient. Sexual interest and feelings will probably come back when the immediate crisis has passed.

♦ *Share your feelings.* Making relationships work is a task we all face, but it can be made more difficult by worries about our worth and attractiveness. Whether you are looking for a new relationship or already have a regular partner, you may find yourself in the position of having to share your sexual feelings with someone, perhaps for the first time.

This sharing may feel awkward at first. Learning how and when to talk about sexual issues may not come easily. You may feel shy or nervous about exploring new and different ways of finding sexual pleasure. You may wait for your partner to make the first move while your partner is waiting for you to make the advances. This familiar waiting game is often misunderstood as rejection by both people. It may be frightening to think of breaking the silence yourself. Yet a good move is to make the first move. Try sharing some of the myths or expectations you grew up with about sexuality. Often this is humorous and may break the ice in starting a frank discussion about your sexual needs and concerns. Try not to make broad, generalized statements. Talk about what is important to *you* and about how *you* feel. The payoff is greater understanding of each other's needs and concerns, and that is worth the effort.

♦ *Expect the unexpected.* The first time you have sex after treatment, physical limitations or fears about your performance, appearance or rejection may keep you from focusing on the sheer pleasure of physical contact. On the other hand, you may be surprised by unfamiliar pleasurable sensations. If you expect some changes as part of the natural recovery process, they will be less likely to distract you from sexual pleasure if they do happen.

♦ *Give yourself time.* You and your partner may be frightened of, or even repulsed by, scars, unfamiliar appliances or other physical changes. That's natural too. But such feelings are usually temporary. Talking about them is often the first step to mutual support and acceptance. Don't pressure yourself about having to "work on sex." A satisfactory and enjoyable sex life will happen one step at a time. You may want to spend some time by yourself exploring your body, becoming familiar with changes and rediscovering your unique body texture and sensations. Once you feel relaxed doing this, move on to mutual body exploration with a partner.

♦ *Take the pressure off intercourse.* Almost all of us were brought up to believe that intercourse is the only real or appropriate way of expressing ourselves sexually. Yet sexual expression can encompass many forms of touching and pleasuring that are satisfying psychologically and physically.

When you resume sexual activity, try spending some time in pleasurable activities—touching, fondling, kissing and being close—without having intercourse. Re-experience the pleasure of playing, of holding and of being held without having to worry about erections and orgasms. When you feel comfortable, proceed at your own pace to other ways of being sexual, including intercourse if you like.

Experiment and explore to discover what feels best and what is acceptable. If radiation therapy, for example, has made intercourse painful, try oral or manual stimulation to orgasm, or intercourse between thighs or breasts. If you are exhausted by the disease or movement is painful, just cuddling or lying quietly next to your partner might be a satisfying form of intimacy.

♦ *Don't let your diagnosis dictate what you can do sexually.* Your sexuality cannot be "diagnosed." You will never know what pleasures you are capable of experiencing if you don't explore. Try new positions, new touches and above all new attitudes. Your brain is your best and most important sex organ. And its ability to experience sensation is virtually limitless.

♦ *Plan sex around your changing energy levels.* Life with cancer can be exhausting.

Fatigue, depression and just feeling sick are almost normal for cancer patients at certain times. The amount of energy you have for all kinds of activities, including sex, can vary from day to day or week to week. So plan sexual activities to coincide with the times when you think you will feel best.

♦ *Ask for help if you need it.* Don't hesitate to seek counseling or information if you have problems. Help is available from a wide range of sources. If you want to discuss any problems, bring them up with your health care providers. Ask them to recommend competent sex counselors or therapists in your area. There may also be other resources available nearby, such as people who have had both cancer and experience in talking about sexual concerns.

♦ *Be patient.* The important thing is to be patient, with both yourself and your partner. You won't adjust overnight. Give yourself time to explore and share your feelings about your body changes and time to again see yourself as a desirable sexual being. When *you* can accept the way your body looks and recognize your potential for sexual pleasure, it will be easier to imagine someone else doing the same.

The satisfaction and good feelings—emotional and physical—that can come from a sexual relationship require patience, communication, respect, cooperation and a willingness to remember that in some respects the relationship must be learned all over again, physically if not emotionally.

Everything may not work properly at first. Everything may not be enjoyable at first. But have the courage and confidence to keep trying.

24
STAYING PHYSICALLY FIT

Ernest H. Rosenbaum, MD, and Malin Dollinger, MD

If you were involved with an exercise program before you became ill, you will probably be open to the idea of getting involved in an active program all through your recovery. But if you have never been involved in an organized exercise routine you may need some encouragement. Welcome this encouragement if you get it. If you don't get it, seek it out, because getting and staying physically fit should be one of your most important goals.

WHY YOU SHOULD EXERCISE

Physical fitness is healthy for everyone, of course. But it is essential for all cancer patients. Even though it's hard to find the energy to exercise when you are sick, the benefits of keeping your body in an active state are too great to ignore. When you participate in a daily exercise program:

1. You will improve your prognosis If you are in good physical condition, you may tolerate therapy better. This, in turn, may allow you to have more aggressive treatments and so stand a better chance of remission or cure. It is well known that successful treatment and an improved prognosis depend directly on physical status. The simple truth is that if you are physically fit, you may live longer and enjoy a more active life.

2. You will stop your muscles from wasting away When we are healthy, we all usually exercise our muscles one way or

another—by walking up and down stairs, doing housework, going shopping, taking part in athletic activities like golf and tennis or simply by walking as we go about our business. Even a low level of activity helps to maintain muscle tone and strength. But during an acute or chronic illness, prolonged bedrest is often necessary. Muscles shrink in size and strength when they're not used for a long time. An exercise program will make sure that doesn't happen to you.

3. You will recover faster If you do not exercise after surgery or while you're undergoing radiotherapy or chemotherapy, your muscles will get weaker and weaker. The tissues that may be broken down by therapy will not be repaired as quickly as they should be. By exercising, you can help your tissues rebound and you can minimize any deterioration in your joints. You might also help prevent complications such as bone softening, blood clots and bedsores. And, not least, you'll get some relief from the boredom and depression that often come with being confined to bed.

WHEN TO START

Become physically active as soon as possible after treatment. It is now the general practice within one day of surgery to get out of bed and at least sit in a chair. Even this minimal activity helps reduce the loss of muscle mass and increase strength.

True, pain can limit physical exercise

after a mastectomy, bowel surgery or some other major operation. And you may be depressed by a change in your body image and not feel like doing anything. You may need help to get going. But with appropriate timing, you should turn your attention to rehabilitation.

In the Hospital At least a gentle exercise program should begin while you are still in the hospital. This may involve simple muscle tightening while you lie in bed or passive muscle exercises. As your strength returns, different forms of physical activity—isometric and isotonic exercises and rhythmic repeated movements for various muscles—will help get you on the path to improved fitness. Massage therapy can complement these activities, helping you relax your mind and body and improving your circulation.

You might think all this will involve too much of an effort while you're still in the hospital. But you will feel much more confident when you do go home if you have already started to regain your strength. You will also be less prone to falls or other accidents that might result from a weakened condition.

PLANNING A PROGRAM

Before you leave the hospital, physical therapists can assess your physical condition and come up with an appropriate set of exercises. Everyone has different wants and needs, so programs are usually customized. They will also be flexible, taking your energy level into account. The staff of the Physical Therapy Department can also instruct you, your family and other caregivers on how to proceed with your program at home. Their recommendations on an appropriate program may be essential to your recovery.

Safety Rules When you begin exercising, keep in mind a few simple rules for safety:
♦ Ask your doctor if you're ready to exer-

cise. Let him or her set limits to your activity.
♦ Have someone join you. This will make the exercise more enjoyable and safer, especially when you are just getting out of bed and may feel dizzy.
♦ Stop and rest if you feel tired or if your muscles are sore.
♦ Leave out any exercises that seem too difficult and try them another day when you feel stronger.
♦ Try to repeat each exercise three to five times at first, then gradually increase the repetitions to ten or twenty.
♦ Try to exercise at least twice a day, more often if you feel up to it.

The most important rule is to start out gradually. Don't overdo it. Muscles that haven't been used for days or weeks will strain very easily. Light warmup exercises several times a day will be useful, both as a starting point for your program and as a daily prelude to more vigorous exercises later on.

When you start your exercise program, you might experience some fatigue, dizziness or even nausea. Discuss any problems with your doctor or physical therapist. But these side effects usually pass fairly quickly.

Working Through the Stages A graduated program may take you through three stages:
♦ *Stage 1—Beginning to Move Exercises.* These are simple exercises that help you maintain and increase your range of motion. They don't require much exertion and can be done while you are lying in bed.
♦ *Stage 2—Increased Activity Exercises.* A small weight (up to 2 lbs./1 kg) is used to increase resistance. These exercises can be done when you are spending part of the day out of bed sitting in a chair.
♦ *Stage 3—Up and About Exercises.* These exercises will build up your strength when you are able to stand, walk and spend the whole day out of bed. (For more detailed information, consult

Rehabilitation Exercises for the Cancer Patient, by Ernest Rosenbaum, Francine Manuel, Judith Bray, Isadora Rosenbaum and Arthur Cerf, available from Bull Publishing, PO Box 208, Palo Alto, California 94302.)

Once you are back to your normal level of activity, you will have to establish a set routine so that you do your exercises every day. Try not to miss even one day if you are up and around and active. This will build up your body's reserves so that if you do need a temporary period of bedrest your energy stores won't be depleted.

While you should think of your program as being as much a part of your recovery as visits to the doctor, try to enjoy yourself. Exercising can be a lot of fun. And it can be very stimulating.

If you have days when depression and boredom get you down and exercising seems like too much of a burden, just remind yourself of all the benefits of exercising regularly. Your program will improve your energy level and stamina, improve your appetite, help you relax and help you sleep at night.

The more you exercise, the better you will feel.

25
RELAXATION AND CANCER RECOVERY

Lenore Dollinger, RN, PhD

We are all beginning to recognize that health is a balance of many factors—physical and environmental, emotional and mental, lifestyle habits and spiritual beliefs.

Stress plays a key role in this balance. Stress is well known as a contributing factor in a broad range of disorders. In fact, it's estimated that 50 to 80 percent of illnesses have some stress component. Stress is recognized as a risk factor in addictions, obesity, high blood pressure, peptic ulcer, colitis, asthma, insomnia, migraine headaches, lower back pain and many psychological disorders.

Whether stress is also a risk factor in the development of cancer is unknown. Some people believe it plays a part, others do not. But it certainly *is* a factor in your recovery from the disease.

POSITIVE AND NEGATIVE STRESS

Stress is not always negative. Positive stress allows us to act, think, move and respond to situations with purpose. We wouldn't function without it. The stress I am talking about in relationship to your need for relaxation is what I call *negative* stress.

People with cancer suffer a lot of negative stress. There are many sources:

♦ fear of dying
♦ loss of ability to work, which may lead to financial insecurity
♦ pain
♦ changes in appearance
♦ changes in relationships
♦ mental confusion
♦ "life-and-death" decisions that have to be made
♦ less energy
♦ less mobility
♦ severe physical symptoms
♦ feelings of aloneness
♦ anxiety about medical or surgical procedures
♦ anxiety and nausea before and during chemotherapy

Negative stress is the stress that increases your fears. It makes you feel helpless and unable to function. This is the kind of stress you can't seem to cope with. It is known that negative stress will make it especially hard for you to cooperate and assist in your therapy.

You want to do all that you can to manage this stress.

RELAXING TO REDUCE NEGATIVE STRESS

Relaxation is an excellent way to manage stress. Many people believe that relaxation techniques alone can reduce all levels of stress. This is generally true for people who are *not* in crisis. But people in crisis— and people with cancer often are—have to take practical steps toward stress reduction before a healing relaxation can occur.

Reducing Pain It is pretty well impossible to relax if you are suffering acute or chronic physical and emotional pain. So the most important practical step you can take to reduce stress is to reduce your physical pain. You may have to take pain medication or antianxiety medication at first. But you will notice that as you follow through on a stress-reduction and relaxation program, you will become less and less dependent on these medications. Once the mental and emotional struggle and severe pain have been attended to, then you can get down to the business of deep relaxation.

Enjoying Yourself You can take many other practical steps to reduce stress. Make up your own list, perhaps starting with these suggestions:

♦ exercise appropriate for your condition
♦ listening to music
♦ support groups
♦ sharing feelings with friends and family
♦ adopting a pet
♦ professional counseling
♦ watching funny movies
♦ reading comic or comical books
♦ getting a massage
♦ showing gratitude
♦ helping someone else

You reduce stress by doing those things you need to do—getting second opinions, counseling, controlling your symptoms and sharing your feelings. You also reduce stress by doing the things you enjoy doing—listening to music, going to movies or attending religious services.

Successful methods for stress reduction are different for everyone. One person might meditate quietly, another might run a few miles. Most people find music relaxing, but one person might listen to rock 'n' roll while another listens to Mozart. There is no right way or wrong way.

DEEP RELAXATION TECHNIQUES

The relaxation techniques described here do more than just reduce stress. They bring you into what is called an alpha state. Alpha describes a brainwave pattern that represents a deeply relaxed and meditative state. In this alpha state, stress is reduced enough to increase your sense of well-being, improve your ability to function, and make it easier for you to participate in your own recovery.

Before you can relax enough to be in the alpha state, you must decrease the negative stress you are experiencing. Then you can use several relaxation methods known to produce alpha states—acupressure, meditation and visual imagery.

Getting in the Mood Before using any of these methods, put yourself in a calm and quiet mood. One way to do this is to sit in a chair or lie down. Make sure you are comfortable. Make sure your surroundings are quiet or at least without distraction.

Then start taking very deep breaths. Breathe into your abdomen. You can check this out by resting your hand on your abdomen and feeling your hand go up and down. This is deep abdominal breathing. It's also called hara breathing, a healing kind of breathing that is very relaxing. Do this a number of times slowly and deeply until you feel relaxed.

You might also use a relaxation tape. There are many different tapes and many different ways of relaxing. Sources for these tapes are listed at the end of this chapter. Each tape will give you instructions.

Whatever method you use, once you're in a relaxed state you can go on to actively use one or more of the following techniques:

Acupressure This involves the application

of finger pressure on points where it is believed that our life force or energy comes to the surface of the body. These points are the same ones used in acupuncture.

One acupressure technique you can use

to create deep relaxation is to interweave your fingers and place them over your solar plexus, which is found in the center of your body just below the breastbone. Then sit back and quietly relax. Experience the feeling that you have—a sense of calm or sedation. You will soon be in a very relaxed state.

You might ask a friend or family member to sit at your feet. Have them put a hand under each calf, spreading their fingers. Have them sit there with their hands under your calves for about 15 minutes. This too will put you in a deeply relaxed state.

Meditation This is the act of focusing the thoughts in your mind. Another way of describing it is "engaging in contemplation or reflection." You can do this in many ways. A common way of putting yourself in a meditative state is to focus your attention on a single object. It could be a piece of fruit or the flame of a candle.

Another method is to repeat a sound. A common sound you may be familiar with is "om," which many people use in meditation. You can use any sound you are comfortable with.

Meditation takes practice. When you put yourself in a relaxed state and then meditate, you will notice that your mind tends to be very busy. You will have trouble staying focused. When your mind does start to wander, take a deep, slow breath and let the object or sound you are repeating come into rhythm with your breathing. Then continue.

Visual Imagery Again, put yourself into a relaxed state through deep breathing or a relaxation tape. Then visualize a scene or a color you find very, very relaxing. A peaceful, pleasurable setting might be a warm beach or a lush green meadow or a cool, refreshing mountain lake. It could be an image of floating on a soft white cloud.

Something else that might be relaxing

for you is the color blue (or pink or white). Take this color and visualize yourself being flooded by it and relaxing. There is no right or wrong here. Whatever relaxes you when you visualize it is right for you.

Acupressure, meditation and visual imagery are methods that are known to induce deep relaxation and to create a fertile environment for recovery. You can use all of them or just one. And remember that stress reduction and deep relaxation are two separate actions but can be performed simultaneously.

Using these techniques can help you control pain and increase your sense of well-being. They can also increase your ability to tolerate therapy and improve the quality of your life.

These techniques cannot be overused. You can use them for as long as you are comfortable. But don't struggle to keep doing them. Remember, your goal is to relax; you will notice that the more you do them, the longer you will be comfortable doing them. And once again, remember that there is no right or wrong way. Just "your way."

WHERE TO FIND STRESS MANAGEMENT TAPES

Audiotapes that help you reduce or manage stress have become so popular that many are now available in drugstores and health food stores as well as bookstores and libraries.

You can also order tapes or ask for catalogs by contacting:

The Enterprises Store
1200 N. Lake Avenue
Pasadena, California 91104
(818) 798-7893 or 1-800-826-0364

Gateways Institute
PO Box 1778
Ojai, California 93023
(805) 646-8148

**Jin Shin Do Foundation
for Bodymind Acupressure**
PO Box 1097
Felton, California 95018
(408) 338-9454

Potentials Unlimited, Inc.
4808-H Broadmoor SE
Grand Rapids, Michigan 49508
1-800-221-6121

SelfCare Catalog
PO Box 130
Mandeville, Louisiana 70470-0130
(504) 893-1195

Whole Person Press
PO Box 3151
Duluth, Minnesota 55803
(218) 728-4077

26
WELLNESS: PARTICIPATING IN YOUR FIGHT FOR RECOVERY ON THE PSYCHOSOCIAL FRONT

Harold H. Benjamin, PhD

People with cancer now have a choice. They can choose to be *Patients Active*, a part of the team fighting for their recovery, or they can choose to be *Patients Passive*, handing over responsibility for their recovery to their health care team.

Thirty or 40 years ago, most cancer patients didn't know they had any options. They were Patients Passive and their role was well defined. It included following their physician's instructions, accepting his or her ministrations and, if the patient was so inclined, praying for divine intervention. That was the only role they thought they could play.

But there's a new field of scientific study—an additional method of fighting for recovery—evolving. It's called psychoneuroimmunology, or PNI for short. It is broadly defined as the study of the effect that mental and emotional activity have on physical well-being. It has taught us that patients can play a much larger role in their recovery—a role that may actually affect the outcome of the illness *and will probably improve the quality of life.*

This chapter is about that choice. First, it suggests activities you can do and attitudes you can develop that will help you become a Patient Active. These activities and attitudes have been learned by working with thousands of cancer patients at The Wellness Community.

Second, it explains why someone with cancer who takes specific, conscious, purposeful actions to fight for recovery *will*

improve the quality of his or her life and *may* enhance the possibility of recovery.

There are three important points to consider when thinking about the possibility of recovery:
♦ The stronger the immune system, the more likely the recovery.
♦ The immune system may be enhanced by pleasant emotions.
♦ The immune system may be weakened by long-term, unremitting, unpleasant emotions.

If you understand these statements, everything that follows will be much more meaningful.

The assumptions on which this chapter is based should be emphasized.

First, treatment by a competent medical team is the primary method of fighting to recover from cancer. The psychosocial methods described here are supportive of, and adjunctive to, medical treatment. They are not alternatives.

Second, there really is a choice. But there is no right or wrong choice. There is no choice that is good or bad, brave or cowardly. Every decision you make is the right decision for you. Choose the passive role or the active role. Both will be right. In these matters, you know better than anyone else what is good for you. If you decide to try all or none of the following suggestions, that is the right decision for you. You cannot make a wrong decision.

Another fact that's important for you to know is that if you decide to try any or all of these suggestions and they don't seem to be working, that doesn't mean that you aren't doing them right or that you're not trying hard enough or that you're inadequate in some other way. Be assured that you are doing whatever is to be done as well as "it" can be done.

ATTITUDES AND ACTIVITIES TO HELP YOUR FIGHT

Before reviewing the following suggestions, understand that not all of them apply to everyone with cancer. Nor are they easy to accomplish. They are listed here because we want you to know what methods are available so you can choose what is best for you in your own unique circumstances.

Also keep in mind that although the main purpose of each suggestion is to try to direct the course of your illness toward health by strengthening your immune system, our experience is that a most important benefit to the people who use these suggestions is an improvement in the quality of their lives. And that's reason enough to give them serious consideration.

1. Make plans for the future.

People don't plan for the future if they believe there is no future in their future. If you are not making plans you may be unconsciously giving up. So you may find it helpful to come up with a list of short-term goals and long-range plans. Making plans in itself is a pleasant and positive experience. Why not enjoy yourself while giving yourself hope for the future?

2. Fight unwanted aloneness.

This is easier said than done. People with cancer know that many of their friends and family act differently toward them after the diagnosis. If you find yourself in this situation, then communicate, communicate, communicate. Tell your friends and family what you want and expect of them. When this is discussed openly, some—maybe not all, but some—of them will change. You might also become part of a support group in your area. It may be very important to fight the unwanted aloneness that can be so depressing.

3. Make sure you are not acting like a recluse.

Many people with cancer find it difficult to be with their friends and family in the way they were before the diagnosis. If you are having similar feelings, decide whether that's what you really want. If not, remember that although cancer has brought about physical and emotional changes that may make it more difficult to communicate, you are basically the same person you were before you developed cancer. Revitalizing old relationships is probably easier than you think. Do what you can to renew relationships and not be alone more than you want to be. Tell your friends what you are feeling and ask them to help you not be reclusive. Communicate, communicate, communicate.

4. Regain and maintain as much control over your life as is reasonable.

Most cancer patients have to give up some control over their lives to health professionals, family and friends. So will you, probably. But don't give up more than you need or want to. Make a list of the control you've lost and make a conscious decision about what is reasonable for you to take back. Feeling that you're not in control is a very unpleasant emotion.

5. Use some method to evoke the relaxation response.

The relaxation response is the name used to describe a physical state arrived at by several methods, including acupressure, meditation and directed visualization (*see* Chapter 25). The relaxation response is important to people with cancer because when that state is achieved, the immune system is enhanced for a while. And that may have a beneficial effect on the course of your illness. It is easy to do, takes very little time, has no unpleasant side effects and almost always leaves you feeling more peaceful and relaxed.

We suggest that you choose some method of meditation or directed visualization that suits you and use it regularly. There are those who believe that learning to trigger the relaxation response is the most important part of being a Patient Active.

6. Be careful of the words you use about your illness.

To describe yourself as a victim afflicted with a catastrophic or fatal disease leaves little room for anything but despair—a very unpleasant emotion. So why not use less dramatic and less ominous words? If you persuade yourself by the words you use that you are doomed, you may unconsciously give up. Try to describe your illness and your battle with it with words that are as hopeful as you can make them.

7. Pursue happiness and avoid stress.

This is easy to say but sometimes difficult to do. Remember, pleasant emotions may enhance and unpleasant emotions may suppress the power of the immune system. So do as much as you can to bring about those pleasant emotions and avoid unpleasant ones.

"Not so fast," you say. "That's not so easy. You may not know it, but I'm not feeling great. I have a lot to worry about." And of course you're right. But leaving aside any effects on the immune system, here you have a suggestion that is almost sure to at least improve the quality of your life. It may not be so easy, but isn't an improved quality of life worth the effort?

Trying to increase pleasant emotions and decrease unpleasant ones is probably what we all should be thinking about all

of our lives. But now, if you have cancer, it is particularly important to be *consciously* aware of how and where you spend your time and whether or not you are enjoying yourself as much as possible. The pursuit of happiness is a reasonable part of your fight for recovery.

8. Become partners with your physician.

Some patients want to hear nothing but instructions. Others want to have every bit of information they can get and be involved in the decision-making process. Most physicians are now flexible enough to act in any capacity that is in the best interests of their patients, including acting more as your partner in achieving better health. So decide with your physician what you both want the relationship to be. Communicate, communicate, communicate. A strained relationship with this very important person in your life can bring on unpleasant emotions for both of you.

9. Be with other people who have cancer.

Many people with cancer say that only someone else with the disease truly knows what having cancer feels like and understands the struggle. Being with people who do understand forms an esprit—a camaraderie—that is a most pleasant emotion. It also relieves tension because you can't frighten them as you do your friends and family. You don't have to be constantly on your guard.

If there is no cancer support group in your area, you can find other cancer patients by asking your physician, your local cancer society or other organizations that provide services to people with cancer.

10. Do what you can to keep up hope.

Hopelessness is one of the most unpleasant emotions known to humankind. But when the diagnosis is cancer, many of us believe that there is no hope. That's just not true. There are millions of people in the world today for whom cancer is just a memory. There is no type of cancer that does not have some recovery rate. Forty to 50 percent of all people who develop cancer in the United States will eventually conquer the illness. Others will live long lives controlling the cancer as they would some other chronic disease. Hope is not only desirable but emotionally *reasonable*.

11. It is not necessary to give up intimacy and affection.
If you and your intimate partner want to maintain some type of physical affection after the diagnosis, adjustments can almost always be made to accommodate that desire despite psychological and physical problems. Once again, the solution is communication. Perhaps it won't be easy, but if intimacy has been reduced or eliminated and it's important to you to regain it, make the effort.

WHY YOU SHOULD BECOME A "PATIENT ACTIVE"

To understand fully the implications of these suggestions, it is best to review a few basic facts about cancer.

Cancer cells are not necessarily powerful, dominant engines of destruction. They may be thought of as weak, confused, abnormal cells, which appear in all of our bodies from time to time. Their primary abnormality is that they continue to divide and subdivide long after a normal cell would have stopped. If they continue unchecked, they form a continuously growing clump of cells called a tumor, which, when it becomes large enough, will interfere with the performance of nearby organs.

If these abnormal cells are of the type that can grow only at the place of origin, they form a benign (non-cancerous) tumor that can usually be surgically removed. If they are of the type that can travel and spread to other parts of the body, the illness is categorized as one of the more than 200 illnesses called cancer.

One theory holds that although cancer cells may appear in everyone's body from time to time, all of us do not develop cancer because our immune systems are strong enough to destroy the cancer cells as they appear. That's what the immune system is for. According to this theory, then, for cancer to develop the cancer cell must appear and the immune system must be weak enough not to be able to handle it.

Recovery and the Immune System But how important is the immune system to someone who already has cancer? What part can it play in the fight for recovery? Until recently, the conventional wisdom was that the immune system had no part to play in the fight. That wisdom said that the only way to fight cancer was to try to remove the cancer cells from the body surgically or to kill them with chemicals or radiation.

Then along came immunologists who hypothesized that if the immune system were strengthened by various methods—including the introduction into the body of chemicals such as interleukin-2 and interferon—the system could destroy the cancer cells from within. This investigation continues worldwide with varying degrees of success.

PNI Studies The scientists of particular interest here are those involved in psychoneuroimmunology (PNI). They also believe that if the immune system is strengthened, recovery following conventional medical treatment will be more likely. But they are looking for ways to strengthen the power of the immune system not chemically but by psychological and social (psychosocial) means as an adjunct to conventional medical treament.

As noted, PNI studies have suggested that long-term, unremitting, unpleasant emotions weaken the immune system while pleasant emotions strengthen its power. This information led the scientists to hypothesize that people with cancer can consciously take action to enhance the power of their immune systems, which *may* make the possibility of recovery more likely. In other words, if you increase the number of pleasant emotions and decrease the number of unpleasant emotions, it may help redirect the course of the illness toward health.

Although there is as yet no statistical evidence that enhancing the immune system increases the likelihood of recovery, one recent study at Stanford University found that women with advanced breast cancer who were involved with group therapy as part of their fight for recovery lived twice as long as those who were not. Many observers see this as the first well-conceived study suggesting that being a Patient Active may affect the course of cancer.

KNOWING THAT YOUR CANCER IS NOT YOUR FAULT

If you have cancer, it is important for you to know that no matter what anyone says, you cannot be blamed for the onset of the illness. You may find that hard to believe, especially since there are many so-called experts who, for reasons of their own, try to persuade cancer patients that they developed cancer because they subconsciously wanted to or were in some way negligent or inept in the decisions they made.

Certainly, from all of the foregoing information, it's clear that there is the possibility that lifestyle—such as being under too much stress—just might play a part in the evolution of cancer. But unless you smoked after the Surgeon General's report came out and then developed lung cancer or exposed yourself to too much sun after being warned that it might cause skin cancer or melanoma, *there is no possibility that you can be at fault.*

To believe that you are to blame for your cancer, you must believe that:

♦ something you were doing or not doing was causing cancer cells to grow in your body;

♦ you should have known this was happening;

♦ you should have known how to stop those cancer cells from growing and make them go away; and

♦ you should have done whatever was necessary to make them stop growing and go away.

One can see how ridiculous that is.

Saying that someone with cancer is not to blame for the onset of the illness often prompts the question, "If I didn't cause the cancer, how can I hope to be a part of its cure?" That's like asking, "Since I didn't cause the weeds to grow, how can I kill them?" The answer to both questions is the same. Just as you can kill weeds, you can try to help "kill" the cancer cells even though you didn't cause them to grow. And being a Patient Active just might help kill some of them.

There are also "experts" in alternative care methods who imply that if people with cancer do what those "experts" tell them to do, they are sure to recover. They also hint that if you try to follow their advice and don't seem to be recovering, it's your fault. All that is false.

What is true is that there are many actions people with cancer can take that may have a beneficial effect on the fight for recovery. Unhappily, there is no guarantee that such actions will have the desired result.

Fight for recovery with all your might, if that's what you want. Do everything in your power to make your body the world's most inhospitable place for a cancer cell to live. And if the illness does not seem to be abating, don't let anybody tell you that you aren't doing "it" well enough or that you are not trying hard enough. That's nonsense. Whatever you are doing is right and proper for you. You are doing "it" as well as "it" can be done.

You are the very best "you" that ever was or ever could be.

27
HOME CARE

Malin Dollinger, MD, Ernest H. Rosenbaum, MD, and Isadora Rosenbaum, MA

◇

Most people feel much more comfortable in the warm, familiar surroundings of home than they do in a hospital or convalescent home. Medical facilities naturally seem strange. They are antiseptic, regulated and sometimes forbidding. Yet many cancer patients prolong their hospital stay. Why? Because they—or their families—are afraid they won't get proper treatment at home or be able to cope with home care problems.

These fears are understandable, but they can be overcome. Medical and non-medical crises can be anticipated. And they can often be avoided by training in the elements of home care—for patients and families alike—before discharge from the hospital.

Is Home Care for You? Home care can play a vital part in your rehabilitation. But it isn't for everyone. There are times when going home is just not practical. Not only your physical needs but also the ability of you and your family to cope with the psychological stress of a home care situation have to be assessed.

It is often hard for someone with cancer to endure the indignities that daily dependence on family members can bring. And the stress of having a chronically ill person at home may be too much for a family already stressed by other responsibilities. You may well be better off in a nursing facility.

Home care is a cooperative effort. You, your family and your medical team are all involved and the decision to go home has to be made by all concerned—the attending physician, discharge planners, family members and you.

PLANNING TO GO HOME

The key to successful home care is planning. Problems have to be anticipated. Changes might have to be made in the way your home is organized. You might have to buy or rent special equipment and work out the routines necessary for proper care. All this may seem like a lot of work, maybe even too much of a burden. Yet a comfortable and workable home care environment can be devised. And it can be a helpful step to recovery.

Discharge Planning Once you, your doctor and others make the decision to go home, you should be able to call on the services of a discharge planner. This planner—who may be a medical social worker, public health nurse or discharge coordinator—will help define your needs and match them with the resources available in your community.

Training Depending on the hospital, you, your family and any other potential caregivers might be able to enroll in the home care training programs now provided by many hospitals. These programs are usually taught by nurses and home care planners and take from three to five days to complete.

The first part of the program may be devoted to making sure that home care really is practical and appropriate for you and your family. The rest of the program may combine personal and/or videotape instruction with teaching in the hospital, followed by your practicing the skills to be used at home.

Assessing Your Resources Since the objective of home care is to keep your home life as normal as possible while still providing you with quality medical care, the first step to effective home care is taking a good look both at the support available to you and at the physical layout of your home.

Home care requires a willingness of family and friends to accept the responsibility of helping you on a sustained basis. Some key questions have to be answered.
♦ How much time can your family and friends spare?
♦ How will they balance providing support to you with their work and other responsibilities?
♦ If more than one family member will be providing care, can a rotation schedule be worked out?
♦ Will infants or growing children make other demands that will have to be met?
♦ Can each caregiver have enough free time to maintain his or her own physical and emotional well-being?

In the home, you and the home care planner should look closely at the physical setup. You'll have to pay special attention to the bathroom and bedroom, the location of stairs and the space available for extra equipment. You might have to get rid of scatter rugs or small objects on the floors. Railings might have to be installed and rubber strips attached to the tub and shower to prevent slipping.

Equipment The planner will also help you decide what equipment you will need. Commonly needed aids include:
♦ Hospital beds—manual, semi-electric or electric; safety side-rails; overhead

trapeze bars; overbed tables
♦ Wheelchairs—standard folding or powered chairs
♦ Walking aids—canes, crutches, walkers and folding walkers
♦ Bathroom safety equipment—bath benches, grab bars, shower attachments, elevated toilet seats and toilet assist frames
♦ Patient aids—commode chair, flotation pads, sheepskin pads, transfer lifts and respiratory equipment
♦ Patient care items—foam cushion rings, bedpans, urinals, heel and elbow protectors, sitz baths and incontinence pads and pants.

Most of this equipment should be available through local supply companies. And most medical insurance policies will cover the cost of rental or purchase.

Other Resources The planner can also put you in touch with the home care agencies in your community such as the Visiting Nurses Association and direct you to other community resources. The local chapter of the American or Canadian Cancer Society can also provide information on support groups and organizations devoted to specific problems, such as the United Ostomy Care Association or the Reach for Recovery Program.

GETTING TREATMENT AT HOME

One reason some cancer patients put off going home is that they're worried they'll have to be always going back and forth over long distances for their therapy sessions. This was a legitimate concern not many years ago, but things have changed.

In a way, things have come full-circle. In the first half of this century, medicine had much less to offer in the way of specific therapies than it does now. Before the age of antibiotics, modern diagnostic tools and effective treatment for many now curable diseases, doctors sent their patients to the hospital only when they were extremely ill. Medical care was given primarily in the home or in the doctor's office. But as medical advances and technological developments gradually led to superb diagnostic and treatment methods, hospitals became the primary centers for medical care. People were admitted for complex diagnostic studies and for the initiation of therapy, especially for serious diseases like cancer.

But the pendulum has been swinging away from the hospital as the focus of medical care and back to the home and the doctor's office. Both can be just as effective places for treatment as hospitals are. And both are a lot more convenient.

Doctors have realized for some time that they could deliver the same chemotherapy program they gave in hospitals in the comfort of their own offices where efficient and experienced oncology nurses, lounge chairs and television distraction were available. Patients also found this far more acceptable and desirable than a stay in the hospital, especially for treatment that lasted only four to six hours. After a few years of observation that this office procedure was effective, safe and satisfactory, it was not a radical step to perform the same procedure in a person's home.

Now hospitals are again used mainly for serious, life-threatening medical problems or complications, major surgery or beginning complex therapies that require sophisticated equipment or observation that can't be obtained elsewhere.

The New Home Care Services Home and office care offer significant advantages—lower cost, the avoidance of a strange and unfamiliar environment and especially the ability of a family to offer direct, supportive care.

Home care services are expanding in many areas. Where these services are available, a variety of important treatment procedures—including chemotherapy, antibiotics and total parenteral nutrition—

can be given in the home by an oncology nurse working under the supervision of an oncologist. The ability to give home chemotherapy safely has been greatly improved by the use of implanted venous access devices such as the Hickman, Broviac or Groshong catheters or Infusaport devices.

If you need these services, the nurse can remain with you for as many hours as necessary and your family members can be taught to give other medications to control symptoms and side effects.

Insurance companies and other third party payers are rapidly agreeing to pay for home care in many instances, especially when the cost of performing the service at home is shown to be a lot less than it is at a hospital.

CARING FOR YOUR BODY

Like most people with cancer, you are probably going to have a number of problems in body care. But these too can be anticipated and dealt with before discharge from the hospital. You and your family should be instructed in specific care techniques.

Bowel and Bladder Care You should be given a practical approach to bowel and bladder care. Special attention will be given to the problems of constipation, diarrhea and incontinence. You and your family should have a basic knowledge of laxatives, enemas, catheters and dietary management. (For more detailed information, *see* Chapter 17.)

There are two main problems with the bowels, both uncomfortable but both preventable in many cases:

Constipation Irregular or infrequent bowel movements can be caused by many things—chemotherapy drugs, pain-controlling narcotics, changes in diet or environment or lack of activity.

It can be prevented by adding foods high in fiber and bulk to your diet, such as fruits, vegetables, whole-grain breads and cereals and bran. You should also drink plenty of fluids and be as active as possible. Stool softeners, stimulating laxatives and suppositories can help. More severe constipation can be relieved by enemas (either commercially prepared or a home mixture of 1 tsp./5 mL of table salt and 1 pint/500 mL of tap water). If your white blood cell count or platelet count is severely depressed, talk to your doctor about what to do for constipation.

Diarrhea Unusually frequent and liquid bowel movements can result from chemotherapy, radiotherapy, emotional stress or sensitivity to certain foods. Your doctor can help find the cause and advise you if you need medication.

To relieve the discomfort, restrict yourself to warm fluids so your bowel can rest. Then gradually add foods low in roughage—dry toast, crackers, mashed potatoes, applesauce and rice. As you slowly return to your normal diet, drink plenty of liquids to replace the fluids lost in the diarrhea.

Incontinence If you have a problem controlling urination, two kinds of catheter can be used. Men can use a condom type that fits snugly on the shaft of the penis and is attached to a gravity drainage bag. The other type is a Foley catheter that is inserted directly into the bladder and attached to a bag that is changed regularly.

With either type, it is important to keep the skin clean and dry. With the Foley catheter, special care has to be taken to keep the connections and drainage port free of contamination. A nurse can show you and your family the procedures to follow before you leave the hospital.

Skin Care If you have to remain in bed for long periods, you'll have to pay special attention to the condition of your skin. When some part of the body lies against a surface like a mattress for a long period, nutrients and oxygen can't reach the skin cells. The area breaks down and the skin cells die. This creates pressure sores or bedsores.

Your tailbone, hips, spine, elbows, heels, ankles and shoulder blades are particularly susceptible to these sores. It is especially important to prevent your skin from being damaged by this kind of chafing because the sores can become infected. And weight loss and the side effects of radiation or chemotherapy can lower resistance to infection.

Proper skin care, along with adequate nutrition, helps prevent pressure sores and will also keep you feeling refreshed. A nurse or physical therapist can instruct you and your family in the basic techniques of skin care, such as:

♦ frequent position changes (most important)
♦ dry, wrinkle-free linen
♦ heat
♦ gentle massage
♦ good hygiene
♦ the use of talcum and skin lotions
♦ the use of a foam rubber ("egg crate") mattress or a foam or sheepskin pad to cushion your body and provide better air circulation.

Mouth Care Daily care of your mouth and teeth is always necessary, but cancer treatment can create special problems. Radiotherapy affects the mouth when it is given directly to the area and mouth sores may be a side effect of chemotherapy given for tumors in any part of the body.

You should brush your teeth daily with a soft-bristled brush. You might also floss daily to clean between the teeth, although it could be too irritating to your gums.

Your mouth should also be kept moist, both for oral health and for comfort. If a dry mouth is a problem, your doctor can prescribe an artificial saliva or a saliva stimulant. Rinsing your mouth frequently with water, chewing sugarless gum or sucking on ice chips or sugarless candies can also help keep the mouth moist.

PAIN CONTROL

Patients about to go home from the hospital are often worried about how they will deal with pain. If they've been getting medication from nurses and doctors to relieve pain, they often wonder, "Who will give me the medicine at home?" "What if I run out of medicine?" "Suppose I need an injection?" "What if I'm alone and the pain gets worse?"

The important point to remember is that most pain can be relieved. There are many medications available and one or more of them will certainly help. (For detailed information, *see* Chapter 19.)

Also remember that pain is a complex experience that is not only physical. Psychological and emotional factors play a major role in anyone's response to pain. Chronic pain that is relieved for a while and then returns can be very tiring. That fatigue in turn can make the pain worse. Acute or sudden pain can set off anxieties and fears.

The key to overcoming pain is to feel that you are the expert and you *can* do something about it. Having control over pain helps you relax. Relaxation means less anxiety, and less anxiety means less pain.

Keeping Track of Your Pain The first step in your gaining control over pain will be taken in the hospital when your doctor recommends the type and frequency of medication. You and/or your family should then keep a record of how the medication affects you.

Monitor where the pain is, what it feels like—sharp, dull, intermittent or stabbing—how long it takes the medication to start working, how long the relief lasts and whether there are any side effects. All this information will help your doctor make minor changes in dosage or pre-

scribe other, possibly more effective medication. Keeping track of the effects while you are still in hospital will also prepare you to be self-reliant in pain control once you get home.

Injections You might be prescribed medication in the form of pills, liquids, rectal suppositories or injections. Pills, liquids and suppositories are familiar and usually easy to take. But many people are afraid to give themselves injections.

These fears can be overcome with help and a little training in the proper techniques from hospital staff. After all, many diabetics give themselves injections every day. A nurse can show you and your family how to measure the medication and draw it into the syringe, how to prepare the skin and how to inject the needle. A little practice will be needed before you feel able to give a shot safely and comfortably. But once you know you can do it you will have more confidence that you can control your pain.

Where to Give the Injection The doctor or nurse will also advise you about where to give the injection. Generally, medications that are either irritating to the skin or designed to act quickly are injected deep into the muscle tissue (intramuscular). Non-irritating medications are often injected just below the skin (subcutaneous).

The three common places for intramuscular injections are the upper outer portion of the buttocks, the thigh midway between the hip and the knee, and the upper arm about a third of the way down from the shoulder to the elbow. Subcutaneous injections can be given at many places, the most common being the fleshy part of the upper arm.

Side Effects Pain medications can produce side effects such as nausea or constipation, but both can be treated. It's very important, however, that you tell your doctor about the side effects and let him or her recommend what to do about them. Treating them yourself can cause complications. If you take certain types of bulk laxatives at the same time as narcotic pain medication, for example, the laxative can actually *cause* rather than relieve severe constipation.

EMOTIONAL SUPPORT FOR YOUR FAMILY

When you get home from the hospital, you may be a little frightened. But you'll probably be eager to get back to sleeping in your own bed and returning to your normal routines. Your family will be happy you're coming home, but they'll be worried too. They will wonder about providing you with proper care. They will have to deal with new routines, changing roles, new expectations. Not least, they will have to deal with the many changes of mood and behavior you'll go through as you cope with your illness.

Home care is a major undertaking for family members. They give not only their physical services but also their empathy and compassion. Many people with cancer, because of the intensity of their illness, are often able to give little emotional support in return.

So family members may need special emotional support. They may feel left out of critical decisions, burdened with responsibilities, afraid of what the future will bring. They may feel angry about the disruption of their own lives and guilty for any number of reasons. Family members must be especially helped to not feel guilty for considering their own needs as well as yours and for taking time for their own social and recreational activities. It is also important to include children in discussions appropriate to their age and level of understanding.

The Importance of Communication The emotional needs of everyone can best be met by planning and open communication. If more than one family member is involved in care, a schedule to rotate responsibilities should be arranged. If one person is the main caregiver, he or she has to be allotted some free time for mental and physical well-being. Resentments and fears should be discussed as freely as possible so that frustrations don't simmer and rise to the boiling point. Shared feelings are always easier to handle.

Psychological counseling or support groups made up of families of other cancer patients can also give family members a forum for emotional release. Your doctor, medical social worker or local medical organizations can put family members in touch with appropriate groups.

And if your home situation grows tense or emotionally exhausting, you might consider a temporary stay in a nursing home. Giving family members some respite from the rigors of home care—even for a few days—might let everybody come back to the home care setting in a refreshed and more relaxed frame of mind.

IF THERE'S AN EMERGENCY

One of the biggest fears you and your family may have when planning to go home is what will happen if there's an emergency. Your doctor, home care planner or medical social worker can help you and family members prepare for emergencies. They will go over with you what situations might come up and the procedures for getting help quickly. They can also instruct family members in appropriate first aid procedures.

For your own peace of mind, you should follow a few procedures as soon as you get home:
♦ Prepare a card listing the telephone numbers of your doctor, pharmacy, ambulance service, fire department, police and a close relative or friend. Keep the card by the telephone.

♦ Prepare a self-care card recording important facts about your condition and medications. You may not always be able to reach your own doctor and if you or your family have to explain things to another doctor on call, you may get confused or lose valuable time if vital information isn't at your fingertips. The self-care card should include your name, diagnosis, the treatment you've been getting, which chemotherapy drugs you've been on, any other medications you are taking, any allergies you may have, the names of other doctors involved in your care and your blood type, if available.

What to Do If an emergency does arise, you or your family members should follow three basic principles:
1. Stay calm. Remember that help is always available and will usually arrive within minutes of an emergency call.
2. Determine the problem and call for help. Check the pulse rate to see if it is fast, slow or irregular. Check for breathing problems, changes in mental state, new pain or sudden increases in pain, nausea or vomiting, or injuries from a fall

or other accident. If the symptoms seem to require immediate attention, call the doctor or appropriate emergency service at once.
3. Take appropriate action while waiting for help to arrive. The most common emergencies are heart-related problems, breathing problems, bleeding, broken bones and falls.

Though hospital staff can give family members some training in dealing with these emergencies, the best preparation is the first aid courses offered by the Red Cross or other organizations in the community. These courses will teach family members the technique of cardiopulmonary resuscitation (CPR), the Heimlich maneuver to deal with choking, how to operate oxygen equipment rented for use at home, how to stop serious bleeding and what to do to keep someone comfortable when bones are broken.

The most important thing for family members to keep in mind is, *when in doubt, call for help.* It is far better for a doctor or paramedic to find the situation not as serious as originally thought than to risk the life of a loved one.

28
PLANNING FOR THE FUTURE

Ernest H. Rosenbaum, MD, and Malin Dollinger, MD

"The best way to get something done is to begin."
—*Elmo A. Petterle*

◇

The chances for living a long and healthy life are now greater than ever before. Age is just a number that measures time. As George Burns said, "You're not old until the candles on your birthday cake cost more than the cake."

Today, we have better nutrition, better physical fitness, improved living conditions, new drugs, new advances in medical science such as transplants, bypasses and other life-prolonging discoveries. More and more cancers are becoming curable when they are diagnosed at an early stage. Cancer treatment techniques are constantly being developed and new therapies like immunology and genetic engineering are holding out the prospect of curing more cancers in the future.

Yet living with cancer remains a fearful, anxious time despite all the promise of medical advances. No matter how well informed you are about your cancer or all the therapies that might be used to treat it, you still feel some loss of control over your fate. You put your life in the hands of specialists and live in uncertainty, hopeful one day, gloomy the next.

Although living with uncertainty may seem uncomfortable, it does allow room for hope and positive thoughts. You may discover that life can be more meaningful. Little pleasures can become very important. You may even begin to "stop and smell the roses." Once any anger or bitterness about having cancer is put aside, you will find there is still tremendous room for enjoyment.

And, if you are like many other people faced with uncertainty, you may get your life in focus with more clarity than you have known before. Thinking about their own mortality, perhaps for the first time, many people decide to make plans for the future if the best happens or if the worst happens. In either case, the act of making plans wonderfully concentrates the mind. If you make that decision yourself, the act of planning will let you face the uncertain future with clarity, simplicity and the comforting knowledge that your affairs are in order and that as few things as possible are left undone.

YOUR LEGACY OF LOVE

We all know that at some time death will take us. And each of us makes—or should make—some plans for when the time comes. Most of us buy life insurance to provide financially for the people we love. We make wills so that when death occurs there is a clear plan for the distribution of our earthly possessions.

But beyond these basics, few of us take the time to prepare in detail for the time when we are no longer around. Making such preparations isn't pleasant. In some ways it may be very difficult. It is something that we often put off, partly because we all consider ourselves immortal or too young to worry about death and all its implications.

But avoiding discussing or thinking about it only puts off the kind of planning that really should be done. It just passes a burden on to our survivors. More than 90 percent of survivors in America are unprepared to handle the responsibilities and immediate needs when a loved one dies.

Planning Tools A book by Elmo A. Petterle called *Legacy of Love* (Shelter Publications, PO Box 279, Bolinas, California 94924) is a practical guide on how you can make life easier for the people you leave behind. Its objective is to approach the problem of potential death with compassion and sensitivity. The book was designed for everyone—young, old, rich, poor, married, single, healthy and ill.

It was not written to scare you into thinking that your time is running out because of age or any other reason. It is simply a strategic planning tool, a workbook you fill in yourself. It deals with realities in a very practical and organized way so that your survivors know what they need to know and are properly instructed and prepared for what has to be done.

♦ The book introduces you to the material you will be working on, including how to start planning for your beneficiaries. It gives advice on will preparations, on what you have to do, what the first priorities are and what is not important.

♦ It covers the details on how you wish to be cared for if you become very seriously ill, including a Living Will and Durable Powers of Attorney.

♦ It gives advice and a place to fill out your instructions about your choice of a cemetery or other resting place, mortuary and funeral arrangements, memorial or other types of services, newspaper information and advice on death benefits that are available in the United States.

♦ It provides survivors with a list of immediate after-death contacts and phone numbers in order of importance. This is convenient at a most awkward time.

In their grief, people often don't think clearly and may make errors such as being sold costly funeral services that might directly contradict your wishes, which should be honored.

♦ It also lists the proper contacts to be made within the first 10 days—such as instructions for the post office or motor vehicles departments—and what contacts should be made within the first month—telephone, gas and electric, water companies, waste disposal, newspapers, credit cards, clubs and organizations, cable TV and other organizations that deserve to be listed.

♦ It provides guidance and planning space to be filled out on financial plans, any investments you've made, property and casualty insurance, as well as information about home and personal property insurance. It is amazing how ill informed many people are about life insurance policies, social security benefits, medical insurance, pensions, profit-sharing plans, IRAs and Keogh provisions that have often been made years before. Working through this section may give you a few surprises.

♦ It lets you catalog vital information on banks, savings accounts, loans, safety deposit boxes and so on so that this information is available when it should be.

♦ It gives advice on how to deal with bureaucracies that are often insensitive to the needs of people at such personal times.

♦ It provides necessary information about medical history that may be important to the family, as well as about family history and where personal letters can be found.

There are other tools that can assist you in your planning. One especially helpful book is *The Diagnosis is Cancer*, by Edward J. Larschan, JD, PhD, and Richard Larschan, PhD (Bull Publishing, PO Box 208, Palo Alto, California 94302). This book covers some of the same ground as *Legacy of Love*, but from a different perspective, dealing primarily with the legal arrangements necessary for survivors.

Many people unfortunately procrastinate, but books like *Legacy of Love* and *The Diagnosis is Cancer* give all thoughtful people an opportunity to lessen the pain and suffering of their survivors, simply because they love them.

HOPE AND THE WILL TO LIVE

Like every creature in the animal world, human beings have a fierce instinct for survival. The will to live—that instinct to fight when our lives are threatened by illness or some other crisis—is a natural impulse in all of us.

Yet some people are easily destroyed by the mental and physical effects of disease while others call on inner resources to sustain them through the experience. Why do some people respond positively to suffering while others cannot endure? Maybe the survivors have learned to be resilient by coming through earlier crises, becoming strong, tough and confident in the process. Maybe the small flame of gritty determination that makes us keep struggling at even the lowest ebb just burns brighter in some than in others. But the most important reason may be hope.

Many doctors have seen how two patients of similar ages, with the same diagnosis and degree of illness and the same treatment program experience vast-ly different results. And the only noticeable difference between the two was that one person was pessimistic and the other was optimistic.

Hope, courage, effort, determination, endurance, love and faith all nurture the will to live. And the greatest of these is hope. There may be times when you feel exhausted and overwhelmed by never-ending problems, when you feel ready to give up the struggle to survive. Yet if you have hope you can carry on.

As long as there is even a remote chance for survival, as long as there are even minor improvements, hope can be kindled and nurtured. As long as your family, friends and support team keep a positive attitude, hope can see you through any crises or times of reversal.

But hope has to come mainly from within. You can have hope if you are willing to fight for your life and if you are ready to do everything you can to improve your health. Just as soldiers have a revival of mood and spirit as they march home singing from an exhausting day, so you can find new energies and new strength.

Even at the roughest times, you probably have untapped reserves of physical and emotional strength at your command. Call on them and use them to survive another day. These resources are the foundation and the source of your recovery.

PART III:
DEVELOPMENTS IN ASSESSMENT, DIAGNOSIS AND TREATMENT

29
RISK ASSESSMENT, CANCER SCREENING AND PREVENTION

Ernest H. Rosenbaum, MD, Malin Dollinger, MD, and Guy R. Newell, MD

The number of new cancer cases in the U.S. is now approaching a million cases a year. After heart disease, it remains the second leading cause of death, claiming almost half a million lives in 1986, the last year for which statistics are available.

It is now such a common disease that it is widely described, analyzed and talked about in all the mass media. Much of this media coverage is sensationalized. Reports emphasize newly discovered "causes" of cancer or questionable therapies and "cures." Many stories blow research findings out of all proportion. Media outlets jumped all over very, very preliminary findings on the possibility of an association between coffee drinking and pancreatic cancer, for example. The same media outlets treated the conquest of the centuries-old scourge of smallpox as a minor item on the inside pages.

This kind of coverage has encouraged an attitude of "Oh, what's the use? Everything causes cancer, especially the good things in life. Why bother trying to avoid it? If it happens, it happens."

Some people take a different tack, saying, "Ah, by the time I get it they'll have found a cure." True, new research approaches may hold the keys to reducing the number of cancer deaths or even curing the disease. Genetic research may figure out what turns a cancer cell on and so find a way to turn it off genetically. Biologic research could lead to an antitumor vaccine much like vaccines for measles or other diseases. But results from those researches may be many years away.

What both attitudes ignore is the fact that almost half of all diagnosed cancers can be cured *now*. Worst of all, they ignore the results of many years of research and study showing that many diseases, including cancer, are *preventable*.

Prevention Prevention is especially desirable with a disease like cancer. Think about it. Cancer can change your life drastically. It can be very debilitating, potentially painful, costly to treat and fatal in half of all cases.

The U.S. Surgeon General and the Department of Health and Human Services have proposed a program known as the Year 2000 Goals. The program is designed to reduce cancer deaths by 50 percent by the turn of the century, saving approximately 230,000 lives each year.

The program focuses on state-of-the-art treatments, early detection, screening and prevention. In the short term, it's expected that greater use of state-of-the-art treatments will bring about the greatest reduction in the number of deaths. But screening and prevention will save lives.

Prevention can take two forms:
♦ trying to make sure that cancer will never develop, and
♦ finding cancer in its most curable stage, namely before any symptoms appear.

Both approaches depend on an understanding of the causes of cancer and the risk factors associated with the disease.

RISK FACTORS

As outlined in Chapter 1, the transformation of normal cells into cancerous tumors may be caused by insults or "hits" to the cell's genetic structure. These hits—a combination of heredity, environmental factors and especially lifestyle habits—interact and accumulate over time.

There are hits that initiate cancer—tobacco smoke, x-rays, certain hormones and drugs, sunlight, industrial chemicals and some sexually transmitted viruses. And there are promoters such as alcohol and stress. It takes two hits to damage a cell and affect the DNA. As the hits accumulate, a breaking point is eventually reached and a normal cell mutates, changing into a cell that grows uncontrollably.

Some risk factors we can do nothing about. But most are a matter of choice.

Heredity When there is a family predisposition to cancer, heredity may be the first event that promotes the growth of cancer. A cell may then be changed into a cancer cell by a single hit of a carcinogen. Although a tendency or susceptibility to developing cancer can be inherited under certain conditions, only about 2 percent of malignancies are caused directly by heredity. Most family histories of cancer result from a complex interaction of genes, environment and lifestyle.

Geographic Area People living in areas where there are vitamin or mineral deficiencies such as selenium deficiency may run a higher risk of cancer. The biggest influence of geographic area, however, is on diet, which may also be influenced by cultural habits.

Many studies have been carried out on cancer rates among migrant workers. Two studies looked at Japanese migrants who moved to Hawaii and whose next generation moved to California. The incidence of breast cancer was found to be very low in Japan, probably because of dietary factors. When the same hereditary population moved to Hawaii and adopted some American customs, the incidence of breast cancer rose. When the same genetic population then moved to California and adopted the American-style diet, the cancer rate increased to the same level found in native-born Americans.

Diet High levels of fats—both saturated (hard, mostly animal) and unsaturated (liquid, mostly vegetable oil)—appear to play a role in causing cancers of the colon, rectum, prostate, testes, breast, uterus and gallbladder. Low fiber consumption plays a role in the development of colon and rectal cancers. Even lean people with high-fat and low-fiber diets run increased risks of developing these tumors.

Eating preserved foods, especially smoked or nitrate-cured meats, increases the risk for cancers of the esophagus and stomach.

Low levels of vitamins A and C increase the risk for cancers of the larynx, esophagus, stomach, colon, rectum, prostate, bladder and lung.

Exposure to Environmental Carcinogens Exposure in the workplace to cancer-causing chemicals such as coal products, benzene, cadmium, uranium, asbestos or nickel can greatly increase the risk of developing cancer. Carcinogens are now also showing up in the air, water and soil.

Exposure to Sunlight On sunny and even cloudy days, intense amounts of ultraviolet rays may affect your skin. With the thinning of the protective ozone layer, these rays are becoming even more intense and more dangerous. The sun can cause sunburn, wrinkles, premature skin aging and leathery or rough skin. It can also produce skin cancers such as basal cell carcinoma, squamous cell carcinoma and possibly melanoma.

Sexual Practices Sexual history and habits influence the chance of developing cancer. They can either protect you or promote the growth of tumors. Childbearing reduces the risk of cancers of the ovary, uterus and breast. And women who give birth before age 30 are less likely to develop breast cancer in later life.

The more sex partners you have, the more likely you are to be exposed to sexually transmitted viruses. Some of these can cause cancers of the head and neck, cervix, penis and anus, as well as AIDS and AIDS-related cancers.

Alcohol In about 7 percent of males and 3 percent of females—about 4 percent of people overall—alcohol can lead to cancers in the head and neck, the larynx and possibly the liver and pancreas. Alcohol consumption also has a strong relationship with smoking, a combination that greatly increases the risk for cancers of the mouth, throat and esophagus.

Tobacco Smoke Despite the claims of the tobacco industry, there is no longer any question about the causal relationship between smoking and cancer. The link has been established statistically since 1950, though it was apparent long before that.

In the early years of the century lung cancer was a rare disease. There were probably not more than 400 or 500 cases each year. Some professors of medicine were advising their students as late as 1920 that they might see only one case of lung cancer in their professional careers. But when inhalable Burley Turkish tobaccos (which didn't cause excessive coughing) came on the market in 1912, smoking became much more popular.

By 1950, when the first report relating smoking and lung cancer was published in the *Journal of the American Medical Association*, there were 18,000 lung cancer deaths. By 1982, there were 111,000. In 1990, there were an estimated 160,000 deaths. This death rate has started to decrease in men but is still increasing in women. Lung cancer has replaced breast cancer as the number one cause of cancer deaths in women.

EARLY DETECTION
Despite all the advances in treatment, early detection can probably prevent more cancer deaths than any other approach. If tumors could always be detected and removed when they are tiny, no one would ever have to worry about metastatic disease.

Early detection depends on recognition of cancer's warning signals and prompt medical attention when symptoms appear. But what helps early detection immeasurably is self-examination and simple screening tests performed as part of an annual medical examination.

Self-Examination A simple test to help reduce the risk of breast cancer is breast self-examination. This is a low-risk, noninvasive evaluation that does not involve any radiation exposure or any cost. It's estimated that 90 percent of cancerous tumors can be detected by monthly self-examination. Training programs that teach women how to perform a full examination have had great success.

Men should also practice self-examination, feeling each testicle to detect any lumps every four months. Although testis cancer is uncommon, it is one of the most common cancers in men aged 20 to 35 and is curable, especially when detected early.

With some training and experience, men and women could examine their skin, mouth, thyroid gland, genitals, rectal area and lymph nodes for any suspicious lumps or patches.

Screening During a Checkup
During the yearly physical examination, various cancer-prone organs should be examined. Mammography and chest x-

rays should be used as well as Pap smears and pelvic examinations. This kind of diagnostic screening is particularly important if you come from a family with a history of cancer or if you have ever had cancer yourself. If you have had one cancer you are more likely to get another one, so you should have periodic checkups and evaluations.

RISK ASSESSMENT AND SCREENING

"Screening" someone with a specific complaint such as a breast mass or a digestive problem will obviously lead to more diagnoses of breast or colon cancer than screening apparently normal, healthy people.

But screening apparently healthy people with no specific complaints to see if a cancer might be discovered has become a significant and popular field of activity. These screening programs could lead to earlier treatment and much higher chances for cure. There are two ways of approaching cancer screening: whole populations can be assessed, or the risks faced by individuals can be detailed.

Risk Assessment Some people may be at greater risk to develop cancer. This may be because of their genetic makeup, their exposure to some environmental cancer-causing substance or their having close (first-degree) relatives who have had cancer.

To identify such people, cancer risk assessment programs have been developed at many medical centers. In these programs, the "client" fills out a questionnaire detailing his or her life history, family history, medical history, work history and lifestyle habits. The questionnaire data is fed into a computer and analyzed. A report containing a comprehensive and detailed analysis of the risk of cancer in that particular individual is then produced and given to the "client" and/or a designated physician.

These programs often suggest preventive measures that might be taken, including some medical treatment or lifestyle changes. A history of heavy cigarette smoking, for example, would lead the program to recommend regular chest x-rays and physical examinations, as well as a recommendation to quit smoking. A family history of colon cancer would lead to a recommendation that family members be regularly screened by sigmoidoscopy or colonoscopy at regular intervals and that stools be examined for bleeding.

Quite a few cancer risk assessment programs are available for use by the general population. But it is important to understand that the programs are designed solely to give information about the increased risks for developing specific types of cancer.

Completing a risk assessment questionnaire is *not* a medical procedure and such programs do not constitute the practice of medicine. No physician-patient relationship exists. There is no physical examination, no blood tests or x-rays. Nor is any information provided beyond an estimate of the relative risks of certain types of cancers and general ways in which those risks could be reduced or those cancers detected.

Widespread Screening There is a medical relationship with a physician when apparently healthy people have specific tests done to detect cancer in its early stages. Comprehensive and specific sets of examinations to detect cancer have been developed, most notably by the Strang Clinic in New York City and others.

During these examinations, the doctor's attention is directed to specific sites that may harbor cancer. Which sites depend on the patient's case history. The larynx might be examined with a mirror, the lungs by chest x-ray, the bowel by endoscopy or x-rays and the pelvis by x-ray, ultrasound and physical examination.

Although there has been a great deal of information published on the usefulness of extensive screening of healthy people, the practice has not yet been widely accepted by the medical community nor, especially, by insurance companies and other third party payers.

There has been some acceptance of the concept, though. In 1988, Medicare in the U.S. approved payment for routine mammograms because it has become increasingly clear that for certain age groups this simple procedure can detect breast cancers earlier and in a potentially more curable stage. A mammogram can provide a diagnosis about one year before a tumor could be detected otherwise. But questions of cost-effectiveness continue to be raised.

Is Screening Cost-Effective? A workup to screen for colon cancer might cost $1,000. There might be false negative tests that were really positive. There might be false positives in the stool hidden blood test that would lead to other tests and office visits. A small percentage of cancers might be found, but the yield would not be cost-effective.

Similarly, every woman could have a mammogram annually. But at a cost of up to $175 for each of the hundred million women in the U.S., the total cost of a screening program would be more than $17 billion each year. When you consider that mammography is useful only for tumors a doctor can't feel on physical examination, few tumors are discovered in women with no breast complaints.

On an individual basis, each person certainly merits screening. Anything that creates an earlier diagnosis is to be encouraged. But questions inevitably have been raised about the expense and complexity of screening programs for large groups of people. It has been especially difficult for some insurance companies to justify spending the substantial sums needed to diagnose a small number of cases.

Pap Smear Results All that said, however, screening can obviously make a differ-

ence. Pap smears to screen for cervical cancer are now part of the standard physical examination for 85 percent of women aged 20 to 39. By the turn of the century, the goal is to include the Pap smear in 90 percent of all physical examinations for women 20 to 39 and 80 percent for women in the 40 to 70 age group.

Since the Pap test became widely used, the incidence of cervical cancer has fallen dramatically around the world as more carcinomas in situ have been found. In the U.S., the rate has been cut in half.

Screening Guidelines for Other Tumors
The American Cancer Society as well as professional groups—such as the American College of Physicians, American College of Surgeons, and American College of Obstetricians and Gynecologists—have proposed various recommendations for screening that, although not unanimously approved, are similar.

♦ *Colon cancer* After age 40, a yearly digital rectal examination and test for hidden blood in the stool. After age 50, a sigmoidoscopy/colonoscopy every two or three years and an elective serum chemistry panel and CEA test.

♦ *Lung cancer* An elective yearly chest x-ray after age 40, especially for smokers, and a serum chemistry profile.

♦ *Ovarian cancer* Yearly pelvic examination, pelvic ultrasound and a serum CA-125 test.

♦ *Prostate cancer* Yearly digital rectal examination, rectal ultrasound, serum chemistry profile and a PSA (prostate specific antigen) test.

GUIDELINES FOR PREVENTION

Studies are confirming what doctors and many others knew 20 years ago—lifestyle does make a difference in the development of cancer. With 30 to 35 percent of cancers associated with diet, 30 to 32 percent caused by smoking and 4 percent related to alcohol, almost 70 percent of cancers are the direct result of the lifestyle choices we make.

Two-thirds of cancer cases, then, can be prevented if enough people made different choices. Reducing the number of smokers by 50 percent would save at least 75,000 lives each year. Dietary improvements would save at least 20,000 lives annually. But although many are aware of cancer risk factors, few seem willing to change their habits.

What You Can Do to Reduce Your Risk of Cancer

Diet

1. Reduce your intake of dietary fats—both saturated and unsaturated—from the current estimated level of 40 percent of total calories to between 20 and 30 percent of total calories, and increase your consumption of fiber from 8 to 12 grams to 20 to 30 grams per day.

2. Increase your consumption of fruits and vegetables as well as whole grains. Fruits and vegetables contain vitamin A, vitamin C and vitamin E, as well as the minerals zinc and selenium.

3. Eat cruciferous vegetables—cabbage, cauliflower, broccoli, brussels sprouts, rutabagas and turnips. These are good sources of the beta-carotene and fiber that help reduce the risk of several cancers, especially colon cancer.

4. Reduce your consumption of smoked or charcoal-broiled foods.

5. Drink moderate amounts of alcoholic beverages if you drink any at all. Ideally you should have no more than one drink or 4 oz. (125 mL) of wine per day.

6. Reduce your consumption of red meats and animal fats.

7. Keep physically trim and fit to avoid being overweight. This helps prevent cancer by reducing excesses of hormones that may promote cancer growth. It is as important to exercise as it is to maintain

good nutrition. Even moderate exercise helps to burn fat, make muscles firm and reduce fat bulges.

Lifestyle

1. Don't smoke. If you do smoke, stop.

2. Limit your alcohol intake to one drink a day or less.

3. Don't drink and smoke at the same time. This combination increases the chance for head and neck cancers by about 50 times.

4. Reduce stress or practice stress-reduction management.

5. Protect yourself from sexually transmitted viruses by using condoms when appropriate. There is an increased incidence of cancer in patients with homosexual practices and an increased incidence of cervical and penile cancers in women and men with multiple sexual partners.

Environment

1. Avoid excessive exposure to sunlight. Use sunscreens to reduce the sun's damage to your skin. Lighter complexioned, red-headed, blond or freckled people will need a higher-rated sunscreen—15 to 25—than darker-skinned or black people who have built-in sun protection through melanin in the skin.

2. Reduce or control any exposure to known chemical carcinogens such as benzene and industrial asbestos by using protective techniques. Preferably, avoid contact altogether.

3. Help in any way you can to enact legislation that will establish clean air and water standards.

THE MOST EFFECTIVE PREVENTIVE MEASURE: NOT SMOKING

Every year, over 400,000 Americans die because of smoking. Of these, more than 200,000 die because of cardiovascular disease, 57,000 die from lung diseases such as emphysema, bronchitis and pneumonia and 26,500 die from strokes. About 170,000 die of cancer.

Cancer rates have not increased significantly over the past half century, except for lung cancer. Cure rates have improved steadily from 20 percent to 50 percent, except for lung cancer. Smoking is responsible for 85 percent of lung cancer cases. It is the leading cause of cancers of the larynx and mouth and plays a part in cancers of the stomach, bladder, kidney, pancreas and cervix.

Cigarettes are cancer factories. Cigarette tar contains toxic carcinogens, and many other carcinogens enter cigarettes during production—pesticides and fertilizers in the field and chemicals during processing and manufacturing.

A burning cigarette gives off almost 7,000 chemicals such as carbon monoxide, argon, nitrosamines, benzpyrene, radioactive polonium 210, cadmium, methane, benzene, formaldehyde, vinyl chloride, arsenic and hydrogen cyanide. Over 4,000 of these chemicals are toxic and 43 are known to cause cancer. The carcinogens are also found in the tobacco used in pipes and cigars.

A non-smoker sitting in the same room as a smoker cannot escape at least some of the 4,000 toxic compounds released in tobacco smoke. In his 1989 report, the U.S. Surgeon General estimated that almost 3,000 non-smokers would die each year because of second-hand smoke.

With a "Smoke Free Society" in his 10-year plan, the Surgeon General established a list of short-term objectives for the 1990s:

♦ The proportion of adults who smoke should be reduced to below 25 percent.

♦ The proportion of women who smoke during pregnancy should be no greater than one-half the proportion of women overall who smoke.

♦ The proportion of children and youths aged 12 to 18 years who smoke should be reduced to below 6 percent.

♦ The average tar yield of cigarettes should be reduced to below 10 mg. The other components of cigarette smoke known to cause disease should also be reduced proportionately.

When the Surgeon General first advised about the dangers of smoking in 1964, 52 percent of the American population smoked. The percentage is now down to about 30 percent, with a reduction to about 15 percent being the goal for the year 2000. The major population to be targeted in the current prevention program is young people, who, if they are going to smoke at all, usually begin before age 20.

The Surgeon General's 1989 report emphasized once again that smoking is "the leading preventable cause of death in America."

Smoking has been called "the most deadly form of drug dependence." It is a difficult habit to break. But quitting is possible, as over 35 million ex-smokers in the U.S. alone can confirm.

30
ADVANCES IN CANCER GENETICS

Christopher Benz, MD, Ernest H. Rosenbaum, MD, and Malin Dollinger, MD

◇

Each cell in our bodies contains all of our genetic information in 46 chromosomes, 23 inherited from each parent. Each chromosome contains many thousands of genes, small subdivisions of the material that is the blueprint of life, DNA.

Genes are the carriers of genetic knowledge. A gene is capable of transmitting a single characteristic such as eye color from parent to offspring. There are an estimated 50,000 to 100,000 genes within a human cell. Only about 100 of them are known to regulate cell growth and division.

It has been known for years that one of the causes of cancer is changes or defects in our chromosomes. But only recently have new techniques in molecular biology made it possible to see abnormalities in the chromosomes and their genes, including small mutations in DNA. These new methods, along with other research initiatives, have led to discoveries that have profound implications for the diagnosis, prognosis and treatment of cancer.

TUMOR-CAUSING AND TUMOR-SUPPRESSING GENES

The DNA abnormalities that lead to the development of cancer may occur in either of two types of genes—those that promote cell growth or those that suppress cell growth.

Both types function normally and in a coordinated way during human growth and development. But genetic changes can cause the normally well regulated growth-promoting mechanisms within a cell to become uncontrolled.

Oncogenes One of the more exciting discoveries in recent years is that some of our normal genes may be activated in various ways and transformed into genes capable of changing a normal cell into a cancer cell. These activated and cancer-causing genes are called oncogenes.

An oncogene is activated by a metabolic defect that occurs inside the cell. This defect may be inherited or may spontaneously arise after exposure to a physical or chemical agent (a carcinogen) that damages chromosomes or DNA. Radiation in the form of sunlight or x-rays, chemicals and other environmental factors such as cigarette smoke or asbestos, for example, are all carcinogens that are known to cause cancers with excessive exposure, probably by altering one or more oncogenes.

Defects may often be repaired, but the cell's ability to repair DNA damage weakens with age. The unrepaired persistence of the activated oncogene will predispose a person to develop cancer in the tissue containing that gene.

We all carry unactivated or normal forms of oncogenes in our chromosomes. In the unaltered state, these genes are referred to as proto-oncogenes. They stay dormant or perform useful functions throughout our lives unless they are stimulated, mutated or otherwise activated to become oncogenes. Once activated, they can work with other genes to transform a normal cell into a cancer cell. This is believed to be a multistep process in which the DNA undergoes an initial change, then more decisive changes complete the process of malignant transformation.

While there are several theories about the exact causes of these genetic changes —such as a virus inserting its own DNA into a normal cell's chromosome, a virus acting as a random mutating agent or a single carcinogenic bullet that knocks out a critical gene—the most commonly accepted theory suggests that multiple genetic insults, or hits, are necessary to cause cancer (*see* Chapter 1). A single gene loss can be inherited and lead to family histories of cancer. Other genetic hits may accumulate because of environmental carcinogens or lifestyle indiscretions such as smoking or overeating.

There are approximately 50 known oncogenes. They are often named for the types of cancer they induce in animals, such as *ras* for rat sarcoma. Oncogenes may stimulate other genes by producing increased amounts of special proteins. Some may produce abnormal amounts of growth factors or cellular receptors for growth factors. There is usually more than one oncogene activated in any given tumor and these may coordinate to produce cancer. But exactly how these oncogenes and their protein products cause cancer to develop is still not completely understood.

Tumor-Suppressor Genes As their name implies, tumor-suppressor genes are normally protective, preventing the unregulated growth of a cancer cell. If one of these genes is absent or its protein product is unable to work properly, the cancer-producing action of an undetected oncogene may not be completely suppressed and a tumor may develop.

There are likely many tumor-suppressor genes, but the first to be discovered and characterized was the retinoblastoma (RB) gene. When the RB gene is missing or mutated, uncontrolled cellular growth can occur. This leads to retinoblastomas, rare and often fatal eye cancers occurring in children, as well as other kinds of cancer.

A retinoblastoma develops when there is a DNA abnormality that involves genes from both parents. An abnormality in only one RB gene can result in a susceptibility to develop tumors. This susceptibility can be inherited and exist in all cells throughout the body, explaining why children who are cured of retinoblastoma still have an increased chance of developing another cancer such as sarcoma, leukemia or melanoma later in life.

GENETIC SCREENING, DIAGNOSIS AND TREATMENT PLANNING

Single and multiple genetic defects associated with tumors are now being identified in clinical and laboratory research programs.

It is now possible to identify in any individual whether a specific oncogene has become activated or whether a tumor suppressor gene is defective or absent. It is likely that within a few years these genetic factors will be used routinely to determine both the diagnosis and the prognosis of people with cancer.

Since the presence of certain genetic defects may predispose some cancers to spread, genetic tests can enable physicians to identify individuals who are at higher risk for developing metastases. In these cases, more intensive clinical follow-up can then be offered or more effective adjuvant therapy can be given to improve the chance for cure.

The routine use of specific genetic tests has already begun and the new knowledge about and understanding of cancer genetics is having an influence on cancer therapy.

Screening Techniques that test for genetic defects including activated oncogenes and abnormal tumor-suppressor genes are becoming available for use in selected situations such as detecting familial polyposis of the colon, a benign condition that predisposes some people toward developing colon cancer.

Prenatal tests can detect abnormalities involving the RB tumor-suppressing gene, thereby identifying infants who are at risk for developing malignant disease later in life.

Diagnosis The recent FDA approval of the first DNA probe-based diagnostic test for chronic myelogenous leukemia is a sign that the field of molecular biology has come of age.

The Philadelphia chromosome (Ph1), a specific abnormality in this type of leukemia, was the first well-described chromosomal marker related to a gene rearrangement in cancer. The changes that result in this chromosome transforming a normal cell into a leukemic cell are now known. A proto-oncogene called c-*abl* normally resides on chromosome 9. It is activated—in other words, becomes an oncogene—when it travels to a critical point on chromosome 22. The exchange of genetic material between chromosomes 9 and 22 results in a shortened chromosome 22, the Philadelphia chromosome. It is believed that the activated c-*abl* oncogene produces an increased amount of an enzyme known as protein tyrosine kinase that sends stimulative signals to the cell's nucleus. The result of this persistent signaling is a leukemic cell.

The importance of this from a diagnostic point of view is that a DNA probe is now available that confirms the diagnosis of chronic myelogenous leukemia.

Similar DNA probes are being developed as aids in the diagnosis of different types of leukemia, lymphomas and other cancers. They appear to be able to recognize gene rearrangements and mutations in a high number of breast, ovary and bladder cancers, as well as in other malignancies such as retinoblastomas and sar-

comas. They are also being used to distinguish between malignant, premalignant and benign forms of disease.

Although much research is still needed to improve our understanding and expand the application of DNA probes, genetic techniques such as these will likely be used on a more routine basis in the future to accurately diagnose and classify all malignant diseases.

Treatment Planning Different types of genetic abnormalities may cause the growth-promoting mechanisms within a cell to become uncontrolled. An oncogene may become "amplified," meaning that there is more than one DNA copy of the oncogene, which increases its effect on the cell. Alternatively, a different genetic process can lead to the mutation of a single DNA component, resulting in the loss of a normally functioning growth-suppressor gene.

Such abnormalities in both oncogenes and suppressor genes can lead to uncontrolled cellular growth and are believed to occur in a large percentage of human breast and colon cancers. Since these genetic abnormalities seem to have a bearing on prognosis, their identification can be helpful in planning treatment.

Gene Amplification Some breast cancers are associated with DNA amplification and overexpression of the proto-oncogene called HER-2/*neu* (also c-*erb*B-2). About 25 to 30 percent of breast cancers have multiple DNA copies of this oncogene. Detecting its amplification or the overproduction of its product may be useful clinically. It may help in determining patient prognosis and in deciding, for example, if adjuvant therapy should be given after surgery.

Since 20 to 30 percent of breast cancers recur even though they have apparently good risk factors—such as small tumor size, positive estrogen receptors or negative lymph node involvement—it is hoped that new tests such as those for the HER-2/*neu* oncogene will be able to identify women at an exceptionally high risk for recurrence and for whom additional therapy might increase their chances for cure or prolonged survival.

The HER-2/*neu* oncogene has also been found to be amplified or overexpressed in ovarian, gastric and non–small cell lung cancers. In these cases, there also appears to be a correlation between this abnormality and poor prognosis with increased mortality.

Genetic Losses Recent studies have suggested that one tumor-suppressor gene—p53, found on chromosome 17—is defective or missing in many cases of breast, colon and bladder cancer. Missing segments of other chromosomes have also been identified, suggesting that other tumor-suppressor genes are abnormal in these three common cancers. Losses on chromosomes 9, 11 and 17 occur in bladder cancers, for example, and losses on chromosomes 3, 6 and 11 occur in ovarian cancer.

These findings support the theory that multiple genetic losses and not just a single gene defect lead to cancer progression.

ONCOGENE THERAPIES

With the diagnostic and monitoring potential of cancer genetics already being realized, researchers are now trying to develop therapies to inactivate the oncogenes that turn on tumor cells and to correct defective suppressor genes. Several approaches are being investigated.

Gene Therapy The approach that theoretically could lead to the most specific and curative form of treatment is commonly called gene therapy. This involves replacing a defective oncogene or tumor-suppressor gene with its normal counterpart.

Since retinoblastomas, Wilms' tumors and lung, breast and colon cancers are known to be caused by genetically inacti-

vated tumor-suppressor genes, these cancers might be obvious targets for gene therapy designed to replace abnormal tumor-suppressing genes.

Gene therapy can also take the form of inserting newly designed or foreign (recombinant) genes into bone marrow, blood, skin or other cells removed from a patient. When returned to the patient, these new genes can make therapeutic proteins.

The first attempts at gene therapy for humans, recently undertaken by medical investigators at the National Cancer Institute, are taking this approach. These investigators are trying to make peripheral blood lymphocytes overexpress tumor-fighting lymphokines such as interleukin-2.

There are, however, at least three major technical obstacles that must be overcome before gene therapy will be feasible for the treatment of human cancers:
♦ Tumor cells tend to reject foreign genes even after they are transferred into the cell.
♦ It is not yet possible to get the corrective genes into all the cancer cells in a patient's body.
♦ The amount of protein currently produced in cells bearing a newly transferred gene is still too low to expect complete correction of the tumor-causing defect.

Other Approaches Researchers are investigating anticancer vaccines and antibodies directed against oncoproteins such as HER-2/*neu* and EGFR (epidermal growth factor receptor). The therapeutic use of antibodies—alone or as carriers of powerful cell toxins or radionuclides—has already been shown to interfere with the tumor-causing action of oncoproteins. Such antibodies can selectively inhibit cell growth in cell cultures and in cancer patients and will likely be the most easily realized anti-oncogene therapy.

A different approach involves new drugs that can inactivate oncoproteins such as *ras* or associated enzymes such as protein tyrosine kinases. Yet another approach focuses on antisense oligomers such as those directed against the c-*myc* and c-*myb* transcripts that inhibit the intracellular expression of specific oncogenes.

These approaches all attempt to develop cancer treatments that target specific genetic defects. In theory, such treatments will be able to reduce the uncomfortable and life-threatening side effects now associated with chemotherapy.

Most important, some form of oncogene therapy could potentially be used to prevent tumors in people who are at a higher than normal risk for cancer because of their family history or environmental exposure.

31
PDQ: THE PHYSICIANS DATA QUERY SYSTEM FOR CANCER TREATMENT INFORMATION

Susan Molloy Hubbard, RN, and Vincent T. DeVita, Jr, MD

◇

Successful cancer treatment is often closely linked to care from knowledgeable doctors with experience in the delivery of the best available cancer therapies. Current statistics on cancer mortality suggest that wider use of effective, state-of-the-art cancer treatments could sharply reduce cancer deaths throughout the country over the next decade.

To make information on effective treatments more widely known, the National Cancer Institute (NCI)—the major source of federal funding for cancer research in the United States—has developed a computerized information system called Physicians Data Query, or PDQ. The PDQ system provides doctors with the most current information on the treatment of cancer. It contains up-to-date information on clinical trials that are testing new treatment approaches in patients with cancer. It also has directories of doctors who treat cancer and of hospitals with cancer care programs.

How PDQ Is Organized The PDQ system is composed of computerized information organized in interconnected files that make up a database. The information has been organized into data files for several reasons.

First, portions of the database can be transmitted electronically from one location to another over standard telephone lines, from a computer in a medical library to a computer in a doctor's home or office, for example.

Second, the data files can be frequently updated with new treatment information.

Third, data files can be presented in a format that users can easily search for very specific types of information.

Finally, the files can be interlinked in such a way that users can retrieve information from different files concurrently with a simple command, generally a numbered option from a menu of choices.

THE PDQ CANCER INFORMATION FILE

The PDQ Cancer Information File contains information on:
- prognosis (chance of recovery)
- staging (the extent of spread)
- histopathology (tumor cell type)
- state-of-the-art treatment options (effective or standard)
- promising research studies.

The treatment information in PDQ was written by cancer specialists with input from experts around the country. Treatment guidelines are provided for all major types of cancer—over 78 types in all. Information on the management of patients with rare cancers is being added.

The file also contains information on articles published in the medical literature that have demonstrated the effectiveness of the therapies recommended in PDQ's state-of-the-art statements. Short summaries of these articles can be displayed on the doctor's screen for review.

Because treatment recommendations for a patient with a cancer that has not spread from its site of origin are often quite different from the therapies recommended for a patient whose tumor has spread (metastasized) to other organs, PDQ generally recommends treatments by stage. In certain cancers, however, other factors, such as the location of the tumor or the type of cells that have become cancerous, can be more relevant than the stage in deciding on treatment. In such situations, PDQ provides recommendations by those factors. When there is no effective standard therapy, the PDQ recommendation is for doctors and their patients to consider clinical trials that evaluate new approaches.

Format PDQ's treatment information is provided in two formats:

♦ state-of-the-art statements, which are written for doctors and present information in medical terms that are often very technical; and

♦ patient information summaries, which doctors can share with their patients when discussing their prognosis and treatment options. These summaries are written in simpler language and contain references to printed materials written for cancer patients. The summaries are designed to complement discussion with a doctor rather than serve as a primary source of treatment advice for patients. A doctor will know facts about an individual patient's condition that may affect the selection of treatment.

The diagnosis of cancer and subsequent decisions about therapy can be overwhelming, and patients are often confused and upset. It is important to discuss treatment options with medical experts and with family or close friends. Doctors and patients (and their families) can use the material in the PDQ patient informa-

tion summaries to talk about their disease and treatment options. The treatment recommendations in this book have been written especially for patients and their families based on the treatment information provided in PDQ.

Information on how to care for the side effects of cancer or its treatment, such as pain, digestive problems, nausea and fatigue, are also presented in the PDQ cancer information file. A set of guidelines for early detection of many common cancers is included, as well as information on the design of clinical trials. The information on clinical trials describes what clinical trials are, how they are performed and the purpose of various types of trials.

Updates The cancer information file is updated monthly based on the recom-mendations of the PDQ Editorial Board, a group of 29 prominent doctors with expertise in treating cancer. This board meets once a month to review and discuss new treatment information and to update treatment recommendations. A group of Associate Editors, comprising more than 60 specialists from across the United States and Canada and representing all aspects of cancer treatment, complements and extends the expertise of the core Editorial Board.

THE PDQ PROTOCOL FILE

New cancer treatments must prove to be safe and effective before they can be made widely available. The PDQ protocol file contains descriptions of treatments currently being given to cancer patients in organized clinical research programs called clinical trials.

There are many kinds of clinical trials, ranging from studies of ways to prevent, detect, diagnose, control and treat cancer, to studies of the psychological effects of the disease and ways to improve the patient's comfort and quality of life, including pain control. The more than 1,300 clinical trials in PDQ's protocol file are evaluating new approaches to treatment. Each treatment program in PDQ is designed to answer specific questions and to find better ways to help cancer patients.

All treatment research supported by NCI in clinical trials is listed in the PDQ protocol file. Clinical trials that are being performed with other sources of support can be voluntarily submitted by the doctors performing them and will be listed in PDQ after they are approved by the cancer specialists on the PDQ Editorial Board. The NCI invites all doctors to submit their cancer treatment protocols to PDQ.

Finding the Appropriate Clinical Trial
New treatments often use surgery, radiation therapy and/or chemotherapy alone or in combination. Another area of cancer treatment under evaluation in clinical trials is biological therapy, in which substances that affect the body's natural defense system against disease (biologicals and biological response modifiers) are given as therapies to cancer patients.

The clinical trials in PDQ are classified by:
♦ the primary tumor type—colon or breast cancer, for example;
♦ the type or "modality" of treatment—surgery, radiotherapy, chemotherapy, biological therapy;
♦ the study phase (Phase I, II, III or adjuvant trial); and/or
♦ specific drugs or biologic substances.

Protocol summaries give detailed information on the objectives of the study, patient entry criteria (medical requirements) and details about the treatment regimen, including drug dosages and schedules. Each protocol also provides the names, addresses and phone numbers of the doctors performing the study. Information on protocols is updated monthly.

Searching the Database Doctors may easily search the PDQ protocol file to identify clinical trials for patients with a specific type and stage of cancer as well as

trials being performed in a particular place (one or more cities, states, and/or postal zip codes). The protocol file gives a doctor the latest information on clinical trials being offered anywhere in the United States and includes information on studies being conducted in Canada and several European countries.

With this information, doctors can help patients who want to participate in a clinical trial to become enrolled in one that is suitable for them. Because the descriptions of the clinical trial and the medical requirements of patients who fit into the study are quite technical, a doctor familiar with the patient's case should be the one to make the contact with the doctors listed in PDQ as being directly responsible for the protocol.

Clinical trials show doctors which therapies are more effective. For example, some clinical trials compare the best known surgical treatment with a newer operation to see if one produces more cures and causes fewer side effects than the other. Many standard treatments were first shown to be effective in clinical trials. The state-of-the-art therapies that are recommended in PDQ should be considered a foundation for building new and better treatments. Treatment protocols are designed to take advantage of what has worked in the past and to improve on this foundation.

Taking Part in a Clinical Trial Clinical trials offer patients the most up-to-date care available. Patients who take part in clinical trials have the first opportunity to benefit from new research and can make an important contribution to medical science. The medical requirements for taking part in a trial depend on many factors. Patients who want to know more about clinical trials should talk with their doctors and ask them to print out PDQ's information on the design of clinical trials.

Patients should learn as much as they can about the trials before making up their minds about participating. A cancer specialist is often the best person to counsel a patient about the selection of a standard treatment option or a clinical trial.

Asking the Right Questions The important questions for anyone considering a clinical trial are:
♦ What is the purpose of the study?
♦ What does the study involve? What kinds of tests and treatments are done and how are they done?
♦ What is likely to happen in my case with or without this new research treatment?
♦ What are my other choices and their advantages and disadvantages? Are there standard treatments for my case, and how does the treatment in the study compare with them?
♦ How could the study affect my daily life?
♦ What side effects can I expect from the study?
♦ How long will the study last? Will it require an extra time commitment on my part?
♦ Will I have to be hospitalized? If so, how often and for how long?

♦ Will I have any costs? Will the treatment be free?
♦ If I am harmed as a result of the research, what treatment would I be entitled to?
♦ What type of long-term follow-up care is part of the study?

THE PDQ DIRECTORY

The directory contains the names, addresses, telephone numbers and medical specialties of more than 15,000 doctors who spend the majority of their time treating cancer patients.

The names of the doctors included in the PDQ directory have been compiled from the membership directories of 17 American medical societies. Doctors conducting clinical trials that are included in the PDQ protocol file are also listed in the directory file, as are more than 1,600 health care organizations that have organized programs of cancer care.

The inclusion of individual doctors and organizations in the directory file does not imply endorsement by the National Cancer Institute.

Medical Societies That List Their Physician Members in the PDQ Directory File

American Academy of Dermatology*
American College of Mohs Micrographic Surgery and Cutaneous Oncology
American College of Surgeons*
American Radium Society
American Society of Clinical Oncology
American Society of Colon and Rectal Surgeons
American Society for Head and Neck Surgery
American Society of Hematology
American Society of Pediatric Hematology and Oncology
American Society for Therapeutic Radiology and Oncology
American Urologic Association*
Association of Community Cancer Centers
Society of Gynecologic Oncologists
Society of Head and Neck Surgeons
Society of Pelvic Surgeons
Society of Surgical Oncology
Society of Urologic Oncology

* Doctors who belong to these societies and spend most of their time treating cancer are invited to submit their names for inclusion in the directory. The remaining societies list all of their physician members.

Organizations in the PDQ Directory File

American Association of Cancer Institutes
Association of Community Cancer Centers
Clinical and Comprehensive Cancer Centers funded by the
National Cancer Institute
Clinical Cooperative Groups funded by the National Cancer
Institute and affiliates
Community Clinical Oncology Program (CCOP) grantees
Organizations with hospital cancer programs approved by the
American College of Surgeons' Commission on Cancer

ACCESS TO PDQ INFORMATION

Patients and others who want to know more about cancer and how it is treated can obtain PDQ information from their doctors or by contacting the National Cancer Institute's Cancer Information Service (CIS). This service, staffed by trained counselors, provides answers to questions from the public, cancer patients and their families, as well as health professionals.

Individuals with questions can call toll-free 1-800-4-CANCER (1-800-422-6237) to be connected to the CIS office serving their area. The counselors at this number use PDQ to obtain information on state-of-the-art treatment and clinical trials for callers. The call and the information is free.

Publications The CIS supplies free publications to patients and families with specific questions on cancer and its treatment. The following is a partial list of helpful publications:
♦ *Advanced Cancer: Living Each Day*
♦ *Chemotherapy and You*
♦ *Eating Hints: Recipes and Tips for Better Nutrition During Cancer Treatment*
♦ *Radiation Therapy and You*
♦ *Taking Time: Support for People with Cancer and the People Who Care About Them*
♦ *What Are Clinical Trials All About?*
♦ *When Cancer Recurs: Meeting the Challenge Again*

There are also publications that discuss what patients need to know about specific cancers. For a complete list of publications, write to the National Cancer Institute, Office of Cancer Communications, Building 31, Room 10A24, 9000 Rockville Pike, Bethesda, Maryland 20892.

Computer Access A doctor can access the PDQ database directly. To do so, the doctor needs a computer terminal or a personal computer equipped with a modem and telecommunications software.

These accessories enable the computer terminal to link up with the central computer that contains the PDQ system at the National Library of Medicine (NLM) or a commercial vendor over a standard telephone line. The computer must be able to receive data in ASCII format. Although not essential, it is also highly desirable to have a printer so that a copy of the PDQ data appearing on the screen can be produced for the doctor and patient to review.

Where PDQ Online Is Available PDQ is currently available on the National Library of Medicine's computer network. This system, which is called MEDLARS—Medical Literature Analysis and Retrieval System—is available 24 hours a day, seven days a week to doctors with computers that communicate with the NLM system.

Most medical or hospital libraries that have access to the databases on the National Library of Medicine's MEDLARS system are able to access PDQ. PDQ is particularly easy to use as implemented on the NLM MEDLARS system because it can be searched by making selections from a menu of choices.

To use PDQ, the doctor must have a MEDLARS access code and a PDQ password. A doctor may request an access code by contacting the MEDLARS Management Service Desk at 1-800-638-8480.

Online access to PDQ on the NLM system costs $23.50/hr from 10 a.m to 5 p.m (Eastern Time) and $16.50/hr at all other times, including Saturday and Sunday. These charges are prorated. In other words, if the user is connected to PDQ for only five minutes, he or she will be charged one twelfth the cost of a connect hour. There is no initial fee or subscription charge and a typical search requires only a few minutes of time. An online service operated by the European Organization for Research and Treatment of Cancer (EORTC) in cooperation with NCI makes PDQ treatment information available to European doctors.

Use of PDQ on the NLM system has risen steadily over the four and a half years it has been available. During 1987,

PDQ was used for about 1,700 hours. During 1989, it was used 13,800 hours, making it the second most commonly used database on the NLM system.

Commercial Access Commercial database vendors with medical information systems also provide access to PDQ. More information on these commercial vendors can be obtained from the NCI. Contact the PDQ Coordinator, National Cancer Institute, Building #82, Room 100, Bethesda, Maryland 20892. Or call 301-496-7403 (fax 301-480-8105).

Disc Access PDQ is offered as a CD-ROM. The advantage of a compact disc is that the user does not have to connect with another computer over a telephone line to search the PDQ system. The user merely accesses the information on the CD from his or her computer. However, the user must have a CD-ROM player that can communicate with the user's computer terminal.

Because the treatment information in PDQ changes each month, vendors must regularly send out a new CD to each user. Therefore, CD versions of PDQ are offered by annual subscription. Information on vendors that provide PDQ on CD is also available from the NCI.

Your physician can also get access to PDQ treatment recommendations by fax, via CANCERFAX.

PART IV:
TREATING THE COMMON CANCERS

ADRENAL GLAND

Malin Dollinger, MD

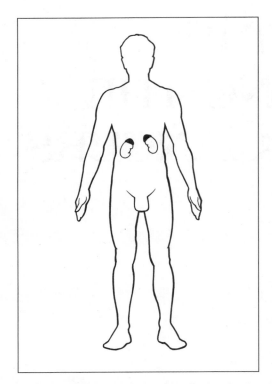

sex hormones in males and females respectively.

When excessive amounts of these hormones are produced, a variety of clinical symptoms can result, including feminization in men, masculinization in women and the signs of excessive hydrocortisone production (Cushing's syndrome). Tumors of the cortex (aldosteronoma) or of the medula (pheochromocytoma) produce excessive amounts of aldosterone or norepinephrine, respectively causing sustained or intermittent hypertension. Tumors that produce more than one hormone are usually malignant.

The vast majority of adrenal tumors are benign, being discovered either because of the effects of hormone overproduction or by virtue of the ability of ultrasound, CT or MRI scanners to detect small adrenal tumors that are usually benign adenomas.

Malignant adrenal tumors are treatable and curable when still confined to the gland.

Tumors of the adrenal glands are fairly rare, but they often attract considerable attention because they can produce an excess of one or more hormones.

The two glands, located just above each kidney (*see* page 377), produce a variety of hormones that are essential for life. The central part of the gland—the medulla—produces norepinephrine (noradrenalin), a substance necessary for the transmission of nerve impulses. The outer part—the cortex—produces three hormones: aldosterone, which regulates salt and water balance; hydrocortisone, which is essential for body metabolism; and androgens and estrogens, which are the

Types Primary tumors of the adrenal glands include a benign tumor (cortical adenoma), which may develop in up to 8 percent of people, often without any symptoms or clinical findings. Other types include adrenocortical carcinoma, pheochromocytoma, neuroblastoma, ganglioneuroma, as well as a variety of other benign tumors. The adrenal gland is also a common site for metastatic cancer, particularly lung and breast cancer and melanomas.

Benign adrenocortical adenomas are generally less than 2 1/2 in. (6 cm) in diameter and, if functional, usually secrete a single hormone, such as hydrocortisone.

The most common malignant tumors, adrenocortical carcinomas, tend to be large and to secrete several hormones. About 30 percent of these are non-functioning, meaning that they do not produce hormones. These tumors are usually recognized only after they have grown to a considerable size.

Pheochromocytomas, tumors of the adrenal medulla, can be either benign (15 percent) or malignant (85 percent). Either type can produce hormones or other substances that may cause significant, severe and sometimes devastating health implications, but only the malignant tumor can spread to other places.

How It Spreads Adrenal tumors can directly invade nearby tissues and spread to regional lymph nodes. The most common sites for metastases are organs within the abdomen, the lungs, liver, bone and the other adrenal gland.

What Causes It Unknown.

RISK FACTORS

People with neurofibromatosis and the Von Hipple-Lindau Syndrome as well as the multiple endocrine neoplasia (MEN I and II) syndromes are prone to develop pheochromocytoma. Patients with MEN I may develop adrenal cortical tumors. They are more common in males than in females. No specific preventive measures exist.

SCREENING

Because these tumors are so rare, no specific screening measures seem appropriate. A physician should suspect some type of adrenal tumor, however, if there are signs of Cushing's syndrome or high blood pressure in the presence of potassium deficiency, as well as unexplained hypertension, especially if it is severe.

Patients with medullary thyroid cancer and hypertension should be screened for pheochromocytoma prior to stressful procedures.

COMMON SIGNS AND SYMPTOMS

Non-functioning tumors—those that don't produce hormones—are normally discovered by CT or MRI, but may have abdominal masses, often with pain, weight loss or evidence of metastasis.

The hormonally active tumors produce a variety of symptoms. Women may have signs of masculinization (virilization) such as excess body and facial hair, a decrease in menstrual periods or enlargement of the clitoris. Breasts can become enlarged in men. Puberty may come early to children. The signs of Cushing's syndrome include swelling of the face and back of the neck, along with bruising and purple lines over the abdomen. Hypertension and signs of diabetes may appear.

People with a pheochromocytoma typically have attacks of anxiety and marked or sustained high blood pressure. Hypertensive crises may occur during minor operations or after a trauma or exercise. The blood pressure may often fall when the person rises from a sitting position. Other symptoms include headaches, sweating, palpitations and a rapid heartbeat.

Pheochromocytomas can produce other hormones besides norepinephrine, including ACTH, epinephrine and dopamine, so these patients may also have Cushing's syndrome. If these tumors occur in both adrenal glands, this may represent a component of multiple endocrine neoplasia (MEN), which includes medullary carcinoma of the thyroid gland (*see* "Thyroid") and parathyroid hyperplasia.

DIAGNOSIS

With the use of ultrasound, CT and MRI scanning, adrenal tumors are being discovered at an earlier stage than they used to be. In fact, a diagnostic dilemma occurs when an adrenal mass is discovered on a routine CT scan. Most of these are fortunately benign adenomas, but a diagnostic work-up should be done to discover if the mass produces hormones or is cancer.

Pheochromocytomas can occur outside the adrenal gland and may be difficult to find. An extensive search is appropriate for anyone with typical signs and symptoms, even if CT scans of the adrenals are negative. Most of these tumors can be identified by MIBG scans.

Blood and Other Tests
♦ Endocrine studies (blood and urine tests).
♦ Serum chemistry profile.

Imaging
♦ CT, MRI or I-131-MIBG scans.
♦ In some cases, selective angiography and adrenal venography.
♦ Chest x-ray or bone scan to detect metastatic lesions.

Endoscopy and Biopsy
♦ A biopsy is necessary for a definitive diagnosis. The primary tumor may be biopsied surgically or with a CT-directed needle biopsy.
♦ Alternatively, an accessible metastasis in the lymph nodes or liver can be biopsied.

STAGING

Adrenocortical carcinoma is staged according to the TNM classification indicating the size of the tumor, the degree of invasion into adjacent tissues and whether it has spread to regional lymph nodes or distant sites.

There is no acceptable staging system for pheochromocytoma other than localized and benign versus malignant and metastatic.

TREATMENT OVERVIEW

Adrenocortical carcinomas are curable if the diagnosis can be made before the tumor is larger than 2 in. (5 cm) or has spread outside the adrenal gland. At the time of diagnosis, however, most people with adrenal cortical carcinomas (70 percent) have Stage III or Stage IV disease. The initial treatment for all stages, even Stage IV, is to surgically remove the entire tumor. Radiation and chemotherapy may be used as adjuvant treatment after surgery.

The 40 percent of these cancers that produce hormones have a better prognosis than those that don't, but this is probably because the symptoms of excess hormone production lead to an earlier diagnosis.

Surgery Removal of the entire tumor is the only treatment that can lead to a cure. This may sometimes also require the removal of the adjacent kidney. As much of the primary tumor as possible is removed, even if all of it can't be, to decrease the amount of hormones produced.

Prolonged remissions have been reported after the removal of metastatic disease in the liver, lung and brain. As with the primary tumor, even if all the metastases cannot be removed, it may still be beneficial to remove most of them, for this will remove the source of the hormones and these cancers may grow slowly.

Surgery to remove pheochromocytomas requires specific preparation and management before, during and after the operation. The management of these tumors is extremely complex, and the surgical and medical teams have to have a thorough familiarity with the very specific medical and pharmacologic measures needed to minimize the risk to the patient and control the anticipated complications. The blood pressure may rise significantly during anesthesia or surgery, causing a life-threatening crisis.

Radiation There may be an adjuvant role for radiation therapy after an early-stage tumor is removed, although this is still investigational. In more advanced disease, radiation therapy may shrink bone metastases.

Chemotherapy The drug mitotane is the only chemotherapeutic agent known to be effective in patients with adrenocortical carcinoma.

TREATMENT BY STAGE AND TYPE

ADRENOCORTICAL CARCINOMA

STAGE I
TNM T1, N0, M0
The tumor is less than 2 in. (5 cm) and does not invade other tissues.

Standard Treatment Complete surgical removal of the tumor.

Five-Year Survival 80 percent

Investigational
♦ Adjuvant radiation therapy.
♦ Adjuvant chemotherapy with mitotane.

STAGE II
TNM T2, N0, M0
The tumor is larger than 2 in. (5 cm) but is still not invasive.

Standard Treatment Complete surgical removal, similar to Stage I.

Five-Year Survival 80 percent

Investigational
♦ Clinical trials of new treatment combinations, especially with radiation therapy and mitotane, are appropriate for some patients.

STAGE III
TNM T1–2, N1, M0 or T3, N0, M0
The tumor has invaded outside the adrenal gland into fat but does not involve adjacent organs (T3), or the regional lymph nodes have become involved (N1).

Standard Treatment The tumor is completely removed, along with any enlarged lymph nodes.

Five-Year Survival 20 to 30 percent

Investigational
♦ Radiation therapy if the tumor cannot be removed but remains localized.
♦ Chemotherapy with mitotane may reduce the amount of hormone produced by the tumor or retard tumor growth.

STAGE IV
TNM Any T, any N, M1 or T3–4, N1, M0

Standard Treatment The goal of treatment for an adrenocortical carcinoma that has spread to adjacent organs (a T4 tumor) or has metastasized to distant sites is palliation rather than cure.

Chemotherapy with mitotane may lead to partial or complete remissions lasting several months. Other treatment options are radiation therapy to bone metastases and/or the surgical removal of localized metastases, particularly those that produce hormones.

Five-Year Survival Less than 1 percent

Investigational
♦ Clinical trials may be appropriate for patients with metastatic disease or with recurrent cancer.
♦ Cisplatin seems to benefit some patients with metastases and is being clinically evaluated.

PHEOCHROMOCYTOMA
LOCALIZED
Localized benign pheochromocytoma is confined to one or both adrenal glands.

Standard Treatment Before treatment, medical management is started with phenoxybenzamine (Dibenzyline) to block the action of the hormones produced by the tumor. Because rather specific, specialized and vital medical management is essential before surgery or any other treatment is given, an endocrinologist is often involved and the surgery is often done in a major medical center.

The standard treatment is the removal of the tumor (adrenalectomy). Besides the essential preoperative management, blood pressure has to be controlled with specific drugs during surgery and prevented from falling after the operation.

Five-Year Survival Over 95 percent

METASTATIC
The pheochromocytoma has spread to nearby lymph nodes or has extended into local tissues.

Standard Treatment If the pheochromocytoma has spread, it is still treated with aggressive surgery to remove all visible evidence of disease. This is to reduce the excess hormone production that causes many of the clinical problems these patients have. Long-term medical management of symptoms using drugs to control the effects of the excess hormones is extremely important. The same medical precautions taken with localized tumors before, during and after surgery are essential.

A variety of chemotherapy combinations have been used, including cyclophosphamide + vincristine + dacarbazine (DTIC), which may produce tumor regression and improve symptoms, biochemical markers and hypertension.

Radiation therapy may improve or palliate local complications caused by metastases.

Five-Year Survival About 40 to 45 percent

Investigational
♦ Clinical trials are under way to attempt to find more effective chemotherapy treatments.
♦ One therapeutic approach for patients whose tumors cannot be removed, have recurred or have metastasized is targeted radiation therapy with I-131-MIBG. This treatment has resulted in the shrinkage of tumors and a reduction in symptoms in some patients.

TREATMENT FOLLOW-UP

For adrenocortical carcinomas, treatment follow-up should include:
♦ Repeat CT or MRI scanning to assess possible recurrence or metastases.
♦ Measurement of specific hormones produced by the tumor.
♦ Studies— liver function tests, chest x-rays—to document the status of metastases.

Follow-up for pheochromocytomas should include:
♦ Measurements of hormones produced by the tumor by plasma and urine tests.
♦ Abdominal CT or MRI scans to assess the status of the primary tumor.
♦ Bone scans, chest x-rays and liver function tests to evaluate the status of metastases.
♦ Routine and regular blood pressure determinations to assess the effects of the hormone produced by the tumor.

RECURRENT CANCER

The selection of treatment for recurrent tumors depends on which therapy was initially used and the site of recurrence. Clinical trials evaluating new chemotherapy drugs should be considered for recurrent adrenocortical carcinoma. Recurrent pheochromocytoma is managed in the same way as metastatic disease.

THE MOST IMPORTANT QUESTIONS YOU CAN ASK

♦ What hormones is my tumor producing?

♦ Should an endocrinologist be involved in my care?

♦ If the tumor cannot be completely removed, would radiation therapy and chemotherapy be helpful?

♦ What is the role of mitotane in my treatment and what are its side effects?

♦ Can I live for a long time even if the tumor can't be removed?

ANUS

Ernest H. Rosenbaum, MD

◇

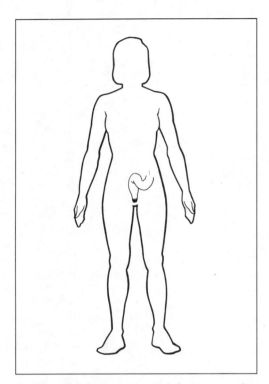

Cancer of the anus—the inch-long muscular tube where the rectum opens into the body surface—is less common than other bowel cancers, accounting for only about 1 to 2 percent of all cancers of the large bowel and its outlet. Fewer than 10,000 cases occur annually in the United States.

Anal cancer is highly treatable and often curable, especially in the early stages. The first sign of the cancer is often bleeding, which may be mistaken for hemorrhoids or benign anal disease. Anal cancers are often discovered by a pathologist in a specimen from a surgical operation done for apparently benign disease.

Types The vast majority—80 to 90 percent—of all primary cancers of the anus develop in the skin and are called squamous cell (epidermoid) carcinomas. These often first appear as an ulcer. An important subset is made up of tumors that arise in the anal lining from embryonic tissue (cloacogenic) or the anal lining of transitional cells (basaloid tumors). There is also a squamous cell tumor within the anal lining (intraepithelial) called Bowen's disease that is a premalignant lesion of the skin around the anus.

Anal cancers can also develop in glandular tissue (adenocarcinoma). Less common lesions include small cell carcinomas, malignant lymphomas, sarcomas, melanomas or Paget's disease, an intraepithelial adenocarcinoma of the mucous or sweat glands. Melanomas have a poor prognosis, since they spread via the bloodstream.

Well-differentiated tumors have a more favorable prognosis than poorly differentiated tumors.

How It Spreads Anal tumors can extend directly into adjacent tissues, including the skin, sphincter muscle, or to local organs such as the prostate, bladder or vagina. Tumor cells can spread via the lymph system to lymph nodes in the groin (if the tumor is below the pectinate line) or to pelvic lymph nodes (if the tumor is above the pectinate line). Metastases can also travel through the bloodstream.

What Causes It Chronic irritation of the anus is a primary cause. People who get anal cancer usually have a history of risk factors, one of which may be related to the human papilloma virus or the trauma of anal intercourse.

RISK FACTORS

At Significantly Higher Risk
♦ This cancer is more common in women over 40.
♦ Primary association with a history of chronic anal irritation—genital warts, abscesses, fistulas, fissures and infections such as chlamydia, trichomonas, genital herpes and gonorrhea.
♦ Associated with venereal warts and the presence of the papilloma virus.
♦ Anal margin cancer (cancer encircling the anus) is more common in men.
♦ Increased incidence in cigarette smokers.
♦ Increased risk in homosexuals, probably related to anal intercourse and infections with a retrovirus such as HIV (human immunodeficiency virus).
♦ Anal cancer may occur along with benign anal disease. It is more common in those with hemorrhoids, anal degenerative skin changes and white plaque (leukoplakia) on the mucous membranes.

SCREENING

A careful anal exam is an important part of a yearly physical. A digital rectal examination and anoscopy should be performed whenever there are rectal symptoms such as pain, bleeding, itching or hemorrhoidal complaints. All hemorrhoids, inflammation and local anal disease should be examined by a physician with a special interest in anal or rectal disease. And all lesions in the area should be biopsied no matter how benign-looking they are.

COMMON SIGNS AND SYMPTOMS

There are often no symptoms of anal cancer in its early stages. But there may be bleeding, discomfort or pressure, pain, itching or a rectal mass. Small amounts of rectal bleeding not associated with anemia are often attributed to hemorrhoids.

Occasionally, a change in bowel habits, diarrhea or constipation may be noted and a bowel obstruction might develop.

There may also be local pain or pressure that is not relieved by a bowel movement.

DIAGNOSIS

Physical Examination
♦ Digital rectal exam or an exam with local or general anesthesia if necessary.
♦ A small anal mass, often like hemorrhoids, may be found. Sometimes the mass protrudes and reaches a significant size.
♦ Physical examination for local invasion into muscle sphincter.
♦ Lymph nodes in the groin may be enlarged, indicating metastases.
♦ Perirectal and mesenteric lymph nodes are involved in 50 percent of patients.

Blood and Other Tests
♦ Complete blood count.
♦ Liver function chemistries (alkaline phosphatase, LDH, SGOT).
♦ Tests of kidney function (creatinine).
♦ Papilloma virus culture or DNA test, if available.
♦ Test for hidden blood in the stools.

Imaging
♦ CT and MRI scans of the pelvis to assess local invasion and whether the iliac and groin (inguinal) lymph nodes are involved (30 percent have inguinal metastases and 10 percent have liver metastases at the time of diagnosis).
♦ Rectal ultrasound may help assess local cancer and lymph node invasion.
♦ Pelvic and abdominal ultrasound.
♦ Abdominal CT scan if the liver is enlarged or if liver function tests are abnormal.
♦ Chest x-ray.

Endoscopy and Biopsy
♦ Anoscopy/proctoscopy under local or general anesthesia if necessary.

STAGING

The stage of anal cancer describes whether the cancer has remained within the anus, has spread to lymph nodes near the anus or has spread to other sites, usually within the abdomen or other organs. The stage as defined by the TNM classification is important in determining the initial treatment options.

TREATMENT OVERVIEW

Surgery, radiotherapy and chemotherapy are all used to treat anal cancer.

The prognosis depends on the size and location of the tumor. The outlook is more favorable if the tumors are small (less than 2 in./5 cm), if there is no lymph node involvement or local extension and if the primary tumor is in the anal margin rather than the anal canal. Primary tumors less than 1 in. (2 cm) in size have a better prognosis, as do tumors that are well-differentiated (more mature) rather than undifferentiated or poorly differentiated.

Options by Size of Tumor The choice of conservative surgery or radiotherapy (with or without chemotherapy) for anal or perianal cancer depends on the size of the tumor, local invasion and/or lymph node involvement. Radical surgery (an abdominal-perineal resection) is often required for larger or more extensive cancers, and will result in a loss of anal function, a colostomy, and urinary and sexual malfunction. It is reserved for larger or residual cancers.

♦ Superficial in situ tumors—those that invade less than 1 in. (2 cm) can be treated with local excision or radiotherapy alone.

♦ Tumors 1 to 2 in. (2 to 5 cm) are *best* treated by chemotherapy (5-fluorouracil + mitomycin-C or 5-FU + cisplatin) plus radiotherapy, leaving surgery for "salvage" therapy. Some physicians still use just radiotherapy, but most oncologists today use combined chemotherapy and radiotherapy.

♦ Tumors larger than 2 in. (5 cm) are treated by chemotherapy, radiotherapy and surgery for residual disease.

♦ If the cancer is confirmed as local or is less than 1 in. (2 cm) in diameter and is well-differentiated, removal of the squamous anal verge or the anal canal will produce a high chance for cure, with 70 to 90 percent surviving five years. Removing the groin lymph nodes as a prophylactic measure does not improve these results and often contributes to lymphedema.

♦ A clinical trial is comparing radiation therapy with radiation plus 5-FU. High-dose radiation therapy alone (greater than 6,000 cGy) may be curative and has a five-year survival of greater than 70 percent and 80 percent control of small local tumors. Patients who relapse may require salvage surgery.

Options by Lymph Node Status The lymph nodes in the groin (inguinal), pelvis and perirectal area may become involved by anal cancer.

♦ When lesions are less than 1 in. (2 cm), nodes are not usually treated.

♦ When primary lesions are between 1 and 2 in. (2 to 5 cm), groin and pelvic nodes are treated prophylactically with radiation therapy.

♦ When lymph nodes can be felt, the treatment is chemotherapy and radiotherapy.

Combined Therapy Information from clinical trials supports the idea of using radiation therapy, or chemotherapy plus radiotherapy for the initial treatment of epidermoid cancer of the anus, reserving surgery for residual disease. Radiation therapy plus chemotherapy has been used as an alternative to surgery for patients with inguinal lymph node metastases.

External radiation therapy with chemotherapy is now the first line of therapy, resulting in a 90 percent local control. An alternative is interstitial implants of iridium with external radiation therapy, without chemotherapy.

The first choice of treatment should be radiotherapy with chemotherapy for small or even large, but not huge, lesions. Whether to give chemotherapy before radiotherapy or simultaneously is now being evaluated.

When all the tumor is eradicated by radiation and chemotherapy, careful follow-up is vital. The lymph nodes in the groin have to be watched carefully, since the most common site of local recurrence is in the pelvis and lymph nodes. If the tumor recurs, salvage surgery will be needed.

Treatment of the less common adeno-carcinoma involving the upper portion of the anus (near the rectum) differs from treatment of squamous carcinoma. For smaller lesions, local excision or fulguration may suffice. For larger lesions, an abdominal-perineal resection may be required. Combined radiotherapy and chemotherapy is not as useful, although rectal adjuvant chemotherapy and radio-therapy programs can be employed. In selected cases, interstitial implants of iridium with external radiation therapy may be an alternative.

TREATMENT BY STAGE

STAGE 0
TNM Tis, N0, M0
Carcinoma in situ—a very early, microscopic, non-invasive cancer that has not spread below the membrane of the first layer of anal tissue.

Standard Treatment Surgical removal of the tumor.

Five-Year Survival 100 percent

STAGE I
TNM T1, N0, M0
A tumor less than 1 in. (2 cm) found only in the anal mucosa with no evidence of spread to lymph nodes or other organs. There is no sphincter muscle involvement.

Standard Treatment Small tumors of the skin around the anus and of the anal margin may be adequately treated by local excision with or without radiation therapy with preservation of the sphincter muscle.

When surgery that will preserve the sphincter is possible, both radiation and chemotherapy can be used before the operation to reduce the size of the tumor. Selected tumors may also be treated by implanting iridium in the tissue. Careful follow-up is mandatory.

When surgery would significantly impair anal sphincter functions, radio-therapy is an effective alternative, usually with chemotherapy.

External radiation therapy for small lesions—with or without chemotherapy—may also be used to avoid surgery and/or avoid a colostomy. Surgery may be neces-sary for large lesions that do not shrink with radiotherapy and chemotherapy.

Combination chemotherapy with 5-fluorouracil (5-FU) + mitomycin-C with primary radiation therapy is more effective for larger lesions than radiation therapy alone in reducing the need for surgery and/or a colostomy. Cisplatin + 5-FU is an alternative treatment with radiotherapy. Both combinations seem to be equally effective.

The former standard approach—an abdominal-perineal resection (APR), which involves removal of the anus and rectum and requires a colostomy—is now rarely used except for recurrent disease. If there is still tumor in the anal canal after non-surgical treatment, the surgery that will be required ranges from a local sphincter preservation operation to a complete abdominal-perineal resection with colostomy.

Five-Year Survival Over 95 percent

STAGE II
TNM T2–3 N0, M0
The tumor is larger than 1 in. (2 cm) and

has spread into the muscle wall of the anus (the sphincter muscle is involved), but does not involve lymph nodes or other adjacent organs.

Standard Treatment Current treatment is combination chemotherapy with 5-FU + mitomycin-C or cisplatin + 5-FU plus radiation therapy. When the response is not complete, the tumor can be removed surgically.

The treatment options for anal cancer involving the sphincter are the same as for Stage I.

Five-Year Survival 75 percent

STAGE IIIA
TNM T4, N0, M0 or T1–3, N1, M0
The cancer has spread to nearby lymph nodes or has spread to nearby organs such as the vagina, urethra or bladder (it is often hard to determine Stage IIIA, since many patients clinically appear to be Stage II).

Standard Treatment Abdominal-perineal resection has been the treatment of choice in the past. Deciding whether to perform this operation may depend on whether the physical examination or the CT or MRI scans find that the perirectal lymph nodes are involved. The need for a biopsy of perirectal lymph nodes to differentiate between Stage II and Stage III disease may not be verifiable without surgery.

Chemotherapy and radiation given before surgery may not only improve the long-term results, but also permit sphincter preserving surgery by shrinking the tumor substantially before the operation.

Five-Year Survival 60 percent

Investigational
♦ Trials to evaluate postoperative external beam radiation to the involved area, which may improve local control and survival, are ongoing.
♦ Chemotherapy after surgery is also being evaluated.

STAGE IIIB
TNM T4, N1, M0 or any T, N2–3, M0
The cancer has spread to the internal iliac and/or groin lymph nodes on one or both sides or has spread to adjacent organs such as the vagina, urethra or bladder. Metastatic disease to the groin (inguinal) nodes is a poor prognostic sign and markedly reduces the chance for cure, although cure is still possible.

Standard Treatment Options include combination chemotherapy and radiation therapy as in Stage I, followed by surgical removal of the remaining disease at the primary site. This may involve either a local excision or an abdominal-perineal resection with colostomy. Removal of superficial and deep inguinal lymph nodes for residual tumor on one or both sides can be done in a separate operation.

Another option is an abdominal-perineal resection of the primary tumor as the initial treatment, with delayed removal of superficial and deep inguinal nodes.

Five-Year Survival 10 percent

STAGE IV
TNM Any T, any N, M1
The cancer has spread to the tail bone (sacrum), to distant lymph nodes within the abdomen far from the original cancer site or to other organs in the body such as the vagina, urethra, bladder, liver and/or lung.

Standard Treatment There is no standard treatment for patients with metastatic anal carcinoma. Relieving the symptoms produced by the primary cancer is the major consideration.

Palliation Treatment options include palliative surgery, palliative radiation and palliative combined chemotherapy and radiation.
♦ Abdominal-perineal resection is sometimes needed to control pain, bleeding or infection caused by tumor breakdown.

♦ Radiation has helped control pain and bleeding. The use of radiosensitizing drugs may improve local control.

♦ Endoscopic laser treatment has been used to reduce local tumor obstruction and also, sometimes, to control bleeding (*see* Chapter 9).

♦ Combination chemotherapy with 5-FU + mitomycin or 5-FU+ cisplatin as well as bleomycin or investigational combinations (see below) can be considered. For those who don't respond to these drugs, cisplatin + 5-FU therapy may be a good salvage program.

Five-Year Survival Unusual

Investigational Various chemotherapy drug combinations are being evaluated, including:

♦ mitomycin + Adriamycin + cisplatin
♦ 5-FU + bleomycin + lomustine (CCNU).

TREATMENT FOLLOW-UP

Careful follow-up is essential. This includes a history and physical examination every two to three months for three years after treatment, then every three to six months for the next three to five years.

♦ Careful observation for signs of enlarged inguinal lymph nodes.

♦ Chest x-rays and liver blood tests (alkaline phosphatase, SGOT) at follow-up visits.

RECURRENT CANCER

For a substantial number of patients, local recurrences of anal cancer after chemotherapy and/or radiation therapy or surgery can occasionally be controlled by various treatments. Surgical removal of the recurrent tumor, the addition of various chemotherapy protocols with or without radiation and the use of radiosensitizers and endoscopic laser treatments can improve the local control.

Current investigational programs—including combinations of mitomycin + cisplatin + Adriamycin and bleomycin + lomustine (CCNU)—have been variably effective in controlling metastatic and/or recurrent disease.

THE MOST IMPORTANT QUESTIONS YOU CAN ASK

♦ How should anal cancer be evaluated?
♦ How do different pathologic types affect prognosis?
♦ How does staging affect prognosis?
♦ Can anal cancer be cured without surgery?
♦ What new advances in therapy are being used to reduce the need for a colostomy?
♦ What are the roles of local radiotherapy and of chemotherapy?

BILE DUCT

Alan P. Venook, MD

◇

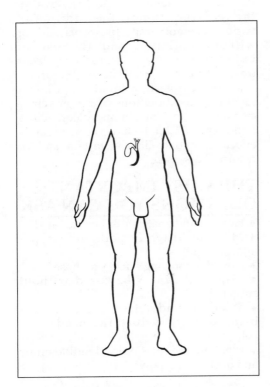

Bile is manufactured in the liver and helps the body digest fats. The bile ducts course throughout the liver collecting bile, then travel beyond the liver to connect with the gall bladder and small intestines (*see* page 336). Bile duct cancers may, therefore, arise in many locations in and around the liver.

Bile duct cancer—also called cholangio-carcinoma—is a rare cancer, and the prognosis depends largely on where the tumor begins and how large it has grown by the time of diagnosis. The only definitive treatment is the complete surgical removal of the tumor, which is not often possible. If the cancer cannot be entirely removed, the principal goals of therapy become the relief of symptoms caused by the accumulation of bile, and relief from pain.

Types The vast majority of these tumors develop in glandular tissue within the bile duct (adenocarcinoma). Other tissue types include squamous carcinomas and sarcomas. The therapy for all types of bile duct cancer is the same, depending on the extent of the tumor at the time of diagnosis.

How It Spreads Bile duct cancer tends to spread into the adjacent liver, along the bile duct surface and through the lymph system to lymph nodes in the region of the liver (porta hepatis). Tumors in the bile duct leading from the gall bladder to the common bile duct (cystic duct) can spread to involve the gall bladder. Ultimately, other lymph nodes may become involved, as well as other organs within the abdomen.

What Causes It The cause is unknown. People with chronic inflammatory processes, such as ulcerative colitis or parasitic infections of the bile ducts, are at higher risk for developing this cancer. But no one cause has been clearly demonstrated.

RISK FACTORS

At Significantly Higher Risk
♦ Chronic infection with the liver fluke Clonorchis sinensis, which is prevalent in parts of Southeast Asia. People may become infected with this parasite by eating raw or pickled freshwater fish from this region. Most people with this infection do not develop cancer, however.
♦ People with chronic ulcerative colitis

have a higher incidence of both benign inflammatory processes of the bile ducts (sclerosing cholangitis) and bile duct cancer.

♦ People with congenital abnormalities of the bile ducts (choledochal cysts) are more likely to develop bile duct cancer.

SCREENING

There are no screening methods to detect bile duct cancer at an early stage.

COMMON SIGNS AND SYMPTOMS

There are no signs or symptoms that indicate bile duct cancer. It usually develops slowly and the symptoms are often very subtle. Jaundice (the skin turning yellow) and itching are the most common signs. Jaundice is caused by the accumulation in the skin of a component of bile (bilirubin) that normally empties into the intestines after traveling through the bile ducts.

Bloating, weight loss, decreased appetite, fever, nausea or an enlarging abdominal mass are all signs that *may* be attributable to bile duct cancer. Pain usually signifies advanced disease.

DIAGNOSIS

Physical Examination

There are no specific findings on physical examination. Even if the findings associated with bile duct cancer are present, other explanations are far more likely. Findings may include:

♦ Jaundice.
♦ Fever.
♦ Tender mass below the ribs on the right side of the abdomen.
♦ Enlarged, hard lymph nodes.
♦ Swelling of the legs (edema) and fluid in the abdomen (ascites).

Blood and Other Tests

Diagnostic tests are usually done to determine the cause of jaundice. These tests may lead to the diagnosis of bile duct cancer, but a simple gallstone or other illnesses can cause the same problems and are much more likely to be the cause of the jaundice.

♦ A complete blood count may reveal a decrease in hemoglobin (anemia). A normal white blood cell count makes an infection in the bile duct (cholangitis) less likely, but an increased white count raises the likelihood of infection or cancer.

♦ Liver function tests may be abnormal, with the likeliest abnormalities being in the serum bilirubin and alkaline phosphatase, reflecting a blockage of flow within the bile duct.

♦ Prothrombin Time and Partial Thromboplastin Time (PT and PTT) are tests of clotting that may reveal a disorder in patients with poor liver function caused by an obstructed bile duct.

Imaging

♦ Abdominal ultrasound images of the gall bladder and bile ducts may reveal an enlargement of the bile ducts behind the blockage, since these channels will enlarge (dilate) when the pressure within the drainage system increases.

♦ PTC (percutaneous transhepatic cholangiography) involves taking an x-ray after a dye has been injected through the skin into the bile ducts. This can make a "road map" of the bile ducts within and outside the liver and may establish the site of the blockage.

♦ ERCP (endoscopic retrograde cholangiopancreatography) may be done to investigate the cause of an elevated bilirubin. This technically difficult procedure involves passing an endoscope through the mouth and into the small intestines. The physician operating this scope (endoscopist) identifies the site within the intestines where the bile and pancreatic ducts empty their contents. By injecting dye into this opening and doing an x-ray, a "road map" of the bile ducts may be made. PTC and ERCP may both be necessary to completely define the site and cause of an obstruction, and will correctly predict the presence of a cancer about 90 percent of the time.

♦ CT scanning assesses the extent of the tumor within the bile duct and its extension into the adjacent liver, lymph nodes or other structures within the abdomen. Often, bile duct cancer is not seen on a CT scan.

♦ Magnetic resonance imaging (MRI) may be helpful in determining if the bile duct cancer can be surgically removed.

♦ If the diagnosis of cancer is confirmed or suspected, a chest x-ray should be done to look for tumor nodules in the lungs that would confirm the distant spread of the cancer.

Endoscopy and Biopsy

♦ Biopsy, either with a fine needle (FNA) or regular needle, can be done through the skin without significant danger or through the scope when ERCP is done. The tumor cells may also be found in the bile; they are characteristic. Their presence may help decide whether surgery should be performed if the other studies also suggest the tumor has spread. It can be difficult to obtain an adequate biopsy sample because the tumors are often small and lie within normal liver tissue.

STAGING

A TNM staging system is used for bile duct cancer, but when deciding which treatment option to use there are really only two stages—localized and unresectable disease.

TREATMENT OVERVIEW

The optimal treatment for bile duct cancer is surgery. Unfortunately, by the time symptoms develop, the cancer has usually spread throughout the bile ducts and into the liver, meaning that the tumor cannot be entirely removed.

Chemotherapy and radiation therapy are occasionally useful to relieve symp-

toms. Although they have not been shown to be effective in curing the cancer, these measures can be taken to maintain the quality of life.

 Surgery The decision to take a surgical approach depends on the overall health of the patient and on the location of the tumor. If a patient is ill from complications of the cancer—jaundice or infection, for example— a drainage tube (stent) should be placed into the bile ducts to treat the complications. The patient then has to be allowed to recover before an operation is attempted.

If the tumor is in either the left or the right bile duct and hasn't spread to the lymph nodes, it may be possible to remove the tumor with its accompanying lobe of the liver because people with normal liver function do not need both lobes.

Tumors involving the junction of the right and left bile ducts (Klatskin tumor) create more problems. The tumor may not have spread, but its removal requires rebuilding the bile ducts. This can be done by removing all of the tumor and attaching a loop of intestine to the liver where the cut end of the bile ducts are draining (called a Roux-en-Y). This is a difficult operation and the overall health of the patient is an important factor in deciding whether to perform it.

Bile duct cancers can also occur at the far end of the duct, near where it empties into the intestine. Removing these tumors may also require a Roux-en-Y, as well as removal of parts of the intestines and pancreas (called a Whipple procedure). This extensive surgery is extremely complicated and has many side effects. It should be done only when a tumor has not spread beyond the local area.

 Chemotherapy Studies have not shown that chemotherapy can prolong survival, but the standard drugs used (mitomycin-C or 5-fluorouracil)

may cause tumors to shrink and help about 25 percent of patients. Even with tumor shrinkage, however, patients may not be better off after chemotherapy. The treatment has side effects and the tumor ultimately regrows.

There may be a role for chemotherapy after surgery, although this has not been studied systematically. In the hopes of finding a better chemotherapy treatment and improving survival, patients should be considered for clinical trials if chemotherapy is planned.

 Radiation Radiation is effective against bile duct cancers and may play a significant role. If the tumor is fairly small, it may be treated with radiation without causing much damage to the surrounding non-cancerous liver tissue.

Treatment may include placing a radiation-containing probe into the bile duct (brachytherapy). This therapy may also apply to patients with a small bit of tumor left after surgery or as a supplemental (adjuvant) therapy when the surgery is thought to have been complete. Studies evaluating the role of radiation therapy are ongoing.

Combined Therapy The combination of radiation and chemotherapy may play a role as adjuvant therapy. This treatment, which should be done as part of a clinical trial, may delay any recurrence of the cancer or even cure people who have already had surgery.

TREATMENT BY STAGE

LOCALIZED

At this stage, the cancer is confined to the bile duct. It is quite rare to find a bile duct cancer at this limited stage, for it would be unlikely to cause an obstruction of the bile flow when it is very small.

Standard Treatment Surgery can be done with hopes of a cure. The extent of surgery necessary depends on the tumor's location and size. It may be possible to remove a tumor limited to a small portion of either the right or left bile duct with its surrounding liver in a routine operation. But cancers involving the bile ducts at their junction within the liver require removal of liver tissue and then the complicated reconstruction of the bile drainage system. Tumors close to the intestine and pancreas may demand even more difficult surgery.

Whatever the extent of the surgery, tubes may have to be left within the bile duct system for a time to insure against bile leakage or the formation of scar tissue within the bile ducts.

It is not known whether drainage tubes should be placed through the bile duct blockage before surgery. If patients are ill because of the obstruction—the bile has become infected, for example—then a stent should be inserted to enable the patient to be in better condition for the surgery. Radiation to the tumor site is an alternative if patients are too sick to have surgery.

Unfortunately, even with meticulous surgery and careful screening, the majority of tumors will regrow within the bile ducts, in the nearby liver tissue or elsewhere in the body. So it is generally agreed that treating the surgical area with radiation after the tumor has been removed is useful in that it may help to destroy any remaining tumor cells.

The chemotherapy drug 5-fluorouracil is often given at the same time as the radiation in an effort to improve the effectiveness of treatment. This combination therapy is felt to be better than other treatments.

Five-Year Survival Up to 25 percent

Investigational Various combinations of surgery, radiation and chemotherapy may be considered. But because this is such a rare disease, it is difficult to study the relative benefits of newer treatments.

UNRESECTABLE

The tumor cannot be removed because it

has spread to local lymph nodes, liver tissue or elsewhere in the body.

Standard Treatment There is no standard treatment, so chemotherapy and/or radiation therapy clinical trials should be considered.

Significant relief of symptoms may be achieved. Patients with symptoms such as itching or infection may benefit from a procedure to create a bypass system for the bile. Such a bypass tube (stent) can be placed through the skin during percutaneous transhepatic cholangiography or through a scope during ERCP.

With the ERCP stent placement, the tube may drain into the intestines and a collecting bag may not be needed. Occasionally, neither of these methods drains the bile successfully. In that case, surgery designed to create a bypass channel may be done.

Two-Year Survival Less than 1 percent

Investigational
♦ Clinical protocols designed to test the additive benefit of radiation and chemotherapy are ongoing.
♦ Newer forms of radiation, such as hyperthermia (the application of heat to the region) are also being studied.
♦ Patients who wish to try chemotherapy may be offered new drugs.

TREATMENT FOLLOW-UP

Careful follow-up is important after the surgical removal of a localized cancer because once a recurrent tumor is large enough to be seen on x-ray, it is probably too large to be cured.
♦ CT scans should be done every two to three months for the first year after curative surgery, since an early recurrence may still be removed if it is small enough at the time of diagnosis.

SUPPORTIVE THERAPY

♦ Problems associated with jaundice can include severe itching and infections in the bile. If the drainage procedures described above are not effective, itching will often be relieved by Benadryl, Atarax or cholestyramine.
♦ Large doses of narcotics may be needed to relieve pain. Such drugs may have excessive side effects, since they are eliminated by the liver, which may not be functioning properly.
♦ Non-steroidal anti-inflammatory drugs may be surprisingly effective even against the pain associated with bile duct cancer.
♦ Frequent small meals may be necessary to get enough nutrition since an abdominal mass may reduce the size of the stomach.
♦ Water pills (diuretics) can reduce fluid in the abdomen or legs. They may cause significant imbalance in kidney function, however, and can create problems if not carefully monitored and adjusted.
♦ Nausea will often be relieved by standard medications, including suppositories.
♦ Loss of appetite may be helped by a drug called Megace.
♦ Sleep disturbances are common, but most sleeping pills are broken down by the liver, so they should be used carefully.

THE MOST IMPORTANT QUESTIONS YOU CAN ASK

♦ Should I see another physician to confirm that this tumor can or cannot be removed?
♦ Can the drainage of my bile ducts be done through my intestines so I won't have to have a tube coming out through my skin?
♦ Am I a candidate for an investigational therapy at another medical center?
♦ How sick will radiation and/or chemotherapy make me, and does the potential benefit make it worthwhile?
♦ Can anything be done to improve the quality of my life?
♦ Is the treatment worthwhile if the tumor is too advanced for surgery?

BLADDER

Alan Yagoda, MD

◇

Bladder tumors account for about 5 percent of new cancers (49,000 cases) in the United States. Bladder cancer ranks as the sixth most common cause of cancer and causes almost 3 percent of cancer deaths, about 9,700. It is the fourth leading cause of cancer deaths in patients over 75. While the average age of people who get bladder cancer is 68, this tumor is found in people as young as 45 to 55 years old.

Its origin is associated with certain chemical substances that induce or promote the growth of cancer (carcinogens). Men get it at a rate three times higher than women because of their greater exposure to such carcinogens in the workplace.

Five-year survival rates over the past 30 years have improved from 50 percent to over 70 percent, partly because the disease is being found in earlier stages when current therapies can be effective. Over 70 percent of cases are now being discovered with local tumors within the bladder. Only 20 percent now have regional disease just outside the bladder, while 3 percent have distant metastases.

Types The urinary tract is lined with what are called transitional cells, and more than 90 percent of bladder cancers originate from these cells. The layer of three to four transitional cells lining the bladder can grow to six, seven or more abnormal layers when they are irritated. Chemical carcinogens, chronic bladder infections, conditions called cystitis cysticia and cystitis glandularis, and chronic and repeated bladder trauma—repeated bladder catheterizations in paraplegics, for example—can cause cell changes that may turn into cancer.

This superficial layer of transitional cells is separated from the bladder muscle (which contracts to expel urine) by a thin, fibrous band called the lamina propria. The lamina propria separates tumors that are invasive (spreading into muscle) from those that are superficial (non-invasive). Treatment options depend on this distinction. Most bladder tumors are superficial and can be treated successfully.

Most of the remaining tumors—either alone or combined with transitional cell carcinoma—develop either in the glandular tissue (adenocarcinoma) or in an embryonic remnant of the gut (urachal tumors, also adenocarcinoma). In men, adenocarcinoma occurs in the urethra and its glands near the prostate. The remaining bladder cancers are squamous cell carcinomas, which are the most frequent type of urethral tumor in women.

There are also non-cancerous tumors called benign papillomas, labeled Ta, Grade I tumors. Fewer than 5 to 10 percent of patients with a benign papilloma will ever develop the more worrisome malignant superficial tumors (carcinoma in situ, or Tis) or muscle invasive tumors. Muscle invasive cancers probably go through a Tis phase, so even though Tis does not invade muscle the potential for invasion is implied. More important, Tis tends to recur again and again. Tis tumors, therefore, indicate an unstable, or sick, bladder lining.

How It Spreads Tumors can grow through the bladder muscle directly into the surrounding fat (perivesical) and into adjacent structures such as the prostate, vagina, rectum, uterus and pelvic bone. They also can directly enter the small blood and lymph vessels that supply the normal bladder wall. When they do, they can spread to local lymph nodes in the pelvis and farther up in the abdomen or be carried by the bloodstream to the lungs, bone and liver.

What Causes It Most of the time we are unaware of exposure to potent bladder carcinogens in our food and water supply, but some materials and the industries that use them have been strongly implicated with an increased risk for development of bladder cancer.

Bladder carcinogens include benzidine, bracken fern (sometimes used in salads), naphthylamines and aromatic amines, nitrosamines, some cancer therapy drugs (cyclophosphamide, Alkeran), various dyes and solvents, chronic abuse of some pain medications such as phenacetin and acetaminophen, and smoking cigarettes.

RISK FACTORS

The United States and Europe have the highest incidence of bladder cancer.

Cigarette smokers develop bladder cancers almost three times as often as non-smokers. Smoking may be responsible for 40 percent of bladder cancers in men and 29 percent in women. This relationship may be due to a substance called 4-ABP, a carcinogen found in tobacco smoke and the blood of smokers and which is known to induce bladder cancer. This substance disappears from blood within 90 to 120 days after a person stops smoking.

The relationship of tumors to the use of artificial sweeteners such as cyclamates and to coffee drinking is very weak. Recent studies have completely failed to find any risk above that of the general population.

Because chemical carcinogens and their breakdown products pass through the kidney down the urinary tract, the whole urothelial tract is exposed to these irritants and is at risk for forming new tumors. This is why people cured of one urothelial tract tumor have to be followed closely throughout their lifetime.

Those with a renal pelvis cancer, for example, are 21 times more at risk to develop another urinary tract tumor compared with the general population. Ten to 20 percent of those with a bladder cancer have been found to develop a superficial urethral tumor.

A good deal of work is now being done to evaluate agents that can prevent the development of such tumors. Much has been written about the testing of certain vitamin A derivatives for preventing tumors and for making early tumors revert back to normal cells. But high doses of the derivatives now marketed (vitamin A itself or beta-carotene) should be avoided, since the doses needed to prevent new tumors produce severe liver toxicity.

At Significantly Higher Risk
♦ Smokers, especially of cigarettes.

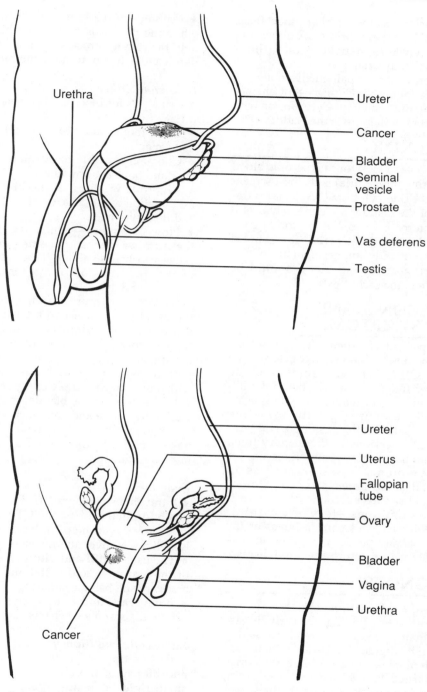

Urethra

Ureter

Cancer

Bladder

Seminal
vesicle

Prostate

Vas deferens

Testis

Ureter

Uterus

Fallopian
tube

Ovary

Bladder

Vagina

Urethra

Cancer

Overall view of pelvic organs showing bladder and surrounding structures

♦ Beauticians, leather workers, machinists and metal workers, printers, rubber and textile workers, truckers and those exposed to industrial dyes.
♦ Abusers of certain pain medications.
♦ People taking alkylating agent chemotherapy drugs, such as Cytoxan, or who have had radiotherapy to the bladder.

SCREENING

A urinalysis to look for microscopic blood in the urine (hematuria) is the best screening test. Urine cytology (PAP) and ultrasound of the bladder are extremely useful in symptomatic cases, but are too insensitive and not cost-effective for general screening. Bladder monoclonal antibodies for testing urine and blood should be available in the early 1990s.

COMMON SIGNS AND SYMPTOMS

Eighty percent of patients first go to their doctor because of blood and/or clots in the urine. Other urinary signs include increased frequency of urination, intermittent hesitancy, urgency, bladder spasms and pain or burning with urination (dysuria), difficulty passing urine and recurrent infections in the urinary tract. There are many more common reasons for such symptoms, however, such as an enlarged or inflamed prostate, stones, injury and various infections.

Late symptoms—loss of weight or appetite, fever, and pain in bones or the rectal, anal and pelvic area, for example—generally indicate more advanced disease.

DIAGNOSIS

Physical Examination
♦ There are few findings for early disease other than a bladder or pelvic mass discovered by digital rectal examination.
♦ With more advanced disease, there may be enlarged lymph nodes in the groin, abdomen or neck, a mass in the lower abdomen or an enlarged liver.

♦ Feeling the bladder with both hands while the patient is under anesthesia can help the staging process by indicating the depth and extent of tumor penetration.

Blood and Other Tests
♦ Urinalysis for blood in the urine (hematuria).
♦ Complete blood count (CBC) to evaluate anemia.
♦ Chemistry profile to evaluate kidney, liver and bone abnormalities.
♦ Vigorous washing of the bladder for examination of the cells (cytology, or PAP) and flow cytometry.
♦ Flow cytometry—which can measure the number of chromosomes in tumor cells—can help evaluate the effectiveness of therapy and tumor aggressiveness more accurately.

Cells having more chromosomes than the usual number of two are called nondiploid or aneuploid cells and have a worse prognosis. The disappearance of aneuploid cells after anticancer drugs are placed inside the bladder is associated with a prolonged complete response.
♦ In the near future, bladder monoclonal antibodies, alone and combined with flow cytometry, should help in screening, diagnosis, predicting the potential for metastases, and therapy.

Imaging
♦ Intravenous pyelogram (IVP).
♦ Abdominal and pelvic CT scans and chest x-rays can help find metastases to lymph nodes, liver and lungs.
♦ The use of MRI and ultrasound images of the abdomen and rectal and urethral areas are still being evaluated.
♦ Bone scans and bone x-rays are used before surgery only when there is bone pain.

Endoscopy and Biopsy
♦ Cystoscopy is the direct visualization and biopsy of the bladder by passing a small rigid or flexible tube through the urethra into the bladder.

STAGING

The TNM staging system is generally used for bladder cancer, although an alternative—the Jewett-Strong-Marshall system—is also used. There are slight differences in the two methods.

A major problem in clinical staging is the inaccuracy rate of 30 to 50 percent in determining precisely the extent of muscle and lymph node involvement when compared with the surgical or pathological staging of a tissue specimen.

In 20 to 40 percent of cases, high-grade (Grade 3) and high-stage (T3 and T4) lesions have lymph node metastases found at the time of surgery.

TREATMENT OVERVIEW

Treatment depends on the stage of disease. For superficial tumors that do not invade muscle, resection (cutting out), fulguration (burning out with heat or laser) or intravesical therapy (placing drugs directly into the bladder by a catheter inserted through the urethra) are the treatment options.

Therapy for muscle invasive lesions (Stages B, C and D) depends on the extent of invasion, the grade of the tumor and how involved the local lymph nodes and the blood vessels of the bladder are.

Surgery Removal of the tumor can often lead to cure. In selected cases where a single, relatively low grade tumor is found without carcinoma in situ, removing the tumor along with the adjacent portion of the bladder wall that guarantees an adequate margin (partial cystectomy) is appropriate.

But if the bladder shows evidence of "instability"—a tendency to continuously form new tumors as shown by the repeated presence of carcinoma in situ—a radical cystectomy is the treatment of choice. Radical cystectomy involves removing the entire bladder, the fat and tissue surrounding the bladder (perivesical) and the pelvic lymph nodes. In men, the prostate and seminal vesicles are removed. In women, the uterus, tubes, ovaries, anterior vaginal wall and urethra are removed.

Cystectomy raises many quality-of-life issues, especially concerning its effect on sexual function because of the nerves controlling penile erection being cut and the need for an ileal conduit (a piece of the gut or small bowel) leading to a large plastic bag outside of the body to collect urine.

Both problems have now been attacked and the various alternatives have to be discussed with a urologist. For instance, newer pouches (Kock, Indiana, Camay, Mainz, etc.) have a large internal reservoir and a small external opening (nipple) that requires self-catheterization to remove urine only two or three times a day. This is much more appealing cosmetically because the external nipple can be left uncovered or be covered with an adhesive bandage. In some cases, a "neopouch" can be used—an attachment of a piece of bowel directly to the urethra—requiring no external pouch or catheterization at all.

Sexual function in males can also be improved by penile implants or by medication injected into the penis before sex.

Radiation External radiation can be used for more advanced stages of bladder cancer. Overall, the five-year survival rate for muscle invasive disease with surgery is 30 to 40 percent; for radical external radiation therapy, 20 to 30 percent.

Chemotherapy When superficial tumors constantly recur, intravesical treatment is tried. This therapy permits direct contact of high concentrations of cytotoxic or immunologic drugs in the bladder, which bathe the superficial cancer cells for one or two hours. People with renal pelvis, ureteral and urethral cancers are not good candidates for intravesical therapy, although a few reports have described limited success.

There have been more studies of chemotherapy with single and combination drug regimens, before and/or after surgery or radiation therapy. If used before surgery (neoadjuvant), the aim is to decrease tumor size, increase the chance for a surgical cystectomy, destroy any tiny metastases that later seed the body but cannot be seen on x-rays or other imaging studies, predict good-risk versus poor-risk cases, lead eventually to bladder preservation (no need for removal of the bladder and creation of a pouch) and, more important, increase survival.

Some studies in limited numbers of patients suggest benefit with neoadjuvant chemotherapy combined with either surgery or radiation therapy, but others have found only increased toxicity. There is an urgent need to confirm the value of preoperative chemotherapy, and clinical trials have been started in the United States and Europe. Until the results are known, preoperative chemotherapy must still be considered investigational.

Patients with large bladder lesions (T4), nodal involvement (N+) or disseminated disease (M+) should be offered chemotherapy.

Laser Therapy Superficial cancers can be treated by laser vaporization-coagulation with Nd:YAG or carbon dioxide (CO_2) lasers.

Combination Therapy Therapy with preoperative and/or postoperative radiation has not been found to be as effective in improving survival as previously thought and has been abandoned in many cancer centers. The real problem after a cystectomy is the appearance of distant metastases in over two-thirds of patients despite excellent local pelvic control of the cancer.

High-grade, high-stage bladder cancers must be thought of as a disseminated disease. More systemic, instead of local, therapy will be required to improve survival.

Biological Therapy The best immunological drug is BCG vaccine (used for tuberculosis vaccination) given by catheter inside the bladder (intravesical) weekly for six consecutive weeks. Cystoscopy and urine cytology with flow cytometry at six weeks after the last dose are used to evaluate effectiveness. If a partial response is seen, that is, fewer lesions are found than previously, another course may be given. BCG is completely effective in more than 60 percent of cases and has been proven to be better than no therapy and all cytotoxic drugs.

People who respond completely to BCG not only have fewer superficial tumor recurrences but also develop fewer muscle invasive cancers requiring surgery. They also live significantly longer than non-responders.

Not all strains of BCG preparations are effective, and toxicity includes temporary local bladder irritation, fever and, in very rare cases, a type of tuberculosis infection that can be treated successfully with anti-tubercular drugs.

TREATMENT BY STAGE

STAGE 0
TNM Tis, N0, M0
Ta, N0, M0
In the Jewett-Strong-Marshall staging system, Stage 0 means the tumor is very superficial and does not even invade the lamina propria. It has not spread to lymph nodes and there are no metastases.

Tumors can be either a papillary exophytic mass (Ta or like a bunch of grapes on a thin stalk) or a flat Tis (Tumor in situ).

There is some controversy about the designation of Grade I (very well-differentiated) Ta lesions, since the malignant potential for spreading into lymph nodes or metastasizing is almost non-existent. Many urologists believe Ta Grade I tumors should be designated as non-cancerous benign papillomas, in contrast to Grades II and III Ta masses that are true cancers having the potential to invade their stalk and travel down into the lamina propria and then into muscle. People who develop one papilloma have about a 30 percent chance of developing another, while those with two or more have a 70 percent chance.

Standard Treatment Surgery is the first treatment of choice and is generally curative. There is almost no requirement for a total cystectomy for benign papillomas. In selected cases, however, a segmental or partial cystectomy may be appropriate.

Intravesical therapy is used for recurrent papillomas, mostly as a preventive agent. Effective anticancer cytotoxic drugs include thiophosphoramide (Thiotepa), doxorubicin (Adriamycin), mitomycin-C and, in Europe, epodyl (Ethoglucid). Complete tumor regression succeeds in 20 to 45 percent of cases. More important, none of these drugs seem to be cross-resistant with each other or with immunological drugs. About 30 percent of patients have complete tumor disappearance.

Patients with diffuse recurrent Tis or who fail one or more trials of intravesical therapy should be considered for cystectomy.

In the United States, external radiotherapy, radiation seeds or needles and intraoperative radiation therapy have not yet been proven effective in controlling or in preventing Stage 0 disease.

Five-Year Survival Over 90 percent

Investigational
♦ New immunological drugs—interferon, interleukin-2, tumor necrosis factor, keyhole-limpet extract—are being evaluated.
♦ New cytotoxic drugs such as epirubicin and mitoxantrone are being tested.

♦ Photodynamic laser therapy uses a photosensitizing material called hematoporphyrin that is similar to that found in red blood cells. Hematoporphyrin is unique in that it goes into all cells but remains for a prolonged time only in cancer cells. A specific wavelength of light generated by a laser will change the hematoporphyrin retained within the cancer cell into a toxic drug. This technique is still experimental and needs much more study before it can be used for carcinoma in situ.

STAGE I or A
TNM T1, N0, M0
The tumor is superficial. It does not invade through the lamina propria and cannot be felt. There is no spread to lymph nodes and no metastases.

Standard Treatment Same as for Stage 0.

Five-Year Survival Over 75 percent

Investigational Same as for Stage 0.

STAGE II or B1
TNM T2, N0, M0
The tumor invades through the lamina propria into the inner half of muscle. Using two hands, the physician can feel the tumor before surgery.

Standard Treatment Surgery via the cytoscope can cure low-grade T2 lesions in highly selected patients. A partial or segmental cystectomy when the bladder is otherwise normal can be curative too. However, staging errors approach 50 percent, and if the T2 tumor is high grade (Grade III) or invades blood vessels it probably should be considered as a higher stage T3 or B2 lesion. In that case, a radical cystectomy is the preferred treatment, as it is for most T2 cancers.

Radiation therapy after complete removal of a T2 tumor with removal of the bladder at first sign of local relapse (salvage cystectomy) is another option that has produced almost similar results.

Five-Year Survival 55 to 70 percent, depending on tumor grade and the accuracy of staging

Investigational
♦ Several new approaches are being explored—interstitial radioactive implants, intraoperative radiation therapy, intravesical hematoporphyrins plus photodynamic laser therapy and hyperthermia with radiation.
♦ Combination of radiation therapy plus chemotherapy with cisplatin, and more recently with three and four drug chemotherapy regimens—called CMV, MCV (followed by radiation plus cisplatin) and M-VAC—look very promising. Some early results have described 60 to 70 percent complete remission rates with bladders being preserved in limited numbers of cases. These rates were discovered clinically (by cystoscopy), however. Only 20 to 30 percent have been found to be truly tumor-free with pathological staging after surgery.

Follow-up has been much too short to determine five-year disease-free survival. Results of new clinical trials will have to be reviewed before these new combinations are accepted as superior to the "gold-standard" of cystectomy.

STAGE III or B2 and C
TNM T3, N0, M0
A tumor that invades deeply into muscle (more than halfway through) is designated as T3a, or B2 by the Jewett-Strong-Marshall system. If it invades into perivesical fat, it is a T3b, or C by the Jewett-Strong-Marshall system.

About 35 percent of clinical Stage III cases show tumor invasion outside the bladder at the time of surgery, so survival statistics vary. For those having tumors outside the bladder, survival is low—about 20 percent—with most relapsing from distant metastases. Survival rates are much better—30 to 50 percent—for true Stage III cases that have a lower grade and

in those cases where the tumor can be downstaged (reduced) after preoperative radiation therapy or chemotherapy alone or after radiation therapy plus cisplatin.

Standard Treatment Cystectomy.

Five-Year Survival 25 to 45 percent

Investigational Treatment for this stage is becoming controversial. Since most patients do not do well with cystectomy alone, many investigators are entering patients into clinical trials that will answer the important question of how effective neoadjuvant therapy is in increasing survival.
♦ Two national protocols under investigation are: chemotherapy with M-VAC versus no chemotherapy before cystectomy; and MCV chemotherapy followed by combined radical (doses of 7,000 cGy) radiation therapy plus cisplatin.

Preliminary results suggest that patients downstaged from a T3 to a much lower stage tumor fare much better. Until results of prospective randomized trials are available, these approaches must still be considered investigational. Patients are urged to participate in these studies so that correct answers to the true value of neoadjuvant therapy can be discovered.

STAGE IV or D
TNM T4, N0, M0
Any T, N1–3, M0
Any T, any N, M1
The tumor invades adjacent organs such as the prostate, uterus and vagina alone (T4a, N0, M0 / D1), or it spreads to the pelvic bone and abdominal wall (T4b, N0, M0 / D1), to pelvic lymph nodes (any T, N1–3, M0 / D1), to abdominal lymph nodes (any T, N4, M0 / D2) or to other organs (any T, any N, M1 / D2).

Almost half of Stage IV cases will be found, during surgery, to have lymph node involvement. The cystectomy fails because metastases occurred before the operation. Over 50 percent of patients with D2 disease die within one year, over 80 percent within two years.

Standard Treatment Patients with extensive nodal disease should first be treated with chemotherapy. Only if the tumor completely disappears should cystectomy be considered as an adjuvant form of therapy.

Cystectomy, with or without radiation therapy, can be beneficial in a very limited number of T4a, N0–1, M0 cases, but if more than microscopic nodal involvement is found, adjuvant chemotherapy could be used. There is still no clear-cut proof that adjuvant chemotherapy is beneficial, but the prognosis for Stage IV is so poor that some form of additional treatment could be tried, preferably within the context of a clinical study.

Five-Year Survival 5 percent

Investigational
♦ Chemotherapy and chemoradiation therapy programs.

RECURRENT OR METASTATIC CANCER

Cisplatin, methotrexate, doxorubicin (Adriamycin) and vinblastine are active single chemotherapy agents and have been combined into a number of programs. Popular regimens include:
♦ methotrexate + vinblastine + Adriamycin + cisplatin (M-VAC) Studies have proven that M-VAC is better than both CISCA and cisplatin alone and is the treatment of choice. Thirty-five to 70 percent of patients will respond, with 15 to 35 percent having a complete tumor regression that sometimes lasts more than five years.

The use of M-VAC is limited, however, by the need to maintain good kidney function (cisplatin and methotrexate are both excreted by the kidney) and the require-

ment that the patients cannot have cardiac abnormalities because of Adriamycin toxicity. CMV can be given to those who cannot take Adriamycin. Even when kidney and heart function are normal, full doses of Adriamycin or M-VAC can result in major complications in almost a quarter of cases.
♦ Investigational studies suggest that toxicity can be decreased and even higher M-VAC doses can be given when combined with granulocyte macrophage-colony stimulating factor (GM-CSF) or granulocyte-colony stimulating factor (G-CSF).
♦ cisplatin + cyclophosphamide + Adriamycin (CISCA)
♦ methotrexate + cisplatin (MP)
♦ cisplatin + methotrexate + vinblastine (CMV or MCV)
♦ Other single drugs that show some anti-tumor activity against bladder cancer include 5-fluorouracil, mitomycin-C, carboplatin and other new platinum derivatives. Therapy remains limited for adenocarcinomas, although some respond to 5-fluorouracil combinations.
♦ Radiation therapy can be palliative for bone and brain metastases.
♦ Immunological agents have not yet been adequately tested for this tumor.

THE MOST IMPORTANT QUESTIONS YOU CAN ASK
♦ What stage is my cancer?
♦ Do I need surgery, and how extensive would it be?
♦ What is the role of radiotherapy or chemotherapy?
♦ When do you place drugs into the bladder instead of doing surgery?
♦ How can I control my urine after my bladder is removed?
♦ How can I function sexually?
♦ If my bladder doesn't have to be removed, how often do I need to have cytoscopy performed?

BRAIN TUMORS: ADULT

Malin Dollinger, MD

◇

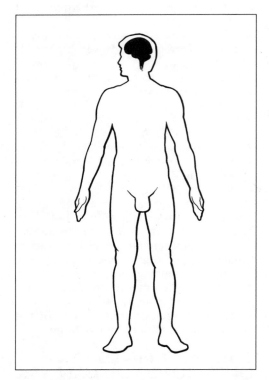

Primary brain tumors—those that arise in the brain rather than spreading there from other areas—make up about 1 percent of all cancers in the United States (12,000 cases a year) and cause about 2.5 percent of cancer deaths. They are the most common solid tumors in children (*see* "Childhood Cancers: Brain Tumors"). In adults, there is a steady rise in incidence with age, the peak occurring between the ages of 50 and 55.

The brain is also a frequent site of metastasis from other tumors, most commonly cancers of the breast, lung and kidney and malignant melanoma. Multiple tumors are more common if they are metastatic, although a single metastasis can occur and may mimic a brain tumor. A previous diagnosis of a cancer elsewhere, however, would make the physician suspect a metastasis rather than a primary brain tumor. The brain can also be involved by the direct extension of nasal tumors.

Types Brain tumors arise from various types of cells in the brain, with tumors of supporting tissues being more common than nerve cell tumors. These tumors tend to be named after the kind of cell they arise in. A tumor of the astrocyte—a neuron-support cell—is referred to as an astrocytoma. A tumor of the cells lining the open areas inside the spinal cord and brain is an ependymoma. A tumor of the neurons may be a ganglioneuroma, neuroblastoma or retinoblastoma. There are more rare tumors of specialized cells within the brain, such as germinoma, pinealoma, chordoma and choroid plexus carcinoma.

What Causes It A high percentage of brain tumors have no known cause. A few unusual diseases have a significant association—such as neurofibromatosis, tuberous sclerosis, familial polyposis and the Osler-Weber-Rendu syndrome—but these are all extremely rare.

A variety of statistical and environmental associations have been made, but except for the known association between vinyl chloride and gliomas, no chemical or environmental agent is definitely linked.

Viruses have been implicated in the development of brain tumors in animals, but direct injection into the brain is needed to produce them. No definite association has been established in humans, although there is an association in patients with the Epstein-Barr (EB) virus and primary brain lymphomas.

The idea of an injury or trauma producing brain tumors is probably the result of coincidence. The trauma may have resulted from a seizure due to the tumor, or minor trauma may produce more clinically significant symptoms if a tumor is already present.

An association between gliomas and diabetes has not been definitely proved. There is a very high risk (over 300 times) for developing primary central nervous system lymphoma in immunosuppressed patients, following organ transplantation or with AIDS.

Multiple meninginomas (tumors of the outer lining of the nervous system) are more common in Israel, perhaps because of the (now-discarded) practice of treating scalp fungus infections (ringworm) with radiotherapy.

SCREENING

There are no useful screening measures in healthy people. If a physician suspects a tumor on the basis of the characteristic clinical signs, careful neurologic evaluation as well as CT scanning will lead to an earlier diagnosis and the best chance for long-term control or cure.

COMMON SIGNS AND SYMPTOMS

There are two broad categories of symptoms. The first results from the increase in pressure in the brain as the tumor expands. The skull is hard and cannot yield, resulting in symptoms such as:

♦ Headache, which is often generalized. It is persistent and worsens with activity such as straining. It is often worse at night or in the early morning.

♦ Vomiting, which may or may not be associated with nausea. It is more common in children than in adults.

♦ Seizures. The onset of seizures in an adult without any history of seizures strongly suggests a brain tumor and appropriate examinations including CT or MRI scans should be done promptly.

♦ Change in mental ability or personality. Sometimes these changes will be obvious to the family and not to the patient, or vice versa.

♦ Lethargy.

The other category of symptoms has to do with the tumor's location and the pressure effects it produces on nearby structures. There are many types of local symptoms, including weakness of various parts of the body, especially an arm or a leg, difficulties in coordination or balance, impairment of memory, various vision defects, speech problems, changes in sensation and, in the case of brain stem tumors, defects in the functioning of nerves that exit from the base of the brain. These symptoms and signs may help determine the tumor's location.

DIAGNOSIS

Often a neurologist or neurosurgeon needs to evaluate the patient. Although an excellent tentative location can be suggested on the basis of a careful history (from the family as well as the patient) and neurologic evaluation, CT and MRI scans will usually confirm the suggested location and enable treatment planning to begin immediately.

Physical Examination
♦ As well as a complete neurologic examination, specific tests such as visual field determinations and hearing tests are sometimes useful.

Blood and Other Tests
♦ Cerebrospinal fluid is obtained by lumbar puncture. It may be examined for markers produced by some tumors or searched for malignant cells from tumors that have a tendency to spread from the brain into the spinal cord or its covering. A lumbar puncture may be risky when

①	Frontal lobe
②	Parietal lobe
③	Temporal lobe
④	Occipital lobe
⑤	Cerebellum
⑥	Brainstem (Pons, Medulla)

Areas in the brain that develop brain tumors

there is increased pressure in the skull, although the risk has been largely removed now that CT or MRI scans can determine if enlargement of the fluid cavities within the brain (ventricles) or major pressure shifts within the brain are present.

Imaging
♦ Radiologic imaging by either CT or MRI. There are advantages and drawbacks to each of these methods, depending on the types of tumors and their locations within the brain.

On CT, for example, gliomas sometimes have abundant blood vessels (vascular) and brighten after intravenous contrast material is injected. Meningiomas also usually enhance with contrast material and, like other brain tumors, may have a characteristic clear zone (edema) around them. They are identified not only by the presence of calcium in the images but also by their location. Oligodendrogliomas and craniopharyngiomas may have both calcification and fluid (cystic) components.

MRI, even without contrast, tends to produce better images of soft tissues than CT, but with MRI it may also be difficult to distinguish between a tumor and surrounding edema (swelling). Some low-grade astrocytomas may not produce a definite diagnostic image on CT scan, but will on MRI. A new family of contrast agents has greatly improved the quality of

MRI images, as contrast (dye) enhancement did with CT.

One or the other of these techniques may be more useful in certain parts of the brain. The decision about which to use has to be made by the radiologist, working with the referring physician. CT and MRI are both satisfactory to follow the course of patients during and after therapy. CT is currently less expensive than MRI.

♦ Myelography (x-ray of the spine, after injection of contrast into the area next to the spinal cord) is occasionally needed to identify the spread of tumors within the central nervous system and to determine the extent of primary tumors of the spinal cord. Despite its near total replacement by MRI, myelography is still occasionally useful for uncovering tumors in the spinal cord and its covering.

♦ Electroencephalogram (EEG) and skull x-rays are often not required, although skull x-rays are occasionally needed to define the relationship of the skull to the tumor in order to plan the entry site for a biopsy or surgery.

♦ X-rays of the blood vessels of the brain (angiography) are infrequently done before surgery to see how close the tumor is to nearby blood vessels. This may assist the neurosurgeon in planning the complete removal of the tumor.

Endoscopy and Biopsy

♦ A tissue diagnosis is desirable and is usually feasible except when critical areas such as the hypothalamus or brain stem are involved. A needle biopsy can be done with very precise positioning of the needle in a process called stereotactic neurosurgery. The needle pathway (trajectory) is determined by computer to reach a target and obtain a tiny bit of the tumor with minimal risk of damage to the brain and surrounding structures, making a biopsy diagnosis possible.

♦ The new imaging techniques may provide a very likely diagnosis before the biopsy, but an exact tissue diagnosis is an important factor in deciding on the best choice of treatment.

STAGING

There is no useful staging system for primary brain tumors. It is difficult to know their exact size after CT or MRI scans and even after surgery. A tumor will often project into the apparently healthy brain tissue surrounding it, and these areas of tumor may be invisible on imaging studies.

Staging systems for medulloblastomas have described a progression of stages that reflect the size of a tumor, local extension and spread of tumor to the cerebrospinal fluid.

TREATMENT OVERVIEW

Brain tumors have a number of features that set them apart from other cancers.

♦ They seldom spread outside the central nervous system.

♦ Even tumors regarded as relatively slow growing or more benign can produce symptoms as severe and life-threatening as malignant tumors. This is because they may occur in a vital area of the brain or because when the tumor reaches a critical size, there is no room for it to expand within the surrounding skull. This puts significant pressure on key structures.

♦ The location of the tumor, as well as its cell type, is an important prognostic factor. A tumor in the brain stem, for example, has a poor prognosis.

♦ The brain has no lymphatic blood vessels to remove the products of tumor dissolution, so the tumor may not appear to shrink on CT or MRI scans even if treatment is successful.

♦ Unless a dramatic, early and sustained improvement occurs after therapy, it may be difficult for a long time to determine the response to treatment. Treatments may themselves produce temporary neurologic deterioration that might take weeks or months to clear.

♦ Most chemotherapy drugs cannot penetrate the blood-brain barrier to reach the brain, although a few agents can.

 Surgery Surgery is the principal treatment for primary brain tumors. With advances in imaging, earlier diagnosis, drugs to decrease brain swelling, sophisticated planning, preoperative and anesthetic management and special microscopes and surgical instruments, it is possible to remove significant amounts of tumor with relative safety.

Modern surgical instruments ensure maximum tumor removal with minimal disruption of normal brain tissue. These include the Cavitron ultrasonic aspirator, which disrupts the tumor by ultrasound and then removes it by suction. Specialized laser instruments have also become useful.

Surgery has a number of roles, including attempts at curative resection, gross total resection, incomplete or subtotal resection or simple biopsy. There are also procedures to relieve pressure, such as placing shunts within the fluid cavities of the brain.

Some tumors, especially those that are histologically benign, can be cured by their complete removal. These include neurofibromas, meningiomas, acoustic schwannomas and low-grade astrocytomas. Sometimes a tumor will be apparently controlled but will then recur. Another operation may be done in an attempt to improve control.

Radiation This is a secondary method of treatment for brain tumors—or a primary method if surgery cannot completely remove the tumor or is not possible. A complex, sophisticated science has developed to attempt to give effective treatment to the area of the tumor, which is usually larger than that which can be seen on CT or MRI.

Great care is taken to minimize the radiation dose to non-cancerous tissue, but there are still potential complications and problems such as swelling of the tumor or surrounding brain, destruction of nerve tissue and late changes in mental function.

Novel ways of giving radiation have recently been developed. More than one treatment may be given in a day (hyperfractionation), temporary or permanent radioactive seeds can be placed within the tumor (interstitial radiation), radiation-sensitizing drugs may be used, as well as other types of radiation beams produced by special sources.

Radiation therapy appears to produce a modest improvement in survival when given after surgery for the more common types of brain tumors.

A very new investigational method called the video tumor fighter involves surgically placing a metallic pellet within the tumor. The pellet is heated by radio waves and, with the aid of a magnetic field, is moved back and forth throughout the tumor to destroy it.

 Chemotherapy Chemotherapy has been used as an adjunct to radiation and surgery, but many chemotherapeutic agents cannot cross the blood-brain barrier. The most commonly used drug is carmustine (BCNU), but others include cisplatin, vincristine, procarbazine, hydroxyurea, cytosine arabinoside, cyclophosphamide, 5-fluorouracil and etoposide.

Novel methods of giving chemotherapy include intra-arterial administration directly into the tumor area, chemotherapy following disruption of the blood-brain barrier by an intra-arterial sugar (mannitol), as well as high-dose chemotherapy with autologous bone marrow rescue.

Giving both radiotherapy and chemotherapy after surgery produces a still greater improvement in survival for some tumors. If the tumor is supplied by excess large blood vessels (hypervascular tumor), therapeutic angiography can block the blood supply. This procedure, called embolization, may make it easier to remove the tumor surgically. It is also used to deliver chemotherapy drugs though a catheter directly into the tumor.

TREATMENT BY TUMOR TYPE

ASTROCYTOMA

These tumors are classified according to grade.

Standard Treatment A Grade I astrocytoma is often curable. Standard treatment is surgery or surgical removal plus radiation therapy if there is known or suspected residual tumor after the operation.

Grade II tumors are less often curable with the same standard treatment of surgery plus radiation therapy. Some investigational protocols currently evaluate the addition of radiation therapy as well as chemotherapy.

The cure rate for Grade III tumors is low, with the standard treatment of surgery plus radiation therapy.

Five-Year Survival About 50 percent for Grade I tumors, about 25 percent for Grade II, and 10 to 20 percent for Grade III tumors

Investigational
♦ Forms of treatment being studied include radiosensitizing drugs, heat therapy (hyperthermia), intraoperative radiation therapy and new chemotherapy drugs and biologic agents.
♦ Clinical study protocols should be considered for tumors that cannot be completely removed.

GLIOBLASTOMA MULTIFORME
Standard Treatment This is a very rapidly growing tumor. The standard treatment is surgery combined with radiation therapy, with or without chemotherapy. Survival is generally poor. Patients are candidates for investigational protocols similar to those for Grade III astrocytomas.

Chemotherapy and improved surgical techniques such as fluorescein mapping of tumor borders and ultrasound intraoperative imaging have been associated with doubling the survival time (once the tumor is diagnosed) and improving the quality of life.

Five-Year Survival Less than 5 percent

BRAIN STEM GLIOMAS
These tumors arise at the base of the brain and in most cases are diagnosed and treated on clinical grounds. A biopsy may be unwise because of the risk of the procedure, although in some specialized centers, sophisticated instruments have allowed for biopsy and radioactive seed implantation without excessive risk.

Standard Treatment Therapy is generally radiation therapy alone. MRI and CT have allowed for detailed visualization of these lesions.

Five-Year Survival 30 to 60 percent

EPENDYMOMA
This slow-growing tumor starts in the membranes lining the cavities of the brain (ventricles).

Standard Treatment This tumor can often be cured if it can be completely removed. Radiation is added if there is known or suspected tumor remaining after surgery.

Five-Year Survival 40 to 60 percent

CRANIOPHARYNGIOMA
These tumors occur more often in children than in adults but are seen at all ages (*see* "Childhood Cancers: Brain Tumors"). They occur in the central portion of the brain and cause increased pressure within the skull (intracranial) as well as various eye symptoms, depending on their size.

Standard Treatment Microsurgery is the standard treatment, if the tumor can be totally removed.

Radiation therapy may be quite effective and may be used in combination with subtotal surgical resection. These decisions depend on clinical and CT and MRI observations.

Five-Year Survival 80 to 90 percent

MEDULLOBLASTOMA

This tumor resembles a similar and much more common tumor of childhood. The peak incidence occurs between the ages of five and nine, with a second peak between the ages of 20 and 30.

Standard Treatment This tumor tends to spread within the central nervous system. Up to one-third of patients have malignant cells in the cerebrospinal fluid or metastasis along the spinal cord. A few patients will have metastasis outside the central nervous system.

Standard treatment consists of surgical removal, if possible, followed by radiation therapy if there are any known or suspected residual tumor cells. This tumor is quite sensitive to radiation therapy.

The entire cranial-spinal axis (brain and spinal cord) has to be treated.

This tumor is sensitive to a variety of chemotherapeutic agents. Clinical trials are trying to improve the effectiveness of chemotherapy by using drug combinations; already, several combinations have been reported to produce improvement.

Five-Year Survival About 50 percent

MENINGIOMA

This tumor arises in the covering of the brain and may be discovered because of seizures or dementia. Pressure symptoms may develop when it grows. Compression of adjacent brain tissue and cranial nerves as well as skull changes may occur. Since meningiomas can exist in a variety of locations, the symptoms can vary considerably.

Standard Treatment During surgery, as much of the tumor as possible is removed. If all the tumor cannot be removed, radiation therapy is given.

Five-Year Survival Over 90 percent (most are permanently cured) if all the tumor can be removed by initial surgery, 60 to 80 percent if not

OLIGODENDROGLIOMA

These tumors occur most often in people between 30 and 50 years old and grow more slowly than most other primary brain tumors. They usually have a long history of minimal symptoms before diagnosis. Seizures occur in about 80 percent of patients.

Standard Treatment Surgical removal is the standard therapy, followed by radiation therapy, because the tumor usually infiltrates the surrounding brain even when this is not clearly visible to the surgeon.

These tumors frequently recur in the previous site of surgery and a second operation may be necessary.

Five-Year Survival 90 percent

PRIMARY CENTRAL NERVOUS SYSTEM LYMPHOMA

These tumors are especially seen in patients whose immune systems have been suppressed. This may be because of inherited immunosuppressive diseases, after therapy for organ transplantation or other acquired conditions that suppress immunity such as tuberculosis, blood vessel inflammation (vasculitis), lupus erythematosus and Epstein-Barr (EB) virus infection. Primary lymphoma of the central nervous system has lately become a common manifestation of AIDS.

Standard Treatment The role of surgery is usually to establish a tissue diagnosis, since there are usually multiple lesions that are inaccessible and surgery is not curative.

Radiation produces improvement, but relapse may occur in one to two years. Studies are evaluating various chemotherapy combinations. It is clear that remissions can be produced, but it is not yet known which therapy is the most effective.

Five-Year Survival Unusual

SUPPORTIVE THERAPY

Anyone being treated for a brain tumor needs measures to combat not only the symptoms associated with the primary tumor but also the side effects of treatment.
♦ Nausea and headaches produced by the tumor may require antinausea medication and pain medication.
♦ Swelling of the brain around the tumor is common. This may be a reaction to the tumor and produces an effect on the brain equivalent to a lesion much larger than the tumor itself. Corticosteroid hormones, such as prednisone or dexamethasone (Decadron), will usually decrease the swelling and will often reduce the symptoms of the tumor quickly. This rapid reduction in symptoms is often a good prognostic sign, but is not associated with any actual effect on the tumor.

These medications are usually continued through the completion of radiation therapy and then are reduced as low as possible. They can often be discontinued. A few patients, however, need a very low maintenance dose of corticosteroid hormones even if the tumor is not active or has been controlled. In such cases, some of the original symptoms, such as headache, nausea or neurologic abnormalities, may recur if the steroid hormones are discontinued.
♦ A significant number of patients with brain tumors will require antiseizure medi-

cation (anticonvulsants), most commonly Dilantin and phenobarbital. These are usually given for at least six months and often indefinitely. The dosages are determined by control of the symptoms, as well as by drug blood levels, which are measured regularly. The dosage required to control seizures varies from patient to patient.
♦ Neurologic status may change or deteriorate because of a cascade of secondary effects on the brain rather than because of tumor growth. Factors causing apparent neurologic deterioration may include lowering the steroid dosage too rapidly, mineral or electrolyte imbalance, complications such as infections or metabolic problems, other medications, particularly for pain, and also the effects of radiation therapy. Tumor destruction from radiation may briefly produce waste products that may irritate the brain.

Because the brain lacks lymphatic blood vessels, there is no efficient method of removing the waste materials of tumor destruction. This is why tumors that may be responding to treatment may not appear to change in size. Many patients improve neurologically, even though the mass noted on CT or MRI scans may not appreciably change in size over a long time. The residual mass may be destroyed tumor and/or scar tissue or cystic structures resulting from treatment, without any tumor necessarily being present.
♦ Some patients who will eventually show improvement appear to become worse near the end of the first course of chemotherapy. This may be due to the tumor increasing in size slightly before being destroyed by chemotherapy, and may also be related to some of the factors noted, especially the lack of an efficient mechanism for removing tumor wastes and the swelling around the tumor produced by irritation from these wastes.

The minimal swelling in the tumor and its surroundings may produce a more significant increase in symptoms than would a tumor elsewhere in the body because the rigid skull prevents any increase in size without compression of other parts of the brain, producing even more symptoms. This may explain why the dosage of corticosteroids cannot be lowered below a certain "threshold" level in some patients.

"Remote" effects of cancer on the nervous system There are a number of clinical syndromes and patterns of neurologic malfunction that occur in patients with cancer without the cancer actually involving the brain or spinal cord. These are called remote (paraneoplastic) effects and most involve some type of muscle weakness or degeneration and sometimes sensory loss (numbness).

What causes these effects is not known for certain. It has been suggested that some toxic material from the tumor could be involved. Alternative explanations include an autoimmune response produced by the tumor or some hidden viral infection. Such known diseases as endocrine malfunction, vascular disorders, infections, nutritional deficiency and complications of cancer treatment should be excluded.

Most of these remote disorders have no successful treatment and may or may not improve even if the tumor related to them is successfully treated.

TREATING TUMORS OF THE SPINAL CORD

Many of the tumors mentioned previously may occur in the portion of the central nervous system below the brain stem, inside the spine. Most primary spinal cord tumors are benign but produce pressure symptoms because of compression of the cord and the nerve roots emerging from it.

The symptoms and signs of these tumors include:
♦ Decrease in sensation or strength in the trunk or extremities.
♦ Band-like pain that seems to surround the chest or abdomen like a belt.

♦ Weakness and wasting of muscles as well as lack of ability to feel temperature changes and pain (these symptoms are related to tumors in the central spinal cord).
♦ Problems with bladder or rectal muscle control.
♦ Impotence.

Standard Treatment An effort is made to remove as much of the tumor as possible without destroying vital nerve structures. MRI imaging is becoming more valuable for accurately evaluating spinal cord tumors, replacing the use of a myelogram (injection of dye into the spinal canal). It is essential to know the exact extent of the tumor, as it has to be approached surgically by removing part of the bone covering the spinal canal (laminectomy).
♦ Radiation therapy is generally recommended after surgery if the tumor could not be completely removed, although the dosage is limited because of the risk of damage to the spinal cord.
♦ Although there are no significant studies of chemotherapy for primary spinal cord tumors, if the tumor can't be completely removed it would be appropriate to consider the use of the same drugs active against brain tumors of similar types.
♦ Cancers arising elsewhere can metastasize to the spine or spinal cord and produce pressure symptoms such as pain, weakness or loss of sensation (numbness). Diagnostic methods are similar to those for primary spinal cord tumors.
♦ If there are sufficient pressure symptoms, especially weakness of the arms or legs, and the tumor is not known to be very sensitive to radiotherapy (lymphoma, myeloma), immediate surgery is usually required to prevent more weakness and paralysis. Since it is seldom possible to remove all the tumor surgically, these patients are also given radiation therapy to the involved area of the spine.

METASTATIC CANCER TO THE CENTRAL NERVOUS SYSTEM

One of the serious complications of cancer anywhere in the body is metastasis to the brain. This occurs in anywhere from a quarter to a third of all patients with cancer.

Brain metastases are more often multiple, so the finding of two or more brain lesions suggests that they are metastatic and not primary tumors. Primary brain tumors can occasionally arise in several locations, but specific features on MRI or CT scans will usually distinguish them from metastases. A single metastasis may also occur.

Whether a specific tissue diagnosis (biopsy) is necessary depends on the clinical situation. In a patient with a primary tumor that commonly metastasizes to the brain—such as lung cancer, breast cancer or malignant melanoma, especially if it occurs within two years of the primary diagnosis—and the primary stage was advanced, the finding of two or more lesions typical of brain metastasis on MRI or CT scans may be quite adequate to permit definitive therapy.

Conversely, in a patient who had a localized-stage primary tumor many years earlier, the development of multiple brain lesions and especially a single brain lesion may generate a search for a new primary cancer or a primary brain tumor.

Symptoms The symptoms are similar to those of primary brain tumors, including headache and various neurologic disturbances such as weakness, confusion, personality change or seizures.

It is important to rule out other causes of these symptoms, especially severe headache. Other diseases such as infections and various cerebrovascular events (strokes) such as hemorrhage or thrombosis may produce symptoms resembling those of brain tumors.

Diagnosis In evaluating these symptoms, similar diagnostic measures to those used with primary brain tumors are employed, including careful neurologic examination and CT or MRI scans. In a patient with a known diagnosis of malignancy, the CT scan is usually an early study done for evaluation of severe headache or other symptoms. The finding of brain metastases will radically change the intent and direction of therapy. This complication generally takes precedence over almost any other complication in a cancer patient. MRI is better able to visualize very small brain metastases than is CT.

Standard Treatment Initial therapy usually includes corticosteroid hormones such as Decadron. A rapid improvement suggests that subsequent radiation therapy will be effective. More aggressive and urgent measures are sometimes needed if the symptoms are severe, and these include special types of sugar (mannitol) given intravenously to reduce brain swelling. If seizures are a problem, hospitalization and/or antiseizure medication may be needed.

The role of surgery in the management of brain metastasis is generally confined to the removal of single metastatic lesions, especially if a long interval has occurred since the primary cancer was diagnosed and treated and there is hope that this is a "solitary" metastasis.

Surgery may also be done when the diagnosis is not known for certain, when a metastasis is present in an area producing severe or dangerous symptoms and when hemorrhage or infection within a tumor in the brain has to be controlled. Occasionally patients may need a specialized device (Ommaya reservoir) to administer drugs into the cerebrospinal fluid. This is a small rubber balloon with an attached tube that is placed under the scalp to provide easy access to the cerebrospinal fluid and avoid repeated lumbar punctures.

Much more often there are multiple metastatic lesions in the brain and only a short time has elapsed since the initial tumor diagnosis. In this situation, radiation therapy, usually to the entire brain, is the most effective treatment. It is assumed that there may be other lesions in the brain besides those visible on CT or MRI and that these might grow if not treated. Radiation seed implants (brachytherapy) are sometimes used.

The role of chemotherapy in this situation is uncertain. Studies are now attempting to demonstrate a role for chemotherapy as well as for immunotherapy.

Results of Treatment Radiation therapy may often produce modest improvement and add some months or even a few years to survival. The occurrence of brain metastasis in a patient with known cancer, however, generally suggests that survival is limited to a year or less. Exceptions do occur.

Treatment of cancer in most other parts of the body is generally deferred (unless it is in a critical or life-threatening location)

until the brain metastasis can be treated and some improvement shown.

Studies for the aggressive treatment of brain metastasis by combining surgery and radiation therapy, even including reoperation or surgery following radiation treatment, are under way. But unfortunately, trials of aggressive forms of therapy, particularly combined treatments, are difficult because of significantly impaired neurologic functions, tumor elsewhere in the body that is also producing major effects on important organs and other complications of the cancer or other unrelated diseases.

THE MOST IMPORTANT QUESTIONS YOU CAN ASK

♦ What type of brain tumor do I have?
♦ How does it usually behave?
♦ What type of surgery is most useful?
♦ Will I need radiation afterwards?
♦ Is there a role for chemotherapy?
♦ Will my symptoms go away?

BREAST

Malin Dollinger, MD, Ernest H. Rosenbaum, MD, and Christopher Benz, MD

◇

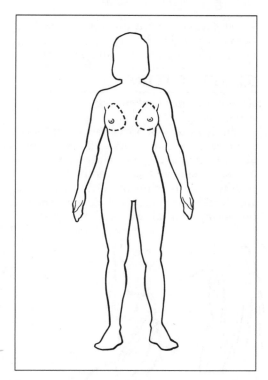

Breast cancer is the most common malignancy in women, affecting about one woman in 9. About 175,000 women will develop breast cancer in the United States in 1991, and about 45,000 will die of it. Breast cancer is most curable when detected in its earliest stages, and there is great interest in screening healthy women— beginning when they are between 30 and 40 years old— with periodic physical examinations, breast self-examination (BSE) and mammography. These measures will detect breast cancers at a much earlier stage, resulting in earlier treatment and a better chance for cure.

For decades, breast cancer was treated by one standard curative surgical procedure—the Halsted radical mastectomy. Women whose cancer was inoperable or who had residual or recurrent local disease were given radiotherapy. Those with metastatic disease were given chemotherapy and radiotherapy. Over the past 20 years, the approach to evaluating and treating breast cancer has changed considerably.

Types Breast cancers are divided generally into two types: lobular cancers that start in the many small sacs in the breast that produce milk; and the much more common ductal cancers that form in the tubes that carry milk from the lobules to the nipple. Within these broad categories, there are over 30 histologic types as seen under the microscope. About half are infiltrating ductal cancers, meaning that they spread through the duct wall. Another 28 percent are combinations of infiltrating ductal cancers and other types, including mucinous, papillary and lobular.

Infiltrating lobular carcinoma (5 to 10 percent of breast cancers), which is often detected as a thickening of the breast tissue rather than as a lump, may be found in many places, not only in the same breast but also in the opposite one.

Other infiltrating cancers include Paget's disease, a cancer that begins in the area of the nipple and is associated with bleeding, redness, itching and burning (this is not the same as Paget's disease of bone, which is a chronic benign process), and inflammatory breast cancer, which shows up as a hot, red, swollen area having the appearance of an infection or inflammation. This sub-type has a worse prognosis, because the red color and warmth of the skin indicate that tumor cells have already spread into many lymphatic vessels.

In situ cancers are confined within the lining of the ducts or lobules. They are not invasive but are believed to be the precursors of invasive cancers. In most cases, they have not yet grown into surrounding tissues and can usually be cured by limited surgery.

Nearly all breast cancers arise from glandular tissue (adenocarcinomas), although other types also occur, including squamous cell carcinomas, sarcomas, carcinosarcomas, cystosarcoma phylloides and sweat gland carcinomas. There are several less common types which have a generally better prognosis than infiltrating ductal cancer such as medullary carcinoma (6 percent of cases), mucinous (2.5 percent) and tubular (1 percent). Each type has prognostic and therapeutic implications.

How It Spreads After cancer starts, it may be several years before a lump appears. There are wide differences in the way a breast cancer behaves. It may remain confined to the breast for a long time, or, in other cases, spread to nearby lymph nodes and distant organs early in the disease.

What Causes It No definite cause has been established, although genetic factors, personal history and diet all play a role.

RISK FACTORS

At Significantly Higher Risk
♦ Increasing age.
♦ Family history of breast cancer, primarily in parents, daughters and sisters, but also in second-degree relatives such as aunts, cousins and grandmothers. This is true for relatives on the father's side as well as the mother's. (Genetic markers are becoming available to screen for some

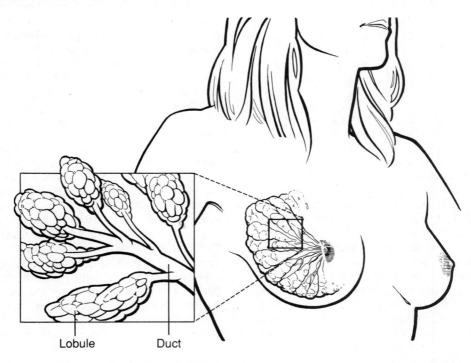

Lobule   Duct

Normal breast structures in which cancers may develop

forms of familial breast cancer.) The risk is about 6 times greater if a mother or sister had breast cancer before menopause, and up to 10 times greater if the cancer was in both breasts. A specific gene for familial breast cancer has been discovered (17q21).

♦ Some premalignant breast lesions may be associated with development of breast cancer, including multiple papillomatosis, atypical hyperplasia and, occasionally, very large cysts in the breast (not the more common and smaller fibrocystic breast condition). Most women with fibrocystic changes are not at increased risk because of them. There is no relation between these palpable breast changes and the risk of cancer.

♦ There is a slightly higher risk for women who have never carried a term pregnancy or who were first pregnant after age 30.

♦ History of previous cancer in one breast, especially if it occurred before menopause.

♦ Early onset of menstruation and late onset of menopause.

♦ Excessive radiation, with an increased risk for women who were given radiation for postpartum mastitis, received prolonged fluoroscopic x-ray evaluations for tuberculosis or were exposed to upper body radiation before the age of 40.

♦ Women with a family history of cancer of the cervix, uterus or colon have a slightly increased risk of developing breast cancer.

♦ Female descendents of European Jews have a higher than normal risk.

♦ Obesity with excess caloric and fat intake (three times the usual risk).

At Lower Risk

♦ Term pregnancy under age 18.
♦ Early menopause.
♦ Surgical removal of the ovaries before age 37.
♦ Japanese ancestry (but not if born in America and adopting American dietary habits).

Factors That May Affect Risk, but Whose Role Is Unclear

♦ Taking female hormones such as post-menopausal estrogens or premenopausal contraceptives. Some studies have suggested an increased risk with early oral contraceptive use or many years of estrogen replacement at menopause. Other studies have *not* shown an increased risk with either oral contraceptive use or estrogen replacement therapy. These findings need further study.

♦ A low-calorie, low-fat (especially animal fat), high-fiber or Oriental-style diet may decrease risk.

Factors Not Related to Breast Cancer

♦ Fibrocystic breasts.
♦ Multiple pregnancies.
♦ Breast feeding.
♦ Coffee or caffeine intake.

SCREENING

A thorough breast examination should be part of every routine physical and be included with a yearly gynecologic check-up. There are two well-proven methods for detecting early breast cancer:

♦ Monthly breast self-examination (BSE) can be taught by trained physicians and nurses. Most communities have centers to teach women how to perform this vital examination. It is far more likely that a woman will detect changes in her breasts earlier and more efficiently than would someone who examines her less frequently.

BSE identifies a significant number of women concerned about breast masses that are not cancer, as 90 percent of breast lumps are benign. But it can detect cancers earlier, when there is a greater chance for cure as well as for breast preservation.

♦ Mammography (low-dose x-ray imaging of the breasts) for apparently healthy women. This low-cost procedure is quick, simple and safe. There is now widespread agreement that it can discov-

Regional lymph nodes important in breast cancer

er cancers up to a year before they can be felt. The American Cancer Society recommends that women have a baseline mammogram done between the ages of 35 and 40, then have mammograms every year or two between 40 and 49 and yearly thereafter. When there is a family history of breast cancer or other risk factors, an earlier baseline mammogram and yearly mammograms after age 40 are recommended.

♦ The smallest lump usually felt is about 1 cm (1/3 in.), and contains 1 billion cancer cells. Routine mammography can detect smaller cancers less than 0.5 cm (1/5 in.). One 1987 study showed that the five-year survival was 22 percent better for cancers diagnosed by mammography compared to cancers diagnosed after a lump appeared. This technique now results in 60 percent of women having negative axillary nodes, compared to 50 percent 10 years ago. Smaller cancers

will also require simpler, less extensive therapy.

Some concern has been expressed about the risk of frequent x-ray imaging, but the potential benefits far outweigh any risk. The mammogram x-ray dose is about one-tenth of that 20 years ago and is less than the cosmic radiation received during an airplane flight. The risk of a mammogram causing a tumor has been compared to the risk of getting lung cancer by smoking one cigarette.

COMMON SIGNS AND SYMPTOMS

Breast lumps are found in most patients, although sometimes the lump is seen only on mammography and no mass can be felt. The cancer is often hard and irregular and may feel different from the rest of the breast. There may also be a persistent lump in the armpit (axilla), a symptom of

244

enlarged lymph glands. Pain in the breast is more often due to a benign condition, but medical evaluation is advised.

Spontaneous discharge from the nipple of one breast may indicate breast cancer but can often be due to a benign condition. Any cancer that first appears in this way is usually very small and has a high cure rate. There may be irregularity or retraction of the breast skin or nipple. Scaling of the nipple may indicate Paget's disease, a form of local nipple cancer.

In advanced cases, there may be significant swelling or distortion of the skin or breast. Skin pores may be accentuated because of lymphatic involvement, creating an appearance resembling the skin of an orange, known medically as peau d'orange. This may indicate the advanced stage called inflammatory breast carcinoma, which may also be signaled by redness, swelling or increased heat in the skin.

Breast cancer may occasionally first appear as metastatic disease, with signs or symptoms related to whatever other organ is involved—pain in an area of bony metastasis, swelling in the neck, lung nodules seen on chest x-rays or liver enlargement.

DIAGNOSIS

It may be difficult to clinically distinguish malignant from benign breast masses such as fibrous tumors (fibroadenomas), fatty collections, inflammatory masses, infections or cysts. In premenopausal patients, it is common for benign lesions to enlarge just before menstrual periods and then shrink.

It is often helpful for the physician to draw an exact diagram with a description of a newly detected mass. Mammography and/or biopsy may be useful, but if these are not done the mass should be re-examined one or two months later if there is any suspicion that it might be cancer. If the mass persists, mammography and biopsy should be considered.

Physical Examination

♦ Physical examination of the breast is conducted with the patient in various positions and with careful recording of any suspicious masses or abnormal findings.
♦ This should be accompanied by a complete physical, including a pelvic examination and evaluation for signs of cancer in other locations such as the skin, lymph nodes and liver.

Blood and Other Tests

♦ Blood counts and chemistry panel to determine organ function and detect metastases, including liver function tests (alkaline phosphatase, LDH and SGOT).
♦ Tumor marker blood tests—including serum carcinoembryonic antigen (CEA) and CA 15-3—may be performed to help determine prognosis and follow the course of the disease.
♦ Tumor tissue tests, including hormone receptors, DNA and other protein markers with potential diagnostic and prognostic value (*see* below).

Imaging

♦ Ultrasound can be useful in detecting and diagnosing breast cysts. The accuracy rate in determining whether a mass is cystic (containing fluid) or solid is at least 95 percent, which may eliminate the need for more complex procedures. Some physicians prefer to withdraw fluid from all cysts (aspiration) whether a mass can be felt or not and to have the fluid examined for abnormal cells. But in some centers a clearly benign cystic lesion on ultrasound is not treated further as long as the ultrasound criteria for a simple cyst diagnosis are met.
♦ Mammography is helpful in evaluating a suspicious mass, especially if it is new, persistent or in a woman whose breasts are larger and more difficult to examine or who has had breast implants. It is also used to locate precisely the position and extent of a known tumor. A two-view mammogram and special views, including magnification,

provide vital information, but a mammogram is not a definitive diagnostic test, since 10 percent of cancers (and a higher percentage in women under 40) may *not* be detectable by this technique. A suspicious mass should be biopsied even if the mammogram does not show cancer.

♦ Mammograms may show microcalcifications characteristic of cancer, although no mass may be present. Biopsy is then done, often guided by the mammogram.

♦ Mammography may also be used for screening or to help detect other masses that cannot be felt; evaluate patients with precancerous conditions; evaluate yearly the opposite breast in patients with known breast cancer, as there is a higher risk of developing cancer there; and evaluate women with metastatic adenocarcinoma from an unknown primary source. This last point is especially important because breast cancer may respond to chemotherapy hormonal management that would not be used to treat other forms of metastatic cancer.

♦ Chest x-ray to assess lungs and ribs for metastases and specialized x-rays of other areas if there are specific bodily complaints.

♦ Bone scan to rule out bone metastases. This is often not necessary with small cancers.

♦ Abdominal CT to evaluate the liver, especially if the serum alkaline phosphatase (a bone and liver enzyme) is elevated.

Endoscopy and Biopsy

♦ Fine needle aspiration (FNA) can determine if a lesion is cystic or solid. If a cyst disappears after draining by a needle and does not recur, no further treatment or evaluation is needed. Tissue should be removed by biopsy for microscopic examination if a mass is still present after fluid is removed, if blood is removed, if abnormal cells are found in the fluid, if no fluid can be aspirated or if the mass returns two weeks later (*see* biopsy diagram, page 248.)

♦ Almost all biopsies of suspicious breast masses used to be open surgical biopsies, but FNA biopsy is being used more often. This simple office procedure can usually give a definitive answer about the possibility of cancer, but interpretation by a specially trained cytologist or pathologist is necessary to evaluate the tissue correctly. About 1 in 20 aspirations does not confirm a malignancy when one is known to be present (false negative), so either a repeat FNA, a needle-guided biopsy or an open surgical biopsy should be done if mammography or physical findings are suspicious and the initial FNA is negative.

♦ Mammography may help guide the surgeon to biopsy the correct area. A benign cyst can overlie a malignancy, and the cyst could be biopsied by mistake, leading to a false sense of security. A mammogram of the biopsy specimen is often done to be sure the suspicious area has been removed.

♦ In stereotactic fine needle biopsy, computer-assisted x-rays allow the biopsy needle to be precisely positioned, especially for smaller lesions or localized microcalcifications.

STAGING

Stage is directly related to prognosis and determines the type of treatment to be offered, especially when several therapies are available. The TNM classification system is used to stage breast cancer according to the size of the primary tumor (T), the involvement of the lymph nodes in the armpit (axillary nodes) next to the affected breast (N) and the presence or absence of metastasis (M). The clinical stages range from Stage I to IV. Stage 0 is in situ cancer, which is still localized to the point of origin and has not yet begun to invade outward or spread. TNM staging for breast cancer is shown on page 256, 257, 260 and 261.

FACTORS AFFECTING PROGNOSIS AND TREATMENT DECISIONS

The prognosis and selection of therapy are influenced by the size, type and stage of the cancer, the microscopic appearance, the involvement of axillary lymph nodes and the number of nodes involved, and the woman's age and her menopausal status (natural or surgically induced) at the time of diagnosis. The larger the cancer, the more likely it has spread to axillary lymph nodes and metastasized.

They are also influenced by several other increasingly important prognostic factors. These tests offer predictive information about the risk of recurrence or metastasis. This may make it possible to identify women with a worse prognosis who should be offered earlier and/or more aggressive therapy. Prognostic markers also help oncologists tailor the most appropriate forms of adjuvant chemotherapy to each individual. These tumor tissue tests include:

♦ The measurement of protein receptors for two types of female hormones that affect breast cancer tissue—estrogen and progesterone. The tumor content of these receptors—positive or negative—correlates with prognosis and response to hormonal therapy.

♦ Flow cytometry for analysis of the tumor's DNA content. The average amount of cellular DNA in the chromosomes of the tumor—DNA ploidy—strongly correlates with the cancer's aggressive activity. Poorly differentiated tumors tend to have abnormal DNA content (aneuploid), and patients with these tumors will not generally do as well as those whose tumors have the correct amount of chromosomal DNA (diploid).

♦ Cell cycle analysis. Both normal and malignant cells go through a complete cell cycle known as mitosis. During one phase of the cycle (the S-phase), new DNA is synthesized in preparation for the division of one cell into two. Flow cytometry as well as other techniques are used to measure the S-phase fraction, or growth rate.

The percentage of tumor cells in this S-phase is an indication of how rapidly a tumor is trying to grow. As might be expected, tumors with a high S-phase fraction—in other words, growing rapidly—have a less favorable prognosis. The S-phase fraction for breast cancer can range from less than 1 percent to more than 20 percent of the cells

♦ Immunohistochemical detection of abnormal tumor proteins, including secreted enzymes and stress proteins. Lower levels of the enzyme cathepsin-D or specific "heat-shock" proteins, for example, are associated with better survival.

There are also abnormal oncogene and growth factor-related products. The product of the HER-2/*neu* oncogene is overproduced in about one-third of breast cancers. The overproduction appears to be associated with earlier tumor relapses and lower survival rates. Another promising marker is the epidermal growth factor (EGF) receptor.

♦ A recent study showed that the number and density of tiny blood vessels in the tumor could be correlated with the risk of metastasis.

Years of clinical testing will be needed to confirm how many of these tests add to our ability to identify individuals with a higher risk of relapse and reduced chances for survival. It is expected, however, that during the next few years many additional tests will be discovered and routinely performed on all breast tumors.

TREATMENT OVERVIEW

It is now standard practice for primary physicians, surgeons, radiation oncologists and medical oncologists to work together to plan and carry out each patient's treatment. Any one of these physicians can assume the role of "quarterback," serving as the leader for decision-making and conveying information to the patient and family and other members of the medical team.

Surgery In the past, the principal role of surgery was to perform a one-step procedure involving a biopsy of a breast mass, followed immediately by a radical mastectomy. A woman would often discover that she had had a mastectomy when she awakened from surgery.

Types of limited surgery, showing typical incisions and amount of tissue removed

Fortunately, in the past 20 years there has been a change to a two- or three-step approach. FNA and a limited biopsy are now done first, allowing for a rational and comprehensive discussion about treatment options with the patient and family. In some states, written information about the various options has to be provided to all patients by law.

Today's surgeon may choose to biopsy the mass with a needle, by incisional biopsy (especially a large mass) or by excisional biopsy, which involves removing the entire mass and is called a lumpectomy or tylec-tomy. Surgeons may also have to biopsy areas already suspected of being a metastasis. The biopsies should obtain enough tissue for hormone receptor analysis, other tumor tests mentioned previously, as well as for routine pathologic evaluation.

If cancer is found on biopsy, there are a number of options. The traditional Halsted radical mastectomy, seldom performed nowadays, meant removing the entire breast, axillary lymph nodes and the chest muscles. Today, a modified radical mastectomy—in which the axillary lymph nodes are removed but the pectoral muscles are not—may be performed in some cases, especially if the cancer is large. The surgeon might also remove just a portion of the breast in a procedure sometimes called a quadrantectomy. These lesser operations, if correctly chosen, have equivalent chances for cure and produce much better cosmetic, functional and psychologic results.

It is now also recognized that axillary lymph nodes are not an effective barrier to tumor spread. The nodes are removed not as a curative measure but mainly to provide information about the risk of recurrence and metastasis and to better define the need for adjuvant therapy. Removing all or some of the lymph nodes in the armpit—called axillary lymph node dissection and sampling, respectively—may be performed with either a separate incision during the primary operation or as a completely separate surgical procedure. Sampling is done in most patients, being omitted only if treatment decisions would not be influenced by the results.

♦ *Breast Reconstruction* Another role for surgery is reconstructing a breast after one has been removed. This is being done more often than it used to be. It is also being done earlier and with techniques that produce a more cosmetically acceptable result. An experienced plastic or reconstructive surgeon may see the patient before primary surgery to give advice and assistance, but is more often consulted near the end of therapy if the patient wants her breast reconstructed.

BREAST RECONSTRUCTION

Women who have had a mastectomy have a number of options to restore a more normal physical appearance, including wearing a breast prosthesis. But breast reconstruction greatly improves an overall feeling of wholeness. It eliminates the need for an external prosthesis and decreases the number of clothing restrictions.

There are now several ways to reconstruct the breast, each with advantages and disadvantages. There are also new ways of reconstructing the nipple. The opposite breast may have to be reshaped or made larger or smaller to provide the best symmetry. A team approach—where the plastic surgeon works with the primary physician, general surgeon and radiation and medical oncologists—generally leads to the most satisfactory appearance.

The first question to be decided is whether to reconstruct the breast immediately after a mastectomy or to delay the procedure.

The immediate approach has the advantage of creating a breast-mound from the beginning, which is less psychologically disruptive ("mourning" for the lost breast). Immediate reconstruction is appropriate in women with small cancers and negative axillary lymph nodes who wish to avoid an extra operation but realize that there is a slightly higher risk of healing problems. But if the tumor is large and a modified radical mastectomy has to be done, immediate reconstruction is not usually performed. The primary goal is curing the cancer. Satisfactory plastic reconstruction is a secondary goal.

The delayed approach has many advantages. It allows the surgical wound to heal. The surgical margins and axillary lymph nodes can also be evaluated by a pathologist, which may let both patient and physician make better decisions about the most appropriate and desirable technique to use.

Reconstruction is also delayed if radiotherapy and chemotherapy are used along with surgery. Both can cause low blood counts and impaired immunity, increasing the risk of infection, slower wound healing and other complications. Reconstruction is usually delayed for four to six weeks after radiation therapy is completed and two to three months after chemotherapy ends.

One-Stage Silicone Breast Prosthesis On rare occasions, a small silicone implant can be placed under the chest wall muscles during the mastectomy operation. This can be done in some small-breasted women who have had a minimal amount of breast tissue removed.

Advantages
♦ Re-establishes a breast mound in a single operation.

Disadvantages
♦ Does not generally produce a breast contour that is as natural-looking as those produced by other techniques.
♦ As with any silicone implant, there is a small risk of infection, which could lead to the implant's temporary removal.
♦ There may be long term side effects of silicone in some patients.
This is under intensive study and should be discussed with your physician.

Tissue Expansion Technique An inflatable silicone prosthesis is placed under the muscles in the chest wall and is gradually inflated with sterile salt water. This is done weekly in the doctor's office. Two to three months are usually needed before the breast reaches the size needed to match the opposite breast. The implant may be used for an extended time or may be exchanged in a simple operation for a permanent prosthesis.

Advantages
♦ The technique is simple and can be done on an outpatient basis under local or general anesthetic.

Disadvantages
♦ Takes a long time to complete.
♦ There is a risk of infection, as in the one-stage procedure.

Latissimus (LATS) Flap Technique This technique became very popular in the late 1970s and early 1980s. It is most useful when the lower chest wall tissues are tight or thin or when there has been some localized radiation damage after the mastectomy.

A silicone breast implant is used along with the broad, fan-shaped back muscle (latissimus dorsi), which is rotated around to the chest wall to replace the tissue removed during the mastectomy.

Advantages
♦ Adds fullness to the lower portion of the breast where it is most needed.
♦ Produces a more natural breast crease.

Disadvantages
♦ Skin from the back may be a different shade or texture.
♦ Creates an additional chest scar and a visible scar on the back.
♦ Transferring back muscles may impair muscle power for some athletic activities.

TRAM (transverse rectus abdominus myocutaneous) Flap Technique This is the most complex of the commonly used techniques and is not appropriate for all patients.

A portion of the vertical muscle in the center of the abdomen (the rectus abdominus) and a large ellipse of skin and fat from the lower abdomen are transferred onto the chest wall and shaped in the form of a breast.

Advantages
♦ Cosmetic results are generally pleasing. Skin transferred from the abdomen to the chest wall is usually a good match in color and texture.
♦ A silicone prosthesis is usually not required.
♦ A "tummy tuck" follows the transfer of skin and fat from the lower abdomen.

Disadvantages
♦ Possible weakness or hernia of the abdominal wall.
♦ Additional scars across the upper breast and lower abdomen.
♦ Involves a major, lengthy surgical procedure.

Microsurgical Free Flap Technique Along with the TRAM flap technique, this is the most recent method of breast reconstruction. Also like the TRAM flap, this procedure is sometimes carried out after simpler techniques have failed. It is performed infrequently and often as a last resort.

Tissue from the center of the abdomen, the back or the buttocks is transferred to the chest wall and shaped like a breast. Blood vessels from the free flap are attached to blood vessels in the chest wall by microsurgical techniques.

Advantages
♦ Similar to TRAM flap.

Disadvantages
♦ Additional scars.
♦ Requires the special skills of a plastic surgeon trained in microsurgery.

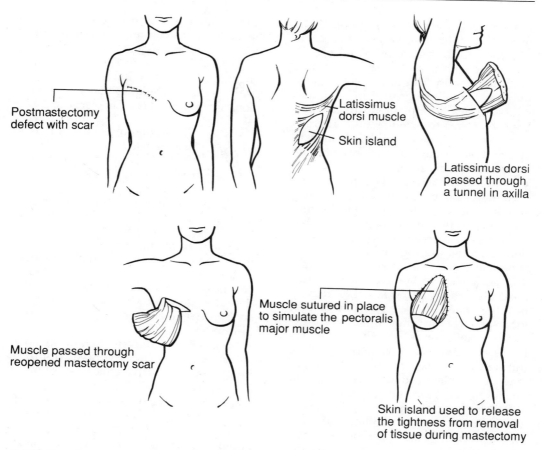

Postmastectomy defect with scar

Latissimus dorsi muscle

Skin island

Latissimus dorsi passed through a tunnel in axilla

Muscle passed through reopened mastectomy scar

Muscle sutured in place to simulate the pectoralis major muscle

Skin island used to release the tightness from removal of tissue during mastectomy

LATS breast reconstruction, using skin flap from back muscle

 Radiation Radiotherapy is a standard treatment for breast cancer, usually after the primary tumor and lymph nodes are removed.

Another use of radiation therapy as primary treatment is in postmastectomy radiation to the chest wall. This may be done if the tumor was found at surgery or after tissue examination to invade the skin or chest wall muscles, if it was very large or if many lymph nodes were involved. The assumption is that there may be hidden tumor cells in the chest wall or armpit (axilla) after surgery that can be eradicat-ed effectively by radiation. In addition to the chest wall, the area treated (the radiation port) sometimes includes the lymph nodes in the armpit or over the collarbone (supraclavicular nodes).

In patients who later develop chest wall recurrence, radiation therapy is often used (if the area was not previously treated with radiation), usually with a wide margin to kill the presumed microscopic tumor implants that could also be nearby. This therapy to localized recurrences may achieve permanent control over the cancer in up to half of patients.

Radiation is given daily, usually five

days a week, over about six weeks. The usual technique involves external beam radiation to the entire involved breast, sometimes with an additional booster dose to the tumor area. This boost may be given by an external beam or with radiation seeds surgically implanted directly into the tumor area (brachytherapy). There is no increased risk of a secondary malignancy or a breast cancer on the opposite side as a result of radiotherapy.

♦ *In Metastatic Disease* Radiation is often used in treating metastatic disease, both to shrink tumors and to relieve local symptoms such as pressure or pain. If metastatic bone lesions occur in a weight-bearing bone such as the leg, for example, the bone may fracture with very little injury. This is called a pathologic fracture. Such areas are usually given radiation to help heal the bone, decrease pain and control local spread of the tumor.

If a bone lesion is extensive, there may be a significant risk of pathologic fracture during the next several months it might take to complete radiation therapy and healing. An orthopedic surgeon is often called in to determine if a fixation device—such as a rod or plate surgically placed over the cancerous bone to stabilize it—should be used to minimize the risk of fracture during this time.

Similarly, pain in the spine or spinal lesions seen on a bone scan or x-ray should be promptly investigated. If a metastatic tumor is present, there may be a risk of compression fractures of the vertebrae (even on simple walking) or of pressure on the spinal cord by the tumor, which can result in paralysis. Tumors that spread to the neck are especially worrisome because compression and fractures there can lead to paralysis of both arms and legs (quadriplegia) as well as loss of bladder and bowel control (incontinence).

Pain is often produced by tumors pressing on nerves, and radiation may help relieve the pain by shrinking these tumors. As is true in other types of cancer,

the radiation dosage has to be kept low in some locations because of the limited tolerance of normal tissues.

Side effects of radiotherapy may include tiredness and skin changes, but with modern techniques major complications are infrequent (*see* Chapters 6 and 17).

 Chemotherapy Chemotherapy may be used either as an adjuvant therapy for high-risk patients following surgery or to treat metastases.

♦ *Adjuvant Therapy* Adjuvant or prophylactic chemotherapy and/or hormonal therapy is now given to most patients after surgery to try to prevent or minimize the growth of microscopic deposits of tumor cells that might grow into a recurrent tumor. Some patients with no obvious metastases at the time of surgery but who are at high risk for such micrometastases may be rendered disease-free.

Some uses of adjuvant therapy are now clearly defined and accepted. In other areas there are differences of opinion. There may be several acceptable alternatives depending on the preferences of physician and patient. Adjuvant therapy is a constantly evolving field, so an experienced and up-to-date medical oncologist should be involved in treatment planning from the time of diagnosis to explain and implement the latest developments.

♦ *In Metastatic Disease* A variety of treatment combinations have a significant chance of causing metastatic tumors to shrink or stop growing. Cure is not usually possible in this situation, although improvement in symptoms and tumor shrinkage may last for months and often many years. More aggressive and effective combinations are being developed in clinical trials.

♦ *Intensity of Treatment* In the past, chemotherapy was often omitted if the white blood cell or platelet counts dropped moderately (even if there were no symptoms or significant risk) or when minor gastrointestinal or other side effects occurred. Sometimes a dose of chemotherapy would be modified or postponed because of holidays or inconvenience. It is now recognized that these practices are unwise.

For metastatic disease and especially for adjuvant treatment, *it is important to give full doses and to avoid postponing regularly scheduled doses for minor reasons or for less than significant toxicity.*

Attempting to be "kind" to a patient by making toxicity as tolerable and minimal as possible can decrease the chances of a good result from the treatment. The kindest thing a physician can do is make sure the dose is as close to the theoretical maximum safe dose as possible and is also given on time. One study of the standard CMF program (Cytoxan + methotrexate + 5-fluorouracil), for example, indicated that if less than 80 percent of the calculated dose was given the results were significantly worse than if 80 percent or more of the planned dose was given according to the therapy schedule.

Hormonal Therapy The lining of the ducts and lobules in the breast change under the influence of hormones, and hormonal manipulation and therapy play an important role in managing breast cancer. A variety of methods were once used to manipulate the hormone balance— removing the ovaries or adrenal glands and sometimes the pituitary gland, for example. Many women responded to these manipulations, others did not. Those who responded not only seemed to have disease that was less aggressive but if they relapsed they could be treated by another hormonal maneuver with an increased chance of response.

More recently, it was discovered that the amount of estrogen and progesterone receptors in a tumor signifies that tumor's dependence on these hormones. This measurement has become important in determining tumor behavior and treatment. Tumors are classified as positive or nega-

tive based on the amount of receptor protein present. Tumors with positive receptors are associated with a better patient prognosis and longer survival.

Estrogen receptors may be found in up to two-thirds of patients, while only 40 to 50 percent have progesterone receptors. Postmenopausal women are more likely than premenopausal women to have receptor-positive tumors.

About half of patients with receptor-positive tumors, especially older, postmenopausal women, will respond to hormonal treatment using a drug such as tamoxifen, which blocks the action of estrogen in the tumor cells. It is taken orally and has few major side effects except for occasional hot flashes. Sometimes the progestational hormone Megace is used, and occasionally the androgenic agent Halotestin. Both are usually given after tamoxifen no longer effectively arrests tumor growth. Another agent, Cytadren, is sometimes used to decrease hormone production, especially if metastatic disease is present. Recently, gonadotropin releasing hormone analogs (lupron or zoladex, for example) have been used in premenopausal women to decrease female hormone production.

Patients whose tumors lack both estrogen and progesterone receptors have a low response rate to hormonal therapy. Therefore, they generally do not receive agents such as tamoxifen on an adjuvant basis or as treatment of metastatic disease.

Since hidden breast cancer cells may remain in the body after initial treatment, *it is extremely important that before any female hormones of any kind are taken by a woman who has had breast cancer, she should discuss the potential risk with her oncologist.*

♦ *Hormonal Therapy in Special Situations* Tamoxifen may be the primary tumor treatment in some very special situations—for elderly patients who cannot have or refuse to have surgery, for example, or for patients with estrogen receptor positive tumors who can't have surgery or chemotherapy because of medical problems. In older patients, especially those over 80, tamoxifen will often shrink tumors. Except in such special circumstances, tamoxifen should not be considered an alternative to established primary therapy.

Investigational Women who have 10 or more positive axillary lymph glands at primary surgery are at very high risk for recurrent disease. Women with Stage IV cancer have a very low cure rate with conventional therapy, including aggressive chemotherapy. The prognosis in both situations might be improved if extremely high doses of chemotherapy could be given, but such doses cannot normally be tolerated because of damage to bone marrow and blood cells. Recent investigational programs have tried to overcome this problem.
♦ The use of autologous bone marrow transplantation (ABMT) for metastatic and even high-risk early-stage breast cancer is currently under study. ABMT is riskier than the usual treatment with chemotherapy. Because the patient's own marrow is used, the risk is not related to the grafting problems seen in allogeneic bone marrow transplants where marrow comes from another donor (*see* Chapter 12). Rather, it relates to the fact that blood counts become very low for many weeks, during which time there is a high risk of bleeding and/or infection. A small percentage of patients (less than 10 percent) will not survive treatment with ABMT.

Clinical studies are trying to determine if the increased chance of long-term disease control offered by ABMT warrants the expense and risk for breast cancer patients. In trials with patients who had advanced metastatic breast cancer, ABMT has produced better response rates than conventional therapy, especially in patients who had not been previously treated for their metastatic disease.

Ribs

Muscle

Side view

Skin

Tissue expander

Inflation port

Breast reconstruction using inflatable tissue expander

About 20-25 percent are free of evidence of disease two years after treatment. Current studies are trying to determine the curative advantage of ABMT as an adjuvant therapy for patients with 10 or more involved lymph nodes. In one study, 80 percent of such patients were free of evidence of disease three years after treatment.

♦ Another technique to combat the life-threatening problem of low blood counts associated with chemotherapy is to give colony-stimulating factors such as GM-CSF. These stimulate the rapid production of blood cells and minimize bone marrow toxicity (*see* Chapter 8). Early results show some promise, but it is too soon to know if the observed response rates will be translated into improved survival. GM-CSF was approved in 1991 for use by community oncologists.

♦ To attempt to *prevent* breast cancer in women at high risk, an investigational trial of tamoxifen is being planned.

TREATMENT BY STAGE

STAGE 0 (in situ)
TNM Tis, N0, M0

Non-invasive or in situ cancers consist of lobular carcinoma in situ and ductal carcinoma in situ (intraductal carcinoma). These cancers are often small and may be discovered incidentally by mammography before a mass can be felt. They may also be in several locations in one or both breasts. In situ cancer can also be found in the presence of invasive cancer, in which case the cancer is staged and treated according to the invasive cancer.

Standard Treatment Both types are generally curable.

♦ For intraductal carcinoma, standard therapy is a wide excision of the tumor with or without low axillary node dissection. It is critical to remove an additional area around the initial biopsy if the edges of the biopsy showed tumor cells. Axillary lymph nodes were usually removed in the past, but several studies have shown that positive nodes are rare for this type of cancer. Accordingly, axillary sampling rather than full dissection is often performed today.

An alternative treatment is complete excisional biopsy with radiation therapy, with or without a simultaneous low axillary dissection. Another option is to remove the entire breast tissue (total mastectomy), with or without axillary dissection.

♦ In situ lobular cancer—a form that more commonly occurs in both breasts—is thought by some to be less malignant, but patients with this lesion have a 25 percent risk of developing some form of invasive cancer over many years.

There is some controversy about management of these patients. Standard treatment can include periodic examinations (including mammography) and follow-up without any additional therapy. This may be adequate if the patient is aware of the long-term risk of developing invasive cancer and will participate in the frequent evaluations. Sometimes biopsies are done on the opposite breast. Axillary lymph node dissection is not necessary.

An alternative is total mastectomy on one or both sides, with or without low axillary dissection. This choice is often appealing to women who don't want to have examinations several times a year, mammograms once or twice a year and the constant worry that invasive cancer may be found during their next visit to the doctor.

Five-Year Survival Over 95 percent

Investigational
♦ More limited surgical procedures such as lumpectomy, especially combined with radiation therapy. Preliminary results suggest that they may be equivalent to more aggressive surgical procedures.
♦ The role of radiation therapy in managing in situ ductal cancer is still controversial and under clinical evaluation.

STAGE I
TNM T1, N0, M0
The tumor is 3/4 in. (2 cm) or less in size, without any evidence of spread to nearby lymph nodes or distant sites.

Standard Treatment This stage is most often curable with surgery. The treatment plan may use radiotherapy and chemotherapy as well as surgery, and has to be tailored to the individual, taking the risks and benefits of each plan into account.

The surgical procedure used depends on the tumor's size and location, the size of the breast and whether the patient prefers a more extensive operation (probably without radiotherapy) or feels strongly about preserving her breast with a more limited procedure. Options include:
♦ Excisional biopsy and/or lumpectomy with a separate axillary node dissection. With a lumpectomy, there is a significant risk of residual microscopic cancer, and radiotherapy is given to the breast to minimize the possibility of residual tumor cells growing. This often requires an external radiation boost or internal implant as well as the usual external beam therapy to the entire breast.
♦ Removal of a larger wedge or portion of the breast, again with an axillary node dissection and radiation to the breast. This has a lower failure rate than lumpectomy

with radiation. For both lumpectomy and wedge resections, the margins *must* be free of cancer. If they are not, there is a much higher local failure rate. Sometimes (less than 10 percent of the time for Stages I and II) a tumor seems small, but with microscopic study is found in multiple sites or is found to be so extensive that a mastectomy may be needed to remove all cancer and improve the chance for cure.
♦ Modified radical or a total mastectomy, with removal of axillary lymph nodes. Radiotherapy is sometimes needed after a modified radical mastectomy in patients at high risk for microscopic residual tumor that could lead to a recurrence in the area of surgery. A patient with tumor at the edge of the surgical specimen may have hidden tumor cells near the incision. Radiotherapy is 90 to 95 percent effective in eliminating these cells and preventing tumor recurrences in the skin of the chest, which is a very troublesome, hard to manage problem that is far easier to prevent.

Removing the tumor and a portion of surrounding tissue while conserving a major part of the breast, usually if followed by radiation therapy, provides a cure rate about the same as the modified radical mastectomy.

The conventional recommendation has been to remove the axillary lymph nodes, since about one-third of patients who do not have obviously enlarged nodes still have microscopic involvement (positive nodes reclassifies the disease as Stage II, a treatment category requiring adjuvant chemotherapy).

Adjuvant Therapy For many years it was not customary to treat Stage I breast cancer with chemotherapy. These patients generally have a good prognosis, with only about one chance in four of further tumor spread. For cancers smaller than 1/2 in. (1 cm) in diameter, the chance of recurrence is less than 10 percent within 10 years of diagnosis. The National Institute of Health Consensus Conference on Treatment of Early Stage Breast Cancer in June 1990 suggested that it is reasonable not to give adjuvant treatment to patients with these very small tumors unless they are part of a clinical trial or high-risk factors are involved.

Recent trials suggest, however, that many other Stage I patients will benefit from adjuvant chemotherapy. Two large trials by the National Surgical Adjuvant Breast Project (NSABP) showed significant benefit at four-year follow-up for estrogen receptor negative patients given chemotherapy and for estrogen receptor positive patients treated with tamoxifen.

Although there is an early benefit for adjuvant treatment in patients with negative axillary lymph nodes, it has not yet been possible to show improvement in survival. It will be several years before it is known what the benefits of such therapy are and which patients should be considered for it. A careful discussion with each patient is appropriate.

Adjuvant therapy with chemotherapy for estrogen receptor negative patients and tamoxifen for estrogen receptor positive patients usually begins within four to six weeks of surgery. There are several effective programs, with other drug combinations and hormonal therapies under clinical evaluation.

Five-Year Survival 85 percent

STAGE II
TNM T0, N1, M0 or T1, N1, M0 or T2, N0, M0 (IIA)

T2, N1, M0 or T3, N0, M0 (IIB)

Stage IIA implies either a small primary lesion (less than 3/4 in./2 cm) and positive axillary lymph nodes or a larger primary lesion (between 2 and 5 cm) without positive nodes.

Stage IIB consists of a primary lesion between 3/4 and 2 in. (2 - 5 cm) and positive axillary nodes or a very large tumor [greater than 2 in.(5 cm)] with no axillary metastases.

Standard Treatment Stage IIA and IIB cancers can often be cured with various surgical procedures. Conservative surgery that removes only a portion of the breast, followed by radiation therapy, may in selected cases [for tumors smaller than 1 1/2 in.(4 cm)] be equivalent to more radical surgery for tumor control.

The same considerations for selection of the surgical procedure apply as in Stage I, including the size of the cancer, the size of the breast and concerns about breast preservation. The indications for axillary dissection are similar to those in Stage I. Surgical options are also similar, namely:
♦ Excisional biopsy or lumpectomy, with an axillary node dissection, followed by radiation therapy to the breast. This is suitable only for a primary tumor no larger than 1 1/2 in. (4 cm) and when there is no tumor at the surgical margin. For tumors larger than 2 in. (5 cm), chemotherapy may be given before surgery.
♦ A wedge or partial breast resection, again with axillary node dissection and postoperative radiation. The limitations on tumor size and tumor-free margins again apply. Radiation therapy consists of external radiation and sometimes an implant or, alternatively, an optional booster dose of external radiation. Local

recurrence rates are lower than with lumpectomy alone.

♦ Modified radical or total mastectomy. In a few patients with large tumors [larger than 1 1/2 in.(4 cm)] or extensive tumors (invasion of the chest wall muscles, for example), conservative surgery is not beneficial. The Halsted radical mastectomy may even be required to remove all of the tumor in some cases, although usually a modified radical mastectomy is sufficient. Post-masectomy chest wall radiation is given in selected patients with muscle invasion, residual tumor in the chest wall, or a high risk for tumor cells close to the surgical margins. Some physicians irradiate patients with more than four positive axillary nodes with very large tumors, or if lymphatic vessels within the breast are involved.

Patient survival with Stage II cancer depends on controlling tumor cells that have likely already spread throughout the body. Starting adjuvant chemotherapy promptly after surgery is critical since the major risk to life is the possibility of hidden metastases. Radiotherapy, which may limit drug dosages, can begin later, as early as three months after chemotherapy has begun or even after six months when chemotherapy has been completed. While radiotherapy to the chest wall decreases the chance of local recurrence it does not affect tumor cells that may be elsewhere in the body. The exact timing of radiotherapy is a question still being addressed by clinical studies.

The Conservative Surgical Option The June 1990 NIH Consensus Conference (*see* "Stage II") held that breast conservation treatment—with close follow-up to detect local recurrences early—is appropriate primary therapy for most women with Stages I and II breast cancers and is preferable because it provides the surgical equivalent to total mastectomy while preserving the breast.

Conservative surgery followed by primary radiation therapy depends upon careful patient selection, however. Not all women with early-stage cancer are good candidates for this approach.

♦ It is appropriate if there is a single, well-defined primary tumor no larger than 1 1/2 in. (4 cm) in diameter [preferably less than 1 1/4 in. (3 cm)] and there are no diffuse microcalcifications.

♦ It is sometimes not used in patients with large breasts (because of concern about the cosmetic result) or those with a large tumor in small breasts where biopsy would produce a significant loss of breast tissue and compromise symmetry.

♦ Conservative surgery plus radiotherapy is not suggested if there are multiple malignant tumors in one breast, widespread microcalcifications on mammography or a history of collagen vascular disease. The latter patients often develop scar tissue (reactive fibrosis) with radiation therapy, undesirable breast changes that might require additional surgery.

♦ Another factor in selecting this option is the location of the primary tumor. Tumors in or near the nipple will require its removal. Sometimes conservative surgery followed by radiation can still be done, but in some cases, extensive disease is found extending along the ducts from the nipple to the base of the breast, which would then require mastectomy. There is no unanimous agreement on the type of surgery needed for cancers near or involving the nipple.

♦ Patients with lesions in the extreme edge of the breast may be better candidates for this option, since if a mastectomy were done, it might require removing additional portions of the chest wall.

♦ A small percentage of patients will develop a recurrence in the breast area following limited surgery to conserve the breast. Mastectomy may still be able to control the disease in most cases.

♦ Radiotherapy should not be given during pregnancy because of the hazard to the fetus.

Adjuvant Chemotherapy After surgical treatment to control local disease in the breast, adjuvant chemotherapy is recommended to reduce the risk of recurrence.

♦ Drug combinations shown to produce a survival advantage include CMF (Cytoxan + methotrexate + 5-fluorouracil (5-FU)) with or without VP (vincristine + prednisone), and CAF (Cytoxan + Adriamycin + 5-FU).

♦ Earlier combinations that have been tried include L-PAM (Alkeran) + 5-FU for premenopausal women and L-PAM + 5-FU + tamoxifen for postmenopausal women with receptor positive tumors. Recent studies suggest that shorter courses of Cytoxan + Adriamycin (AC) may be at least as good as CMF given for six months.

♦ Adriamycin (doxorubicin) can produce cardiac toxicity, a form of heart muscle weakness. This can be disabling and life-threatening, but the risk can be reduced by giving the drug slowly via continuous intravenous infusion over one or more days and by limiting the total dosage. Cardiac studies monitor the heart muscle and provide early warning that the drug must be stopped before any significant damage occurs.

♦ A related drug, mitoxantrone, appears to be nearly as effective and may be associated with less cardiac toxicity. There are also investigational drugs such as ICRF-187 and ADR-529 that may protect against cardiac toxicity.

♦ Adjuvant chemotherapy has been shown to prolong the disease-free interval and survival of Stage II premenopausal patients with positive axillary lymph nodes. The treatment lasts from six to nine months in most programs, but no more than a year.

♦ There may be some benefit in giving adjuvant chemotherapy to postmenopausal women with positive axillary nodes, but the results are less impressive than in premenopausal patients.

♦ Postmenopausal women whose lymph nodes and hormone receptors are both positive are usually given adjuvant tamoxifen therapy, which can be as effective at prolonging disease-free and overall survival as chemotherapy is in premenopausal patients. Tamoxifen is given for at least two years. Recent studies suggest that five or more years may be more beneficial.

♦ It may be more necessary to give chemotherapy in postmenopausal patients with positive nodes and negative hormone receptors. However, many studies suggest that tamoxifen may be beneficial.

♦ Patients with negative lymph nodes and larger (T2 or T3) tumors have the same considerations as those with Stage I cancers. Both premenopausal and postmenopausal patients benefit, but as is true for Stage I cancers, the benefit of hormonal treatment is most significant in women over 50.

Five-Year Survival 66 percent

STAGE IIIA
TNM T0–2, N2, M0 or T3, N1–2, M0
The hallmark of Stage III is a big tumor [over 2 in. (5 cm)] with involvement of the axillary lymph nodes on the same side as the cancer or with fixation of the lymph nodes to one another or to other structures. If the lymph nodes inside the chest are involved or the tumor extends into the chest wall or involves and ulcerates the skin, the lesion is Stage IIIB.

Standard Treatment This stage is generally regarded as operable and is treated aggressively. Control for long periods is possible, but more often than not the tumor ultimately recurs. Treatment plans often use surgery, radiation and chemotherapy in varying sequences.

Initial surgical treatment is a modified radical or radical mastectomy. Several months of chemotherapy may be given before surgery to try to shrink or eliminate the tumor and make it easier to remove surgically, and this may improve survival. Combinations that have been extensively used in this manner include CMF (Cytoxan + methotrexate + 5-FU) and CAF or FAC (Cytoxan + Adriamycin + 5-FU).

Chemotherapy and radiotherapy are generally given after surgery.

Investigational Current clinical trials are exploring the possibility that aggressive chemotherapy including ABMT may enable breast conservation surgery rather than modified radical masectomy.

STAGE IIIB
Any T, N3, M0 or T4, any N, M0
Standard Treatment This stage, which includes inflammatory carcinoma, is generally regarded as inoperable. Surgery is usually limited to the initial diagnostic biopsy, with treatment of the local tumor by chemotherapy or radiation. Chemotherapy is often used because over 50 percent of patients have hidden metastases. If a good response is obtained with chemotherapy and/or radiation, surgery may be helpful to remove residual tumor.

Because all three therapies are used but their best sequence has not yet been determined, newly diagnosed patients with Stage IIIB cancer should be considered for clinical trials. Complex treatment programs involving integrated chemotherapy (with or without autologous bone marrow transplantation) and radiotherapy followed by surgery are under study. If a clinical trial is not available, consideration should be given to one of the current aggressive combined treatment protocols.

Five-Year Survival 41 percent

Investigational Current clinical trials are exploring the possibility that aggressive chemotherapy including ABMT may enable breast conservation surgery rather than modified radical masectomy.

STAGE IV
TNM Any T, any N, M1
There are distant metastases (to bone, liver or lung, for example) or skin and chest wall involvement beyond the breast area.

Standard Treatment Surgery is generally limited to a biopsy to prove the diagnosis and tumor cell type, as well as provide hormone receptor levels. The primary tumor may have to be treated with surgery or radiation, but this problem is generally overshadowed by the need to control metastases.

Chemotherapy and/or hormonal therapy are the principal treatments. Tumor shrinkage is common in about 60 percent of patients, although only in 10 to 20 percent does the tumor completely disappear for a long time.

♦ If the metastasic disease is not immediately life-threatening or doesn't involve such critical internal organs as the liver, hormonal management is usually tried before starting chemotherapy. This may involve tamoxifen or removal of the ovaries for premenopausal patients, and progestins, androgens, Cytadren, estrogens or tamoxifen for postmenopausal patients. Hormonal manipulation may be especially useful for those with predominantly bone metasteses.

♦ If metastases are life-threatening or hormone receptors are negative, chemotherapy combinations similar to those used in earlier stages are given. Again, the risk of Adriamycin-induced cardiac toxicity may limit the amount of drug that can be given.

Five-Year Survival 10 percent

Investigational
♦ All patients are candidates for clinical trials, which may involve new drugs in Phase I, II or III trials, new biologic agents, autologous bone marrow transplantation (ABMT), treatment with monoclonal antibodies, or high-dose chemotherapy with growth factor (such as GM-CSF) support. The use of ABMT for advanced disease shows some early promise (20-25 percent after two years) but the final role of ABMT is uncertain.

BREAST CANCER IN MEN

Male breast cancer is rare, but one out of every 150 cases of breast cancer involves a man, usually one over 60 years old. The cancer is commonly advanced when discovered. There is a higher frequency of Stage III disease, principally because of skin involvement by the tumor.

Although a painless breast lump is the most common sign, most breast lumps in men are benign and are related to some other cause, such as medications or liver disease.

Standard Treatment Both simple and radical mastectomies have been done, but no statement can be made about a standard method. Skin grafting is frequently required.

Radiation therapy is often used postoperatively to decrease the risk of local recurrence. Some centers are now treating male breast cancer patients with chemotherapy or hormonal therapy because nearby lymph nodes are commonly involved and because adjuvant chemotherapy has had such good results in women. Preliminary data are highly encouraging.

It is customary to obtain hormone receptors in these patients, although most male tumors are hormone receptor positive and respond to hormone manipulation, especially tamoxifen.

The generally poor prognosis in male breast cancer may reflect delays in seeking therapy—as long as 10 months—which is perhaps due to low awareness by the public and doctors of the possibility of this diagnosis.

TREATMENT FOLLOW-UP

Careful follow-up after treatment is essential for two purposes—to detect recurrences and to monitor the response to treatment. The standard procedure involves:
♦ Regular physical examinations and mammograms.
♦ Blood chemistry panel (liver, kidneys) and tumor markers (eg CEA, bone, CA15-3) if they were positive initially.
♦ Imaging studies—abdominal CT, MRI, radioisotope scans and x-rays—to look for metastases or assess the status of known metastases.
♦ Bone scans, if the initial bone scan was positive, pain develops or the serum alkaline phosphatase level is elevated.

♦ Chest x-ray and x-rays of positive areas on bone scan.

♦ Special studies such as endoscopy or fine needle aspiration of recurrent masses.

Detecting Recurrence Hidden metastases can lie dormant for a long time after surgery. In unusual cases, recurrences have been noted 15, 20 or even more years after the primary cancer developed. Life-long close and comprehensive follow-up is therefore required to be sure that recurrences are detected and treated early.

During the first two years after initial treatment, the intervals tend to be short—every one to two months. If no evidence of recurrence is found, the intervals are lengthened during the next few years, usually to about every three to six months.

♦ Any abnormal studies, such as bone scans, x-rays (including CT) or blood tests, are repeated at appropriate intervals. Tumor markers such as carcinoembryonic antigen (CEA) and CA 15-3 are often included if they were positive at the time of diagnosis, since they are then useful in detecting the earliest recurrence of metastatic cancer.

Monitoring Response to Treatment For either recurrent or metastatic disease, appropriate studies are done to determine response to treatment. Before any significant change in therapy—a new chemotherapy program, for example—it is essential to establish baseline information, documenting current status by blood tests, examinations, measurements and x-rays.

Objective clinical response is ordinarily defined as at least a 50 percent shrinkage in the greatest diameter of a metastatic lesion.

A metastatic tumor in the lung 1 1/2 in. (4 cm) in diameter would have to shrink to 3/4 in. (2 cm) for this to be called a significant response, with such shrinkage being classified as a partial response. A complete response or remission occurs when all visible and detectable disease disappears.

"Stable disease" suggests disease that does not grow in any area or shrinks by less than 50 percent in diameter (also called minimal response).

Disease progression means that at least one lesion increases in size during treatment.

♦ It is easy to assess lung metastases. Measurements can be made with a ruler held against a chest x-ray.

♦ Lesions in the liver can be monitored by liver function tests, especially the alkaline phosphatase, but also by direct measurement of metastatic tumors seen on abdominal CT or ultrasound images.

♦ Skin lesions and the size of lymph nodes can be measured directly.

♦ Measuring response in bone lesions takes longer and is more difficult because most metastatic breast cancers produce a softening or dissolving of the bone with the appearance of a "lytic" spot that looks like a hole. If treatment is successful, the lytic lesion will fill in with new bone.

For determining the response to chemotherapy or hormonal therapy, a bone lesion that has not received radiation therapy has to be chosen as a marker. Obviously, if a lesion given radiation heals and hormone therapy or chemotherapy is also being given, it would be impossible to know which treatment brought about the healing.

Bone lesions require that an x-ray be done before treatment and another as soon as the treatment has been given an adequate trial.

Following bone scans for evidence of response to treatment may not be as useful as conventional x-rays of lytic bone lesions. Scans may show "hot spots" in any abnormal area, and these spots may also indicate healing. They may also be produced by inflammation, metabolic diseases or severe arthritis. The area could remain positive for months or a few years with successful therapy.

In a few patients with positive bone scans but without any lesions on x-rays, response may be signified by no new lesions developing. If the bone scan is unchanged after six months, especially if pain lessens, the positive areas can be presumed to indicate healing.

♦ In a few breast cancer patients, the bone lesions themselves produce extra bone (blastic lesions) instead of "holes" in the bone (lytic lesions). Here it is not possible to determine healing by looking at x-rays because healing is *also* associated with the laying down of extra bone. Again, healing may be signified by the failure to develop any new lesions elsewhere.

The "Flare" Response Hormone treatment can sometimes produce worse bone pain during the first few weeks of therapy, and the serum calcium level may also rise. This endocrine "flare" may be early evidence that the cancer is responding to the hormone treatments.

If possible, pain medication is given to allow therapy to continue while the elevated calcium level is evaluated and treated. Usually the calcium returns to normal and the pain decreases, confirming a response.

Similarly, the bone scan sometimes becomes temporarily worse in a patient who is clinically improving. The increased uptake on the scan may represent healing of the diseased bone. The x-ray appearance may not change for several months even in patients with a good response to treatment and whose pain has decreased.

RECURRENT CANCER

Recurrent breast cancer may be in the area of the breast surgery or in the chest wall. Alternatively, it may be metastatic disease anywhere in the body.

A recurrence in the skin or chest wall near the surgical site most often indicates that more widespread metastatic disease will occur in the future, although it may be the only site of recurrence in a small group of patients. For these patients, local additional surgery and/or radiation therapy may sometimes be curative.

Most patients with even small local recurrences, however, will eventually develop other areas of metastasis despite aggressive local treatment. After treatment of an isolated local recurrence, only 30 percent of patients have developed *no* other evidence of spread by 5 years, 7 percent by 10 years. These figures apply to patients who develop chest wall recurrence after aggressive surgery such as a modified radical mastectomy. The prognosis is much better if a recurrence occurs in the breast after conservative surgery followed by radiation therapy.

Standard Treatment

♦ If there is no internal disease and recurrence is confined to the area of the original tumor, surgery and/or radiation therapy is used, plus tamoxifen in selected cases.

♦ If there is no life-threatening disease involving major internal organs, if it has been at least two years since mastectomy and if hormone receptors are positive or unknown, the standard treatment is tamoxifen or removal of the ovaries for premenopausal patients, and tamoxifen, estrogens, androgens, Cytadren or progestin therapy for postmenopausal patients.

♦ If patients respond to hormonal treatment and then relapse, other forms of hormonal therapy are used, including androgen therapy, Cytadren, corticosteroids and hypophysectomy.

♦ If major internal organs such as the liver are involved, hormone receptors are negative or it has been less than two years between the primary treatment and the recurrence, chemotherapy is usually given. Standard combinations include CMF, CAF, CMFP and CMFVP (*see* "Stage IIIA" and "Stage IV"). Cyclophosphamide + Adriamycin appears to produce similar results but has been studied less extensively. Other combinations include Mitomycin C + Velban as well as Velban + Adriamycin + thiotepa + Halotestin ("VATH").

Investigational
♦ Tamoxifen in premenopausal women if disease involves no major organs, hormone receptors are positive or unknown, and it has been at least two years since primary therapy (suggesting slow-growing disease).
♦ Combination chemotherapy with or without hormone management for patients who recur after initial response to hormonal manipulation.
♦ If there is major organ involvement and negative hormone receptors or if less than two years has elapsed since primary treatment, clinical trials of combination chemotherapy, newly developed chemotherapy agents and biologic treatment should be considered.
♦ Leuprolide is also undergoing clinical trial as a method of hormonal manipulation.

THE MOST IMPORTANT QUESTIONS YOU CAN ASK
♦ Can I save my breast? Is this wise?
♦ Will I need radiation therapy?
♦ Will the radiation therapy produce any damage to the skin or any deformity? What are the other side effects?
♦ If I need chemotherapy, what are the choices? How long will it last and what are the side effects?
♦ When can I have breast reconstruction done and what are my choices? What will I look like afterwards?
♦ Why do I have to stop taking female hormones?
♦ What can you give me to help me with my hot flashes?
♦ Will I lose my hair? When will I start losing it and how long will it take to come back?
♦ How often do I need to be examined afterwards? What tests will I have?
♦ How often should I have a mammogram?
♦ When will I be sure that my cancer will not come back?

CANCER OF AN UNKNOWN PRIMARY SITE

Raphael Catane, MD

◇

Cancer of an unknown primary site (CUPS) is a metastatic tumor with no obvious source. It is detected by a biopsy that shows cancer from a part of the body that does not produce that type of malignancy, and no site of origin is identified despite a thorough physical examination, blood tests, x-rays and other imaging studies.

No primary site of origin can be identified in 2 to 9 percent of patients diagnosed with metastatic cancer. This is often because the primary tumor is so small that it is undetectable or the primary site is difficult to see directly or by using imaging techniques.

Since by definition the disease is diagnosed at a metastatic stage, the prognosis is generally poor. A significant percentage of patients, however, can have symptoms relieved and can occasionally be cured. For example, germ cell tumors, choriocarcinoma, lymphoma and certain sarcomas are potentially curable even in their metastatic stages. Other tumors such as prostate cancer, breast cancer and endometrial carcinoma are amenable to hormonal therapy.

Unfortunately, the most common origins of CUPS are lung and pancreatic cancers. These two tumors are generally incurable at the metastatic stage, with an average survival of about three or four months and with only 25 percent and 10 percent alive after one and five years respectively.

FINDING THE PRIMARY SITE

In trying to discover the primary site, there are two important considerations.

1. Some primary cancers are much more treatable than others. These include cancers of the breast, prostate, thyroid and ovary, lymphomas (including Hodgkin's disease), as well as germ cell tumors similar to those that develop in the testes. Great efforts are made to determine if one of these is the primary site. Not only is the prognosis much better with these types of cancer, but the treatment has to be specific for that cancer. The usual non-specific combination chemotherapy programs for CUPS have a low rate of response.

2. There are important clues your doctor can use to discover the primary site.

♦ One clue is the location of the metastases. A woman with a tumor that develops in glands (adenocarcinoma) and is found in the lymph nodes of the armpit, for example, is more likely to have carcinoma of the breast. Mammograms are always required, especially if the breast examination is negative. Such women are treated for breast cancer.

♦ The most common sites of CUPS are metastases to the lung, lymph nodes, bones and liver. When CUPS is found in the upper part of the body (above the diaphragm), the most common source is the lung. When it appears in the liver, the usual primary site is the gastrointestinal tract, including the pancreas.

♦ Another clue is the type of pathology. If a person has epidermoid carcinoma in lymph glands high in the neck, for example, the primary site is most often in the nasopharynx, the throat or the tonsils. Special endoscopic procedures and biopsies can be used to look for the primary site and even if it is not found, such people are often treated with the chemotherapy programs for head and neck cancer. (Involved high cervical nodes usually means head and neck can-cer, but if low cervical nodes are involved the cancer could also be breast, lung, lymphoma, melanoma or other tumors.)

Esophagus

Soft tissue sarcoma

Lung

Liver

Pancreas

Colon

Melanoma

Rectum

Prostate

Anus

Testicle

Uterus

Ovary

Possible primary sources of cancer first diagnosed in a metastatic site

TABLE 1: TREATABLE CANCERS OF UNKNOWN PRIMARY SITE

Potentially curable	Chance of significant remission
Germ cell tumors	Breast cancer
Hodgkin's disease	Some lymphomas
Lymphosarcoma	Ovarian cancer
Trophoblastic tumors	Head and neck cancer
Thyroid cancer	Small cell lung cancer
Ovarian cancer	Prostate cancer

DIAGNOSIS

People with CUPS undergo certain standard methods of medical evaluation to discover the primary site (if possible) and other potential areas of spread. Evaluation will include a history as well as a specific work-up for the major potential sites of the cancer's origin that can be treated—breast cancer, germ cell tumors, lymphomas and cancers of the head and neck, lung (especially small cell), prostate, thyroid and ovary. A consensus about the minimal investigation that has to be performed includes the following.

Physical Examination

♦ When CUPS is found in high cervical lymph nodes, a thorough examination of the nasopharynx, throat and upper respiratory tract should be done, usually by an ear, nose and throat specialist.

♦ A gynecological examination, including a rectal examination, Pap smear and a pelvic ultrasound or CT, should be done for any woman with CUPS, especially if the inguinal (groin) lymph nodes are enlarged or there is fluid in the abdomen (ascites).

Blood and Other Tests

♦ Complete blood counts.

♦ Urinalysis to check for blood.

♦ Test for hidden (occult) blood in the stool.

♦ Blood chemistry tests to assess liver and kidney function.

♦ Tests for serum tumor markers that may be elevated with specific cancers, such as CEA (colon), CA-125 (ovary), CA 15-3 (breast), CA 19-9 (pancreas), prostatic acid phosphatase and prostatic specific antigen (prostate), alpha-fetoprotein (hepatoma, germ cell tumors) and βHCG (choriocarcinoma, germ cell tumors).

Imaging

♦ Chest x-ray may reveal the most common tumor origin, carcinoma of the lung. It is often impossible, however, to distinguish between a primary lung cancer and a metastatic lesion within the chest. Sometimes chest CT is also helpful.

♦ Mammograms for all women diagnosed with CUPS. Fifty percent of females with isolated metastases in the lymph nodes in the armpit will have a breast cancer primary. This will not always be seen on a mammogram, however (a false negative result).

♦ It is not helpful to do extensive x-rays—bowel x-rays, for example—to look for a primary site unless there is a specific complaint in that area, such as constipation or gastrointestinal bleeding.

The following imaging study is frequently done:

♦ Abdominal CT scan, especially if there are metastases in the liver. The scan may reveal the presence of the second most common malignancy causing CUPS, pancreatic cancer.

The following imaging studies are occasionally done:

♦ CT, MRI and ultrasound studies of the area of known tumor and likely primary sites.

♦ Nuclear scans of bone, liver and thyroid.

♦ Lymphangiogram if lymphoma is suspected.

Endoscopy and Biopsy

♦ Endoscopic evaluation of the colon, urinary tract and lung is performed when indicated by results of the previous studies.

♦ Biopsies by fine needle aspiration to establish pathologic diagnosis: breast, prostate, pancreas, bone marrow (may need special studies on biopsy: hormone receptors, DNA, other studies).

SPECIAL PATHOLOGIC METHODS

The pathologist has a crucial role in the diagnosis, evaluating the biopsy specimen and determining not only if it is malignant but, on the basis of his or her experience and the tissue's appearance under the microscope, the most likely source.

The pathologist is often consulted before the biopsy is done because some special immunohistochemistry studies require frozen tissue or tissue may have to be specially prepared for examination by an electron microscope. These methods were not generally available even five years ago. They offer a significant advantage in obtaining an accurate diagnosis of the primary site of origin.

Immunohistochemistry Along with the usual tissue stains used to examine the tumor tissue under the microscope, special stains using monoclonal antibodies are directed against specific tumor antigens. These can often determine the likely primary site, thereby allowing therapy to be more specific and improving the chance of remission or even cure.

TABLE 2: SPECIAL STAINS USED FOR SPECIFIC TISSUES

♦ The presence of keratin, a protein found in epithelium (surface tissue), indicates the tumor is a carcinoma rather than a sarcoma or lymphoma.

♦ S-100, a protein found in neuroectodermal tissues, is useful in the diagnosis of melanomas or nerve tumors.

♦ Neuron-specific enolase is positive in small cell (oat cell) lung cancer.

♦ Leukocyte-common antigen found on the surface of leukocytes is positive in leukemia and lymphoma.

♦ Prostate-specific antigen and prostatic acid phosphatase stains are positive in prostate cancer.

♦ Human chorionic gonadotropin is often positive in germ cell tumors such as testis cancer and in choriocarcinoma.

♦ Alpha-fetoprotein is present in primary liver cancer and certain germ cell tumors.

♦ Estrogen receptors are present in breast cancer and cancer of the lining of the uterus (endometrial cancer). Finding estrogen receptors not only helps in the diagnosis but suggests that hormonal therapy may be useful.

Many new tissue stains are being developed and are rapidly enlarging the diagnostic capability of the modern pathologist.

Electron Microscopy (EM) Regular microscopes magnify tissues up to 1,000 times. The electron microscope can magnify tissues 50,000 to 100,000 times. Very small structures inside and on the surfaces of cells, often characteristic of certain types of cancer cells, can be seen. There are structures characteristic of squamous cell cancers, cancers of neuroendocrine origin, muscle tumors and most melanomas. Besides suggesting likely sites, EM studies are useful in eliminating certain tumor types.

STAGING

The actual tumor origin is the most important thing in planning treatment and assessing the prognosis, but staging also has some value. It has been suggested that doctors caring for patients with CUPS should refrain from extensive investigations, since the cost of the evaluation financially and with respect to time and discomfort is not worth the results and may not affect survival anyway.

The results of exhaustive tests are also

sometimes misleading. The tests may sometimes seem to show a positive finding when none is really there (false positive) or may instead fail to show an abnormality that is present but not detectable (false negative).

TREATMENT OVERVIEW

There is no generally recommended treatment for *all* patients with CUPS. Whenever there is a likely primary origin, based on the opinion of the pathologist as well as the clinical, laboratory and imaging studies, the treatment will be given according to that probable diagnosis.

The prognosis for people with CUPS is highly variable because so many different tumors may be involved.

Standard Treatment While no specific standard therapy is generally agreed upon for people with CUPS with no definable primary sources, these patients are sometimes treated with combination chemotherapy programs. If the disease appears to be localized, complete surgical removal or radical radiotherapy may occasionally result in a cure. But when the tumor has spread, investigational protocols might be considered.

Investigational
♦ Combination chemotherapy (frequently including cisplatin).
♦ Hormonal therapy.
♦ New chemotherapeutic agents such as carboplatin (paraplatin) alone or in combination with other drugs.

TREATMENT FOR SPECIFIC PRESENTATIONS

Certain rules have been recommended for a number of specific presentations of CUPS.

"MIDLINE" TUMORS
These tumors originate in the middle part of the body such as the mediastinum (chest) or midabdominal lymph nodes.

Some people with these tumors who are under 50 years of age, have multiple lung and lymph node metastases and tumors that grow rapidly, respond well to combination chemotherapy that contains cisplatin or carboplatin.

Sixty percent of the patients in one such group had a significant response to therapy and 15 percent were apparently cured. Many of them were found to have blood or tissue markers (HCG or AFP) suggesting that they actually had a germ cell tumor.

CUPS IN THE NECK LYMPH NODES
When epidermoid (squamous) carcinoma is found in the neck (upper cervical) lymph nodes, patients should be treated as if they had a tumor of the upper respiratory area even though a thorough ear, nose and throat evaluation—including blind biopsies of the base of the tongue and the nasopharynx—may have been negative.

Treatment will include:
♦ Radical radiotherapy to the cervical lymph nodes.
♦ Surgery to remove the lymph node group involved.
♦ A combination of surgery and radiotherapy.
♦ Chemotherapy, usually with a cisplatin combination.

CUPS IN THE ARMPIT LYMPH NODES
In males, the most likely diagnosis is incurable lung cancer.

In females, 50 percent may have a treatable breast cancer. Treatment will emphasize:
♦ Surgery, including removal of all axillary nodes in the involved site.
♦ Partial or total mastectomy.
♦ Radiation to the axilla and the breast, if not removed.
♦ Hormonal therapy, especially if hormone receptors are present.
♦ Chemotherapy should be considered as suggested for breast cancer.

CUPS IN A SINGLE LYMPH NODE

Any single lymph node site may represent melanoma. A cure may be achieved in 15 percent of cases by completely removing the involved lymph node, even when the primary site is never found.

MULTIPLE SKELETAL LESIONS

In males, a prostatic cancer should be suspected. If there are no other clues, hormonal therapy might be given, because it will be beneficial for a cancer with a prostatic origin and is quite harmless.

In females, breast cancer is a possibility. In both sexes, a thyroid cancer should be kept in mind, since both tumors may be treated effectively even in the metastatic stage (by hormonal therapy and chemotherapy for breast cancer and with radioiodine for thyroid cancer). Metastatic thyroid cancer that does not resemble normal thyroid tissue (poorly differentiated or undifferentiated), however, can seldom be treated with radioactive iodine.

THE MOST IMPORTANT QUESTIONS YOU CAN ASK

♦ How much investigation is really needed to increase my chance of survival or to improve my quality of life?
♦ Has the pathologist used any of the special studies described here?
♦ What is the most probable diagnosis?
♦ Can I benefit from surgery, radiotherapy, chemotherapy or hormonal therapy?

CARCINOIDS OF THE GASTROINTESTINAL TRACT

Ernest H. Rosenbaum, MD, and Malin Dollinger, MD

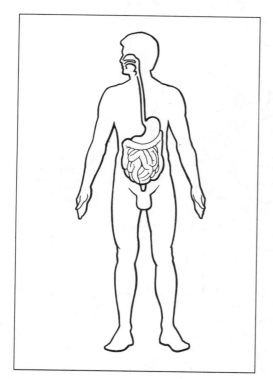

Carcinoid tumors are unusual cancers. Although they can develop in other organs, especially the lung, they generally arise in the intestinal tract, including the stomach, small bowel, appendix and rectum. They are the most common tumors of the appendix, occurring in one out of every 200 appendectomies. They make up 30 percent of small bowel tumors but less than 2 percent of all gastrointestinal malignancies.

In their early stages, carcinoid tumors are highly treatable and often curable. They are usually slow growing and behave like benign tumors. The risk of metastasis is related to the size of the primary tumor.

Carcinoids may occur in multiple sites (about 20 percent have multiple tumors) and, except for those of rectal origin, may produce an endocrine substance called serotonin. In most cases there are no symptoms, so many carcinoid tumors are discovered incidentally during abdominal operations performed for other reasons. The survival of most people with carcinoid tumors is quite good, although symptoms may develop when the tumor cannot be removed, when it recurs after treatment or when there is metastatic disease.

Types There are no meaningful cell type (histologic) variations that help predict the clinical course of these tumors. Carcinoids are broadly classified as neuroendocrine or APUD (amine precursor uptake and decarboxylation) tumors. The APUD type is associated with the MEN (multiple endocrine neoplasia) type I syndrome (pancreas islet cell carcinoid). Malignant carcinoids may produce at least two hormones, serotonin and bradykinin, but many carcinoid tumors are nonfunctional and do not release any substances.

How It Spreads Carcinoid tumors spread by direct invasion of underlying layers of tissue (submucosally). They can also spread via lymphatics to regional lymph nodes and through the blood stream to the liver, lungs or other organs.

The site of origin and size of the primary tumor are important in determining whether the carcinoid tumor is likely to spread. A tumor less than 1/2 in. (1 cm) rarely metastasizes. But 88 percent of

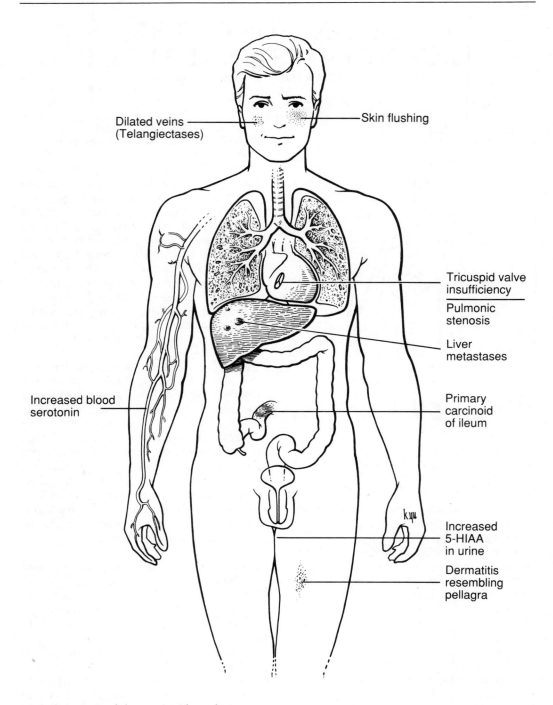

Dilated veins
(Telangiectases)

Skin flushing

Tricuspid valve
insufficiency

Pulmonic
stenosis

Liver
metastases

Increased blood
serotonin

Primary
carcinoid
of ileum

Increased
5-HIAA
in urine

Dermatitis
resembling
pellagra

Manifestations of the carcinoid syndrome

patients with tumors larger than 3/4 in. (2 cm) have metastases, and 18 percent of these develop the carcinoid syndrome (*see* "Common Signs and Symptoms").

What Causes It Unknown

RISK FACTORS

None known.

SCREENING

There are no effective screening methods.

COMMON SIGNS AND SYMPTOMS

Symptoms are unusual in the early stages. When symptoms do occur, the tumor has already spread in 90 percent of patients. The most common symptoms are periodic abdominal pain, intermittent intestinal obstruction (intussusception) and kinking of the bowel. Gastrointestinal bleeding is uncommon and ulcerations of the tumor are rare.

In addition to the symptoms caused by the tumor, there may be symptoms of the carcinoid syndrome. This is characterized by facial flushing, wheezing, diarrhea and cardiac valvular disease. It is caused by abnormal amounts of the two hormones produced by malignant carcinoids, serotonin and bradykinin, and other biologically active substances. The syndrome occurs in about 10 percent of patients with carcinoid tumor, almost always because of carcinoid metastases in the liver.

DIAGNOSIS

Physical Examination
♦ Abdominal mass and enlarged liver.
♦ Prominent skin veins (telangiectasis).
♦ Signs of the carcinoid syndrome—hypertension, heart murmur, wheezing on expiration and flushing of the skin.

Blood and Other Tests
♦ Metastatic carcinoid tumors may be diagnosed by elevated levels of 24-hour urinary 5-hydroxyindolacetic acid (5-HIAA), a metabolic product of the serotonin produced by the tumor, and an elevated serum serotonin level. False positive 5-HIAA tests can be caused by foods such as bananas, avocados and pineapple and by certain drugs.

Imaging
♦ X-rays of the chest and gastrointestinal tract (small bowel and barium enema).
♦ CT scan of the abdomen to detect liver metastases.

Endoscopy and Biopsy
♦ Liver biopsy, if indicated.

STAGING

There is no accepted staging system for carcinoids.

TREATMENT OVERVIEW

Surgery is the standard therapy, but the extent of spread is important in deciding the initial treatment options.

Surgery Surgical removal of the tumor is the standard treatment for cure. If the primary tumor is localized and can be removed, the five-year survival rate is in the range of 70 to 90 percent. Since carcinoid tumors are usually slow growing, even patients with tumors that can't be removed have an average survival of several years. Surgery often offers excellent relief from symptoms, for example, by removing the liver metastases causing the carcinoid syndrome or bypassing intestinal obstructions. Such surgery may add years to a patient's life, an uncommon result of surgery for other types of liver metastases.

Radiation Radiation therapy has a limited role for localized tumors that can't be removed surgically and may also be used for palliative treatment of metastases.

 Chemotherapy There has been modest success with chemotherapy. Drug combinations of 5-fluorouracil with Adriamycin, dacarbazine (DTIC) and streptozotocin have had responses of less than 30 percent.

Palliation Drugs such as Periactin, alpha and beta adrenergic blocking agents, chlorpromazine and corticosteroids may be used to alleviate the symptoms related to the carcinoid syndrome.

A new drug, Sandostatin (Octreotide), was recently found to be very effective in preventing the secretion of serotonin and can help relieve symptoms of the carcinoid syndrome. Interferon-alpha was also reported to alleviate symptoms and occasionally to cause tumor shrinkage.

TREATMENT OF LOCALIZED TUMORS BY SITE

APPENDICEAL CARCINOID

Appendiceal tumors account for 22 percent of all carcinoids. They are treated by appendectomy and, in fact, are usually diagnosed for the first time at surgery. Lesions less than 5/8 in. (1.5 cm) in diameter are essentially 100 percent curable.

Appendiceal tumors larger than 3/4 in. (2 cm) are rare and treated like a carcinoma of the colon. For these larger tumors, removal of the right side of the colon and the lymphatics is recommended.

Five-Year Survival 99 to 100 percent

RECTAL CARCINOID

These account for a quarter of all carcinoids. Rectal carcinoids less than 1/2 in. (1 cm) can be treated adequately by local excision (fulguration), with cure rates approaching 100 percent.

Carcinoid lesions larger than 3/4 in. (2 cm) are treated surgically. As with carcinoma, an abdominal perineal resection may be necessary, but sphincter-preserving surgery may be performed in some cases.

Lesions between 1/2 and 3/4 in. (1 to 2 cm) receive individualized treatment depending on extent of invasion. The cure rate is excellent.

Five-Year Survival 76 to 83 percent

SMALL BOWEL CARCINOIDS

Small bowel tumors make up 28 percent of all carcinoids. Conservative local excision is sufficient for tumors less than 1/2 in. (1 cm) in diameter. For larger tumors, a wedge of the tissues supporting the bowel (mesentery) containing the regional lymph nodes should also be removed.

Anyone with a tumor larger than 3/4 in. (2 cm) should be followed closely for a minimum of 10 years. The follow-up program should include an annual CT scan of the abdomen and annual or semiannual measurements of urinary 5-HIAA and/or serum serotonin levels.

Five-Year Survival 54 percent

TREATMENT OF INVASIVE AND METASTATIC CARCINOIDS

REGIONAL GASTROINTESTINAL CARCINOIDS

Carcinoid tumors with regional metastasis or local extension should be treated by aggressive surgery. If all visible malignant disease can be removed, long-term survival rates will be excellent.

No surgical adjuvant treatment is known to be helpful.

If the regional disease can't be removed, palliative surgery—to remove all the accessible disease, for example—should be carried out.

Chemotherapy is not required until significant symptoms occur, for these patients frequently have many months or even years of comfortable life without further treatment.

METASTATIC CARCINOID TUMORS

A number of standard treatment options are available for metastatic carcinoid tumors.

Surgery This may sometimes be of considerable value when there are large liver metastases involving surgically accessible areas of the liver. Liver metastases that recur after surgery should be considered for another resection if they are in an area where the operation can be done with minimal complications.

♦ For very carefully selected patients with slow-growing disease and symptomatic carcinoid heart disease, heart valve replacement may be indicated.

♦ For patients with bulky or symptomatic liver metastases, one treatment option is tying off the hepatic artery and giving chemotherapy. This can lead to substantial tumor degeneration. It can also cause severe toxic effects—abdominal pain, fever, nausea and a short-term worsening of the syndrome—but many patients do experience subsequent relief from symptoms.

Radiation The role of radiation therapy in managing carcinoid tumors with distant metastasis is restricted to relief from symptoms, most commonly of bone involvement. However, localized metastasis will occasionally respond to radiation therapy.

Supportive Therapy There are a number of ways to manage symptoms from metastatic disease with medication.

♦ Diarrhea will frequently respond to standard antidiarrheal medications such as Lomotil and to dietary changes such as restricting consumption of eggs, milk and cheese.

♦ The somostatin analogue (Octreotide, Sandostatin) has recently been shown to be useful in improving symptoms of the carcinoid syndrome and may be life-saving in carcinoid crisis (sudden exacerbation of symptoms).

♦ Interferon-alpha preparations may have a role in controlling symptoms of the carcinoid syndrome and/or in arresting tumor growth.

♦ Monoamine oxidase inhibitors such as procarbazine (Matulane) and tranylcypromine sulfate (Parnate) are drugs to be avoided. They will exacerbate the carcinoid syndrome by inhibiting the breakdown of serotonin.

♦ Acute symptoms—carcinoid crisis—may be controlled by prednisone, adrenergic blocking agents and histamine antagonists. Some specific drugs are to be avoided in these patients because of the risk of causing the release of these active substances. This is especially true during surgery and in the treatment of low blood pressure.

Chemotherapy Although activity with a variety of single agents and drug combinations has been reported—5-fluorouracil (5-FU) + doxorubicin (Adriamycin) + dacarbazine (DTIC) and 5-FU + streptozotocin—response rates seldom exceed 30 percent. Complete responses are uncommon, and the duration of the response may be short.

Chemotherapy should be used for palliation in patients with symptoms.

Investigational

♦ Protocols using chemotherapy combinations may be considered (*see* "Recurrent Cancer"). One study showed a 50 percent better average survival with 5-FU + streptozotocin than with 5-FU + Adriamycin, but further studies are needed to confirm results and prove that the improved survival is significant.

TREATMENT FOLLOW-UP

Patients should be evaluated every 6 to 12 months. The evaluation should include:
♦ Physical examination.
♦ 24-hour urine 5-HIAA levels.
♦ Serum serotonin level.
♦ Chest x-ray.
♦ Abdominal CT scan, if required.

RECURRENT CANCER

The prognosis for any treated carcinoid patient with a progressing, recurring or relapsing disease is poor. The selection of further treatment depends on many factors, including the therapy initially used, the site of the recurrence and individual considerations.

Since some tumors grow rather slowly, attempts to remove them again or multiple operations to remove liver metastases or slowly growing tumors are worthy of consideration. Reducing tumor volume may provide long-term relief of symptoms.

Investigational treatments are appropriate and should be considered when standard treatment fails.

THE MOST IMPORTANT QUESTIONS YOU CAN ASK

♦ How are carcinoids different from the usual cancers of the bowel?
♦ What tests are needed to follow my progress after surgery?
♦ What does a rising urine 5-HIAA or serum serotonin mean?
♦ What are the toxic side effects of chemotherapy?
♦ What is the role of repeated surgeries for recurrent carcinoid cancers?

CERVIX

Jeffrey L. Stern, MD

◇

Invasive cervical cancer accounts for 2.5 percent of all cancers that afflict women in the United States. About 13,500 cases of invasive carcinoma of the cervix are diagnosed in the United States each year, while there are at least 50,000 new cases of a pre-invasive cancer—known as carcinoma in situ—where the cancer cells are confined to the surface skin of the cervix.

But since 1940, there has been a steady decrease in the incidence of carcinoma of the cervix because most women with no symptoms are screened with cervical and vaginal Pap smears. The probability at birth that a white woman will eventually develop cervical cancer dropped from 1.1 percent in 1975 to 0.7 percent in 1985. Similarly, for black women the probability dropped from 2.3 percent in 1975 to 1.6 percent in 1985.

Types Over 90 percent of cervical carcinomas start in the surface cells lining the cervix and are called squamous cell carcinoma. About 5 to 9 percent start in glandular tissue (adenocarcinoma). Adenocarcinomas are more difficult to diagnose, but they are treated the same way as squamous cell carcinomas and the survival rate, stage for stage, is similar.

There are several types of adenocarcinoma. About 60 percent are the endocervical cell type, 10 percent are each of endometrioid and clear cell carcinomas and 20 percent are adenosquamous carcinoma.

There are two rare types of cervical carcinoma known as small cell carcinoma and cervical sarcoma. Both have a poor prognosis.

How It Spreads Most scientists believe that cervical warts or pre-invasive cervical cancer may develop over a period of months or years after the cervix is infected with the human papilloma virus (HPV). This early tumor—known as mild dysplasia or cervical intraepithelial neoplasia (CIN) Grade 1—can progress to moderate dysplasia (CIN-2), then to severe dysplasia and carcinoma in situ (CIN-3) and eventually to invasive carcinoma. Most physicians believe that about two thirds of all cases of severe dysplasia progress to invasive cancer if left untreated. This transformation takes anywhere from 3 to 30 years, about 10 years on the average.

Once the cervical cancer becomes invasive, it can spread locally to the upper vagina and into the tissues surrounding the upper vagina and the cervix (the parametrium). Eventually it grows toward the pelvic sidewall, obstructing the tubes (ureters) that drain urine from the kidney to the bladder. It can also spread to the bladder and rectum.

Cervical tumor cells can invade the lymphatic system and spread to the lymph nodes in the pelvic wall. Eventually they may spread to the iliac lymph nodes higher in the pelvis, the aortic lymph nodes, the nodes above the collarbone and occasionally to the groin nodes.

Metastases can also spread through the bloodstream to the outer vagina, vulva, lungs, liver and brain. Invasion of the pelvic nerves is common in advanced cases. There may also be spread within the abdomen when the tumor penetrates the full thickness of the cervix.

What Causes It There is much evidence that cervical carcinoma is venereal in origin. Most researchers believe that the human papilloma virus is either the cause or a strong cofactor in the development of pre-invasive and invasive carcinomas of the cervix, as well as pre-invasive and invasive squamous cell cancer of the vagina and vulva. Ninety to 95 percent of squamous cell carcinomas of the cervix contain human papilloma virus DNA.

The virus is a sexually transmitted disease. There are more than 50 types of human papilloma virus (HPV) that infect humans. Types 6 and 11 usually cause warts, while types 16, 18, 31 and 33 usually result in high-grade cervical dysplasia (CIN-2 and 3) and carcinomas. The virus infects the tissues of the lower genital tract and may produce obvious genital warts or mild, moderate or severe dysplasia and

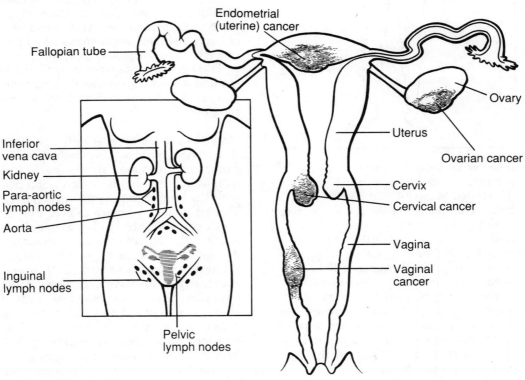

Cancers of female pelvic organs

carcinoma in situ. Genital warts are associated with cervical, vaginal and vulvar dysplasia and invasive carcinoma in about 25 percent of cases.

RISK FACTORS

The average age of women with invasive cervical cancer in the United States is between 45 and 50, but the average age of women with carcinoma in situ is between 25 and 35. The difference is attributed to the long latent period of progression of an in situ to an invasive cervical cancer.

The risk factors for pre-invasive cervical cancer (cervical dysplasia) and cervical cancer are the same. Circumcision is no longer believed to lower the risk of cervical carcinoma.

At Significantly Higher Risk
♦ Suppression of the immune system from corticosteroids, kidney transplants, therapy for other cancers, or AIDS.
♦ A history of genital warts.
♦ A history of herpes simplex virus infection.
♦ Low socioeconomic status.
♦ Early age at first intercourse.
♦ Multiple sexual partners.
♦ Women whose male partner(s) either have or have had penile warts, have had multiple sexual partners or whose previous partners had cervical cancer.

At Slightly Higher Risk
♦ Multiple pregnancies.
♦ Cigarette smoking.

SCREENING

The American College of Obstetricians and Gynecologists recommends that a Pap smear be done for all women by age 18 or who are sexually active, regardless of age. Women who have multiple sexual partners should be screened annually, but those in long-term, stable relationships who have had negative Pap smears three years in a row may be screened less often.

A major problem with the Pap smear is that it is often thought to be normal when it is actually abnormal. The pathologist examining the cells can make an error, the health care provider may not sample the cervix adequately or an infection might obscure the results. The estimated false negative rate is about 20 percent, half of which can be attributed to faulty sampling techniques.

Adenocarcinomas and adenosquamous carcinomas are also more difficult to detect on Pap smears since they start high up in the cervical canal and may not be sampled by the Pap smear. Because of the high false negative rate, routine annual screening is strongly recommended to decrease the likelihood that cervical warts, dysplasia or cancer will be missed.

COMMON SIGNS AND SYMPTOMS

In many cases—and in almost all cases of carcinoma in situ—there are no symptoms. The most common symptoms that do appear include abnormal vaginal bleeding or discharge, bleeding after intercourse and pain.

DIAGNOSIS

Physical Examination
Most women with cervical cancer will have a normal general physical examination.
♦ Careful evaluation of the vulva, urethra and vagina.
♦ Lymph nodes in the groin and above the collarbone should be examined to detect any enlargement.
♦ Examination of the abdomen to look for an enlarged liver, a mass or excessive abdominal fluid (ascites).
♦ A gynecologic pelvic and rectal examination is important to detect disease in the tissue surrounding the cervix and vagina and the pelvic lymph nodes.

Blood and Other Tests
♦ Complete blood count.
♦ Liver function chemistries.

♦ Kidney function chemistries.

♦ The levels of the serum squamous cell carcinoma antigen (SCCA) and the serum carcinoembryonic antigen (CEA) in the blood should be measured. SCCA is elevated in 50 percent of all women with cervical cancer. CEA is elevated in about 20 percent of all cervical carcinomas. Although CEA and SCCA are not accurate enough to use for screening, they are useful to monitor the response to treatment and for follow-up to detect recurrent disease.

Imaging
♦ Chest x-ray.
♦ CT and MRI scans of the abdomen and pelvis.

Endoscopy and Biopsy
♦ Cystoscopy.
♦ Sigmoidoscopy.
♦ All women with an abnormal Pap smear or cervical lesions should undergo an office colposcopic examination. A colposcope is an instrument that can magnify the cervix from 7.5 to 15 times.
♦ The definitive diagnosis is made on a biopsy. Early cancers are occasionally diagnosed by a large biopsy of the cervix, known as a cone biopsy. A cervical conization should be done when colposcopy cannot determine if there is not an invasive cancer, when there are no obvious lesions on the cervix and the Pap smear is consistently abnormal, when a colposcopically directed biopsy does not adequately account for abnormal cells found on a Pap smear, when a diagnosis of microinvasion (early invasion) is found on the biopsy or when a cervical intraepithelial neoplasia is identified by a scraping from the cervical canal (endocervical curettage).

STAGING

Most gynecologic oncologists use the FIGO (International Federation of Gynecologists and Obstetricians) classification. This divides the disease into five stages, with further divisions in each stage. A carcinoma in situ is Stage 0. The cancer is confined to the cervix in Stage I and, in Stage II, either extends beyond the cervix but not to the pelvic sidewall or involves the vagina but not the lower third. A Stage III carcinoma extends to the pelvic sidewall, involves the lower third of the vagina or obstructs one or both of the ureters. In Stage IV, the cancer has spread to distant organs beyond the true pelvis or involves the lining of the bladder or rectum.

TREATMENT OVERVIEW

Squamous cell carcinoma and adenocarcinoma are generally treated in similar ways. Radical surgery and radiation therapy are equally effective treatments for early stage disease (Stage Ia, Ib and small IIa).

For carcinomas more advanced than Stage IIa, treatment is with radiation therapy alone or radiotherapy and chemotherapy. Higher stages are generally treated with higher doses of radiation therapy as well.

 Surgery For younger women surgery is usually recommended because it allows the ovaries to still function and it avoids the atrophy of the upper vagina and the vaginal scarring that can result from radiation. There is also a small chance that women who survive many years after radiation therapy will develop a second malignancy in the radiated area.

Radical exenterative surgery—removal of the rectum and/or bladder and the cervix, uterus and vagina—is reserved for recurrent carcinoma confined to the central pelvis.

Surgery may also be used to stage the disease, since other methods, even using CT and MRI scans, are notoriously inaccurate in detecting lymph node metastasis and intra-abdominal spread in the more advanced stages. Unfortunately, there is no reliable way to diagnose microscopic metastases to the pelvic and para-aortic nodes without removing them. So gyneco-logic oncologists will occasionally recommend a surgical staging procedure before any radiation therapy is given to evaluate the intra-abdominal surfaces and the status of the pelvic and aortic lymph nodes.

Surgical staging is done through an approach outside the lining of the abdominal cavity. This does not involve the manipulation of the intra-abdominal organs as much as an intra-abdominal operation and results in fewer complications following radiation therapy.

The incidence of cancerous pelvic and para-aortic nodes increases with more advanced disease and there may be a survival advantage to removing the involved nodes. About a third of the time, women with microscopic metastases to the pelvic and aortic nodes can be cured if the nodes are removed and radiation therapy is then given.

Women with positive para-aortic nodes may have distant metastases to the lymph nodes above the collarbone (10 to 20 percent of cases). If the neck nodes are positive, then only palliative therapy is warranted.

 Radiation Several radiation techniques may be used depending on the stage of the disease— external beam therapy or the insertion of radioactive substances into the cervix (intracavitary radiation) or into the tumor (interstitial radiation).

Women with metastatic cancer of the para-aortic lymph nodes are usually treated with external beam radiation.

 Chemotherapy This treatment is currently being investigated for women at high risk for recurrent disease (regardless of the stage) or for those with multiple pelvic lymph node or aortic lymph node metastases. It is also being used simultaneously with radiation therapy in women with large cancers. These studies are too recent to determine the effectiveness of chemotherapy.

TREATMENT BY STAGE

STAGE 0 (*Squamous cell carcinoma*)
Carcinoma in situ (intraepithelial carcinoma).

Standard Treatment There are four treatment options for this early-stage tumor.

Freezing the cervix (cryotherapy) can be performed in the doctor's office and has a negligible complication rate.

Laser therapy is usually done for larger lesions.

A cervical conization not only is for cure but is often performed in women in whom colposcopy cannot distinguish between dysplasia and an underlying invasive carcinoma.

For women who have completed their childbearing or have several recurrences, the removal of the uterus and cervix (hysterectomy) is often recommended.

STAGE 0 (*Adenocarcinoma*)

Standard Treatment Adenocarcinoma in situ (confined to the surface of the cervix) is often difficult to diagnose. The diagnosis is usually made with a cervical biopsy or an endocervical curettage. In all cases a conization is required to rule out a truly invasive lesion.

For women who want to remain able to have children, a cone biopsy may cure the disease if the surgical margins, or edges, do not show any evidence of disease. Even so, adenocarcinoma in situ or an invasive adenocarcinoma is occasionally found in the residual cervix even if the cone biopsy has negative margins.

For those who have completed childbearing, the treatment of choice is a simple hysterectomy.

Five-Year Survival 100 percent

STAGE Ia1
Stage I is a cancer confined to the cervix. Stage Ia involves a carcinoma of the cervix diagnosed only microscopically. This is

further divided into two stages based on the depth of invasion of the cervix. In Stage Ia1, there is only minimal, microscopic invasion.

Standard Treatment Women with this stage of disease are usually treated with a cone biopsy or a hysterectomy.

Five-Year Survival 100 percent

STAGE Ia2
The depth of invasion is less than 5 mm from the surface and less than 7 mm wide.

Standard Treatment When the depth of invasion is less than 3 mm from the surface and there is no vascular space involvement, an abdominal hysterectomy is usually performed. It is not necessary to remove the ovaries in younger women. Five-year survival is 100 percent.

Women with cancer invading greater than 3 mm into the cervix or with cancer less than that, but with blood vessel involvement are treated like women with Stage Ib disease.

Five-Year Survival 80 to 90 percent

Investigational Cervical conization may cure women with lesions that invade less than 3 mm of the cervix and have no blood vessel involvement if the edges, or margins, of the cone biopsy do not have evidence of disease. This is appropriate therapy for women who want to preserve their fertility or avoid a hysterectomy.

STAGE Ib
Lesions are larger than in Stage Ia2 but are still confined to the cervix.

Standard Treatment There are two options for treatment. A radical hysterectomy may be done, with removal of the pelvic lymph nodes on both sides. An alternative is external beam radiation (total dose of 4,000 cGy given in divided doses five days a week for five weeks) followed two weeks

later by an intracavitary cesium insertion for two days and usually by a second one two weeks later. Both options result in an equal rate of cure. The choice depends on available local expertise, the age of the patient and her medical condition.

Small lesions are usually operated on while large ones are treated with radiation. Women who have metastatic disease in the removed pelvic lymph nodes are frequently treated with five weeks of external beam radiation therapy to the pelvis following surgery.

Large lesions confined to the cervix may be treated with external beam radiation five days a week for five weeks, followed by a cesium insertion two weeks later, followed six weeks after that by an abdominal hysterectomy and surgical staging.

Five-Year Survival 80 to 90 percent

STAGE IIa
A Stage II cancer is one that either extends beyond the cervix (but not to the pelvic sidewall) or involves the vagina (but not the lower third). In Stage IIa there is no obvious involvement of the tissue surrounding the cervix (parametrial), but there is involvement of the upper two thirds of the vagina.

Standard Treatment Treatment with either a radical hysterectomy and removal of the pelvic lymph nodes or external beam radiation therapy followed by either one or two insertions of intracavitary cesium is standard.

Women with large lesions of the cervix are sometimes managed with preoperative radiation therapy (4,000 cGy external beam radiation therapy, given in divided doses over five weeks, followed two weeks later by a 72-hour cesium insertion), followed by an abdominal hysterectomy and selective node sampling.

Women who have metastatic disease in the pelvic lymph nodes are often given five weeks of external beam radiation therapy to the pelvis after surgery.

Five-Year Survival Approaching 75 to 80 percent

STAGE IIb
There is obvious parametrial involvement, but no extension to the pelvic sidewall.

Standard Treatment External beam radiation therapy may be given in divided doses over five weeks, followed by two 36- to 48-hour cesium insertions two weeks apart.

Five-Year Survival 66 to 80 percent

Investigational
♦ Radiation therapy given at the same time as chemotherapy (cisplatin + 5-fluorouracil + mitomycin-C or bleomycin + mitomycin-C).
♦ Interstitial radiation therapy—with radioactive iridium temporarily implanted directly into the tumor—is being investigated.
♦ Hyperthermia, a technique using radiation therapy and heat, is also being studied.

STAGE IIIa or IIIb
Stage III is defined as a carcinoma that extends to the pelvic sidewall, involves the lower third of the vagina or obstructs one or both ureters. Stage IIIa means there is no extension to the pelvic sidewall, but the tumor involves the lower third of the vagina. In Stage IIIb, there is extension to the pelvic sidewall, obstruction of one or both ureters, or there is a non-functioning kidney.

Standard Treatment External beam radiation therapy followed by two cesium insertions is the standard therapy.

Five-Year Survival 60 percent

Investigational Same as for Stage IIb.

STAGE IVa
Stage IV is defined as cancer that has spread to distant organs beyond the true pelvis or involves the lining of the bladder or rectum. Stage IVa means that a biopsy has shown that either the lining of the bladder or the rectum have become involved.

Standard Treatment This stage is usually treated with radiation therapy or by the surgical removal of the uterus, the vagina and the bladder and/or rectum (pelvic exenteration).

Five-Year Survival 20 to 30 percent

Investigational Radiation therapy given in conjunction with chemotherapy.

STAGE IVb
In Stage IVb there is spread to distant organs.

Standard Treatment Radiation may be used to relieve the symptoms of pelvic disease or isolated distant metastases.

Several chemotherapy drugs are useful for treating cervical cancer, but they are rarely curative. They include cisplatin or carboplatin, which has a response rate of 15 to 25 percent, and ifosfamide, which has a response rate of 30 percent.

Combination chemotherapy, including cisplatin + etoposide + bleomycin, has a response rate of 50 percent. Other drug combinations that have been used in women with metastatic disease include mitomycin-C + 5-fluorouracil + cisplatin, Velban + bleomycin + cisplatin and cisplatin or carboplatin + ifosfamide.

Investigational Many of the drugs used in the standard treatment are being tested in different combinations and doses.

TREATMENT FOLLOW-UP
A Pap smear and a careful examination of the pelvis, abdomen and lymph nodes is performed every three months for the first two years after treatment, and then every six months for three more years.

♦ Routine chest x-rays and pelvic and abdominal CT scans are not warranted in the absence of symptoms.

♦ The serum levels of carcinoembryonic antigen and/or squamous cell carcinoma antigen in the blood will often be measured at each visit if they were elevated before treatment.

RECURRENT CANCER

Symptoms of recurrent cervical carcinoma may include vaginal bleeding or discharge, pain in the pelvis, back or legs, leg swelling (edema), chronic cough and weight loss.

♦ If radiation was not given previously, recurrences that are confined to the pelvis may be treated with external beam radiation and intracavitary or interstitial radiation therapy.

♦ If radiation therapy was already given, the only option is the removal of the vagina, uterus and the bladder and/or rectum with the creation of an artificial bladder—a pelvic exenteration. The five-year survival rate after a pelvic exenteration is about 50 percent.

♦ Women with recurrent tumors that can't be surgically removed or with metastatic disease are usually treated with chemotherapy. Commonly used drugs include single agent cisplatin or carboplatin. Other regimens include cisplatin or carboplatin + ifosfamide, vincristine + mitomycin-C + bleomycin + cisplatin and bleomycin + mitomycin-C + 5-fluorouracil.

♦ Those with unresectable pelvic disease may be re-irradiated with or without heat or given pelvic arterial chemotherapy.

THE MOST IMPORTANT QUESTIONS YOU CAN ASK

♦ What qualifications do you have for treating cancer? Will a specialist in gynecologic oncology be involved in my care?

♦ What is the advantage of surgery versus radiation therapy?

♦ Why or why won't a staging surgery be performed?

♦ Is adjuvant chemotherapy with radiation therapy beneficial?

CHILDHOOD CANCERS

Jerry Z. Finklestein, MD

◇

Cancer in children is a rare disease. For every 120 adults who develop cancer there is one child. Yet next to accidents, cancer is the second most common cause of death in children between the ages of one and 14. In the United States, about 10,000 new cases of cancer are diagnosed in children under 18 each year.

Childhood cancers are different from those in adults. The growth pattern is different and the tumors react differently to treatment. Most important, the problems seen in a child differ from those of an adult.

Fortunately, with the development of new drugs, new treatment methods, better diagnostic tools and the involvement of multidisciplinary medical teams, the outlook for childhood cancers has improved dramatically over the past few decades. More and more children with cancer are now being cured.

Types The most common childhood cancer is leukemia, accounting for about one-third of all cancers seen. The most common types in children are acute lymphoblastic leukemia and, less frequently, acute non-lymphocytic leukemia. A smaller number of children may develop chronic granulo-cytic leukemia.

Brain tumors—gliomas, medulloblastomas and ependymomas—are the second most common type of cancer in children. A new term has recently been designated for certain types of brain tumors—PNET, which stands for primitive neuro-ectodermal tumors.

Some cancers that occur in children are rare in adults. A cancer of the sympathetic nervous system known as neuroblastoma may occur in the adrenal glands located on top of the kidneys or may originate anywhere there is a particular kind of nerve ending known as a sympathetic nerve ending—the chest, the abdomen, the pelvis and, rarely, other sites. A cancer of the kidney known as Wilms' tumor is also particular to children, occurring most commonly in children two to four years old and rarely in those over 16. It may occur in one or both kidneys.

Other childhood tumors that are uncommon in adults are a tumor of the back of the eye called retinoblastoma; a muscle tumor called rhabdomyosarcoma; teratomas, which are tumors of young cells known as germ cells; and a tumor of the liver known as hepatoblastoma.

Bone tumors such as osteogenic sarcoma, Ewing's sarcoma or chondrosarcoma occur in children, particularly teenagers. Histiocytosis X or Langerhans cell histiocytosis is not a malignancy but is often cared for by physicians who specialize in pediatric cancer therapy.

Children, like adults, develop lymphomas known as Hodgkin's disease and non-Hodgkin's lymphoma. They may also have tumors of the liver (hepatomas), skin cancer (melanoma, which is rare) and cancers of the thyroid, adrenal glands and blood vessels.

Over 80 percent of cancers in adults develop in the glands or lining tissues of the breast, lung, intestinal or urinary tract and are called carcinomas. But over 90 percent of cancers of children are malignancies of muscle, bone, supporting tissues or blood vessels and are called sarcomas. The types of cancer seen in children, therefore, differ from those in adults not only in name but in their microscopic appearance.

What Causes It We do not know why children develop cancer. Occasionally there are clues from the environment or from a genetic inheritance pattern that a child may be at risk. But specific causes have not been identified. However, children with certain diseases do have an increased incidence of cancer (*see* "Risk Factors").

For more than 25 years there have been reports of "clusters" or concentrations of childhood cancer developing in certain geographic areas. There were clusters of children with leukemia in Niles, Illinois, in 1963, for example, and another in Woburn, Massachusetts, in 1979. But physicians have not been able to figure out the significance of these clusters.

It is believed that children are more likely than adults to develop leukemia as a result of exposure to radiation. Children exposed to the radiation of the atomic bomb blasts in Japan had an increased risk of acute leukemia in childhood, with the peak occurring about five years after exposure. The incidence of leukemia in children exposed to radiation after the accident in Chernobyl, USSR, remains to be seen.

Years ago, children received radiation therapy for enlargement of the thymus (an organ just under the breast bone) and for skin diseases such as ringworm of the scalp. We now know that this radiation can cause cancer anywhere from 6 to 35 years later. (Radiation treatment is useful in the treatment of many cancers in children, but there is risk that children cured of their first cancer may develop a second one partly related to the use of radiation therapy.)

A number of cancer-causing chemicals or industrial processes are all around us, though their role in causing childhood cancers has not been identified.

There has also been recent publicity about electromagnetic waves produced by high-tension power lines as a possible cause of cancer in children. Various reports have either supported or refuted that information, and further research is being done in the United States to determine whether such electromagnetic waves do in fact play a role.

For parents it is frustrating to acknowledge that there is very little we can do to protect our children from an environmental or genetic factor. Research is continuing, however, and one day we shall probably have better means of protection.

RISK FACTORS

The cancer rate for Afro-American children in the United States is about 80 percent of that seen in white children; children who are black do not have the same incidence of common cancers such as acute lymphocytic leukemia and lymphomas as children who are white. Black children rarely have Ewing's sarcoma, but there is a suggestion that they have a higher incidence of Wilms' tumor, retinoblastoma and the bone tumor known as osteogenic sarcoma.

Several cancers in children—leukemias and Wilms' tumors, for example—peak in incidence between the ages of two and four years. Others, such as lymphomas and bone cancer, have a peak incidence in older children.

At Significantly Higher Risk
♦ Previous exposure to radiation.
♦ Children who do not have an iris—the colored circle in their eye—have a higher incidence of developing the kidney cancer called Wilms' tumor.
♦ Children whose body is bigger on one side than the other (hemihypertrophy) have a higher incidence of Wilms' tumor.
♦ Males with an undescended testicle (cryptorchidism) are at higher risk for testicular cancer.
♦ Children with the skin disease xeroderma pigmentosum have a higher risk of developing skin cancer.
♦ Children with the immune disorder ataxia telangiectasia, Down's syndrome, Fanconi's anemia and Bloom's syndrome are at higher risk for developing leukemia.

SCREENING

A number of tests screen for cancer in adults but very few such tests exist for children. In Japan, Quebec and some other parts of North America, there is an attempt to screen the urine of very young children to detect the presence of abnormal amounts of the chemical group known as catecholamines in the hope that earlier detection of neuroblastoma will result in an improved cure rate.

The child with a risk factor for developing cancer should be evaluated carefully by his or her physician. The screening may be as simple as a blood test in an identical twin of a child with leukemia or a series of ultrasound examinations of the abdomen for many years in a child with hemihypertrophy.

COMMON SIGNS AND SYMPTOMS

Many of the symptoms and signs of childhood cancers are very common and only health professionals with sufficient training will be able to tell whether a complaint is due to a normal childhood disease or a rare disease such as cancer.

Tiredness and paleness are usually the result of nothing more than the flu but could also signal the onset of leukemia. Fever is often noted in a child with an infection, but recurrent fever, especially with bone pain, may be a symptom of leukemia or a bone tumor.

Children who have headaches with vomiting may have nothing more than an upset stomach, but recurrent headaches with vomiting that do not to go away with time require a physician to make sure there isn't a brain tumor.

Children who have a mass in their abdomen are probably just constipated, but the mass could be Wilms' tumor, neuroblastoma, lymphoma or a liver tumor. Lumps in the neck are usually due to an infection, but if they don't respond to antibiotics, a lymphoma is a possibility. Drainage from the ear is usually due to an ear infection and only rarely due to some tumor.

Weight loss is rare in a young child, although it is something teenagers often desire. If the weight loss is not controlled, however, there may be psychological reasons involved or a lymphoma such as Hodgkin's disease.

Obviously, children's complaints are usually the result of normal childhood diseases. But when parents are concerned that their child has a persistent problem, then without question they should take him or her to the doctor. The findings of a physical examination may suggest that special tests are necessary to discover whether the child does in fact have a cancer.

Some signs and symptoms are not common, however. Any newborn child with a cat's eye—a white dot in the center of the eye—should be seen by a physician, since the dot may indicate a retinoblastoma. It is also very rare for children to have blood in their urine, so any child with this complaint should be seen by a physician. Blood in the urine may be the result of an infection, but may also be caused by Wilms' tumor.

DIAGNOSIS

Physical Examination
♦ A complete physical examination should include the groin area, the testicles, the skin and the nervous system. A rectal examination may also be performed to rule out a tumor in that area.
♦ Enlarged liver and/or spleen or a mass in the abdomen may indicate a tumor.
♦ Lumps in the neck that are firm, non-movable and have not responded to antibiotics may be due to lymphomas, leukemias and other cancers.
♦ The eyes may be examined, a procedure that requires the child's cooperation. A special instrument for looking into the eyes (ophthalmoscope) lets the physician see if there is increased pressure in the brain, which is often due to a brain tumor.

Blood and Other Tests
♦ A simple blood test examining the red cells, white cells and platelets will usually let the doctor decide whether acute leukemia is a serious possibility.
♦ Other tests such as a urine test will be helpful in cases of suspected neuroblastoma.

Imaging
♦ X-rays and CT and MRI scans help the physician decide whether there are tumors in the brain, chest, abdomen or extremities.

Endoscopy and Biopsy
♦ Some suspected tumors may have to be biopsied for a definitive diagnosis.

STAGING

Many so-called solid tumors of childhood—those that do not develop in the blood—are often staged by a system that classifies the disease by whether it can be completely removed surgically. The involvement of lymph nodes and spread to distant sites are also considered. Greatly simplified, Stage I usually refers to local disease that can be entirely removed by a surgeon. Stage II could still be a local disease that may also be removed but has extended beyond the immediate area of the tumor. Stage III disease tends to be more extensive but localized in one particular region of the body, and Stage IV disease is widespread, having spread though the blood or lymphatic system to produce new tumors (metastases) in other organs.

Leukemia is often defined according to its potential for relapse as low risk, average risk and high risk. The child with low-risk leukemia has an excellent chance of responding to therapy in the long term and the best chance of being cured. On the other hand, a child with high-risk leukemia may still respond to therapy and may still be cured, although he or she may need more intensive treatment.

TREATMENT OVERVIEW

The treatment of a child's cancer may involve surgery, chemotherapy, radiation therapy, immunotherapy and various supportive measures.

The special problems seen with childhood cancers mean that a child should not be treated only by an individual physician. A team approach is required, with physicians assisted by many specialists including psychologists and experts in nursing, social services, nutrition, physiotherapy, occupational therapy, pharmacy and other fields. They should all be involved in designing the appropriate treatment and support program for the child and his or her family.

This kind of multidisciplinary approach

can be accomplished only in a "center of excellence," an approved pediatric cancer specialty unit. In the United States and Canada there are two cooperative groups known as The Children's Cancer Study Group and The Pediatric Oncology Group. Physicians and hospitals associated with these groups treat the majority of children with cancer in these countries. There are also certain well-known and highly specialized hospitals in both countries in which physicians independently treat children with cancer.

When a child is diagnosed with cancer in most of these centers, his or her case is presented to a Tumor Board, a meeting of physician specialists, subspecialists and other members of the treatment team who evaluate the child, discuss the options and agree to a proposed treatment plan.

(For treatment of osteogenic sarcoma, rhabdomyosarcoma and Ewing's sarcoma, *see* "Sarcomas of Bone and Soft Tissue." For treatment of acute leukemia, *see* "Leukemia.")

Clinical Trials Cancer in children is rare. Each year in the United States, slightly over 3,000 children develop leukemia, 2,000 develop various kinds of brain tumors, fewer than 500 develop Wilms' tumor or rhabdomyosarcoma and fewer than 250 develop retinoblastoma. Obviously, if progress is to be made on more effective treatment methods, physicians throughout the nation have to work closely together in designing therapies.

Accordingly, all children with cancer who are treated in a center of excellence are asked to participate in a clinical research program. It is because of these programs that we have made such gratifying progress in the treatment of childhood cancer over the past few decades. Parents and their children are encouraged to participate in them.

Phase III Trials A child may be a candidate for a research program known as a clinical protocol, which will compare one form of treatment to another. The research protocol will be explained and parents will be asked to agree to participate with their child in the program.

The program may involve "randomization," meaning that which of the several potentially effective treatments the child receives will be decided by chance. Parents are often upset when they learn that if they participate in a research program the decision about which treatment their child will receive will not be chosen by their child's physician. But parents should understand that their child's physician would not participate in the program unless he or she were comfortable that *all* the various treatment choices are reasonable, appropriate and offer the child an excellent chance of attaining a response.

The initial treatment programs designed to answer which treatment program is best are often known as Phase III studies. Sometimes a research protocol is not available, and then the physician chooses the best-known effective treatment available for the disease and presents it as the proposed treatment plan.

Most children respond very well to the initial treatment of their cancer. The opportunity to cure a child with cancer may be as high as 80 to 90 percent for some children with acute lymphoblastic leukemia and Wilms' tumor, but unfortunately less in most other tumors. The patient's physician will be able to describe in detail the chances of the child being cured and the details of the treatment being proposed to attain that goal.

Phase II Trials Unfortunately, not all children respond to therapy. Even those who do may relapse. These children may still have their disease controlled and occasionally cured.

Children with recurrent disease are often asked to participate in Phase II protocols, treatment programs in which the dose and many of the side effects of a particular drug or treatment are known. The goal of treatment is to determine how effective the treatment is for certain kinds of childhood cancer.

If this kind of study is available and the child and parents are asked to participate, the physician will describe in detail the proposed treatment, the risks involved and the possible advantages of the child working with the physician in this research approach.

Phase I Trials Occasionally there are drugs to be tested in children for the first time. Research protocols involving new drugs are called Phase I studies. The goal is to find the appropriate dose to be used, with the hope that the children will respond to the treatment.

Investigational Treatments There is a long list of investigational protocols for most childhood cancers. These protocols are devised after close cooperation and collaboration among investigators working in groups such as The Children's Cancer Study Group or Pediatric Oncology Group or at specific centers of excellence.

The protocols may involve new drugs that have rarely been used in children, such as interferon or IL-2 (interleukin-2). Or they may involve new types of radiation therapy such as high-dose radiation given in a series of small doses (fractionated radiotherapy).

Most pediatric cancer experts do not consider such programs experimental but rather investigational. They consider these protocols an opportunity for the child and his or her family to participate on the frontier of medicine. A child with cancer should be treated with the methods being devised today that will possibly improve the chances for a cure tomorrow, not with yesterday's methods that need to be improved.

Bone Marrow Transplantation Several treatment programs for childhood cancer use the concept of bone marrow transplantation, although this is still considered an investigational treatment under evaluation (*see* Chapter 12).

Allogeneic bone marrow transplantation—which involves giving the child who has cancer bone marrow taken from a donor, ideally a close relative such as a brother or a sister—is being used very often in children with acute non-lymphoblastic (mycloid) leukemia. It is also used quite frequently in children with acute lymphoblastic leukemia who have had a relapse.

In autologous bone marrow transplantation, the patient's own bone marrow is used. A portion of the bone marrow is stored in the laboratory while the patient receives treatment, and then returned in the form of an intravenous infusion of bone marrow cells. These cells circulate throughout the body and settle into the bone marrow compartment from which they came. They subsequently grow and regenerate the bone marrow.

Newer approaches have also recently been devised. It is now known that bone marrow cells may circulate throughout the blood, and machines that can remove some of the circulating cells are being developed, raising the possibility of removing bone marrow cells from a vein rather than by drawing them out of bones through a needle.

In high-dose rescue therapy—also known as autologous rescue—the patient's bone marrow cells are stored while high-dose chemotherapy is given. The cells are then reinfused. The higher doses of chemotherapy may kill cancer cells more effectively but might also seriously damage the bone marrow if rescue therapy were not performed.

SUPPORTIVE THERAPY

Throughout the course of the child's treatment, there will be a need for many kinds of support therapies.

◆ Transfusions of blood products, platelets and white cells may be needed.

◆ Infections are common in children and may require specific antibiotics. Exposure to contagious disease is likely to occur, so the child may require specific gamma globulin.

◆ Supportive measures can include nutritional support such as artificial feedings through a vein (hyperalimentation). Getting access to a vein may be a problem so central venous catheters are often used, such as the Broviac or Hickman catheters or the Port-a-Cath.

◆ Physiotherapists will help children who have motor function problems because of tumors in the central nervous system.

◆ Drugs, other agents and psychological support techniques may be necessary to help children with anticipatory nausea, or nausea and vomiting after radiation or chemotherapy treatments.

TREATMENT FOLLOW-UP

Whatever the treatment a child with cancer is receiving, he or she will be followed closely by the pediatric oncologist, other physician specialists and the multidisciplinary team assembled to work with both the child and the family.

Since the child will be on a research protocol in most cases, the physician will be able to outline for the parents an organized plan for follow-up evaluations. These may include specific liver function tests, urine tests for children with neuroblastoma, specific x-rays, psychologic testing or other tests that can help follow the progress and effects of the disease and the response to treatment.

Even when a child finishes a course of treatment, he or she will require long-term follow-up by a pediatric cancer expert. This is not only because some treatments have long-term side effects, but also because children who are cured of a first cancer do have a small risk of developing

a second one. So even the child who finishes therapy and is apparently cured should be followed by a specialist for the rest of his or her life.

SOME OF THE MOST IMPORTANT QUESTIONS (AND ANSWERS) FOR YOU AND YOUR CHILD

FOR THE CHILD

◆ *What do I have?*
It is now known that children do better when they are told the truth about their illness. We no longer hide from them the fact that they have cancer. We explain the nature of their disease, tell them about the therapy and ask them to work with physicians and other experts to help them reach a cure. Honesty is the best way to help a child with cancer face the serious problems of the disease.

◆ *Why did this happen?*
We do not know why children develop cancer. Although there are sometimes environmental or genetic clues that a child may be at risk, specific causes have not been found in the same way we can say that streptococcus bacteria causes a sore throat.
It is important for the child—and the parents—to realize that having cancer is not a punishment. Cancer occurs in children throughout the world. Parents especially should not feel guilty. Their strength and optimism is needed by their child, who is facing a serious disease and requires their support to conquer the cancer and win the battle for his or her life.

◆ *Will my hair grow back?*
Most children lose their hair temporarily after chemotherapy. In rare cases, such as when very intensive radiation treatments are used, hair may not grow back. But in most cases the child develops a beautiful head of hair after the temporary period of baldness. Many children use wigs to help them with their self-image during these periods.

♦ *What will happen with the acne and chubby face I have when I'm getting prednisone treatment?*

Prednisone and other steroids such as Decadron do cause a temporary gain in weight and may cause facial acne. Once these drugs are stopped the weight gain and the puffiness of the face disappear and the skin improves dramatically. There are very few if any permanent side effects of these treatments. Occasionally stretch marks may be seen in the abdomen, but otherwise the child's complexion and facial configuration do return to normal.

FOR THE PARENT

♦ *When will I get my child back?*

When a child is diagnosed as having cancer, he or she may experience a change in personality. The child's spirit, temperament and behavior pattern may change substantially. The initial treatment may require a long period of hospitalization and even if the child is seen as an outpatient there are frequent visits that may include uncomfortable injections. It may take a while before the family pattern gets back to normal. Parents have to be patient. It may take several months before their child's behavior returns to what it was before the illness.

♦ *How about school?*

For a child, school is the normal working environment. Just as an adult wishes to return to work and continue his or her normal activities, so too the child wishes to get back to the normal routine. Multidisciplinary programs will offer the family support to work with the school system so that the child with cancer can re-enter his or her normal environment. School administrators, teachers and others are becoming more familiar with the fact that children in their classrooms may be undergoing cancer therapy. For the most part, school personnel are understanding. They can develop flexible schedules that permit the child to take advantage of the maximum number of educational opportunities while continuing with treatment programs.

♦ *How can we help relieve the nausea, vomiting and other side effects of chemotherapy?*

Unfortunately, many cancer chemotherapy drugs cause nausea, vomiting, mouth sores, constipation, skin rashes, sore eyes and generally a lower resistance to infection. Physicians can offer other medications that will help the child tolerate some of these side effects. The medications themselves will often cause tiredness. Prompt attention should be given to the constipation caused by vincristine.

♦ *What are the long-term effects of therapy?*

A number of long-term effects of childhood cancer therapy are currently being studied. Radiation therapy to the brain may leave some children with certain deficits in intellectual or motor development, which is why psychometric testing is so important as part of the general treatment follow-up.

Some children may have growth problems. Some may have an organ abnormality because of the effects of radiation therapy or surgery. Rehabilitation may be necessary, such as a new bladder to urinate or an artificial limb. Some drugs also affect the way organs such as the lungs and heart work. Children with cancer may have to be followed for many years to discover whether some of the treatments used to cure the disease will result in organ problems later on in life.

♦ *What are the chances for my child being cured?*

A physician will be able to explain to the child and the parents the chances of attaining not only remission—control of the disease—but actual cure. These "chances" are statistical averages, however, and children are not statistics. A family can concentrate on the negative or on the positive. As long as there is an opportunity for a cure, it makes more sense to concentrate on the positive and focus the family's energy on the possibility that their child will be cured and will grow up and live a normal life span. Most children with cancer *are* cured and become healthy adults, parents and productive members of society.

◆ *What happens if my child does not respond?*

There are children who do not respond to treatment and unfortunately the disease may take their life. If it appears that this is going to happen, the child's physician will be the first to explain to the parents the nature of the problem and the reason why it looks as though the child is not going to have his or her life saved. The health care team will make sure that the child is comfortable and treated in a humane, caring manner. The physician and other members of the multidisciplinary team will work with the family to provide emotional, psychological and spiritual support.

"CLIMBING THE MOUNTAIN"

For the child with cancer and his or her parents there are two basic choices. They can choose the pessimistic road, which goes downhill and expects that the cancer will cause the child to die. They can choose the optimistic road, an admittedly uphill road leading to the top of a mountain.

The curves in the mountain road are many. They are the many problems that have to be handled during treatment, which may include:

◆ Recurrent admission to the hospital for fevers and infections requiring intravenous antibiotics.

◆ Side effects of chemotherapy such as hair loss, nausea, vomiting, mouth ulcers, stomach ulcers, blood in the urine and rectal ulcers.

◆ Side effects of radiation therapy such as hair loss, skin irritation, nausea, vomiting and fatigue.

◆ Side effects of surgery including discomfort and organs that do not work in a normal way.

◆ Allergic reactions to blood, blood products or antibiotics.

◆ Changes in plans to attend school or social functions or to go on family trips.

◆ Therapies that are only partially successful.

◆ Special kinds of treatment such as investigational protocols or bone marrow transplantation.

Each and every one of these problems or curves can be difficult to manage. But each and every one has been managed successfully by other children and other families of children who have cancer. Sometimes, a curve can't be maneuvered and it is necessary to move onto the pessimistic road. But for most children with cancer, the curves can be managed and the climb up the mountain is successful. Treatment may be for six months or a year or even two, three or more years, but the top of the mountain can be reached and on the top there is a straight path. The sky is blue and the sun is shining.

The goal for all children with cancer is that they will be cured. More and more children with cancer are attaining this goal and are growing up to be healthy adults. So children and their parents should be optimistic. Knowing that cure is a possibility, each child and his or her family should plan on climbing the mountain and reaching the top, which is flooded with blue sky and sunshine.

CHILDHOOD CANCERS: BRAIN TUMORS
Malin Dollinger, MD

Primary brain tumors—those that start in the brain rather than spreading there from other parts of the body—are the most common "solid" tumors children get. They pose a major treatment challenge that has to be met by the coordinated efforts of a variety of health care professionals, including specialists in pediatric neurosurgery, radiation therapy and oncology, as well as neuroradiologists and neuropathologists. Significant emotional stresses and problems may occur, requiring intervention by specialized health care professionals.

Many tumors are controllable or curable with treatment, and over half of the children diagnosed with brain tumors will live more than five years. Every child's therapy should be aggressively planned with the intent to cure if possible. This is true even in situations where the same tumor occurring in an adult would not likely be cured.

As is true of all pediatric cancers, but especially with brain tumors, most advances in treatment have been produced by clinical trials of new methods. Various major cancer centers and cooperative groups such as the Pediatric Oncology Group and the Children's Cancer Study Group have clinical treatment protocols available for many tumors, and consideration should be given to enrolling children in such trials. They generally represent the most advanced and promising methods of treatment.

Types Brain tumors are classified by the appearance of their cells under the microscope (histopathology) and their location in the brain. The types that occur in children are usually similar to those seen in adults, although there are a few types that

are much more common in children.

There is a structure in the back part of the brain, a roof-like membrane called the tentorium. This is just above the cerebellum (the portion of the brain having to do with balance and coordination) and the brain stem. There are significant differences in the types of tumors occurring above and below this membrane, as well as in the methods used to make a diagnosis and follow the results of therapy.

About half the brain tumors in children occur below the tentorium, most being in the cerebellum or the nearby cavity called the fourth ventricle. This area of the brain is the posterior fossa. Tumors in the region include astrocytomas, medulloblastomas and ependymoma.

The area above the tentorium, which makes up most of the brain, is called the supratentorial region. Tumors in this area include astrocytomas, cerebral neuroblastomas, ependymoma, craniopharyngioma, meningioma, germ cell tumors, optic nerve glioma, pineal tumors and choroid plexus tumors.

There may be many different names for these tumors, especially as newer classification systems are more descriptive or accurate.

How It Spreads Brain tumors rarely spread outside the central nervous system, but can spread within the brain and the spinal cord.

What Causes It Unknown, although some genetic disorders have been associated with an increased risk.

SCREENING

There are no effective screening measures.

COMMON SIGNS AND SYMPTOMS

Symptoms related to the increased pressure in the brain as the tumor expands include headache, nausea, vomiting (which may or may not not accompany nausea) and seizures. Symptoms related to the tumor's location and the pressure it puts on nearby structures include weakness or changes in sensation in various parts of the body, difficulties in coordination or balance, and vision and speech problems.

DIAGNOSIS

Physical Examination

♦ Complete neurologic examination.
♦ Evaluation for optic tract glioma includes neuro-ophthalmological testing, including visual fields. Subtle changes in the tumor that may not be apparent with CT or MRI scanning can be measured in this way. Young children may have a test called visual-evoked response for diagnosis and follow-up.

Blood and Other Tests

♦ Bone marrow may be analyzed for tumors that spread outside the central nervous system (medulloblastoma, pineal tumors).
♦ For tumors that may spread to the spinal cord or through the cerebrospinal fluid (medulloblastoma, ependymoma, intracranial germ cell tumors, pineal tumors, cerebral neuroblastoma—PNET), spinal fluid should be examined for malignant cells.
♦ For intracranial germ cell tumors, tumor markers including alpha-fetoprotein (AFP) and human chorionic gonadotropin (HCG) are measured. The same markers are also measured in pineal tumors to exclude the possibility of a malignant germ cell tumor.
♦ For pineal tumors, cerebrospinal fluid cytology, sugar and protein.

Imaging

♦ Imaging has been conventionally done by CT for the brain and myelography for the spinal cord. Recently, MRI imaging with gadolinium enhancement has been shown to be extremely sensitive, useful and simpler.
♦ Images of the entire brain and spinal cord should be done for tumors that may spread to the spinal cord (medulloblastoma, ependymoma, intracranial germ cell tumors, pineal tumors, cerebral neuroblastoma—PNET).
♦ Bone scans are usually done in medulloblastoma because this tumor may spread outside the central nervous system, especially to bone.

Endoscopy and Biopsy

♦ Tumors of the brain stem, the medulla and the pons (brain stem glioma) are not usually biopsied. The procedure is risky and there is little benefit since they cannot be removed surgically (radiation therapy is the standard treatment). In a few circumstances, however, stereotactic needle biopsy techniques may enable biopsy to be done when it could have an effect on treatment—for example, if it is not certain that a mass in this area is malignant, if the tumor grows outwards and protrudes into the ventricles or if there is a need to remove part of the tumor because of pressure symptoms.
♦ Biopsy of optic tract glioma is not always possible because it is difficult to expose the area surgically.

STAGING

There are no generally useful staging systems for most brain tumors, although some are classified according to grade. With brain stem glioma, for example, tumors in the higher region—the midbrain—are more likely to be lower grade and have a higher chance of long-term survival than tumors lower down in the pons and the medulla (40 percent versus less than 20 percent).

A variety of staging systems have been used for medulloblastoma. The Pediatric Oncology Group and the Children's Cancer Study Group have divided this tumor into low and high stages. Essentially, low-stage implies smaller tumors without metastasis, in which the tumor remaining after surgery is smaller than 1.5 cubic cm. High-stage refers to larger tumors with evidence of metastatic spread or brain stem involvement and tumor over 1.5 cubic cm remaining after surgery.

TREATMENT OVERVIEW

Treatment includes surgery, with or without radiation therapy. Radiation therapy of pediatric brain tumors is very complex and should be carried out in facilities with extensive experience.

Chemotherapy has recently shown some activity in adults with recurrent brain tumors, and there has been some enthusiasm for treating childhood brain tumors with chemotherapy as well. This is especially so because children under three are very susceptible to growth limitations, especially the hindering of normal brain development, produced by radiation therapy. There is great interest in using chemotherapy initially in children under three to allow radiation therapy to be delayed until a time when it might not be as harmful.

Clinical Trials All children with brain tumors should be considered for entry into clinical trials. This form of cancer is rare in children and trials offer the advantage of the pooled experience of pediatric cancer centers around the country.

Pediatric clinical trials are designed in two ways. One method divides the children into two groups, with one receiving the best currently accepted standard treatment and the other receiving the new therapy that appears promising. The other method is to evaluate a single new treatment in all patients and then compare the results with those obtained with existing therapy, often in the same institution.

TREATMENT BY TUMOR TYPE

MEDULLOBLASTOMA

This is also called primitive neuroectodermal tumor (PNET). It arises in the cerebellum and may spread to adjacent tissues. It also can spread via the cerebrospinal fluid to the rest of the brain or the spinal cord.

Standard Treatment An attempt is made to surgically remove as much tumor as possible. Studies are done during and after the operation to define the risk of relapse, and treatment is given according to the best estimate of low-stage or high-stage disease.

For low-stage disease, standard therapy after surgery is a high dose of radiation to the tumor area and a lower dose to the entire brain and spine. The dosage required is under study in a clinical protocol. This type of radiation is extremely problematic because of concern about failure of treatment and the recurrence of tumor at the junction between adjacent radiation ports. Lowering the dosage of radiation to reduce problems with nervous system development significantly reduces the chance for cure. Children under three should be entered in studies that use chemotherapy and probably delayed or modified radiation therapy.

Treatment of high-stage disease involves chemotherapy in addition to surgery and the radiation therapy usually given in low-stage disease.

Patients at high risk for progression of disease after standard treatment—those with locally extensive disease, tumor that cannot be completely removed and those with metastatic disease—should be placed in the high-stage group and be considered for entry into a clinical trial to find the best sequence and type of chemotherapy.

Five-Year Survival About 50 percent

Recurrent Cancer Medulloblastoma that recurs after radiotherapy should be considered for treatment with active chemotherapy agents such as vincristine, cyclophosphamide and cisplatin. Fewer than one-third of patients respond and long-term control of disease is unusual, so if relapse occurs after these treatments, children should be considered for entry into clinical trials of new agents.

CEREBELLAR ASTROCYTOMA

These are generally low-grade tumors in the cerebellum. Spread is unusual. The tumors can be divided into good-risk and poor-risk groups after review of the histopathology.

Standard Treatment The primary treatment is surgical removal of the tumor. In contrast to most other brain tumors, some patients with microscopic and even larger residual tumor after surgery may survive a long time without any symptoms or tumor growth even without postoperative therapy. This may be significant because a second operation may produce neurologic problems.

The use of radiation therapy after surgery is under considerable discussion. Some radiation oncologists treat all patients with residual disease, others withhold treatment until the tumor starts to grow.

Chemotherapy may be useful to delay radiation therapy in young children with tumors that cannot be completely removed.

Ten-Year Survival About 80 percent

Recurrent Cancer Cerebellar astrocytoma that recurs is treated, if possible, with another surgery. If this is not possible, local radiation is used. If it recurs in an area where it can't be removed and has already received maximum radiation, chemotherapy should be considered. Since there is little information available about the role of chemotherapy, Phase I

and Phase II clinical studies should be considered.

INFRATENTORIAL EPENDYMOMA

These tumors arise from the cells lining the fourth ventricle (a cavity within the brain), as well as those lining a cavity in the center of the spinal cord. They can occur anywhere in the brain or spinal cord, but 60 percent of them start in the back part of the brain, the posterior fossa. The prognosis depends on the grade and size of the tumor and the degree of spread.

Standard Treatment High-dose radiation to the back part of the brain is the usual treatment. Radiotherapy to the entire brain and spinal cord is controversial, being used most commonly in high-grade tumors.

There is no clear benefit for adjuvant chemotherapy, although consideration should be given to using chemotherapy to delay or modify radiation therapy in very young children.

Five-Year Survival 25 to 60 percent

Investigational
♦ Surgery followed by radiation therapy.

Recurrent Cancer This tumor is seldom controlled permanently if it recurs after surgery and radiotherapy. About one-third of patients respond to cisplatin, so Phase I and II clinical trials should be considered.

BRAIN STEM GLIOMA

Tumors arising in the brain stem are often astrocytomas, a tumor of neuron-support cells. These are also referred to as brain stem gliomas. They may be low-, intermediate- or high-grade.

Standard Treatment The usual treatment is high-dose radiation therapy (over 5,500 cGy). Higher doses may be possible using twice-daily (hyperfractionated) treatment. Some current trials use still higher doses.

Some current trials use still higher doses.

The role of chemotherapy is not well known and occasional patients may have to be approached surgically. Children younger than three may be given chemotherapy to delay or modify radiation therapy to reduce the risk of neurologic impairment.

Two-Year Survival Less than 25 percent

Investigational
♦ The use of chemotherapy before the standard radiotherapy treatment.

Recurrent Cancer There is no standard therapy for recurrent brain stem glioma. These children cannot have surgery, have already received maximum radiation therapy, and there are no standard chemotherapy drugs that have significant results. They should be entered in a Phase I or Phase II clinical protocol drug trial.

CEREBRAL ASTROCYTOMA
LOW GRADE
These tumors may sometimes be completely removed surgically, in which case they have a favorable prognosis. These tumors spread by extension to the adjacent brain and sometimes occur in multiple sites.

Standard Treatment The treatment for low-grade supratentorial astrocytoma is surgery. If the tumor cannot be completely removed, radiotherapy is given after the operation. In some centers, radiotherapy is withheld until progression of disease is shown. The role of chemotherapy is not known.

Five-Year Survival 50 to 80 percent

Recurrent Cancer Patients may benefit from chemotherapy if tumors recur after maximum surgery and radiation therapy. No standard agents have a high degree of response, although cyclophosphamide, cisplatin and the nitrosoureas may be useful. Consideration should be given to clinical trials.

CEREBRAL ASTROCYTOMA
HIGH GRADE
Sometimes called anaplastic astrocytoma or glioblastoma multiforme, these tumors often grow rapidly and involve significant portions of the brain.

Standard Treatment Treatment includes surgery, radiation therapy and chemotherapy. Radiation is given after as complete a surgical resection as possible to an area that encompasses the entire tumor and sometimes the whole brain.

A Children's Cooperative Group study with radiation therapy and three chemotherapy agents (vincristine + lomustine + prednisone) produced a 40 percent survival of three years compared with 13 percent for children treated with radiation therapy alone. Again, children under the age of three may receive chemotherapy to delay or modify radiotherapy. A number of clinical trials are evaluating the role of chemotherapy.

Two-Year Survival Less than 25 percent. The prognosis may be better if the tumor can be totally removed. Younger patients and those with lower grade tumors may do better.

Recurrent Cancer Chemotherapy is given if relapse occurs after radiation therapy. Since no standard agents have a high degree of activity, entry on a clinical trial should be considered.

SUPRATENTORIAL EPENDYMOMA
These ependymomas arise outside the posterior fossa (back of the brain), usually within and adjacent to the ventricles.

Standard Treatment Surgery followed by radiation therapy. In low-grade tumors, the primary tumor area is given radiation. With high-grade tumors, the entire brain and spinal cord are treated.

Adjuvant chemotherapy has not been

used, although consideration should be given to its use in very young children to delay or modify radiation therapy.

Two-Year Survival About 40 percent

Investigational
♦ Various radiotherapy trials, with and without chemotherapy.

Recurrent Cancer This tumor is seldom controlled if it recurs after surgery and radiation therapy, although one-third of patients respond to cisplatin. Phase I and II clinical studies should be considered.

CRANIOPHARYNGIOMA
These benign tumors arise in the central portion of the brain and produce problems primarily because of their location. Since they are benign, metastasis is unknown.

Standard Treatment Surgery or radiation therapy or a combination of the two produces a high rate of long-term control in most patients. There is no reported role for chemotherapy.

Ten-Year Survival About 80 percent

INTRACRANIAL GERM CELL TUMOR
Germ cell brain tumors—there are a number of sub-types—usually arise in the central portion of the brain. Under the microscope, they resemble more common germ cell tumors of the testis and ovary. The prognosis relates to the cell type and is especially favorable in patients with germinoma.

Standard Treatment The role of surgery is usually a biopsy to establish the diagnosis, since the location of these tumors usually prevents complete removal. Germinoma is treated with radiation therapy to the brain and spinal cord, with high doses to the tumor and somewhat lower doses to the rest of the nerve tissue. This treatment often produces a cure.

Local radiation therapy or chemotherapy before surgery has produced some encouraging responses, but the definitive role of chemotherapy is not yet known.

Advanced or disseminated germinomas, as well as the various germ cell tumors other than germinoma, are usually treated with radiation to the brain and spinal cord. There are several views about the dosage and areas that should be treated.

Non-germinoma germ cell tumors may respond to a variety of chemotherapeutic agents, including bleomycin, cisplatin, etoposide, cyclophosphamide and vincristine. The role of adjuvant chemotherapy, in addition to radiation, is not yet determined for these tumors that arise within the brain, although chemotherapy is extremely effective in these tumors elsewhere in the body.

Survival Variable

Recurrent Cancer Intracerebral germ cell tumors may be responsive to the same type of chemotherapy combinations used against germ cell tumors in other locations—PVB (cisplatin + vinblastine + bleomycin) and VAC (vincristine + dactinomycin + cyclophosphamide).

If the tumor recurs after treatment with these programs, Phase I and II clinical studies should be used to try to find agents that may be useful in treating this tumor, which is often responsive to chemotherapy.

PINEAL TUMORS
This undifferentiated tumor resembles medulloblastoma, but it develops in the region of the pineal gland in the center of the brain. The prognosis depends upon the size of tumor and its degree of spread.

Standard Treatment The usual treatment is radiation therapy. There is some controversy about the possibility of surgical removal, although biopsy is recommended whenever possible to establish a diagnosis. A high dose of radiation is given to the tumor, with a lower dose to the brain and spinal cord.

Studies are exploring the role of chemotherapy for poorly differentiated pineal tumors, although well-differentiated tumors may be treated with simple local radiation therapy. Young children may be given chemotherapy to delay or modify the radiation treatments.

Two-Year Survival Less than 50 percent

OPTIC TRACT GLIOMA
These tumors grow along the optic tracts of the brain that carry visual impulses. They are low-grade and slow-growing astrocytomas that produce visual symptoms.

Standard Treatment Radiation therapy is the usual treatment for optic tract gliomas that are growing. Some tumors that do not appear to be growing and have no symptoms may be observed without treatment.

Chemotherapy has not been used as an adjuvant to radiation therapy as part of standard treatment, but the previous considerations about the risks of radiation in children under the age of three apply. The use of vincristine and dactinomycin has enabled radiation therapy to be delayed in more than 80 percent of children and is being further evaluated.

Five-Year Survival Over 50 percent

CEREBRAL NEUROBLASTOMA—
*Supratentorial Primitive Neuro-
ectodermal Tumor (PNET)*
There are a variety of names for these tumors. They are poorly differentiated tumors, which microscopically may have

features of various primitive tumors of other cell types. Prognosis depends upon the extent of disease.

Standard Treatment The usual treatment is high-dose radiation therapy. Many radiation oncologists also radiate the entire brain and spinal cord because of this tumor's tendency to spread to the rest of the central nervous system through the cerebrospinal fluid. Chemotherapy is being studied as a possible way to delay radiation therapy until the child is older.

Two-Year Survival 30 to 50 percent

TREATMENT FOLLOW-UP

♦ Repeated clinical evaluation, emphasizing initial neurologic signs and symptoms.
♦ Repeated CT or MRI scanning.
♦ Repeated studies of any other abnormal tests, such as cerebrospinal fluid or visual fields.

THE MOST IMPORTANT QUESTIONS YOU CAN ASK

♦ What type of brain tumor does my child have?
♦ How does it usually behave?
♦ What is the chance of cure?
♦ What is the standard treatment and how successful is it?
♦ Should radiotherapy be used? When?
♦ Should chemotherapy be used? When?
♦ If the treatment is not completely effective or my child relapses later, what else can be done?

CHILDHOOD CANCERS: RETINOBLASTOMA

Jerry Z. Finklestein, MD

Retinoblastoma is a malignant tumor of the retina, the membrane at the back of the eyeball. About 200 children in the United States develop this cancer each year, most diagnosed before they reach the age of three. Twenty to 30 percent have tumors in both eyes. Most children with retinoblastoma have localized disease and are cured.

How It Spreads The tumor may be confined to the retina or extend directly to other parts of the eye. In its later stages, it may spread to the central nervous system or other parts of the body.

What Causes It There are hereditary and non-hereditary forms of retinoblastoma. In 40 percent of cases, there is an inherited abnormality, with the normal tumor-suppressing retinoblastoma gene missing. When a child has disease in only one eye, this abnormality may or may not be present. When there is disease in both eyes, it is almost always the hereditary form. The families of children with retinoblastoma should have genetic counseling.

DIAGNOSIS

Most children in the U.S. are diagnosed while the tumor remains within the eye. The tumor is detected by shining a light into a child's eye and looking for what is called a cat's eye—a white spot in place of the dark pupil. There may also be symptoms such as poor vision or obvious malfunctioning of the eye.

It is important for children with retinoblastoma to be seen in a specialized center where physicians have experience in evaluating the size of the tumor and the extent of the disease. The investigation involves specialized types of x-rays, ultrasound and other advanced imaging techniques such as MRI.

STAGING

Several staging systems are used, but for purposes of treatment retinoblastoma is divided into intraocular (within the eye) and extraocular (spread beyond the eye) disease.

TREATMENT OVERVIEW

Standard Treatment In some cases, it may be possible to destroy the tumor within the eye by using light treatments (photocoagulation), freezing (cryotherapy) or laser therapy. Treatment may, however, include an enucleation, meaning that the eye is removed and eventually replaced with an artificial eye. High-dose radiation also has a role.

Which of these procedures is used depends on the size of the tumor and whether the child has potentially useful vision.

The use of chemotherapy requires additional investigation, although tumors generally respond in a satisfactory manner to a number of chemotherapy drugs.

Five-Year Survival Over 90 percent if disease is confined to the eye; less than 10 percent if it has spread beyond the eye.

TREATMENT FOLLOW-UP

Children with retinoblastoma, especially the hereditary form, have an increased risk for developing other malignancies later in life and so should be followed closely. Up to 8 percent, for example, may develop bone tumors after 18 years, and the percentage may be higher with longer follow-up. Second cancers may develop spontaneously or be the result of treatment. Two-thirds of second cancers occur in tissue that has been irradiated.

CHILDHOOD CANCERS: SOFT TISSUE AND BONE SARCOMAS

Malin Dollinger, MD

Soft tissue sarcomas in children have many similarities to the comparable tumors in adults. They have a similar classification, similar appearance under the microscope (histology) and often behave in the same way. There are many differences, however.

Some soft tissue sarcomas that are common in children are rare in adults, for example. In children, the most common soft tissue sarcoma is rhabdomyosarcoma, a malignant tumor of skeletal muscle that can develop in the head and neck region, the genitourinary tract, limbs or other parts of the body. In treating soft tissue tumors in children, there is an especially important role for primary surgery and reoperation if necessary. Surgical margins should ideally be free of tumor because of the potentially harmful long-term side effects when radiation therapy is given to infants and very young children. However, this need not always be so (especially with rhabdomyosarcoma), because of the newer treatments available for childhood cancer.

Soft tissue sarcomas are often curable if they are localized. The prognosis is generally better for children than for adults. In adolescents, the behavior of these tumors more closely resembles that of adults than of young children. (*See* "Sarcomas of Soft Tissue and Bone" for additional information, including symptoms and diagnostic procedures.)

Types Rhabdomyosarcoma is the most common soft tissue sarcoma in children, accounting for about half of all cases and for 8 to 13 percent of malignant solid tumors in children. Other soft tissue sarcomas—including those that arise in connective tissue (fibrosarcoma), membranes lining joints (synovial sarcoma), nerve structures (neurofibrosarcoma), smooth muscles (leiomyosarcoma) and fat (liposarcoma)—account for about 3 percent of all cases of childhood malignancy. The bone tumor osteosarcoma accounts for about 5 percent of all childhood tumors.

STAGING

Most childhood sarcomas can be divided into two broad stages—localized and metastatic—but are generally classified according to the system used for rhabdomyosarcoma. This tumor is divided into four clinical groups according to the extent of the disease and whether the tumor can be removed.

TREATMENT OVERVIEW

As in adult sarcomas, a team approach is vital, with surgical, radiation and pediatric oncologists being involved, along with the primary physician, rehabilitation specialists and social workers. Therapy is often delivered in the context of a clinical trial at a major medical center with expertise in treating children.

The treatment must be highly individualized because the behavior of the tumor and the prognosis vary greatly according to patient age, cell type and the tumor's primary site and extent and because there may be risks of long-term side effects of treatment. Certain soft tissue sarcomas in infants and young children—including fibrosarcoma, hemangiopericytoma and alveolar soft part sarcoma—have special treatment considerations.

Localized Disease The standard treatment for localized tumors is surgery. Radiation therapy may be appropriate if the surgical margins still contain tumor cells, but every effort is made to achieve local control with surgery because of the long-term risks of radiation therapy in young children.

Chemotherapy and radiation may be used depending on the location and type of tumor. In some cases, clinical trials of new therapies may offer the best chance for success.

Metastatic Disease Aggressive surgery is used to control the primary tumor as well as the metastases if they can be removed. When tumor remains after surgery, radiation therapy as well as combination chemotherapy (using the drugs vincristine, doxorubicin, dactinomycin and cyclophosphamide) may be given. Clinical trials may be appropriate.

Survival with metastatic soft tissue sarcomas (usually to lungs) is poor, but an aggressive approach to treating metastases may significantly prolong survival.

Recurrent Disease Recurrent soft tissue sarcomas have a generally poor prognosis, but aggressive therapy is appropriate, including surgical re-excision, radiation therapy and chemotherapy. The choice of treatment depends on the site of recurrence, earlier therapy, individual patient considerations and the availability of a clinical trial.

SURVIVAL ESTIMATES FOR LOCALIZED SOFT TISSUE SARCOMAS IN CHILDREN

Fibrosarcoma	83–92 percent under age 5, 60 percent over age 5
Neurofibrosarcoma *(malignant schwannoma)*	Very good with complete surgical excision, poor with incomplete surgical excision
Malignant fibrous Histiocytoma	Over 50 percent
Leiomyosarcoma	Fair with gastro-intestinal tumors, poor in other locations
Liposarcoma	Very good
Synovial sarcoma	45–70 percent
Hemangiopericytoma	Excellent in young children, 30–70 percent in older children
Alveolar soft part sarcoma	50 percent

Recurrent Disease Recurrent soft tissue sarcomas have a generally poor prognosis, but aggressive therapy is appropriate, including surgical re-excision, radiation therapy and chemotherapy. The choice of treatment depends on the site of recurrence, earlier therapy, individual patient considerations and the availability of a clinical trial.

The Role of Adjuvant Therapy Adjuvant chemotherapy or radiotherapy has no *established* role in childhood soft tissue sarcomas that have been totally removed (except for rhabdomyosarcomas). Radiotherapy is used in older children if microscopic disease remains after surgery, especially after a second operation to remove microscopic disease left behind after the first.

RHABDOMYOSARCOMA

This sarcoma comprises roughly 10 percent of all cancers in children under 15. There have been enough cases that large clinical trials have defined the optimum work-up and staging and the role of surgery, local radiotherapy and chemotherapy.

Because of difficulties in microscopic diagnosis of this tumor even by experienced pathologists, immunohistochemical stains are now essential to diagnose many cases. Electron microscopic study has also been a definitive diagnostic test.

The single most important predictor of survival is the initial extent of disease. MRI is very useful for determining the extent of disease before surgery and is better than CT for this purpose.

The treatment is usually surgical removal, radiation to control residual tumor and systemic chemotherapy. Chemotherapy for residual disease—especially with the drug ifosfamide—is under study, but the role of adjuvant chemotherapy has now been established for this pediatric soft tissue sarcoma.

TREATMENT BY GROUP

GROUP I

No evidence of tumor remaining after surgery.

Standard Treatment Surgery, followed by chemotherapy. Those with unfavorable types also receive radiotherapy. Adjuvant therapy may consist of vincristine and dactinomycin for one year plus cyclophosphamide for two years. Clinical trials are varying the chemotherapeutic agents and the schedule of administration.

Five-Year Survival 80 percent

GROUP II

Microscopic tumor remaining after surgery.

Standard Treatment Surgery followed by radiation therapy and chemotherapy with vincristine and dactinomycin. Current clinical trials are studing the addiction of doxorubicin for favorable histology and Adriamycin + cisplatin for unfavorable histology.

Five-Year Survival 70 percent

GROUP III

Tumors cannot be completely removed by surgery. Children with this group can still be cured if the tumor starts in a favorable place.

Standard Treatment Surgery, usually a biopsy, is followed by radiation therapy and chemotherapy. Some children need additional treatment such as extensive radiotherapy.

Standard chemotherapy consists of vincristine + dactinomycin + doxorubicin + cyclophosphamide. Clinical trials are evaluating additional chemotherapy with cisplatin, etoposide and dacarbazine, higher dosages of chemotherapy and autologous bone marrow transplantation.

Children with poor-prognosis tumors should be considered for clinical trials of autologous bone marrow transplantation following surgery, radiotherapy and chemotherapy.

Five-Year Survival 60 percent

GROUP IV

Tumors have spread beyond the place of origin (metastasized).

Standard Treatment Same as for Group III.

Five-Year Survival 30 percent

RECURRENT CANCER

The prognosis is poor, and these children should be considered for clinical trials of new therapies.

EWING'S SARCOMA

This is the second most common malignant bone tumor in children. It may extend into the soft tissues around the bones. The most frequent symptom is pain and/or a swelling.

A conventional x-ray is the most reliable method of finding this tumor, while MRI is the most useful way to determine the extent of its spread to soft tissue and bone marrow. Pathologic review of the tumor, with the use of electron microscopy and immunohistochemical stains if needed, is extremely valuable. Ninety percent of these tumors have a chromosome abnormality that can be verified using fresh tumor tissue.

Cure requires that the primary tumor and all known or potential microscopic metastases be eliminated. These have been the major obstacle to cure. Treatment and outcome depend on where the tumor starts and whether metastases are detectable.

The primary treatment is radiotherapy, but sometimes the primary tumor can be surgically excised. Several chemotherapy regimens have been used, but most patients are treated with vincristine + doxorubicin + dactinomycin + cyclophosphamide. Most reports show a survival greater than 50 percent.

TREATMENT BY STAGE

LOCALIZED

The tumor has not spread beyond the site of origin.

Standard Treatment The prognosis depends on the site of origin as well as the possibility of metastases. Since at least 90 percent of patients will have hidden metastases despite having apparently localized disease, multi-drug chemotherapy is recommended for *all* patients.

The treatment is complex, using surgery, radiation therapy and chemotherapy, and depends to some extent on the location of the site of origin. It is best managed by physicians expert in the treatment of this tumor. All patients should be considered for entry into clinical trials.

After the diagnostic surgical biopsy, treatment programs include:
♦ Chemotherapy.
♦ Chemotherapy with clinical trials of additional radiotherapy.
♦ Chemotherapy, followed by surgery to remove expendable bones.

METASTATIC

The most common locations for metastases are the lungs, other bones and the bone marrow.

Standard Treatment Metastatic disease is treated with chemotherapy combinations using doxorubicin, cyclophosphamide, vincristine, dactinomycin, as well as other agents. Newer protocols may use ifosfamide and etoposide. Radiotherapy may also be given to involved areas.

The prognosis is poor although patients with lung diseases may have a better prognosis.

Investigational

♦ Recent research has investigated treatment concepts such as decreasing the dose or volume of radiotherapy, the contribution of surgical removal, the use of preoperative chemotherapy and the value of using two newer chemotherapeutic agents (ifosfamide and etosposide) as part of primary treatment.

RECURRENT CANCER

The prognosis is poor for recurrent disease, especially if the relapse occurs while the initial course of chemotherapy is being given. Treatment depends on the site of recurrence, earlier therapy and individual factors.

OSTEOSARCOMA

Osteosarcomas are tumors that begin in

bones. They are most common in adolescents, especially between the ages of 10 and 25 years. The most common sites of origin are just above or below the knee and in the upper arm.

About 1 percent of adults with Paget's disease (a benign bone disease) develop osteosarcoma, and there is an increased incidence following radiation and in people who have had retinoblastoma. With new information about chromosomal changes, DNA analysis may prove valuable in determining prognosis. A new diagnostic technique analyzes the tumor's reactivity with antibody against a substance called osteonectin.

Common symptoms are a mass or lump in an arm or leg, pain, or a fracture that occurs without obvious injury or with trivial injury. In the absence of symptoms, the tumor is sometimes diagnosed by the chance finding of lesions in the bone or lungs by x-ray. CT and MRI scans are useful in determining the extent of the primary tumor and the degree of soft tissue involvement.

A team of physicians experienced in treating this malignancy, including orthopedic surgeons, pathologists and radiologists, is essential, as certain nonmalignant bone diseases can resemble osteosarcoma on x-ray or under the microscope.

Staging depends on the grade, extension beyond the bone and the presence of metastases.

The prognosis depends on the histology, patient age, the tumor's size and location, duration of symptoms, and blood tests (LDH and alkaline phosphatase). If there are metastases, the prognosis depends on the ability to remove them surgically (especially isolated lung metastases).

The use of adjuvant chemotherapy has dramatically improved the prognosis of adolescents, increasing disease-free survival to 80 percent.

TREATMENT BY STAGE

LOCALIZED

This is highly treatable and often curable. The prognosis depends in part on where the tumor arose.

Standard Treatment Standard methods include:
♦ Surgery to remove the entire tumor (including limb-sparing procedures), followed by adjuvant chemotherapy. Wide surgical resection or amputation is needed to achieve local control. Limb salvage procedures are becoming more important.
♦ Preoperative chemotherapy, then surgery, then additional chemotherapy. Chemotherapy before surgery (neoadjuvant) uses high-dose methotrexate with leucovorin, sometimes with the addition of doxorubicin, bleomycin, cyclophosphamide, dactinomycin and cisplatin. If there is a poor initial reponse to chemotherapy, changing drugs in an attempt to improve the response does not improve survival.
♦ Chemotherapy and high-dose radiotherapy if the primary tumor cannot be removed.

Two-Year Survival 40 to 90 percent

METASTATIC

This is treatable and occasionally curable.

Standard Treatment Options include:
♦ Surgery to remove the primary tumor and, when possible, metastases, followed by combination chemotherapy with drugs such as high-dose methotrexate with leucovorin, doxorubicin, cyclophosphamide, cisplatin, bleomycin, dactinomycin and ifosfamide.
♦ Chemotherapy before the surgical removal of the primary tumor and lung metastases, followed by more chemotherapy.

Two-Year Survival 30 to 60 percent

Investigational Current research is evaluating:

♦ The role of limb-sparing surgical procedures.

♦ The role of preoperative chemotherapy in possibly increasing the numbers of patients who can subsequently have a limb-sparing procedure.

♦ The role of immediate surgery versus chemotherapy before surgery (neo-adjuvant) followed by delayed surgery.

RECURRENT CANCER

Recurrent disease can occasionally be cured by removing multiple lung metas-tases, if metastases are confined to the lungs. Otherwise, the prognosis is poor and clinical trials are appropriate.

THE MOST IMPORTANT QUESTIONS YOU CAN ASK

♦ Can I save my limb?

♦ How sick will I become from chemotherapy? Will I lose my hair?

♦ What is my chance of survival?

♦ Will this treatment allow me to continue in school?

COLON AND RECTUM

Ernest H. Rosenbaum, MD, and Malin Dollinger, MD

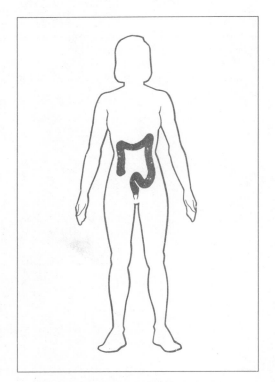

Cancer of the large bowel, or colon and rectum—the last 7 ft. ((2 m) of the intestine—is a highly treatable and often curable disease when it is localized and diagnosed in its early stages. But when it spreads through the bowel wall to lymph nodes or nearby organs, the chances for cure are reduced.

Fifteen percent of all cancers in the United States involve either the colon or the rectum. An estimated 157,000 colorectal cancers will be diagnosed in 1991, 112,000 in the colon and 45,000 in the rectum. Taken together, they are second only to lung cancer as a cause of cancer deaths in the United States (60,750 deaths).

These tumors are so common because about half the population over 40 are thought to have clumps of tissues protruding from the inner layer (mucosa) of the colon or rectum. These mushroom-like growths are called polyps, and while most are benign, one type—adenomatous polyps—may be precursors to cancer. About 90 percent of colorectal cancers arise from these polyps, and a person with a colorectal adenoma runs three times the risk of developing colorectal cancer. Overall, the lifetime risk of developing colorectal cancer is 6 percent (one out of every 20 Americans).

The colon and the rectum look similar and are connected to each other—the rectum is the final 5 in. (12 cm) of the colon above the anus—but there are *major differences* in the way colon and rectal tumors are treated.

Almost half of all patients with colorectal cancer can be cured with surgery, the primary treatment method. Adjuvant chemotherapy can improve the survival for colorectal cancer. Adjuvant radiotherapy and chemotherapy can be used to improve survival for rectal cancer, which is not the case with colon cancer.

The chance for cure is clearly related to how far the tumor has invaded through the bowel wall and whether it has spread to the nearby lymph nodes. For those people whose lymph nodes are invaded by cancer, a major problem is that the tumor can come back after surgery. Recurrent cancer is the ultimate cause of death in one-third of cases.

Types Most colorectal cancers develop in the glands of the inner lining or mucosa and are called adenocarcinomas.

Other kinds of tumors—lymphomas, melanomas and carcinoids—occur much less frequently.

How It Spreads Colorectal cancer spreads directly from the mucosa or inner lining through the muscle wall of the bowel and into adjacent tissues. The tumor may metastasize through the lymphatic system to nearby lymph nodes, to the liver through the portal vein and, less frequently, by the bloodstream to the bones or lungs.

What Causes It Environmental factors contributing to the development of colorectal cancers include diet (high in saturated fat, low in fiber and possibly low in calcium) and lack of exercise. It is most common in industrialized countries with high standards of living. It is becoming more common in Japan as consumption of fats increases.

One percent of colon cancers are related to an inherited condition called familial polyposis in which multiple polyps begin to appear in childhood and adolescence. Given enough time, most affected individuals will develop cancer.

Several genetic factors linked to colorectal cancer have been found. *Ras* gene mutations, largely in the *Ki-ras* gene resulting from environmental causes rather than being passed on genetically, are found in half of all people with colorectal adenomas and cancers. The tumor-suppressor gene p53 on chromosome 17 seems to be inactivated in most cases. A second tumor-suppressor gene—called "DCC", for Deleted in Colon Cancer—has been found on chromosome 18, and other genetic abnormalities have been found on chromosome 5. These may be important for tumor suppression. Once a polyp has one of these chromosome changes, other "hits" to the cell may cause cancers to develop.

RISK FACTORS

At Significantly Higher Risk

♦ Advancing age, usually over age 40.
♦ Family history of colorectal cancer, especially among first-degree relatives (Lynch syndrome Type I). The risk is two to three times the risk of an average person.
♦ "Cancer Family Syndrome" (Lynch syndrome Type II), with a higher risk for colon cancer and other adenocarcinomas such as cancers of the ovary, endometrium, breast and pancreas.
♦ A personal or family history of multiple adenomatous polyps after age 10 (familial polyposis).
♦ Previous polyps of the colon and rectum.
♦ Inflammatory bowel disease such as ulcerative colitis and ileitis (Crohn's disease). With ulcerative colitis, the risk of cancer is about 20 times the average. Cancer may also develop in the flat surface of the mucosa rather than in polyps. Increased risk for ulcerative colitis occurs in gynecologic cancer, prostate or pelvic cancer, and pelvic cancer following radiation therapy.
♦ Diets high in fat and low in fiber and (possibly) calcium. Animal rather than vegetable fat is believed responsible. A recent study indicated that women eating red meat (beef, lamb and pork) daily had 2 1/2 times the risk of those who eat red meat less than once a month. Those eating fish and chicken without the skin were at lesser risk.
♦ High consumption of charcoal-broiled foods.
♦ Inactivity and constipation.
♦ Asbestos and glue workers.
♦ European (Ashkenazy) Jews.

At Lower than Average Risk

♦ Seventh Day Adventists, lacto-vegetarians who do not drink alcohol or smoke, and Mormons, who abstain from alcohol, tobacco, coffee and tea and eat meat in moderation.
♦ Mediterranean and lower European (Sephardic) Jews.
♦ Hispanics.

SCREENING

Since this cancer is highly curable in the early stages, several techniques for early detection are recommended. These apply to the general population but are especially recommended for people with first-degree relatives with colorectal cancer.

Screening for adenomas that may become carcinomas after 10 or 15 years should begin at age 40, with screening for cancer beginning at age 50. A digital rectal examination should be an annual routine for those over 40, along with testing stools for hidden blood. About 3 percent will have a positive hidden blood test, and anywhere from 20 to 50 percent of these will be positive for polyps or cancer (10 percent will have cancer, 20 to 30 percent will have adenomas). These tests have rates of 2 percent false positives and 30 percent false negatives. False negatives are high because colorectal cancers bleed intermittently and the test may be done between bleedings.

The chance of a false positive test can be reduced by not consuming red meat, vitamin C and iron—avoiding cantaloupe, broccoli, parsnips, cauliflower, mushrooms, potatoes, cucumbers, red radishes and horseradish—for 24 hours before the test. A newer test called HemoQuant has fewer false positive results.

The sigmoid colon and rectum should be examined with a flexible or rigid tube (sigmoidoscopy) every three to five years after age 50 (after two negative sigmoidoscopies one year apart). Colonoscopy will examine the entire colon. It takes about five years for an adenomatous polyp to grow to the size where a cancerous change may occur.

Measuring the level of the carcinoembryonic antigen (CEA) in the blood can detect a few early cancer cases, but it is not a good test for screening.

It is hoped that genetic studies will improve screening for people at high risk for developing rectal cancer.

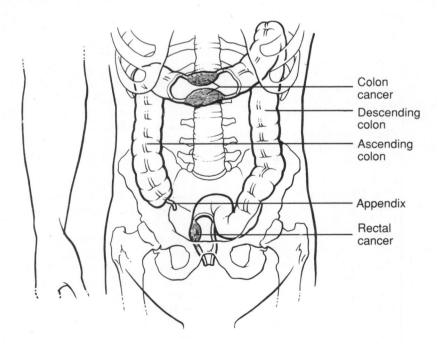

Colon cancer

Descending colon

Ascending colon

Appendix

Rectal cancer

Colon and Rectal Cancers

Screening is costly but effective. Finding colorectal cancer before it invades tissues or spreads to lymph nodes will improve the cure rate. The American death rate from this cancer fell 5.5 percent from 1973 to 1985, but there are still 60,000 deaths per year.

COMMON SIGNS AND SYMPTOMS

Colon cancer symptoms depend on the location of the tumor—right colon or left colon.

Cancers of the larger and more pliable right colon frequently bleed, causing anemia, but do not usually block the colon because the stool is still liquid in the right side of the colon.

Cancers in the left colon may obstruct the bowel, causing a change in bowel habits and stool size. There may be dark red rectal bleeding or blood in the stools, which may be long and narrow.

Cancers in the rectum may cause an obstruction, causing a change in bowel habits (including constipation) and in the size of stools, which may become long and narrow. There may also be rectal bleeding. Other symptoms include abdominal or pelvic pain, gas, vomiting, persistent constipation or diarrhea, weight loss and weakness. Pain is a worrisome problem with rectal cancer, since it often means the tumor is growing into nerves.

DIAGNOSIS

Physical Examination
♦ Digital rectal examination to feel for lumps.
♦ Abdominal exam for a mass or an enlarged liver (hepatomegaly).
♦ Enlarged lymph nodes over the left collarbone and in the groin (inguinal) area.

Blood and Other Tests
♦ Test for hidden blood in the stools (stool tests for bleeding may be negative in half of colorectal cancer cases).
♦ Complete blood count (CBC).

♦ Urinalysis.
♦ Serum chemistry profile, including liver enzymes, cholesterol, calcium, sugar, uric acid and serum iron or ferritin (for anemia).
♦ Test for carcinoembryonic antigen (CEA), a serum tumor marker that may be elevated with primary or recurrent colorectal cancer. Very high levels of CEA may indicate more advanced disease. The CEA level should be measured before surgery and, if elevated, periodically (every 3 - 4 months) after surgery.
♦ Beta-2 microglobulin or CA 19-9 may be a sensitive indicator for tumor bulk and may indicate metastases when the CEA level is normal.

Imaging
♦ Barium enema x-ray.
♦ Ultrasound of the abdomen and, if indicated, within the rectum. Endorectal ultrasonography can accurately show tumor invasion and enlarged lymph nodes outside the rectum, but cannot indicate if enlarged lymph nodes actually contain metastatic tumor.
♦ Abdominal CT and MRI scans to identify distant metastases before surgery.
♦ Chest x-ray may reveal lung metastases.
♦ PET (positron emission tomography) scanning, if available (experimental) can help assess the early response of liver metastases to chemotherapy by showing changes in sugar metabolism.
♦ Radioimaging body scan before surgery with CYT-103 monoclonal radiolabeled iridium antibodies may help detect hidden metastatic disease in about 12 percent of cases. This experimental method can complement CT scans, increasing their diagnostic sensitivity for finding hidden metastatic sites in the pelvis, liver and other areas. Other monoclonal antibody and imaging tests are being developed.
♦ Studies with anti-CEA monoclonal antibodies have shown a high accuracy in detecting tumors smaller than 1/2 in. (1 cm). This may be helpful to the surgeon.

Endoscopy and Biopsy

♦ Examination of the entire colon with a colonoscope (colonoscopy), or the lower part of the colon and rectum with a flexible tube (proctosigmoidoscopy) and biopsy of any mass found.

♦ If there is a rectal mass, a bladder evaluation cystoscopy and IVP (intravenous pyelogram).

STAGING

The stage of colorectal cancer describes whether the cancer has remained within the bowel or has spread to other sites. As with all cancers, the appropriate therapy can be decided only when the stage of the cancer has been defined.

There have been a number of staging systems for colorectal cancer. The original system developed by Dr. Dukes in 1932 has been modified several times. Since 1985, a staging system based on the Tumor/Nodes/Metastases (TNM) classification that corresponds directly with the Dukes system has been used. This allows an improved definition for the number of lymph nodes involved, a factor that can affect the prognosis. The 1990 National Cancer Institute Consensus Panel recommended using the TNM system to help identify people at highest risk because it better describes the tumor size and degree of invasion and the number of lymph nodes involved.

TREATMENT OVERVIEW

Surgery is the primary treatment, resulting in the cure of about 50 percent of patients. Adjuvant chemotherapy (for colorectal cancers) and radiation therapy (for rectal cancers) will probably increase survival. Most researchers now believe that adjuvant radiotherapy decreases local rectal recurrence without any improvement in survival. Combined radiotherapy and chemotherapy increases disease-free survival for rectal cancer more than radiotherapy alone and probably long-term survival as well It should be recommended for people with high-risk tumors who are not candidates for participation in clinical trials.

The prognosis depends on how far the tumor has penetrated through the bowel wall or to adjacent structures and on whether the cancer has spread to local lymph nodes. In node-negative patients, local recurrence is about 5 to 10 percent for Stage I and 25 to 30 percent for Stage II.

Recent studies indicate that the number of local lymph nodes involved is important. When one to four nodes are involved, survival is significantly better than when more than four nodes are involved.

There are several conditions found at the time of diagnosis of *colon* cancer that suggest an unfavorable outcome:

♦ The tumor has penetrated the bowel wall.

♦ The tumor has perforated the bowel wall.

There are several features of *rectal* cancer that suggest an unfavorable outcome:

♦ The tumor is fixed, has invaded, or adheres to other parts of the pelvis or adjacent tissues.

♦ The tumor has perforated the bowel wall.

♦ The tumor is deeply ulcerated.

♦ The tumor penetrates through the bowel wall or encircles the rectal wall.

♦ The tumor is larger than 2 1/2 in. (6 cm).

Poor prognostic factors for both colon *and* rectal cancer include:

♦ Pelvic nodes (rectal) or abdominal nodes (colon) are involved.

♦ There is a large bowel or rectal obstruction.

♦ The veins or lymphatic vessels of the bowel have been invaded.

♦ The tumor cells are poorly differentiated under the microscope.

♦ The chromosome pattern is abnormal.

♦ The level of carcinoembryonic antigen (CEA) in the blood is high before surgery.

♦ The cancer cell DNA is abnormal (investigational).

Caution is needed when planning treatment for colon or rectal cancers because the rectum lacks the covering layer of the bowel (the serosa). Thus, treatment of these tumors differs.

COLON

Surgery Tumors of the colon should be removed whenever practical, even if there are metastases, because complications—blockage of the bowel or bleeding—will inevitably develop.

The standard operation is designed to remove the portion of the bowel with the tumor along with the entire lymph node drainage. This requires removing the vessels that supply blood to a considerable portion of the bowel, so most of the time about one-third to one-half of the colon is removed even if the tumor itself is relatively small. This procedure is easier, safer and more likely to provide surgical margins—areas around the tumor—that are free of cancer. The bowel is then reconnected (anastomosis).

Sometimes, in patients who have tumors in the left side of the colon and who have a partial or complete obstruction, reconnecting the bowel is not possible because there is too much stool or contamination in the area. These patients receive a temporary colostomy, which is removed 6 to 10 weeks later (see Chapter 21).

Local excision may be used for small lesions or the removal of polyps, with a wedge resection for larger tumors.

 Radiation Therapy In selected cases of invasive cecal tumors (where the small bowel joins the colon), radiotherapy may help reduce local recurrences. Palliative radiation is primarily used for localized metastatic tumors and painful liver metastases.

Chemotherapy For metastatic colon cancer, 5-fluorouracil (5-FU) can be used as a single agent (given by rapid injection or continuous infusion) or as part of combination chemotherapy.

For over 25 years, adjuvant chemotherapy trials have tried to improve the surgical cure rate of colon cancer. 5-FU has been combined with other agents such as leucovorin and/or levamisole. Combination therapy is better than 5-FU alone, and recent reports show an increase in survival and a decrease in recurrence.

Trials for Stage II are comparing 5-FU + leucovorin and 5-FU + leucovorin + levamisole, a drug that works as a "biochemical immune modulator" to make 5-FU more effective at killing cancer cells. Levamisole + 5-FU helps restore macrophage and T lymphocyte function in patients whose immune systems may be suppressed.

For people with Stage III (Dukes' C) colon cancer with positive lymph nodes who are unable to enter a clinical adjuvant trial, the combination of levamisole and 5-FU has shown a clear benefit, with reduced rates of both recurrence and death.

Reports on using 5-FU and interferon-alpha (chemoimmunotherapy) for metastatic colon cancer (Stage IV) have shown an increased response rate, and new studies are trying to confirm these preliminary reports. This combination program has increased toxicity, however, with such side effects as fatigue, fever, diarrhea and sore mouth.

 Laser Therapy In certain cases, treatment with lasers may be appropriate for people with colon cancer, primarily for palliation. These cutting beams of light can reduce the bulk of a tumor causing an obstruction in the bowel and can also be used to stop bleeding. Lasers have not been as successful at relieving pain (see Chapter 9).

COLON CANCER TREATMENT BY STAGE

STAGE 0 (Dukes' Stage 0)
TNM Tis (Tumor or carcinoma in situ)
This is a very early cancer that has not spread below the limiting membrane of the first layer of colon tissue (mucosa).

Standard Treatment Treatment may be local excision of the tumor or polyp or a "wedge resection" involving the removal of a portion of the colon. Standard surgery, however, involves removing the tumor along with at least a 2 in.(5 cm) margin of normal colon on either side of the tumor site, and the nearby lymph nodes and veins. Because of the way blood is supplied to the colon, it is necessary to remove either the entire right side or the entire left side of the colon. This decreases the chance for local recurrence and increases the safety of the operation.

Five-Year Survival 95 percent. This should be 100 percent curable with earlier detection.

STAGE I (Dukes' A, B1)
TNM T1-2 N0, M0
The cancer is confined to the lining or muscular wall of the colon and has not yet spread anywhere else.

Standard Treatment This stage is highly curable. Radical surgery is the primary treatment and results in a high cure rate. According to the 1990 Consensus Conference on Colon Cancer, no adjuvant therapy is warranted for this stage because of the low risk for recurrence.

Five-Year Survival 85 to 95 percent, depending on whether the muscular wall has been invaded.

STAGE II (Dukes' B2 or B3)
TNM T3-4, N0, M0
The cancer has spread through the muscular wall of the intestine or has extended to adjacent organs through the structures, but has not spread to lymph nodes. Dukes' B2 extends through the bowel wall; B3 involves adjacent structures.

Mucosa
Submucosa
Muscularis
Serosa

STAGE I

Negative lymph nodes

Cancers

A   B₁

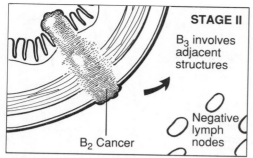

STAGE II

B_3 involves adjacent structures

Negative lymph nodes

B_2 Cancer

Standard Treatment Surgical removal of the primary tumor, with or without adjuvant chemotherapy. Specific adjuvant therapy cannot be recommended for intermediate risk tumors outside a clinical trial. But since a significant percentage of Stage II patients will develop recurrences, they should be considered candidates for clinical trials of adjuvant therapy. Higher-risk tumors are those where there is bowel wall perforation, involvement of adjacent structures and abnormal chromosomes (an aneuploid tumor).

Current adjuvant chemotherapy programs include 5-FU + leucovorin or 5-FU + levamisole. The side effects of treatment with 5-FU + levamisole are few and are primarily associated with 5-FU. Levamisole alone has mild toxicity, mainly gastrointestinal, causing nausea, vomiting, diarrhea or upset stomach, as well as neurotoxicity. Alcohol is to be avoided, as levamisole has an Antabuse-like effect. 5-FU + leucovorin may cause severe diarrhea without low white blood cell counts, and fluids may have to be replaced intravenously in the hospital because of dehydration.

Five-Year Survival 30 to 70 percent, depending on whether adjacent tissues are involved.

Investigational
♦ Adjuvant chemotherapy clinical trials of various combinations including 5-FU and leucovorin or chemoimmunotherapy with 5-FU and levamisole.
♦ Evaluation of the combination of 5-FU + levamisole for Stage II (Dukes' B2)

patients will need another one or two years of study to determine its effectiveness. The number of patients treated so far with the combination has been too low to provide a final answer.
♦ 5-FU + PALA (an immune adjuvant drug) or 5-FU and leucovorin may be given for one year after surgery.
♦ Postoperative local radiation therapy may help control tumors that have spread to tissues adjacent to the colon or lesions in the pelvis.

STAGE III (Dukes' C1, 2,3)
TNM Any T, N1-3, M0
The cancer has spread outside the intestine to one or more lymph nodes near the bowel. Dukes' C1 is within the bowel wall, C2 is through the bowel wall, and C3 involves adjacent structures.

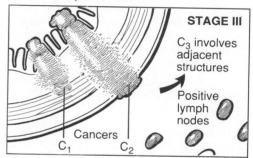

STAGE III

C_3 involves adjacent structures

Positive lymph nodes

Cancers
C_1 C_2

Standard Treatment This stage is highly treatable and often curable with standard therapy, but patients should be considered candidates for adjuvant clinical trials.

The standard treatment is to remove a wide section of the colon and rejoin the remaining ends (anastomosis), followed by adjuvant chemotherapy with 5-FU + levamisole. Clinical trials of new treatments are also appropriate.

More than half the patients with colon cancer have tumors that penetrate the serosa (B2) or have positive lymph nodes (C). It is estimated that about 20 to 25 percent of those with Dukes' B2 and 40 to 90 percent of those with Dukes' C who are treated with surgery will have recurrences and so need adjuvant chemotherapy.

Dukes' C patients now commonly receive a combination of levamisole + 5-

FU (which was recommended by the National Institute of Health's Consensus Conference on Colon Cancer in May 1990). One study of treatment with levamisole + 5-FU for Dukes' C starting within five weeks of surgery did show decreased recurrences and prolonged survival. Another trial showed a 41 percent decrease in the rate of recurrence and a 33 percent decrease in the death rate.

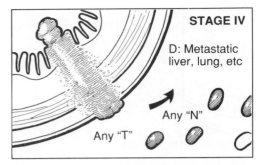

STAGE IV

D: Metastatic liver, lung, etc

Any "N"

Any "T"

Five-Year Survival 10 to 60 percent with positive regional lymph nodes, 40 to 60 percent when the tumor is within the bowel wall (C1), 20 to 40 percent when the tumor extends through the bowel wall (C2), 10 to 30 percent when adjacent structures are involved (C3). These data do not reflect adjuvant therapy programs.

The Consensus Conference used positive lymph nodes for determining prognosis with previous therapy. If one to four nodes are positive, 55 to 60 percent may be cured. When five or more nodes are positive, only 33 percent will be cured. Adjuvant therapy will improve all the old prognostic figures.

Investigational
♦ Adjuvant chemoimmunotherapy trial comparing 5-FU + PALA with 5-FU + levamisole and 5-FU + levamisole or interferon.
♦ Trials to see if 5-FU + leucovorin + PALA is superior to conventional therapy are ongoing.
♦ *See* also Stage II.

STAGE IV (Dukes' D)
TNM Any T, any N, M1
The cancer has spread beyond the colon to distant sites or organs, possibly including the liver or lungs.

Standard Treatment Cancer at this stage is not usually curable, but removal of a large section of the colon and reconnection of the bowel is still the standard treatment so that major problems such as obstruction, bleeding or bowel perfora-

tion can be avoided. In some cases, tumors that are blocking the colon may be bypassed.

It should be noted that 80 percent of colon cancer patients die of liver failure. And, if there are metastases in only a portion of the liver, removal of the metastases by removing part of the liver can cure 20 to 40 percent of such patients. The prognosis is better if there are fewer lesions—one lesion is better than three—and there is *no* survival benefit unless all lesions are removed. Non-curative surgery has the same prognosis as no surgery at all. In selected cases, both the colon cancer and the liver metastases (if there are three or fewer) can be removed at the same surgery.

Liver metastases may be reduced if chemotherapy, with 5-FUDR (floxuridine) delivered by infusion pump through the main hepatic artery, is given after surgery. (*see* Chapter 5)

There are new and innovative treatment methods. Treating liver metastases with intra-arterial chemotherapy—5-FUDR—by infusion pump can improve the response rate to about 50 percent. But several studies have shown side effects—increased liver toxicity, scarring of the bile duct (biliary sclerosis) and liver function abnormalities, gastritis, diarrhea and pain—that required dose reductions in about 40 to 50 percent of patients (see "Metastatic Cancer"). Recent studies have reduced toxicity by alternating 5-FU and 5-FUDR therapy. Response to 5-FUDR intra-arterial therapy often occurs even in patients who failed to respond to intravenous 5-FU or who are no longer responding.

The infusion can be delivered on an outpatient basis by a surgically implanted pump (Infusaid) connected to the hepatic artery. Although the response rate is high, increased survival has not yet been proven.

Hepatic artery 5-FUDR given through a catheter inserted through the skin into an artery in the arm or groin also has a high response rate. This method isolates the blood supply to the cancer and then releases chemotherapy into the isolated area. There may be local toxicity, including liver function abnormalities and biliary tract scarring (sclerosis).

 Palliation Radiation therapy may be given to help control the size of the tumor and/or pain, and both radiation and chemotherapy with 5-FU alone or 5-FU + leucovorin may be used for palliation of advanced cancer.

The 5-FU + leucovorin combination usually provides little benefit, however, to someone who has relapsed after treatment with 5-FU alone. The current treatment recommendation is to begin therapy with 5-FU + leucovorin or an investigational protocol. Other drugs with some anticancer activity that might be considered include mitomycin-C, BCNU, CCNU and the experimental ICRF-159 (Razoxane).

Another method of delivering 5-FU is by continuous intravenous infusion using a portable or bedside pump. A study comparing intermittent direct 5-FU injections with continuous long-term (two to four weeks) low-dose infusions showed a high response rate for the infusion, although the survival outcomes were identical. A later report showed a 45 percent response rate to 5-FU infusion in patients who were resistant to other therapy.

Five-Year Survival 5 percent, rising to 20 to 30 percent if liver metastases can be removed surgically.

Investigational
♦ Chemoembolization is a method of treating liver metastases. This process involves injecting and filling the artery leading to the tumor with a plastic-sponge mixture containing chemotherapy (see "Metastatic Cancer").
♦ Biological therapies using specific antibodies are being evaluated, with several protocols under investigation especially using interferon just before 5-FU + leucovorin. Injections of 5 to 10 million units of interferon three times a week in conjunction with 5-FU by infusion and direct injection has shown a high response rate (greater than 50 percent). This therapy may not be effective if it is used after the disease has progressed on 5-FU.
♦ Trials are comparing 5-FU + PALA versus 5-FU + interferon-alpha versus 5-FU + leucovorin. PALA + 5-FU has been reported to have responses better than 5-FU alone.
♦ Trials with monoclonal antibodies (MAbs) are now being started, with MAbs against colon cancer tagged to a radioisotope being used to locate hidden cancer sites before and during surgery. Preliminary results seem promising, although the eventual role of MAbs is yet to be determined. (*see* summary of Consensus Conference on Colon and Rectal Cancer, on page 324)

TREATMENT FOLLOW-UP

Recommendations for following patients after treatment to detect recurrences include:
♦ History and physical examination every two to three months.
♦ Chest x-ray every 6 to 12 months for three to five years.
♦ CT scans of the abdomen and pelvis twice a year for one to two years, then yearly as required.
♦ Barium enema as required.
♦ Complete blood count and serum chemistry profile every 3 months.
♦ Measurement of the CEA level in the blood every 6 to 12 weeks for 3 to 5 years, since a rise in the level may occur before other clinical, x-ray or laboratory tests show

recurrence. If the CEA rises above normal, about one third of patients may have a recurrent tumor that can be totally removed with surgery and so may be cured.

♦ Periodic proctosigmoidoscopy or colonoscopy at least every year, or more often, depending on staging. If there are polyps, colonoscopy should be done one to three times a year. There is three to four times the risk of developing new tumors.

Recommendations for follow-up after the successful surgical removal of Dukes' A, B and C tumors include:

♦ History and physical examination every three months for detection of tumor recurrence.

♦ Complete blood count, serum chemistry profile and CEA tests every three months.

♦ Colonoscopy (rather than a barium enema) every year to detect recurrent or new polyps or cancer.

♦ Since family members share the same genes and/or diet, first-degree relatives should be tested for hidden blood in the stool and have colonoscopy after age 30.

RECURRENT COLON CANCER

Cancer may recur in the colon or any part of the body, including the liver or lungs. Unfortunately, those who have a recurrence will usually die of cancer.

Treatment for recurrent colon cancer is essentially the same as for Stage IV, although therapy also depends on the site of the recurrence.

♦ When there is only one area of recurrence such as the liver or lung and surgery is possible, the lesion should be removed to increase the chance of cure or prolong survival.

♦ Occasionally, the cancer will come back only where sections of the bowel have been sewn together. These local suture line recurrences can be removed with a reasonable chance for cure.

♦ Chemotherapy with single drugs (10 to 20 percent response), combinations (30 to 40 percent response) or investigational drugs have been used for palliation.

♦ Trials involving the administration of the drugs into an artery with implantable infusion pumps and access devices have been conducted for recurrence in the liver.

Investigational

♦ Recent chemotherapy programs show an improved response rate and may improve survival. Promising developments include: 5-FU + leucovorin, 5-FU + interferon-alpha, 5-FU + PALA, 5-FU + levamisole and 5-FU + levamisole and leucovorin or interferon or PALA.

♦ Dosages of chemotherapy drugs may be significantly increased with the use of hematopoietic growth factors (GM-CSF).

♦ Studies are evaluating adjuvant radiation therapy with chemotherapy and monoclonal antibodies directed against colon associated antigens.

THE MOST IMPORTANT QUESTIONS YOU CAN ASK

♦ What are the symptoms of colon cancer?
♦ Does rectal bleeding always suggest colon cancer?
♦ What are the guidelines for screening for colon cancer?
♦ Can I live a normal life after colon surgery?
♦ Should radiotherapy be used for colon cancer?
♦ What is a good nutritional support dietary program?
♦ When is surgery effective for colon cancer that has spread to the liver or lungs?
♦ When will I know if I am cured? What kind of follow-up will you be doing after my therapy?
♦ What is the role of adjuvant chemotherapy and of chemotherapy for metastatic disease after a colostomy?
♦ How does the immunochemotherapy combination approach work? Can it cure colon cancer?
♦ Can laser treatment cure colon cancer?

RECTUM

Surgery State-of-the-art treatment for localized rectal cancer involves removing the tumor with at least 3/4 in. (2 cm) of normal tissue on either side of it as well as the regional lymph nodes. The surgeon and the surgical pathologist should examine the rectal margins in the surgical specimen for the presence or absence of tumor. If the tumor is small, it may be removed with a local wedge resection.

In some patients with a tumor that is low in the rectum, high-dose radiation given before the operation may reduce the size of the tumor, allowing it to be removed while still leaving enough bowel below the tumor site for the surgeon to sew the bowel back together. This will spare the rectum and the sphincter muscle, thereby avoiding the need for a colostomy in up to 85 percent of patients with rectal cancer.

Mortality for this operation is less than 7 percent, but there is a 25 to 40 percent incidence of impotence or urologic problems. About 10 to 15 percent of patients have a late local recurrence of cancer in the pelvis, particularly when sphincter-preserving operations have been used for low-lying tumors.

But the main concern should be removing all the tumor and a reasonable margin on either side—which leads to cure—rather than preserving the sphincter.

In rare cases of non-invasive tumors—those confined to the top layers of the rectal lining (mucosa and submucosa)—it is sometimes possible to remove the tumor from below, entering through the anus and using a cold probe (cryotherapy), electrofulguration or simple excision of the tumor without removing part of the bowel. Radiotherapy before or after the operation may decrease the incidence of local pelvic recurrence.

In tumors that are very low in the rectum—within 2 to 2 1/2 in. (5 to 6 cm) of the anus—once the tumor and its lower edge have been removed there is no rectum left to sew back together. In these cases the surgeon performs an abdominal perineal resection, the standard treatment for invasive cancer. The rectum and the anus with all its muscular attachments are removed, leaving the patient with a permanent colostomy (*see* Chapter 21).

Ongoing clinical trials are attempting to identify patients who may be spared this extensive surgery. This investigative approach treats selected patients with a local excision of the tumor (as long as the margins show no evidence of cancer), along with radiation to the pelvis and often chemotherapy as well.

A novel stapling device to join the ends of the bowel may sometimes allow the surgeon to perform what is called a low anterior resection in some patients with low rectal cancers. This will also help avoid a colostomy.

Where there is no evidence of gross pelvic disease after local excision with negative margins, adjuvant pelvic radiation may be an alternative to abdominal perineal resection. This may help reduce local recurrence, which is associated with significant symptoms. Follow-up studies are in progress.

Radiation Therapy Radiation given before or after surgery has been used to treat rectal cancer. High-dose preoperative therapy in selected high-risk cases—selection depends on the size and location of the tumor—will improve survival, reduce local recurrence and allow the sphincter to be preserved even in low rectal cancers.

Placing the radiation source inside the rectum (intraluminal radiation therapy) may result in a high cure rate in some cases, as with a well-differentiated tumor less than 3 to 4 cm above the sphincter, for example. This may preserve the sphincter.

Adjuvant Radiation Therapy Radiation therapy given after surgery may be more effective in rectal cancer than in colon cancer because of the increased tendency for tumors to grow back locally. Several trials of adjuvant radiation and chemotherapy after an abdominal perineal resection have suggested a decrease in the rate of local recurrence with a small increase in disease-free and overall survival.

Adjuvant Chemotherapy Stage I (Dukes' A and B1) tumors have a high cure rate with surgery alone and there is no need for adjuvant chemotherapy for these stages. But for more advanced tumors (Dukes' B2 and C), the use of chemotherapy alone has shown some improvement in survival. Combination therapy, using chemotherapy plus radiation, is better than either therapy alone and should be started within 6 weeks of surgery.

Combined Therapy Disease-free survival has recently been extended in patients with Dukes' B2 and C rectal cancer treated with both chemotherapy and radiation, compared with those treated with radiation therapy alone.

Clinical trials are now evaluating 5-fluorouracil (5-FU) with radiation therapy or 5-FU + leucovorin or levamisole or both for Stages II and III (Dukes' B2 and C) rectal cancer. Combined chemotherapy and radiation therapy have been reported to improve disease-free and overall survival, with clear benefit having been shown for combination therapy with 5-FU given before and during radiotherapy.

Palliation With advanced cancer that cannot be cured, radiation therapy may be used for palliation in most cases when it was not used before or after surgery to remove the tumor. 5-FU is often used with radiotherapy.

Short-term palliation may also be achieved with chemotherapy in about 20 percent of patients, although there is little evidence that chemotherapy significantly improves survival for those with advanced (Dukes' D) disease.

Laser therapy may be a very effective way to relieve an obstruction or control localized bleeding (*see* Chapter 9).

RECTAL CANCER: TREATMENT BY STAGE

STAGE 0
TNM Tis (Tumor in situ)
This superficial, non-invasive carcinoma in situ is a very early cancer that has not spread below the membrane (macosa) of the first layer of rectal tissue.

Standard Treatment Because of its superficial nature, limited rather than radical surgery, as well as other procedures, may be used. Surgery may involve only cutting out the tumor itself (enucleation) of the tumor and a small wedge of tissue.

Other options include electrocoagulation and external or internal (inside the rectum) radiation therapy for rectal sphincter preservation.

Five-Year Survival Over 95 percent.

STAGE I (*see* Stage I colon cancer diagram) **(Dukes' A, BI)**
TNM T12, N0, M0
The cancer is confined to the lining or muscular wall of the rectum and has not yet spread anywhere else. In Dukes' A, the tumor is limited to the mucosa. In Dukes' B1, it is within the bowel wall.

Standard Treatment Surgery will generally result in a cure.

When the tumor is in the upper rectum, a wide margin of tissue may be removed and the bowel reconnected (anastomosis).

When the tumor is near the anus, an abdominal perineal resection and colostomy is the standard treatment. Local transanal resection can be done in selected patients.

Radiation inside the bowel (intraluminal) may be used in selected patients. This technique requires special equipment and experience, but the results are equivalent to surgery and can preserve the sphincter muscle.

There is a 5 to 10 percent chance of a local recurrence with this stage of cancer.

Five-Year Survival 85 to 95 percent (95 percent for Dukes' A, 85 to 90 percent for Dukes' B1).

Investigational Results from clinical trials of radiation therapy and electrocoagulation are promising.

STAGE II (*see* Stage II colon diagram) **(Dukes' B2, B3)**
TNM T34 N0, M0
The cancer has penetrated all layers of the bowel wall with or without extension to adjacent tissues (uterus, ovaries or prostate), but has not spread to lymph nodes. Dukes' B2 extends through the bowel wall: B3 involves adjacent structures such as the uterus, ovaries, bladder or prostate.

Standard Treatment Stage II rectal cancer is highly treatable and often curable. There are several options for treatment, including:
♦ Removal of a wide margin of tissue and reconnection of the bowel to the rectum (anastomosis) when the tumor is in the upper rectum.
♦ The same surgical procedure followed by chemotherapy and radiation therapy, which has shown an increased disease-free survival compared with surgery alone or surgery and radiation. 5-FU and radiation can improve remission and prolong survival.

♦ An abdominal perineal resection and colostomy, with or without adjuvant radiation and chemotherapy, for tumors near the anus.
♦ Those with B2 tumors will benefit from adjuvant chemotherapy if they have features that point to a recurrence (abnormal chromosomes by DNA analysis, invasion of the outside wall, perforation, adhesion to organs or invasion of adjacent organs).
♦ For B3 lesions, the pelvic organs (bladder, uterus or prostate) may be removed (pelvic exenteration) when that is necessary to remove all the cancer, with or without adjuvant chemotherapy.
♦ Adding postoperative radiation and chemotherapy will reduce pelvic recurrences and improve chances of survival (there is 25 to 30 percent chance of local recurrence with this stage).
♦ For tumors near the anus, radiation therapy followed by surgery may allow sphincter function to be preserved.

Preoperative or postoperative radiation therapy has resulted in fewer local recurrences but has never been definitely shown to affect survival.

Five-Year Survival 30 to 70 percent (50 to 70 percent for Dukes' B2, 30 percent for Dukes' B3).

Investigational New adjuvant programs may increase survival by 10 to 15 percent.
♦ Adjuvant 5-FU + leucovorin and radiotherapy.
♦ 5-FU + levamisole and 5-FU + PALA, an immune adjuvant drug that increases the effectiveness of 5-FU.
♦ Giving radiation during surgery (intraoperative radiation therapy) is being evaluated for locally advanced disease.

STAGE III (*see* Stage III colon diagram) **(Dukes' C1, 2, 3)**
TNM Any T, N1-3, M0
The cancer has spread within or outside the rectum and one or more lymph nodes

are involved. A Dukes' C1 tumor is within the bowel wall, C2 is through the bowel wall and C3 involves adjacent structures.

Standard Treatment The number of lymph nodes that are positive for cancer needs to be known because patients with one to four positive nodes have a better prognosis than those with five or more involved nodes.

The standard therapy for a tumor near the anus is an abdominal perineal resection with or without adjuvant chemotherapy and/or radiotherapy.

For tumors in the upper rectum far from the anus, a wide margin of tissue may be removed and the bowel reconnected to the anus, with or without adjuvant chemotherapy and radiation therapy.

Removal of the pelvic organs (pelvic exenteration) may be necessary to remove all the cancer and may be followed by adjuvant chemotherapy and/or radiation therapy when the level of penetration has reached the C3 stage.

For tumors near the anus, radiation therapy followed by surgery may allow the sphincter function to be preserved.

There is a 50 percent chance of recurrence with this stage of disease.

The 1990 consensus conference on colon and rectal cancers noted that if one to four lymph nodes are positive, 55 to 60 percent will be cured. If five or more are positive, only 33 percent will be cured. Current adjuvant therapy will improve all of the old prognostic figures.

Five-Year Survival Up to 60 percent (40 to 50 percent for Dukes' C1, 15 to 25 percent for C2, 10 to 20 percent for C3). These data do *not* reflect current adjuvant therapy programs.

Investigational
♦ Survival rates may be increased by 10 to 15 percent with new adjuvant chemotherapy programs such as 5-FU + leucovorin and/or radiation therapy.

♦ Intraoperative radiation therapy (IORT) is also being evaluated in patients with locally advanced disease.
♦ 5-FU + levamisole and 5-FU + PALA are being evaluated.

STAGE IV (Dukes' D)
TNM Any T, any N, M1
The cancer has spread outside the rectum to distant areas, including organs such as the liver or lungs.

Standard Treatment This stage of cancer is largely incurable. Treatment is directed basically toward palliation, although there can be long-term disease-free survival if isolated metastases in the liver or lung can be removed.

Treatment options include:
♦ Palliative removal of the primary tumor in some cases, with radiation therapy for local disease that can't be removed.
♦ Removal of isolated liver, ovary or lung metastases for possible cure. Liver metastases (if there are three or fewer) can be removed at the same surgery to remove the rectal cancer in selected cases.
♦ Patients can be treated either with chemotherapy programs such as 5-FU alone or 5-FU combined with leucovorin or interferon or be considered candidates for clinical trials for new chemotherapy or biological agents. Mitomycin-C, BCNU and CCNU have been used, with a mild response.
♦ Palliative chemotherapy, possibly with the continuous infusion of a low daily dose of 5-FU.
♦ There are a number of other standard and investigational methods of treating Stage IV (Dukes' D) rectal cancer. These closely resemble those described earlier for colon cancer on pages 314 - 315 which should be consulted.

Five-Year Survival Less than 5 percent (*see* summary of Consensus Conference on Colon and Rectal Cancer, on page 324).

TREATMENT FOLLOW-UP

Rectal cancer has a much higher rate of local recurrence than colon cancer. Close follow-up may lead to the earlier diagnosis of recurrent disease and improved treatment. After treatment for rectal cancer, follow-up should include:

♦ Physical examination every two to three months for at least five years.
♦ Chest x-ray every 6 to 12 months for three to five years as indicated.
♦ Abdominal and pelvic CT scans twice a year for one to two years, then yearly.
♦ Serum chemistry profiles and CEA levels every 6 to 12 weeks (when operated on for a rising CEA level, 30 to 40 percent may have a recurrent rectal cancer which may be successfully removed for cure).
♦ Barium enema as indicated.
♦ Sigmoidoscopic examinations every 3-6 months and yearly colonoscopy.

RECURRENT RECTAL CANCER

Rectal cancer can recur locally or often in the liver or lungs, and it is important to determine if the recurrence is only local or metastatic. Treatment depends on the site of recurrence as defined by physical and x-ray examinations and scans.

♦ If local disease can be removed, there is a potential chance for cure.
♦ Often the recurrence can be in one area such as the rectal area, liver or lung, where surgical removal may possibly lead to a cure or significantly prolonged survival.
♦ Alternatively, intra-arterial chemotherapy with an implantable portable pump can sometimes give significant palliation (*see* "STAGE IV").
♦ Hepatic intra-arterial chemotherapy with 5-FUDR for liver metastases has been studied. This approach has been shown to produce a higher overall response rate without significant improvement in survival. In several studies, there is increased local toxicity including liver function abnormalities and biliary sclerosis (*see* "STAGE IV").

♦ As in Stage IV, chemotherapy with single-agent 5-FU or 5-FU in combination with leucovorin, or with interferon with or without leucovorin (investigational), may improve survival and achieve significant palliation. Various doses are used. Lower-dose leucovorin + 5-FU has the same response and survival as high-dose leucovorin + 5-FU. 5-FU + levamisole has no role in recurrent colorectal cancer.

Standard Treatment Removal of liver metastases may be done in selected cases. The five-year survival rate for patients with solitary metastases exceeds 20 percent. The chances for cure are improved when there are only two or three metastases to be removed. Non-curative removal provides no benefits to patients who have no symptoms, since survival is not affected.

Both palliative radiation therapy and palliative chemotherapy may be given for recurrent disease.

Investigational
♦ Biologic therapy with 5-FU + interferon, monoclonal antibodies or interleukin-2.
♦ 5-FU + PALA, Phase I and II agents.

THE MOST IMPORTANT QUESTIONS YOU CAN ASK

♦ How does the Dukes' staging affect my prognosis?
♦ How extensive does my surgery need to be? Will I need a colostomy?
♦ How do you know who needs adjuvant chemotherapy?
♦ When should radiotherapy be used?
♦ What is the role of combination chemotherapy and radiotherapy?
♦ How can one screen for rectal cancer? What should family members do if there is a history of colorectal cancer in a close relative?

CONSENSUS CONFERENCE ON COLON AND RECTAL CANCER:

SUMMARY

A Consensus Conference on Colon and Rectal Cancer was held at the National Institute of Health in April 1990. The treatment recommendations of the panel were:

1.Stage I Colon and Rectal

No adjuvant therapy is warranted, since there is a low risk of recurrence.

2.Stage II Colon

Specific adjuvant therapy cannot be recommended for intermediate-risk tumors outside a clinical trial. Those with larger tumors (T3 or T4), an elevated preoperative CEA level, poorly differentiated tumors and abnormal DNA, are candidates for adjuvant chemotherapy.

3.Stage III Colon

There is a high risk for recurrence, and treatement with levamisole and 5-FU is recommended.

4.Stages II and III Rectal

Adjuvant combined radiotherapy and chemotherapy is recommended postoperatively. This will improve local control and survival.

5.Future Research

Further clinical trials focussing on adjuvant chemotherapy and immunotherapy are needed both to improve the effectiveness of current treatments and try to understand drug and immune mechanisms. Studies are also needed to determine the optimum role of radiotherapy in rectal cancer.

FOR DIETARY PREVENTION OF COLORECTAL CANCER

RECOMMENDATIONS

♦ The diet should stress high fiber and low fat.

♦ Increased growth rate of colon membrane cells may precede colon cancer. Chemoprevention is being tested with micronutrients—vitamins and minerals.

♦ Calcium may help by regulating cell overgrowth.

♦ Other factors are stool acidity (pH) and the effect of bile and fatty acids on the colon's lining (mucosa). Depending on acidity, calcium may help regulate the cancer-promoting role of bile acids and fatty acids.

♦ A woman's trial has shown a 2 1/2 times normal risk of colon cancer when red meat (pork, beef, lamb) is eaten daily (animal fats) rather than a few times a month (vegetable fat was not a risk factor).

♦ 1,200 - 2,000 mg daily calcium intake (in skim milk or substitute, food or pills) to help reduce colorectal cell growth, especially if a polyp has already been found.

♦ Eat the most colorful fresh fruit and vegetables, which may contain chemopreventive agents (vitamins, minerals and fiber). Cruciferous vegetables such as broccoli and brussel sprouts are especially important.

♦ Bran (oat or wheat) has a role in high fiber diets but the results are uncertain. Recent studies show that fiber probably plays a role in colon cancer prevention.

♦Wheat bran supplements may help inhibit polyp formation, but this has to be confirmed. It is possible that fiber in natural foods (fruits and vegetables) are better for cancer prevention.

ESOPHAGUS

Ernest H. Rosenbaum, MD, Carlos Pellegrini, MD, T. Stanley Meyler, MD,
Lawrence Margolis, MD, and Malin Dollinger, MD

◇

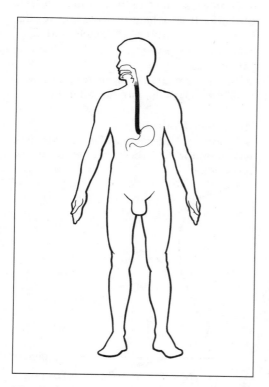

The first recorded case of esophageal cancer was described in China 2,000 years ago. It was called *ye ge*, which seems to have been a polite way of referring to difficult swallowing (dysphagia) and belching. It is a treatable and sometimes curable cancer, although most patients have a poor prognosis because the cancer is usually advanced by the time symptoms appear.

Special attention to good nutrition is an important part of treatment, especially since people in good physical condition with minimal weight loss have a better prognosis. Overall five-year survival is about 10 percent; only 25 to 40 percent of cases are amenable to surgery. Earlier diagnosis and treatment can improve survival. Recent improvements in radiation therapy and chemotherapy results are somewhat encouraging.

Esophageal cancer is relatively uncommon in the United States, affecting about 10,900 Americans each year, with an estimated 9,500 deaths in 1991. It is responsible for 1.5 percent of all cancers in the U.S. and 7 percent of gastrointestinal cancers.

Types Sixty percent of esophageal cancers appear in the cells lining the esophageal tube (squamous cells), usually in the upper two-thirds of the esophagus. About 40 percent develop in the glands (adenocarcinoma) in the lower third. One to 2 percent are relatively rare tumors, such as melanoma, primary lymphomas or tumors in the smooth muscles, among others.

How It Spreads Carcinoma of the esophagus usually starts on the surface layer, invades the surrounding tissue and grows to cause an obstruction that makes swallowing difficult. It spreads through the lymph system to lymph nodes. The most common sites for metastases are the lymph nodes, lungs, liver, brain, adrenal glands and bones.

What Causes It Alcohol and tobacco abuse are the most common causes in North America. Contributing factors in other parts of the world include exposure to environmental carcinogens such as nitrosamines and diets deficient in riboflavin, magnesium, nicotinic acid and zinc. Betel nut chewing and bidi smoking are major factors in India.

Who Gets It Esophageal cancer is much more prevalent in China, Singapore, South Aftica, Iran, Finland, Curacao and parts of Africa than in North America. On this continent, it is most prevalent among men over sixty, smokers, drinkers and blacks. In the United States, men with esophageal cancer outnumber women by 3-to-1 and blacks outnumber whites 3.5- to-1.

RISK FACTORS

At Significantly Higher Risk
♦ Men over 60.
♦ Long-term drinkers, especially in whites.
♦ Long-term smokers (more common in blacks than in whites).
♦ Smokers who drink alcohol (more common in blacks than in whites).

♦ Individuals with muscle spasm (achalasia) or chronic stricture.
♦ Barrett's esophagus with esophagitis—inflammation of the esophagus related to a chronic backup of stomach acid with bile (gastric reflux) causing "heartburn." This may also develop from a malfunction of the gastroesophageal valve that results in backup (reflux) of stomach acid. The male-to-female ratio is 5-to-1 for adenocarcinoma.
♦ Long-term drinkers of very hot tea, which damages the esophageal lining.

At Lower Risk
♦ Mormons and Seventh Day Adventists who monitor their diets and neither drink nor smoke.

Cancer incidence	Divisions of esophagus
15%	Upper 1/3
40%	Middle 1/3
45%	Lower 1/3

The esophagus and nearby organs

SCREENING

Screening programs aren't common in North America because of the low incidence of esophageal cancer. But high-risk individuals (such as those with Barrett's esophagus) can be screened every 3 to 12 months by passing a brush through a nasogastric tube or by endoscopy. Cell analysis (cytology) has a 75 percent detection rate and may be considered for patients with Barrett's esophagus.

COMMON SIGNS AND SYMPTOMS

The most common symptom of esophageal cancer—occurring in 90 percent of patients—is difficulty or pain in swallowing foods and liquids (dysphagia). Other symptoms include weight loss, which can be severe (cachexia), heartburn, hoarseness, pain in the throat or back, vocal cord paralysis, pneumonia and coughing up blood.

DIAGNOSIS

Physical Examination
♦ Enlarged lymph nodes, particularly over the left collarbone.
♦ The vocal cords may be less mobile or paralyzed.
♦ Tapping the spinal area may cause pain in the vertebrae.
♦ Thickening and scaling of the palms and soles.

Blood and Other Tests
♦ Cells for analysis similar to a Pap smear cytology may be scraped off a swallowed balloon or obtained with a brush inserted through an endoscope or a nasogastric tube.
♦ Blood counts and serum chemistry profile.
♦ Serum liver function tests to measure alkaline phosphatase and LDH. Elevated levels may suggest metastases to liver or bone.

♦ An elevated CEA (carcinoembryonic antigen) may indicate liver metastases.
♦ Analysis of cell DNA and DNA histograms are under evaluation as investigational diagnostic tools and may help identify patients with Barrett's esophagus who are about to develop cancer. Preliminary data suggest that a tumor with abnormal chromosomes has a poorer prognosis.

Imaging
♦ A barium swallow and x-ray of the esophagus may reveal a tumor.
♦ A chest x-ray can detect masses in the midchest area and the lungs.
♦ CT scans of the whole lung (mediastinum) and abdomen (liver) will define the size and lateral extent of the tumor so that the stage can be identified accurately. (CT scans will also highlight lymph nodes, although these may not be cancerous.)
♦ Esophageal endoscopic ultrasound of the surrounding tissue will assess the size and depth of the tumor's invasion of the esophagus and evaluate the status of nearby lymph nodes.

Endoscopy and Biopsy
♦ Esophagoscopy is the key test because it allows both visualization and biopsy. A flexible fiberoptic tube is passed through the mouth and down the esophagus. A piece of tissue may be removed with forceps (punch biopsy and cytology). About 25 to 40 percent of patients have a narrowing of the esophagus, which does not permit an endoscope to be passed, so an esophageal dilation may be needed.
♦ A mediastinoscopy (inspection of center of the chest through a thin telescope) may be needed occasionally to assist in staging, for biopsy and to help decide on surgery.

STAGING

The esophagus is not an accessible organ. Although CT and MRI are very helpful, clinical evaluation and staging are difficult. Clinical staging is correct only about half the time, so biopsy and other invasive procedures are usually necessary. The TNM classification system is used to describe the stage.

TREATMENT OVERVIEW

All forms of treatment—radiation therapy, surgery, laser therapy, combination chemotherapy—have been of modest help.

Cancers in the lower two-thirds of the esophagus are generally treated with surgery. Tumors in the upper third (which may have invaded the trachea or larynx) seem to respond better to radiation, but patients with cancers in that area have a poorer prognosis. Unfortunately, 80 to 90 percent of patients have local tissue or lymph node invasion. Nutritional support is necessary. Those with more than a 10 percent weight loss have a poorer prognosis, with an average survival of six months.

 Surgery Since most patients in North America have advanced (Stage III) esophageal cancer before diagnosis, only 25 to 40 percent have tumors that can be removed in an attempt at cure. Before surgery, an evaluation for metastases is performed.

Radical surgery for cure involves removing the entire esophagus (or a good part of it) and the surrounding tissues and lymph nodes. If the lesion is in the lower esophagus near the stomach, the top of the stomach has to be removed as well. Once the esophagus is removed, the stomach can be brought all the way up to bridge the gap (esophagogastrostomy). A portion of the colon may be used instead. This operation is rather demanding of both patient and surgeon. It should be performed only in major medical centers because complex care will be needed during and after surgery.

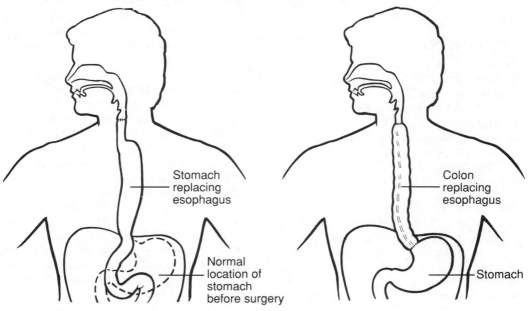

STOMACH "PULL-UP"   COLONIC RECONSTRUCTION

Two types of surgery to replace a cancerous portion of the esophagus

Mortality ranges from 5 to 10 percent, but the removal of the esophagus relieves swallowing problems in over 90 percent of patients and is the only method with a chance of cure.

Tumors in the upper half of the esophagus have usually invaded the trachea or larynx, so reconstruction (with a high risk of complications) will be required.

♦ *Palliative surgery* Bypassing the tumor and creating a new swallowing tube may help some patients whose tumors have invaded the trachea, but otherwise this operation is not recommended for relief of symptoms. A prosthetic indwelling (Celestin) tube inserted through the esophagus may ease swallowing for four to six months. In general, surgery may improve swallowing better than radiotherapy, although the results of chemotherapy and radiation are equal to surgery.

Laser therapy, administered through a flexible tube inserted through the mouth, may open (evaporate) the blockage and relieve dysphagia temporarily. The procedure usually has to be repeated every four to six weeks.

For Barrett's esophagitis with a symptomatic reflux that persists despite potent antacids, H-2 blockers or omeprazole, some medical centers are now investigating antireflux surgery, which may help control symptoms and prevent chronic reflux. Whether this will prevent cancer has not been proven. In patients with progressive Barrett's esophagus who have abnormal changes in the cells that indicate cancer might develop (mucosal dysplasia), the esophagus may be removed as a prophylactic measure.

Combined Therapy Surgery is now often used in combination with chemotherapy and radiation therapy. Combined therapy helps prevent the cancer from recurring and slows the spread of metastases. Chemotherapy may be given before surgery to try to decrease the size of the tumor and reduce metastases, although no randomized trials have shown that chemotherapy and radiation followed by surgery is superior to surgery alone.

 Radiation Therapy The earlier the cancer is diagnosed, the better the results of radiation therapy. Radiation may cure a small number of selected patients, but lesions must be no larger than five centimeters. Generally, radiotherapy is used preoperatively or for relief of symptoms. It is used for palliation if the tumor is larger than 2 in. (5 cm) or if there are distant metastases.

Preoperative radiation can eliminate almost one-third of esophageal cancers but will make only 40 to 67 per cent of tumors operable. Very precise treatment planning with use of an x-ray simulator is important for the best results, with CT scans used to plan treatments accurately.

Chemotherapy with 5-fluorouracil (5-FU) and cisplatin may improve the effect of radiation, although adenocarcinoma (Barrett's esophagus) may not be as sensitive to radiotherapy and chemotherapy. Several investigative programs are currently being tried using multidrug chemotherapy, including 5-FU, VP-16 and/or mitomycin-C with radiation therapy.

Intraluminal radiation using a radiation source placed inside the esophagus (brachytherapy) may complement external radiation. The average five-year survival is 5 to 10 percent for radiation treatment alone.

Adjuvant Chemotherapy Chemotherapy alone is of little benefit. But 5-FU + cisplatin chemotherapy before surgery, will reduce the size of the tumor, allowing a more complete resection (Stages I and II) and may eliminate small metastases. Other chemotherapy programs (5-FU + mitomycin-C, 5-FU + cisplatin or cisplatin + Velban or Vindesine) have shown response to treatment. Studies thus far suggest that carboplatin is less effective than cisplatin and should not be substituted, although it is less toxic.

The role of chemotherapy and radiation therapy is being evaluated. To date, there is modest increased survival from chemotherapy and radiation therapy versus radiation therapy alone. Recent studies of 5-FU + mitomycin-C with radiotherapy have shown an improved survival for Stages I and II disease with almost twice the survival as radiotherapy alone.

 Laser Therapy Endoscopic laser therapy (ELT) has been used over the past few years to relieve swallowing problems. Lasers can vaporize the tumor and cut a hole through a blockage in the esophagus, although the hole will last only a few weeks to three months. The procedure can be repeated to keep the obstruction open, but repeated laser treatments may be more difficult.

Esophageal dilation with ELT can be used to reopen the food channel when surgery or radiation therapy are not practical or when treatment with mechanical methods (by balloon dilators or mercury-filled rubber dilators) fails. Esophageal rupture is a possible complication of dilation.

With laser therapy there are dangers of perforation, bleeding and fistula formation. Lasers can also treat tumors only inside the esophagus, not tumors outside the esophageal wall (*see* Chapter 9).

TREATMENT BY STAGE

STAGE 0
TNM Tis (Tumor in situ)
This very early cancer has not spread below the lining of the first layer of esophageal tissue. It is unusual for cancer to be found at this stage in Western countries, though it's not unusual in China, where esophageal cancer is seen frequently and screening programs are common.

Standard Treatment Early-stage esophageal cancer can be cured with surgery. Radiotherapy could be an option in poor-risk patients.

Five-Year Survival The prognosis is excellent if the tumor is treated surgically or with radiotherapy.

STAGE I
TNM TI, N0, M0
The tumor involves less than 2 in. (5 cm) of the esophagus, does not penetrate the muscular wall, and there is no spread to lymph nodes, adjacent structures or other organs. While patients may have some difficulty swallowing, there is no obstruction of the esophagus.

Standard Treatment Stage I cancer is treatable and occasionally curable. Surgical removal of the tumor is the treatment of choice, with the highest success rate for cancer in the lower third of the esophagus. About 4 in. (10 cm) of the esophagus and the adjacent lymph nodes are removed. With surgery, there is a 5 to 10 percent mortality rate and a 15 to 30 percent complication rate.

Radiation therapy may effectively control and sometimes cure small tumors. Side effects of radiation therapy can include a short-term inflammation of the esophagus and the development of a benign stricture (30 percent), which can be dilated.

There is no standard chemotherapy, but recent studies suggest that combined radiation and chemotherapy (with 5-FU + cisplatin or 5-FU + mitomycin-C) may possibly achieve a clinical remission and cure for Stages I or II cancers. This may be in conjunction with or instead of surgery.

Palliation Surgery and radiation therapy can relieve swallowing problems in about 80 percent of cases.

Five-Year Survival 30 to 50 percent

Investigational
♦ Protocols using combinations of chemotherapy and radiosensitizers, along with radiation therapy before or after surgery, are being evaluated.

STAGE II
TNM T2, N+, M0
The tumor involves more than 2 in. (5 cm) of the esophagus and may involve the entire circumference in one area, causing blockage problems. The cancer has not spread to adjacent organs but may have spread to regional lymph nodes. Most cancers larger than 2 in. (5 cm) have positive lymph nodes.

Standard Treatment Combination therapy with radiation (6,000 cGy) and a chemotherapy infusion of 5-FU and mitomycin-C or cisplatin has produced local response rates of up to 80 percent. About 20 percent of patients had complete remission locally, meaning that no tumor was found at surgery. There is an average survival of one and a half years and up to 3 years for patients who experienced complete remission before surgery.

Surgery holds out some potential for cure, but there is high operative mortality. Stomach reflux and inflammation are common side effects. It should also be noted that because the esophagus has unusual lymphatic drainage, metastatic tumors may be found quite distant from the primary tumor.

Palliation Successful surgery will alleviate swallowing problems for two to three months in 90 percent of patients; radiation therapy will provide relief for 70 percent. Overall survival is about 11 months.

External beam radiation therapy may be palliative for larger tumors or with celiac lymph node involvement (for the lower esophagus) and supraclavicular lymph node involvement (for the upper esophagus).

A radiation source (iridium) may be inserted into the esophagus and left at the tumor site for several hours (intraluminal brachytherapy). Side effects can include inflammation of the esophagus (but rarely the heart or spinal cord), bleeding or a hole from the esophagus into the lungs (esophagobronchial fistula). This may also happen as part of the disease process, especially for the middle third of the esophagus.

Five-Year Survival 10 to 15 percent

Investigational
♦ Radiation therapy given for two weeks before surgical removal of the esophagus may eliminate some of the tumor cells that have spread and make some inoperable tumors operable.
♦ There are several trials being conducted using combinations of chemotherapy (5-FU and cisplatin) and radiosensitizers along with radiation before or after surgery.
♦ Various chemotherapy programs to increase resectability are being evaluated. Chemotherapy may not increase the number of tumors that are operable, but those who respond to chemotherapy live longer than those who don't (12 months versus 6.2 months).
♦ A new laser approach—photodynamic therapy—involves the injection of a substance that makes tissue more sensitive to light. This is followed by the burning of a hole with a laser through the esophageal obstruction. This is safe and may temporarily help to control tumors and allow eating. (*See* Chapter 9.)

STAGE III
TNM T3–T4, any N, and M0
The tumor has spread outside the esophagus and there is extensive lymph node involvement, but there are no metastases.

Standard Treatment Multiple approaches are used with Stage III cancer. Radiation therapy and chemotherapy are used for palliation (5-FU + cisplatin, 5-FU, 5-FU + cisplatin + Adriamycin or 5-FU + mitomycin-C).

Nutrition is a major concern, because patients cannot swallow. A nutritional support program should be instituted with an enteral feeding tube or hyperalimentation. Lasers may be used to open up a blocked esophagus or an eating tube may be inserted.

Five-Year Survival Less than 10 percent when the cancer has spread to adjacent structures but not to other organs

Investigational
♦ Various combinations of chemotherapy, radiation and surgery may be attempted. Radiation and chemotherapy without surgery is being evaluated for patients who are inoperable, have refused surgery or are over 80 years old.
♦ 5-FU + interferon-alpha has shown significant activity.
♦ One study showed improved survival for patients with non-resectable tumors if radiation, chemotherapy and heat treatments (hyperthermia) were given after part of the esophagus was removed.
♦ Laser therapy may be used to reduce obstruction (photodynamic protoporphyrin therapy and dilation). Patients with severe weight loss or anorexia are generally poor risks for therapy.

STAGE IV
TNM Any T, any N, M1
The tumor has spread to other organs (distant metastases).

Standard Treatment There is no standard treatment for Stage IV esophageal cancer. Standard palliative approaches—including external radiation with chemotherapy, with or without the insertion of an eating tube and dilation—are used. All patients may be considered candidates for investi-

gational protocols evaluating new approaches to treatment, including promising chemotherapy combinations.

Five-Year Survival Unusual

Investigational
♦ Chemotherapy and radiotherapy treatments as outlined in Stages II and III.

SUPPORTIVE THERAPY
People with esophageal tumors often have a poor nutritional status. Attempts to correct weight loss may help reduce the complications of surgery, radiotherapy, chemotherapy and combined treatments.
♦ A nasogastric feeding tube (if there is no obstruction) or a gastrojejunostomy may be used for enteral nutrition.
♦ Parenteral hyperalimentation may be necessary for support during therapy.
♦ Esophageal dilation with or without laser therapy to maintain an open esophagus may help maintain nutrition.

TREATMENT FOLLOW-UP
Patients who have had treatment for cure should visit their physician every few months for close follow-up. The adequacy of treatment can be assessed and any needed palliative treatment—radiation or laser therapy—can begin.

RECURRENT CANCER
All such patients may be treated with standard or palliative chemotherapy described for Stages II and III or should be considered candidates for clinical trials.

Palliation is difficult and nutritional support and pain control are helpful.

PREVENTION
♦ Avoid drinking alcohol and smoking.
♦ For Barrett's esophagus, it is important to try to heal the esophagitis and prevent the reflux of stomach acids. Reflux may

be managed by using H-2 blockers to relieve symptoms, by changing the pressure in the lower esophagus with metoclopramide (Reglan) and by not eating for several hours before sleep. Losec (omeprazole), a new drug that has antisecretory properties that suppress gastric acid, may not only help heal esophagitis but also may heal or normalize a Barrett's esophagus. Dietary restrictions—avoiding fats, chocolate and peppermint—opiates, calcium-channel blockers and anticholinergic drugs may also help control reflux.

THE MOST IMPORTANT QUESTIONS YOU CAN ASK

♦ What are the criteria for surgery? for radiation therapy?

♦ How does the stage of disease relate to the chance for cure?

♦ How does squamous cell cancer differ from adenocarcinoma of the esophagus?

♦ What is the role, treatment and prognosis of radiation therapy, the role of surgery, and chemotherapy in treatment of cancer of the esophagus?

♦ How can I obtain nutritional support ?

GALL BLADDER

Alan P. Venook, MD

◇

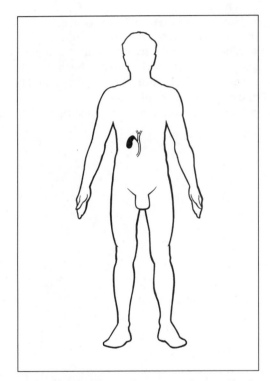

The gall bladder stores bile, which aids in the digestion of fat-containing foods. It is a non-essential organ and can be removed without significant consequences. Gall bladder cancer—also called carcinoma of the gall bladder—is extremely rare. And unless it is very small and found when the gall bladder is removed for other reasons, the treatment now available is not particularly effective.

Because it is so uncommon and because its symptoms mirror those of far more common ailments, cancer of the gall bladder is usually not found until it is at an advanced stage and cannot be surgically removed. In the advanced stages, pain

relief and the restoration of normal bile flow from the liver into the intestines are the principal goals of therapy.

Types The majority of gall bladder tumors are found in glandular tissue within the gall bladder (adenocarcinoma). Others originate in the connective tissue (sarcoma) or other tissues (squamous carcinoma). The management for all gall bladder cancer types is the same, always depending upon the extent of the tumor at the time of diagnosis.

How It Spreads Gall bladder cancer tends to spread to nearby organs and tissues such as the liver or intestines. It also spreads through the lymph system to lymph nodes in the region of the liver (porta hepatis). Ultimately, other lymph nodes and organs can become involved.

What Causes It No one factor has been clearly shown to cause gall bladder cancer. Although it occurs most often in people with gallstone disease, it is extremely rare even in such patients. It is not known if bouts of gallstones predispose people to developing this cancer.

RISK FACTORS

At Significantly Higher Risk
♦ About 85 percent of people with gall bladder cancer have a history of gallstones (cholelithiasis). Sometimes, although not often, the gall bladder becomes hardened (calcified) from repeated inflammation as gallstones are passed. People with this "porcelain gall bladder" have a higher risk of developing this cancer than do others. The typical patient with gall bladder

cancer is an elderly woman with a history of gall bladder problems.

At Slightly Higher Risk
♦ Gallstone disease without a "porcelain gall bladder."

SCREENING

No screening tests are available to detect this cancer at an early stage. But, since the gall bladder isn't essential, people with a calcified gall bladder may consider having it removed as a preventive measure.

COMMON SIGNS AND SYMPTOMS

There are no clinical signs or symptoms characteristic of gall bladder cancer. Jaundice (the skin turning yellow), bloating, abdominal pain, weight loss, decreasing appetite, fever, nausea or an enlarging abdominal mass are all signs that *may* be attributable to gall bladder cancer. Frequently, jaundice is a late development and the other symptoms have been present for a long time. Itching may result from the buildup in the skin of a derivative of bile, bilirubin, which turns the skin yellow. This symptom usually reflects advanced disease.

DIAGNOSIS

Physical Examination
There are no specific findings for gall bladder cancer on physical examination. Even if the following are found, gall bladder cancer would still not be the prime suspect because it is so uncommon:
♦ Fever.
♦ Tender mass below the ribs on the right side of the abdomen.
♦ Enlarged, hard lymph nodes.
♦ Jaundice (the skin turning yellow).
♦ Swelling of the legs (edema).

Blood and Other Tests
Diagnostic tests are notoriously inaccurate in their ability to pinpoint gall bladder can-

cer before surgery. A standard evaluation, however, would include:
♦ A complete blood test, which may be normal or may reveal a decrease in hemoglobin (anemia). The white blood cell count may be normal or increased.
♦ Liver function tests may be abnormal. The most likely abnormalities are in the serum bilirubin and alkaline phosphatase, indicating a blockage in the bile duct leaving either the liver or the gall bladder.
♦ Prothrombin Time and Partial Thromboplastin Time (PT and PTT) are tests of clotting that may reveal a disorder in patients with poor liver function related to a blocked bile duct.

Imaging
♦ An abdominal ultrasound study to view the gall bladder area without exposure to x-rays can confirm that the gall bladder wall has thickened and provide information about the size and characteristics of any mass in the region.
♦ Swallowing pills with dye that travels to the gall bladder, enabling it to be seen on x-ray (oral cholecystography), or the injection of dye into the bile ducts through the skin followed by an x-ray of the area (percutaneous cholangiography) may be done because of symptoms or an elevated serum bilirubin level. While both studies may document an abnormality within the bile ducts or gall bladder, neither can reliably distinguish between inflammation of the gall bladder (cholecystitis) and gall bladder cancer.
♦ A CT scan may help determine the extent of the tumor within the gall bladder bed and the possible involvement of other organs.
♦ Magnetic resonance imaging (MRI) may be helpful in determining if the cancer can be surgically removed, but it is usually not necessary because the CT scan shows similar information.
♦ If the diagnosis of cancer is confirmed or suspected, a chest x-ray should be obtained. A finding of tumor nodules in

the lungs would mean that the disease is already metastatic.

Endoscopy and Biopsy
♦ If cancer is suspected in a situation not involving gall bladder surgery for other reasons, a biopsy, either with a fine needle (FNA) or regular needle, is always required. This can be done through the skin without significant danger.

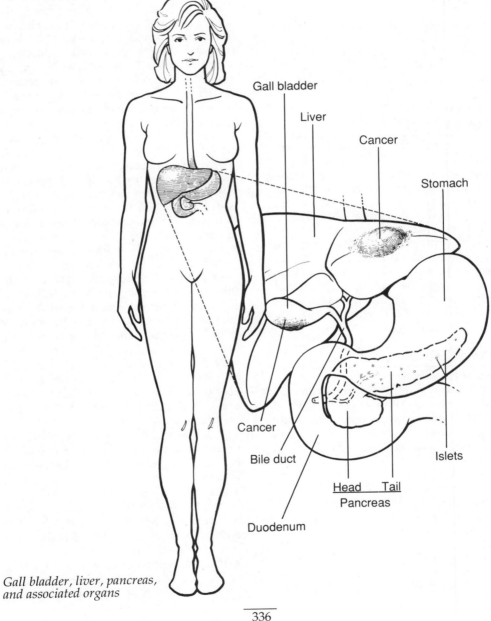

Gall bladder
Liver
Cancer
Stomach
Cancer
Bile duct
Head   Tail
Pancreas
Duodenum
Islets

Gall bladder, liver, pancreas, and associated organs

STAGING

A TNM staging system exists for gall bladder cancer, but for the purposes of deciding on which therapeutic option to use there are only three stages—localized resectable, localized unresectable and advanced disease.

TREATMENT OVERVIEW

Gall bladder cancer can be cured only when it is localized enough to be removed surgically. Unfortunately, virtually the only people with such localized disease are those whose cancer is found unexpectedly when the gall bladder is removed for other reasons.

The goal of the diagnostic work-up is to determine if the cancer can be entirely removed. This is rarely possible because the tumor usually spreads to local regions early in its course. More effective chemotherapy and radiation therapy than are available today are under investigation. These treatments are occasionally useful to relieve symptoms related to the cancer. Although patients with advanced gall bladder cancer have a poor prognosis, measures can be taken to maintain the quality of life.

Surgery Surgery is the only possible cure. If there is no distant tumor spread, the gall bladder as well as the draining lymph nodes and a wedge of normal underlying liver tissue may be removed. This may cure a patient, can help relieve symptoms and may improve the quality of life.

If a gall bladder cancer is found unexpectedly in the pathology specimen after surgery performed for problems not thought to involve cancer, a second operation may be required. If the tumor is limited to only the superficial layers of the gall bladder, observation may be adequate. If the cancer has spread into the surrounding tissues, lymph nodes or blood vessels,

however, a second operation may be performed to remove other tissues that may be involved.

When the tumor cannot fully be removed, it may still be necessary to create a drainage system for the bile from the obstructed gall bladder or bile ducts. This may require surgery, although draining of the gall bladder by a tube placed through the skin by a radiologist or through a tube in the stomach and small intestines usually suffices.

The presence of tumor anywhere else in the body—in the lung, bone or lymph nodes, for example—is a clear indication that surgery will not be curative. If the disease has already spread, there is rarely a need to remove a gall bladder cancer, for such surgery involves a difficult recovery period and so may be more damaging to the patient.

Chemotherapy Studies have not yet shown that chemotherapy can prolong the survival of patients with gallbladder cancer. The standard drugs used—5-fluorouracil or mitomycin-C—may cause tumor shrinkage in about 25 percent of patients. Even with tumor shrinkage, however, patients may be in a worse condition afterward because the tumor usually regrows quickly and the treatments have some side effects.

There is no proven role for adjuvant chemotherapy after a cancerous gall bladder has been removed, but it is logical to consider chemotherapy. In the hopes of finding drugs that may work better than the chemotherapy now used, patients should be entered into a clinical trial if chemotherapy is planned.

 Radiation The usefulness of radiation in gall bladder cancer is limited by the damage it causes to the surrounding non-cancerous liver tissue. Radiation may help patients who have small bits of tumor remaining after surgery or in those who have had large tumors removed.

Patients who are not candidates for surgery may also benefit from radiation to the gall bladder area, although they are still likely to have recurrent tumors. The toxicity of such radiation may also worsen existing symptoms such as nausea and loss of appetite.

Combined Therapy The combination of external beam radiation and chemotherapy may play a role after surgery, perhaps prolonging the period before the cancer returns or even curing people who have undergone surgery without complete tumor removal. This treatment, however, is still being studied.

TREATMENT BY STAGE
LOCALIZED RESECTABLE
In this stage, the cancer is confined to the superficial layers (mucosa and submucosa) of the gall bladder. Cancers at this limited stage are generally found when the gall bladder is removed because of other problems.

Standard Treatment Experts disagree over the extent of surgery needed for a localized gall bladder cancer. Studies are ongoing, but most experts would recommend:
♦ removal of the gall bladder
♦ a lymph node dissection of all the draining lymphatic vessels in the region
♦ the removal of a wedge of about 1 1/2 in. (4 cm) of apparently normal liver.

Such surgery is the most likely treatment to render a patient cancer-free. If the cancer is not recognized until after surgery, the need for a second operation is considered. A patient with a truly limited cancer (superficial) may just be observed closely, but because of the poor prognosis should the cancer recur, it is difficult to argue against the aggressive approach outlined above.

Five-Year Survival About 80 percent. Those with cancers that are still very small but cause symptoms have a somewhat lover five-year survival rate.

Investigational
♦ There is no certain role for adjuvant chemotherapy. Although chemotherapy such as 5-fluorouracil (5-FU) or mitomycin-C is often recommended, no studies have shown that the chance of cure can be increased.
♦ Radiation is often given to the liver area after surgery but has never been proven to be beneficial.
♦ The use of a combination of 5-FU and radiation therapy following complete removal of the cancer is now being studied.

LOCALIZED UNRESECTABLE
Despite being a localized mass, the tumor cannot be removed because of the particular way it has spread to local lymph nodes or adjacent liver tissue.

Standard Treatment There is no standard treatment. Patients should be considered for clinical trials aimed at prolonging survival and relieving the symptoms associated with the tumor.

Two-Year Survival Less than 5 percent

Investigational
♦ Protocols designed to test the additive benefit of combining radiation with chemotherapy are ongoing and should be offered to patients with this condition.

ADVANCED
The cancer has metastisized to distant sites.

Standard Treatment No standard therapy is known to prolong survival in patients with advanced gall bladder cancer. The usual approach is a trial of chemotherapy with a single agent such as 5-FU or mitomycin-C. Even if the tumor shrinks, patients may not benefit because of the side effects of the chemotherapy and because the tumor usually regrows very quickly.

Two-Year Survival Less than 1 percent

Investigational
♦ Combination chemotherapy or new drugs may prove to be better in the treatment of advanced gall bladder cancer than therapies now available. Because the side effects are likely to be greater than those caused by single-agent chemotherapy, such treatment should be done in a clinical protocol.

TREATMENT FOLLOW-UP

Careful follow-up is important after the removal of a localized gall bladder cancer, although once a recurrent tumor is large enough to be seen on an x-ray it is probably too large to be cured. Follow-up should include:
♦ CT scans every two to three months for the first year after surgery, since another small tumor may still be resectable at the time of diagnosis.

SUPPORTIVE THERAPY

♦ Symptoms associated with jaundice can include severe itching and a general sense of poor health. These symptoms can generally be managed with a drainage procedure to bypass the blockage in the biliary tract. This procedure may include placing of a tube through the skin or through the stomach. Surgery is rarely necessary to bypass an obstruction. If

such drainage is ineffective, itching may be relieved by the use of Benadryl, Atarax or cholestyramine.
♦ Pain relief may require large doses of medication. Narcotics must be used carefully, however, since they may have excessive side effects and are metabolized by the liver, which may not be working properly.
♦ Non-steroidal anti-inflammatory drugs may be surprisingly effective even against the severe pain associated with gall bladder cancer.
♦ The use of water pills to reduce fluid in the abdomen or legs may be helpful, but may cause significant imbalance in kidney function and can create major problems if not monitored carefully.
♦ Nausea can be treated with standard medications, including suppositories.
♦ Sleep disturbances are common, but sleeping pills should be used carefully since most are metabolized by the liver.
♦ Frequent small meals may be necessary since an abdominal mass may encroach on the size of the stomach.
♦ Patients with the severe loss of appetite may be helped by a drug called Megace.

THE MOST IMPORTANT QUESTIONS YOU CAN ASK

♦ Should I see another physician to confirm that this tumor is or is not resectable for cure?
♦ Could I benefit from an investigational therapy available at another institution?
♦ How sick will the proposed chemotherapy make me relative to its potential benefit?
♦ Can anything be done to improve the quality of my life?

HEAD AND NECK

James T. Helsper, MD, and Malin Dollinger, MD

———◇———

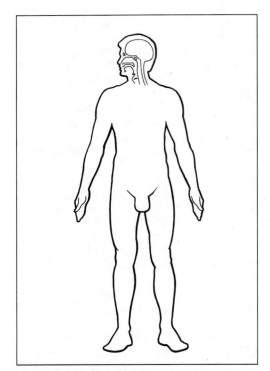

Taken together, head and neck cancers account for 5 to 10 percent of all malignancies. These cancers are more common in men by a ratio of 3 to 1 and are much more common in people over 50. They have a rather good cure rate if they are found early, evaluated adequately and treated with the best available therapy. All three main treatment methods—surgery, radiotherapy and chemotherapy—are used.

There are about 40,000 new cases in the United States each year, and about one third of head and neck cancer patients die of their disease. The use of chemotherapy (such as cisplatin + 5-fluorouracil or low-dose 5-fluorouracil continuous infusion) as an adjuvant to surgery and radiotherapy has produced a definite improvement

in response rates, which may mean a better cure rate in the future.

The broad category of head and neck cancers includes tumors in several areas.

♦ Lip and oral cavity. This includes the lips, tongue, the inside lining of the cheeks (buccal mucosa), the floor of the mouth, the gums (gingiva) and the hard palate.

♦ Paranasal sinuses and nasal cavity. Sinuses are found below and above the eyes and behind the nose.

♦ Salivary glands. These glands produce saliva to moisten our mouth and help us chew food.

♦ Oropharynx. This is the upper part of the throat that can be seen when you say "ahhh." It also includes the tonsils.

♦ Nasopharynx. The nasopharynx is behind the nose and above the oropharynx. It cannot be seen directly.

♦ Hypopharynx. This is the lower part of the throat (pharynx) where food goes just before we swallow it.

♦ Larynx. The larynx (voice box) is in the front of the neck in the region of the Adam's apple.

♦ Metastatic squamous cell cancer to cervical (neck) lymph nodes. If a cancer that is discovered in lymph nodes in the upper part of the neck is squamous cell (or epidermoid), it is usually a metastasis from a head and neck cancer. Unless some other primary source can be found (such as lung cancer), this tumor is generally treated as a head and neck cancer (*see also* "Cancer of Unknown Primary Site").

The most common locations for head and neck cancers—almost half of all cases—are the mouth and throat (oral cavity and oropharynx). About a third are in the larynx.

These cancers and their treatment can have serious results. Because they tend to

Side view of head showing potential cancer sites

involve the upper digestive tract and the upper respiratory tract, these tumors can interfere with eating and breathing. Laryngeal cancer directly affects speech. Several sensory functions are located here—vision, hearing, smell and taste—and the loss or malfunction of any of them is significant.

Successful treatment must, therefore, not only include an attempt to eradicate all the cancer but also take into account:
♦ The need for adequate function—swallowing, eating, speech—after treatment.
♦ A satisfactory cosmetic result. It is as important to consider reconstruction, rehabilitation and prostheses as it is to achieve an adequate surgical removal.

Many health care workers are essential to success. In addition to the head and neck (or ear, nose and throat) surgeon, the treatment team may include the primary physician, radiation and medical oncologists, dentists, rehabilitation specialists, plastic surgeons, dieticians, pathologists, radiologists, oncology nurses and social workers. The patient and his or her family, friends and employer are all involved in the recovery process.

RISK FACTORS

The use of tobacco and/or alcohol is the most important contributing factor. Smokers and drinkers who fail to stop after treatment for a primary head and neck cancer are at significant risk of developing another cancer. In fact, anyone with a head and neck cancer is somewhat more likely to develop another, although giving a new drug called 13-cis-retinoic acid to such patients has decreased the chance of their developing a second primary tumor.

♦ Poor oral hygiene, poorly fitting dentures or broken teeth cause chronic irritation of oral membranes.

♦ Wood dust inhalation (furniture workers) is related to nasal cavity cancer.

♦ Betel nut chewing (India) is related to cancer of the lining of cheek.

♦ Increased carcinoma of nasopharynx among southern Chinese (environmental not genetic).

♦ Epstein-Barr virus (EBV) infection is associated with nasopharyngeal cancer.

♦ Chronic iron deficiency in women is associated with tongue and postcricoid carcinoma.

♦ Nickel exposure is associated with paranasal sinus cancer.

SCREENING

Screening is not generally practiced in North America. There are three approaches to early detection.

♦ Your awareness of typical signs and symptoms and your calling them to the attention of your physician.

♦ A careful examination of the head and neck by your doctor, including an examination of the larynx with the aid of a mirror (indirect laryngoscopy).

♦ Your dentist is in an excellent position to call your attention to suspicious lesions in the mouth such as the premalignant lesion called leukoplakia (white patches). Many oral cancers are discovered by dentists.

COMMON SIGNS AND SYMPTOMS

These tumors can appear as ulcerations of the mucous membranes with hard, rolled edges, or less commonly as protruding growths that look like small mushrooms. Specific symptoms depend on the location.

♦ *Mouth and oral cavity:* a swelling or ulcer that doesn't heal.

♦ *Nose and sinuses:* pain, swelling, bloody nasal discharge, nasal obstruction, double vision or chronic sinus trouble that does not respond to antibiotics.

♦ *Salivary glands:* painless swelling and paralysis of one side of the face.

♦ *Oropharynx:* difficulty or pain on swallowing and ear pain. May also have no symptoms.

♦ *Hypopharynx:* difficulty swallowing, ear pain and enlarged lymph nodes in the neck. May have no symptoms.

♦ *Nasopharynx:* bloody nasal discharge or nasal obstruction, decreased hearing, nerve signs (double vision, pain, hoarseness) or enlarged lymph nodes in the neck.

♦ *Larynx:* persistent hoarseness, difficulty breathing, pain.

♦ *Metastatic squamous cell cancer:* swollen, painless lymph nodes in the neck.

DIAGNOSIS

Specific tests depend on the location of the cancer.

Physical Examination

♦ Inspection of the oral and nasal cavities, using mirrors and telescopes.

♦ Examination of suspicious lesions with the fingers (palpation), as well as examination of the back of the tongue.

Blood and Other Tests

♦ Epstein-Barr (EB) virus antibody measurements may be helpful in diagnosing hidden nasopharyngeal primary cancer in patients with metastatic cancer in the cervical lymph nodes.

Imaging
♦ X-rays of the sinuses and skull.
♦ CT and MRI scans, barium swallow, laryngogram and chest x-ray.

Endoscopy and Biopsy
♦ Biopsy of suspicious lesions.
♦ In cases of metastatic cancer in cervical lymph nodes, biopsy of apparently normal tissues in the tonsils, throat and nasopharynx may discover the site of origin.

STAGING

Head and neck cancers are staged according to the TNM system. Accuracy of staging is especially critical, since a slight difference in the location and size of the tumor has a significant effect on the therapy chosen, the extent of surgery and the prognosis.

Accurate staging requires visual inspection, x-rays, appropriate biopsies, blood tests (such as complete blood counts and liver tests) and careful palpation and measurement of enlarged lymph nodes. The mobility of enlarged nodes should be determined since a lymph node that cannot be moved back and forth may contain cancer that has spread to adjacent tissues. Sometimes examination under anesthesia is needed to directly inspect inaccessible areas such as the larynx, nasopharynx, and oropharynx, as well as to perform necessary biopsies.

TNM STAGE GROUPING
Stage I T1, N0, M0
Stage II T2, N0, M0
Stage III T3, N0, M0
T1–3, N1, M0
Stage IV T4, N0 or N1, M0
Any T, N2-3, M0
Any T, any N, M1

For most subsites there are also other TNM categories that define the tumor more precisely.

STAGING OUTLINE

Oral cavity, oropharynx
(tumor can be seen directly)

Tx	Tumor cannot be measured
T0	No evidence of primary tumors
Tis	Carcinoma in situ
T1	Tumor no larger than 3/4 in. (2 cm)
T2˙	Tumor 3/4 –1 1/2 in. (2–4 cm)
T3	Tumor over 1 1/2 in. (4 cm)
T4	Massive tumor, over 1 1/2 in. (4 cm) with extension to adjacent structures

Nasopharynx, hypopharynx, larynx
(tumor cannot be seen directly)

} SAME

Tumor confined to one site
Involves more than one site at origin
Tumor extends beyond primary site

} SAME

NX	Nodes cannot be measured	
N0	No involved lymph nodes	
N1	Single involved node, same side, less than 1 1/4 in. (3 cm)	
N2	Single involved node, same side,	
	N2a	one node, 1 1/4 –2 1/2 in. (3–6 cm)
	N2b	multiple nodes, none over 2 1/2 in. (6 cm)
N3	Massive involved lymph nodes	
	N3a	a node over 2 1/2 in. (6 cm) on same side
	N3b	nodes on both sides
	N3c	nodes only on opposite side

LIP AND MOUTH (ORAL CAVITY)

These cancers can be treated with surgery, radiation therapy or a combination of both depending on the location and size of the tumor and whether it has spread to lymph nodes. Reconstruction and rehabilitation are essential parts of the treatment plan.

Early cancers (Stages I and II) of the lip and oral cavity are highly curable by surgery or radiation therapy, with the choice depending on the anticipated functional and cosmetic results.

Advanced cancers (Stages III and IV) are usually treated with a combination of surgery and radiotherapy. A few patients with small T3 lesions who have no involved lymph nodes larger than 3/4 in. (2 cm) might receive either surgery or radiation. Patients with these stages commonly develop recurrences near the primary tumor or metastatic disease after treatment and should be considered for clinical trials involving radiation modifiers or the use of combination chemotherapy in addition to surgery and/or radiation. Patients whose tumors grow into blood vessels have a worse prognosis.

TREATMENT OVERVIEW

♦ If surgery is the chosen method, the tumor must be removed along with the areas in the neck where it usually first spreads, to provide a margin of safety. The chosen surgeon must be able to reconstruct the area, working with dentists who are specialists in reconstructing portions of teeth that have had to be removed to provide the best chance of cure. This helps return the patient to the most normal quality of life.

♦ If the cervical nodes are involved, all the lymph nodes on that side of the neck usually have to be removed (radical neck dissection).

♦ Radiation therapy for lip or oral cancer can be with either external beams or occasionally the implantation of radioactive

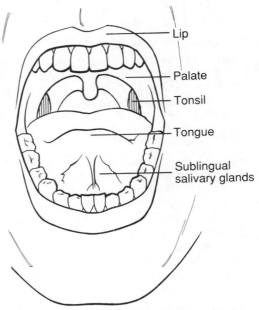

Mouth structures that may develop cancer

seeds into the tumor site for a specified time to give a calculated dose of radiation. Either method can be used alone, but most centers use the two in combination.

♦ Surgery to remove a tumor of the tongue often requires removing a generous portion of the tongue to provide a margin of safety. Surprisingly, there is very little effect on speech and swallowing, although as the tumors grow, a larger portion of the tongue has to be removed and speech becomes more of a problem. A speech therapist may be needed for proper rehabilitation.

♦ Cancer of the space around the teeth usually requires the removal of some of the teeth as well as the primary cancer site in the gingiva (gums). The dental prosthodontist creates a specialized plate for complete rehabilitation.

♦ Occasionally, when the cancer involves the upper gums it may be necessary to remove a portion of the sinus. The prosthodontist is again needed for reconstruction.

♦ For larger cancers that have a lower cure rate with surgery alone, treatment combines all three methods—chemotherapy, followed by surgery, followed by radiation therapy.

TREATMENT BY LOCATION AND STAGE

STAGE I
Standard Treatment

♦ *Lip:* Surgery or radiotherapy, depending on cosmetic and functional results.
♦ *Front of tongue:* Wide local excision. For larger lesions, either surgery or radiotherapy.
♦ *Inside of cheek:* Surgery for small lesions (with graft, if needed) or radiotherapy for larger lesions.
♦ *Floor of mouth:* Surgery or radiotherapy.
♦ *Lower gums:* Surgery, possibly with removal of some bone and the use of a skin graft. Radiotherapy results are usually not as good as surgery.
♦ *Behind wisdom teeth (retromolar trigone):* Can usually be controlled by external radiotherapy. Alternatively, surgical removal, including part of jawbone.
♦ *Upper gums and hard palate:* Surgery, with postoperative radiation if needed.

Five-Year Survival 90 to 100 percent (lip and upper gums), 96 percent (tongue), over 90 percent (inside of cheek), 90 percent (lower gums), 88 percent (floor of mouth)

STAGE II
Standard Treatment

♦ *Lip:* Surgery alone, if simple closure is satisfactory. If surgery has to be complex, radiotherapy produces better cosmetic and functional results.
♦ *Front of tongue:* Radiotherapy initially for smaller lesions to attempt to preserve speech and swallowing. Surgery is used later if tumor remains or recurs. Both

surgery and radiotherapy are used for tumors that are growing deeper.
♦ *Inside of cheek:* Small T2 lesions are treated with radiotherapy, larger T2 lesions with surgery, radiotherapy or both.
♦ *Floor of mouth:* For small T2 lesions, surgery if the tumor is attached to bone and radiotherapy if lesions involve the tongue. Both surgery and radiotherapy can be used for large T2 lesions. The choice depends on the expected disability from surgery. For larger lesions, radiotherapy may be used postoperatively.
♦ *Lower gums:* Small lesions treated with surgery, sometimes requiring removal of some bone as well as a skin graft. Radiotherapy has been used, but results are generally not as good as with surgery alone.
♦ *Behind wisdom teeth:* Same as Stage I.

Five-Year Survival 90 percent (lip, inside of cheek and lower gums), 70 percent (tongue and floor of mouth)

STAGE III
Standard Treatment Surgery and/or

radiotherapy is used, depending on the location of the tumor. Chemotherapy before either surgery or radiotherapy (neoadjuvant) has been used to shrink large tumors and improve the possibility of successful treatment with surgery or radiation. Patients with advanced lesions should have radiotherapy to lymph nodes or surgery to remove them.

♦ *Lip:* Combination of surgery and radiotherapy. Alternatively, these patients are appropriate candidates for clinical trials.
♦ *Front of tongue:* Radiotherapy (may include implant) for less extensive lesions, and surgery with postoperative radiotherapy for more extensive lesions.
♦ *Inside of cheek:* Radical surgery alone, radiotherapy alone or both in sequence. Clinical trials involve adding chemotherapy.
♦ *Floor of mouth:* Extensive surgery or radiotherapy (may include implant).
♦ *Lower gums:* Combined radiotherapy and radical surgery.

♦ *Behind wisdom teeth:* Surgery followed by radiotherapy. Clinical trials involve adding chemotherapy.

♦ *Upper gums:* Superficial lesions are treated with radiotherapy alone. Deep lesions also require surgery.

♦ *Hard palate:* Same as upper gums.

Five-Year Survival 50 percent (lip and inside of cheek), 50 to 60 percent (tongue), 70 percent (floor of mouth), 90 percent (lower gums), 80 percent (hard palate and upper gums)

STAGE IV

Standard Treatment Surgery and/or radiotherapy, depending on the location of the tumor. Neoadjuvant chemotherapy has been used to shrink tumors and improve the possibility of successful treatment with surgery or radiation. Patients with advanced lesions should have radiotherapy to lymph nodes or surgery to remove them.

Clinical trials involving adjuvant chemotherapy are in progress and are appropriate for all sites.

♦ *Lip:* Combined surgery and radiotherapy. Both sides of the neck have to be treated.

♦ *Front of tongue:* Extensive surgery with postoperative radiotherapy for selected patients. For very advanced lesions, radiotherapy alone for palliation.

♦ *Inside of cheek:* Radical surgery, radiotherapy or both in sequence.

♦ *Floor of mouth:* Combination of surgery and radiotherapy. If there are large (over 2 in./5 cm) fixed nodes, radiotherapy is given preoperatively.

♦ *Lower gums:* Advanced tumors are poorly controlled with surgery, radiotherapy or both.

♦ *Behind wisdom teeth:* Surgery followed by radiotherapy.

♦ *Upper gums:* Surgery and radiotherapy.

♦ *Hard palate:* Surgery and radiotherapy.

Five-Year Survival Less than 30 percent for all locations

RECURRENT CANCER

Treatment depends on the location and size of the recurrent tumor, as well as the nature of the original treatment. If radiotherapy was used initially, surgery is preferred. If surgery was used initially, radiotherapy or a combination of both may be used. Because results are poor after using the "other" treatment for a recurrence, clinical trials using chemotherapy or hyperthermia should be considered.

PARANASAL SINUS AND NASAL CAVITY

These cancers are often diagnosed late because they have symptoms resembling chronic sinusitis. They can easily spread throughout the sinus area, and cure rates are generally less than 50 percent. Local growth into vital areas is a more common cause of death than metastases.

There are six sinuses, two just below the eyes (maxillary), two above the eyes (frontal) and two in the center, behind the nose (ethmoid and sphenoid). The maxillary sinus is the one most commonly involved, and cancer there can be difficult to diagnose. It may be necessary to expose the maxillary sinus through a small opening in the mouth above the canine teeth in the upper jaw.

TREATMENT OVERVIEW

Treatment of these tumors is very complex and requires very precise pretreatment evaluation and planning. Most patients require a combination of radiotherapy and surgery.

♦ Since lymph nodes are involved in only about 20 percent of cases, surgery or radiotherapy to the lymph nodes in the neck is used only if these nodes contain tumor.

♦ For patients who have tumors that can be removed at surgery, the surgery is followed by radiotherapy. In some centers, all Stage II and III tumors are treated with radiotherapy before surgery.

♦ Sometimes it is necessary to surgically explore the area of the tumor to see if definitive surgery can be done. If the tumor extends to areas that would be difficult or hazardous to remove surgically, then the treatment is usually radiotherapy.

♦ The radiotherapy dosage must be quite high in all cases.

♦ If the disease recurs, chemotherapy may improve the quality of life and the length of survival.

♦ All patients are candidates for clinical trials of new therapies.

STAGE I
Standard Treatment Surgery is used for small tumors of the lower part of the maxillary sinus. If the tumor extends near the surgical margin, radiotherapy is then given.

For ethmoid sinus cancer, which is usually advanced, extensive surgery (if possible) is followed by radiotherapy. If the cancer cannot be removed, radiotherapy is used alone. Sphenoid sinus cancers are treated with radiotherapy, similar to nasopharyngeal cancers. Nasal cavity cancers are treated with either surgery or radiotherapy.

Occasionally, melanomas and some sarcomas—such as cancers of cartilage (chondrosarcomas) and bone (osteosarcomas or Ewing's sarcoma, a rare type of bone cancer)—occur in this area. Melanomas and sarcomas are surgically excised if possible.

There is also a special kind of tumor in this area called an inverting papil-loma. This is most often described as benign, but some consider it a low-grade cancer because it tends to grow aggressively and because it requires therapy similar to that for cancer. Inverting papillomas are treated with surgery, with radical additional surgery if they recur.

There is also a condition called midline granuloma. Although not classified as cancer, in some cases this is thought to represent a rare kind of lymphoma. Midline granulomas are treated with radiotherapy.

Five-Year Survival 60 to 70 percent

STAGE II
Standard Treatment
♦ *Maxillary sinus:* Surgery and high-dose radiotherapy (pre- or postoperative).
♦ *Ethmoid sinus:* Radiotherapy is generally preferred. Localized lesions can be removed surgically (radical surgery), but radiotherapy is needed afterwards.
♦ *Sphenoid sinus:* Same as nasopharyngeal tumors, using radiotherapy.
♦ *Nasal cavity:* Surgery or radiotherapy for tumors of the septum, radiotherapy elsewhere.
♦ *Inverting papilloma:* Same as Stage I. Radiotherapy may be needed if further surgery is unsuccessful.
♦ *Melanomas and sarcomas:* Surgery if possible.
♦ *Midline granuloma:* Radiotherapy.
♦ *Nasal vestibule (front part of nasal cavity):* Surgery if no deformity is expected or there is no need for reconstruction. Otherwise, radiotherapy.

Five-Year Survival 60 to 70 percent

STAGE III
Standard Treatment
♦ *Maxillary sinus:* Surgery with high-dose pre- or postoperative radiotherapy.
♦ *Ethmoid sinus:* Extensive surgery followed by radiotherapy.
♦ *Sphenoid sinus:* Radiotherapy.
♦ *Nasal cavity:* Surgery or radiotherapy alone. Usually postoperative radiotherapy is preferred.

♦ *Inverting papilloma:* Same as Stage II. Radiotherapy may be needed if further surgery is unsuccessful.

♦ *Melanomas and sarcomas:* Surgery if possible, otherwise radiotherapy.

♦ *Midline granuloma:* Radiotherapy.

♦ *Nasal vestibule:* Radiation first and surgery later if needed.

Clinical trials are in progress for ethmoid sinus and nasal cavity tumors, using chemotherapy combinations in addition to surgery or radiotherapy.

Five-Year Survival 25 to 35 percent

STAGE IV

Standard Treatment Chemotherapy is given before surgery or radiotherapy in an attempt to shrink tumors and make them more treatable. This should be considered for each of the sites below except inverting papilloma and midline lethal granuloma.

♦ *Maxillary sinus:* If the tumor is extensive, surgery may not be appropriate and radiotherapy is used. Sinus drainage must be established first.

♦ *Ethmoid sinus:* Extensive surgery with pre- or postoperative radiotherapy.

♦ *Sphenoid sinus:* Same as nasopharyngeal cancers.

♦ *Nasal cavity:* Surgery or radiotherapy alone or combined.

♦ *Inverting papilloma:* Surgery. Radiotherapy or radical surgery may eventually be necessary.

♦ *Melanomas and sarcomas:* Surgery if possible, but radiation and chemotherapy should be considered.

♦ *Midline granuloma:* Radiotherapy.

♦ *Nasal vestibule:* Radiation if possible and surgery if unsuccessful.

Clinical trials for maxillary sinus, ethmoid sinus and nasal cavity tumors are evaluating chemotherapy combinations in addition to surgery or radiotherapy.

Five-Year Survival 10 to 25 percent

RECURRENT CANCER

Chemotherapy is given if there is a recurrence in the original area following surgery or radiotherapy or of there are distant metastases. Chemotherapy is promising, with effective palliation, improved quality of life and improved survival for patients who respond.

♦ *Maxillary sinus:* Radiotherapy, or extensive surgery followed by radiotherapy.

♦ *Ethmoid sinus:* After limited surgery, extensive surgery, radiotherapy or both.

♦ *Sphenoid sinus:* Radiotherapy. If unsuccessful, chemotherapy.

♦ *Nasal cavity:* If it recurs after radiotherapy, extensive surgery. If it recurs after surgery, radiotherapy. If recurrent after both, then chemotherapy.

♦ *Inverting papilloma:* Same as previous stages.

♦ *Melanomas and sarcomas:* Surgery if possible and chemotherapy directed at the specific cell type.

♦ *Nasal vestibule:* If radiotherapy fails, surgery is appropriate. If surgery fails, radiotherapy or a combination of further surgery and radiotherapy. If these fail, chemotherapy may be given.

For maxillary sinus, ethmoid sinus and nasal tumors, clinical trials using chemotherapy should be considered.

SALIVARY GLANDS

There are four kinds of salivary glands. The parotid glands are in front of each ear (enlarged in mumps), the submaxillary (or submandibular) glands are just below the lower jaw bones, the sublingual glands are under the tongue, and many small, minor salivary glands line the mouth, nose and throat.

There are both benign and malignant tumors of these glands, although the term benign may be misleading. These "benign" tumors rarely if ever metastasize, but their growth can be fairly aggressive and the surgery needed to control them may resemble that needed for malignant tumors of the same gland. There have been cases in which benign salivary gland tumors have caused death by recurring and invading the tissues of the face or brain.

There are at least six kinds of malignant tumors and about the same number of benign ones. The treatment is different for each kind of tumor, so expert pathologic study is necessary.

Twenty-five percent of parotid tumors, 40 percent of submandibular tumors, 95 percent of sublingual tumors and 50 percent of minor salivary gland tumors are malignant.

The most common site of malignant tumors is in the parotid glands. The most common site of tumors of the minor salivary gland tumors is in the palate. These tumors can also occur anywhere in the mouth, the pharynx, larynx and paranasal sinusus.

Salivary gland cancers are caused mainly by the heavy use of tobacco. Increased incidence is also associated with previous radiation exposure to the head and neck. Radiotherapy was used to treat acne during the 1930s, 1940s and 1950s, with a resulting five to eight times higher risk.

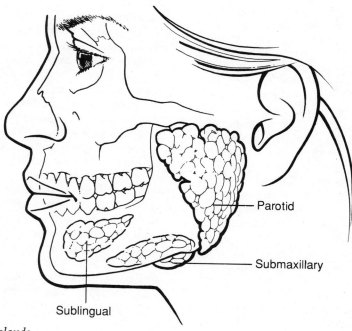

Major salivary glands

TREATMENT OVERVIEW

Early-stage, low-grade salivary gland tumors, especially tumors of the parotid gland, are usually curable by surgery. Large, bulky or high-grade tumors have a poorer prognosis and often receive postoperative radiotherapy. Tumors that cannot be completely removed surgically or that recur may respond to chemotherapy.

Prognosis also depends on which gland is involved, the microscopic pattern, the grade of malignancy, the stage and whether the tumor has extended to involve the skin, lymph nodes, nerves or distant sites.

♦ Minimum therapy for low-grade malignancies of a portion of the parotid gland is a superficial parotidectomy. Great care is taken to preserve the facial nerve that goes through the middle of this gland and controls the muscles on that side of the face. This surgery is very delicate.

For other kinds of parotid tumors, a total parotidectomy is needed to obtain a safe margin around the tumor because it frequently grows microscopically far beyond where it is visible to the surgeon.

♦ Postoperative radiotherapy is being used more and more, especially for lesions that are high grade or have close margins. This seems to improve the cure rate. Fast neutron beam radiation therapy—available in a limited number of centers—has been effective in the treatment of inoperable, unresectable and recurrent tumors, and may be more effective than conventional x-ray therapy.

♦ There is no established role for chemotherapy, but it is sometimes used in special circumstances when radiation or surgery are refused, or for recurrent or unresponsive tumors.

♦ In high-grade cancer, radiation therapy is almost always added. The surgery is often more extensive and may require removal of the facial nerve.

♦ When the tumor has spread to lymph nodes in the neck, an additional operation—called a radical neck dissection—is needed to remove these nodes. One possible result is a drooped shoulder, as well as a flattening of the side of the neck. This must be considered a small price to pay to have a better chance of permanently controlling the cancer.

♦ Chemotherapy is sometimes considered when surgery or radiotherapy are refused or have already been used as much as they can be. Prospects for cure in this situation are low and prolonging life is the goal of therapy.

♦ For patients whose disease has spread beyond the neck, no curative treatment is available.

♦ There are several investigational protocols in use, including chemotherapy, radiation therapy with neutron beams, or radiation accompanied by anticancer drugs such as doxorubicin, cisplatin, paraplatin, cyclophosphamide and 5-fluorouracil.

TREATMENT BY STAGE

STAGE I
Standard Treatment

♦ For low-grade tumors, surgery alone. Radiotherapy may be an alternative if surgery would cause significant cosmetic or functional problems. Radiotherapy is also used after surgery if the margins are involved. Fast neutron beam radiotherapy may be used for tumors that have spread to lymph nodes.

♦ For high-grade tumors, surgery alone, although adjuvant radiotherapy may also be given (especially with positive surgical margins). If the tumor cannot be removed, radiotherapy may be used for palliation. If the tumor has spread to the neck lymph nodes, these nodes should be removed.

Local recurrence may be reduced by adjuvant radiotherapy. Neutron beam radiation is under clinical evaluation, and recent studies indicate that these tumors may also respond to chemotherapy.

Five-Year Survival 90 percent

STAGE II
Standard Treatment
♦ For low-grade tumors, surgery alone, with the same considerations as Stage I. Radical surgery is generally required.
♦ For high-grade tumors, same considerations as Stage I. Postoperative radiotherapy is used to reduce the local recurrence rate if the surgical margins are positive or the nerves or soft tissues of the neck are involved.

Five-Year Survival 55 percent

STAGE III
Standard Treatment
♦ For low-grade tumors, same as Stages I and II.
♦ For high-grade tumors, same considerations as Stages I and II. Chemotherapy should be considered when surgery or radiation is refused or for recurrent or unresponsive tumors.

Studies are trying to improve local control with fast neutron beam therapy, radiosensitizers and chemotherapy.

Five-Year Survival 45 percent

STAGE IV
Standard Treatment There is no curative standard therapy for this stage, in which the tumor has spread to distant sites, so consideration should be given to investigational protocols such as combination chemotherapy, conventional radiotherapy or fast neutron beam therapy.

Metastatic disease can be treated with combinations of doxorubicin, cisplatin, cyclophosphamide and 5-fluorouracil.

Five-Year Survival 10 percent

RECURRENT CANCER
The prognosis is poor regardless of the cell type or stage. Treatment depends on the specific cancer, earlier treatment, area of recurrence and the medical problems of the patient. Surgery is often the first choice, followed by radiation. Investigational treatments are appropriate and should be considered.

OROPHARYNX

Almost all cases of oropharyngeal cancer are related to cigarette smoking or other forms of tobacco use such as pipe smoking and tobacco chewing. Heavy alcohol consumption along with tobacco use increases the risk. Poor oral hygiene or bad teeth can also contribute to cancer. Most oropharyngeal cancers occur in men, although as more women are smoking they now have a higher chance of developing these cancers.

TREATMENT OVERVIEW
♦ This cancer rarely spreads early in its course, but often spreads later. Should the primary site not be controlled and it recurs there, the rest of the body should be evaluated for tumor spread.

♦ The prognosis seems to decrease as the cancer moves back from the lips. The lips have the best prognosis, the tongue second, the area behind the wisdom teeth (retromolar trigone) third. The prognosis is poorest in the hypopharynx. Patients whose tumors grow into blood vessels have a worse prognosis.
♦ A multi-disciplinary approach provides the best chance for cure. The team usually consists of a head and neck surgeon, radiation and medical oncologists, an oral prosthodontist (a dentist experienced in dental reconstruction). Since these tumors often extend into areas that are not easily seen (upwards into the nasopharynx and downwards into the hypopharynx), these areas have to be evaluated before treat-

ment is started. It is often necessary to examine the patient when he or she is anesthetized, using small scopes to see and map the extent of the tumor.

♦ The risk of having a second primary cancer is as high as 15 percent, so endoscopic examinations of the nasopharynx, hypopharynx and esophagus (triple endoscopy) are done to detect other cancers.

♦ A useful maneuver with large tumors is to mark the edge with an India ink tattoo. In patients who receive radiotherapy or chemotherapy to shrink the tumor before surgery, the surgeon will be able to tell precisely where the edge of the tumor was and remove all the tissue originally involved.

♦ No single treatment program offers a clear-cut survival advantage over others. Various choices are possible and the decision will depend on a review of each case, the type and stage of the cancer, the physical and emotional condition of the patient, as well as the experience of the physicians and the facilities available.

TREATMENT BY STAGE

STAGE I

Standard Treatment The choice is determined by the anticipated functional and cosmetic results. Radiation therapy is commonly used. Surgery is equally successful. Either might be used in locations such as the tonsil, where function is expected to be normal after surgery. In areas such as the base of the tongue, radiation is preferred, since surgery would result in major functional problems. Radiation protocols using hyperfractionation (more than one treatment daily) should be considered.

Five-Year Survival 60 to 70 percent, depending on the site

STAGE II

Standard Treatment If radiation is used, the technique is individualized by a radiation oncologist experienced in treatment

of tumors of this area. Radiation implants may be needed. Surgery is an alternative, and the same considerations apply as for Stage I about when surgery or radiotherapy are preferred. The same choice of hyperfractionated radiotherapy applies.

Five-Year Survival 50 percent when the tumor is in the tonsil or back of the tongue

STAGE III

Standard Treatment The preferred treatment usually combines surgery with postoperative radiotherapy. There are new surgical techniques for removal of the tumor and reconstruction. Radiation implants and hyperfractionation techniques are becoming more useful.

All patients in this stage are candidates for neoadjuvant chemotherapy trials.

Five-Year Survival 20 percent (back of the tongue) to 30 percent (tonsil)

STAGE IV

Standard Treatment As in Stage III, aggressive combined surgical and radiotherapy treatments by physicians experienced in treating this type of cancer are necessary. If the tumor can't be removed, radiotherapy is used. Chemotherapy (neoadjuvant) has been used to shrink tumors and make them easier to treat with surgery or radiation.

Clinical trials are combining chemotherapy or radiation sensitizers with radiotherapy or radiation protocols using hyperfractionation or radiation implants.

Follow-up is essential, and should be done monthly for one year, every two months for the next year, every three months the next and then every six months.

Five-Year Survival 14 percent (tonsil) to 20 percent (back of the tongue)

RECURRENT CANCER

Standard therapy is surgery (if possible) if radiotherapy was used originally. If surgery was used before, then radiotherapy is given for recurrent tumors provided it is safe to give more. If surgery was used first, additional surgery is sometimes possible.

Chemotherapy can be used in combination with surgery or radiotherapy. Chemotherapy is also used for metastatic disease or if there is a recurrence that can no longer be treated with surgery or radiation.

The same follow-up is required as for Stage IV.

SUPPORTIVE THERAPY

An essential part of the treatment is the need for rehabilitation after aggressive surgery and radiation. The patient must be motivated and total rehabilitation requires a team approach, with speech therapists, social workers, physical therapists, prosthodontists, occupational therapists and nurses all playing important roles.

Cosmetic appearance, swallowing, speech, chewing and psychological functioning have to be considered. The family is extremely important in supporting the patient during and after therapy. Some functions and appearances may be different, but the *person* is the same.

NASOPHARYNX

The nasopharynx is right behind the nose and above the oropharynx. It cannot be seen directly. It is shaped somewhat like a box. On the sides are the eustachian tubes that adjust the air pressure in our middle ears. At the top is the sphenoid sinus.

Cancers of the nasopharynx are different from other head and neck cancers in that there does not appear to be a link with alcohol and tobacco use and they occur 10 to 20 years earlier (one group in young adulthood and another between 50 and 70 years). The Epstein-Barr (EB) virus has been implicated in most patients. Blood tests available for anti-EB virus antibodies aid in diagnosis as well as screening of high-risk groups.

The most common first sign is a mass in the neck (a lymph node metastasis). At least 80 percent of patients will have some evidence of spread to these lymph nodes, some only microscopically. Other symptoms are hearing loss or signs of middle ear infection, nasal obstruction or nosebleeds, ringing in the ears, inability to equalize the air pressure between the ears, and cranial nerve problems.

Evaluation of patients includes a very careful physical examination, as well as endoscopic examinations of the nose and throat. This is the most likely primary site for the "unknown primary" cancer diagnosed in enlarged lymph nodes in the neck. Most of these cancers are the squamous cell type. The diagnosis is best made by biopsy of the primary site in the nasopharynx and not the enlarged neck lymph nodes. If the primary tumor is not seen and random biopsies of the nasopharynx are negative, then a needle biopsy of the enlarged lymph nodes in the neck is done.

Once the diagnosis has been made by biopsy, CT and MRI scans are essential in determining stage, for the tumor cannot be seen directly. A chest x-ray is usually done because there may be lung metastases. Liver scans and bone scans may also be needed to search for metastases. Staging is difficult to determine exactly. Most patients are probably in Stage IV at the time of diagnosis.

Various factors appear to affect prognosis, including bone involvement, the presence of pain, the length of time symptoms have been present and the location of lymph nodes involved by tumor. Patients who have evidence of Epstein-Barr virus infection (as shown by a blood test) have a poorer prognosis after treatment.

TREATMENT OVERVIEW

Small cancers of the nasopharynx are curable by radiotherapy in 80 to 90 percent of cases. Moderately advanced tumors that have not spread to the lymph nodes in the neck can be cured in 50 to 70 percent of cases. Advanced tumors, especially with extension to other structures such as bone or cranial nerves, are difficult to control.

♦ In patients with extension of tumor into the skull bones or involving cranial nerves, the use of surgery is rarely of help and is seldom attempted.

♦ Radiotherapy is used for treatment of neck metastases. Surgery is usually used only for lymph nodes that do not disappear after radiotherapy or that reappear. Radiation implants may be used in certain selected situations.

♦ Once treatment is completed, extensive follow-up is essential. This includes physical examination, x-rays and scans, blood tests, tests of thyroid and pituitary function, attention to dental and oral hygiene, jaw exercises and evaluation of vision and hearing.

STAGES I and II

Standard Treatment High-dose radiotherapy to the primary area and both sides of the neck.

Five-Year Survival 65 to 95 percent (Stage I), 50 to 65 percent (Stage II)

STAGE III

Standard Treatment Same as for Stages I and II, but surgical neck dissection may be needed if enlarged lymph nodes in the neck either do not completely disappear after radiotherapy or recur.

Neoadjuvant chemotherapy is being studied in clinical trials to shrink tumors and make them easier to treat with radiotherapy or surgery. Clinical trials are also evaluating chemotherapy as an adjuvant after radiotherapy or as combined treatment.

Five-Year Survival 30 to 60 percent

STAGE IV

Standard Treatment High-dose radiotherapy to the primary area and the neck. Surgical neck dissection is done for persistent or recurrent enlarged lymph nodes.

Clinical trials of chemotherapy similar to Stage III are in progress.

Five-Year Survival 5 to 40 percent

RECURRENT CANCER

Selected patients may be given additional radiotherapy, both external beam and implants. Some may be candidates for surgical removal of recurrent tumors.

Metastatic disease and local recurrences not treatable by surgery or radiation may be treated with chemotherapy. Clinical trials are evaluating chemotherapy as well as interferon.

HYPOPHARYNX

The hypopharynx is below the oropharynx. It is the place the food first passes through when we swallow. There are three areas in the hypopharynx :

♦ postcricoid area (junction of pharynx and esophagus);

♦ pyriform sinus; and

♦ posterior (back) pharyngeal wall.

This area is best examined with mirrors, fingers or scopes that can be passed into the mouth. Almost all of the cancers in this area are squamous (or epidermoid) cancers arising in the mucous membranes. A few cancers are of minor salivary gland origin.

These cancers first spread by direct invasion, growing down from the surface membranes into the next layer (the submucosa), then into the muscles and finally into the tissues that surround the pharynx. Further spread is to the lymph nodes in the neck (even at this stage the cancer may still be curable), then to the lungs and elsewhere in the body (where the chance of cure is very remote).

Sometimes these cancers begin with a white plaque or coating on the membrane (leukoplakia), a premalignant condition similar to that found in the mouth, but many cancers begin without any preliminary change. Not all white patches are leukoplakia, and biopsy is necessary to rule out other causes, such as fungal infections or a disease called lichen planus.

Other cancers may occur elsewhere in the head and neck at the same time or later, so the larynx, pharynx, nasopharynx and the entire oral cavity should be searched. The esophagus should also be evaluated. CT and MRI scans are useful in establishing the extent of the disease. Since treatment will vary depending on the stage and extent of disease, it is very important to establish the stage precisely before therapy is begun.

Symptoms generally occur late and spread tends to occur early, so the survival rates for cancers in this area are lower than for other sites in the head and neck.

No single therapeutic approach offers an advantage over the others, so treatment decisions depend on a careful review of each case with attention to the stage, the physical condition, age and emotional status of the patient, the experience of the physicians and the treatment facilities available.

TREATMENT BY STAGE

STAGE I
Standard Treatment Except for rare very small T1 cancers, treatment is primarily surgery, usually followed by radiotherapy. Since early symptoms are rare, fewer than 2 percent of patients are diagnosed when their tumors are small, protrude from the surface and are treatable with radiotherapy alone.

Standard treatment is laryngopharyngectomy and neck dissection. In selected cases, only part of the larynx has to be removed and the voice can be preserved. In larger (T2) tumors, post-operative radiotherapy is used.

There are several approaches to the use of radiation therapy. Some treatment centers give it preoperatively. Others also treat an extended area of potential spread of tumor, including both sides of the neck.

Five-Year Survival 50 to 80 percent

STAGE II
Standard Treatment Therapy is similar to that for Stage I. Treatments being studied include neoadjuvant chemotherapy to shrink tumors and improve the ability to treat them with surgery or radiotherapy. Such neoadjuvant chemotherapy protocols are in common use because of the low survival rate.

Five-Year Survival 50 to 60 percent

STAGE III
Standard Treatment Treatment is complex. Extensive surgery is done, which requires reconstructive procedures using portions of the stomach or small bowel. Radiotherapy is given postoperatively. Surgical and radiotherapy methods and programs, as well as the time schedules involved, vary among treatment centers but give similar results. Patients should be managed by surgeons and radiation oncologists experienced in these complex procedures and treatments.

Patients should be considered for clinical trials evaluating adjuvant or neoadjuvant chemotherapy.

Five-Year Survival 30 to 50 percent

STAGE IV

Standard Treatment If the tumor can be removed, similar considerations and methods to those for Stage III are used. If it can't, radiotherapy is used.

Chemotherapy and radiation sensitizers with the radiotherapy are under clinical evaluation. There are also radiotherapy protocols evaluating hyperfractionation schedules (more than one treatment daily).

Careful and frequent post-treatment follow-up is essential.

Five-Year Survival 15 to 25 percent

RECURRENT CANCER

If radiotherapy was originally used, the standard treatment is surgery if it is possible. If surgery was used originally, then radiotherapy is given unless previous radiotherapy dosage precludes additional treatment. Additional surgery may be possible. Chemotherapy protocols are under clinical evaluation.

LARYNX

The larynx, or voice box, is divided into three regions. From the top down, these are:

♦ The supraglottic larynx. This includes the epiglottis (a flap that keeps food from going into the lungs), the false vocal cords, ventricles, aryepiglottic folds and arytenoids. Tumors of this area cause sore throat, painful swallowing and sometimes a change in voice quality.

♦ The glottis. This includes the true vocal cords and the anterior (front) and posterior (back) commissures. Tumors here may involve one or both vocal cords or may extend out on either side of them. Tumors are usually detected early because they cause hoarseness. Because of these early symptoms and the lack of lymphatic channels where cancer can spread, the cure rate is very good.

♦ The subglottis. This area is below the true vocal cords and extends downwards to about the first tracheal ring (cartilage ring around the trachea). Tumors here are rare.

Almost all cancers of the larynx arise from the lining membrane (mucosa) and are called squamous cell cancers. Salivary gland cancers and other types can also occur in this area.

Cancers spread by growing directly into surrounding tissues and then to lymph nodes in the neck, usually on the same side as where the tumor started. They may still be curable at this stage, but not when they have spread elsewhere.

Common symptoms can include persistent sore throat or hoarseness, difficulty in swallowing, the feeling of something in the throat, a change in voice quality and the appearance of a lump in the neck.

A complete diagnostic examination includes examination with tongue blade, mirrors and scopes, physical examination to rule out other areas of spread and determine the tolerance and precautions for therapy, x-ray barium swallow to show if there is any distortion of the esophagus, CT or MRI scan to outline the tumor and show its extent, chest x-ray to rule out spread to the lungs and biopsy of the lesion to establish the diagnosis.

It is also usually necessary for the larynx to be examined under anesthesia with the aid of a laryngoscope. The area of cancer can be carefully examined and additional biopsies taken to establish the extent of tumor involvement.

TREATMENT OVERVIEW

Small cancers of the larynx have a good prognosis. If there is no spread to lymph nodes, the cure rate is 75 to 95 percent. Although most early lesions can be cured by radiotherapy or surgery, radiotherapy is often chosen first in an attempt to preserve a better voice. Surgery is used later if the tumor recurs. Laser excision surgery is also used.

♦ Locally advanced lesions, especially with large involved lymph nodes, are poorly controlled by either method of treatment or by both methods used together. Distant metastasis is common.

♦ Intermediate-sized cancers require individual decision making about the most appropriate treatment. Factors such as the site, stage, degree of lymph node involvement and general status of the patient will influence the type of therapy chosen.

♦ Second primaries have been reported in up to a quarter of these patients.

♦ Most recurrences occur in the first two to three years, and close follow-up is essential so that cure may still be possible. Examinations as well as previously abnormal staging studies are repeated to document the progress of treatment or detect recurrence.

♦ Because of other illnesses related to smoking and alcohol use, many patients die from illnesses other than the cancer.

♦ Small localized superficial cancers can be successfully treated with radiotherapy alone, surgery alone or laser excision. Radiation tends to be used first to try to preserve the voice. There are also some surgical procedures for small cancers that preserve the voice.

♦ Advanced cancers are often treated by a combination of surgery and radiotherapy. Because the cure rate is low, consideration should be given to clinical trials evaluating chemotherapy, hyperfractionated (several doses a day) radiotherapy, radiation sensitizers or particle beam radiotherapy.

♦ Most subglottic cancers are treated with combined surgery and radiotherapy.

TREATMENT BY STAGE

STAGE I
Standard Treatment
♦ *Supraglottis:* External beam radiotherapy alone or supraglottic laryngectomy. There are frequent problems with the functioning of the larynx after the latter procedure.

♦ *Glottis:* Radiotherapy. Selected patients with small (T1) superficial lesions can have a portion of the vocal cord removed. Partial or sometimes total laryngectomy may be done depending on the tumor's location and size. Laser excision is under clinical evaluation.

♦ *Subglottis:* Radiotherapy alone, with surgery used for recurrence.

Five-Year Survival 75 to 95 percent

STAGE II
Standard Treatment
♦ *Supraglottis:* External beam radiation therapy is used for smaller tumors, which preserves the voice. Another option is a supraglottic laryngectomy or total laryngectomy, depending on the location of the lesion and the status of the patient. Care is needed when selecting this option to ensure adequate lung and swallowing function after surgery.

If a patient is not cured by radiation given as the primary treatment, surgery is then used in an attempt to cure. If surgery is the primary treatment, postoperative radiotherapy is used if tumor is found in surgical margins or lymph nodes in the neck.

♦ *Glottis:* Radiotherapy or surgery (partial or total laryngectomy).

♦ *Subglottis:* Radiotherapy (with voice preservation), with surgery reserved for patients whose tumors recur or those who might not have adequate follow-up evaluation.

Five-Year Survival 55 to 65 percent (supraglottis), 60 to 80 percent (glottis), 30 to 40 percent (subglottis)

STAGE III
Standard Treatment
♦ *Supraglottis:* Standard therapy is surgery with postoperative radiotherapy, but many centers are now treating some patients with external beam radiotherapy initially, depending on the tumor location

and patient status. The voice is preserved in about half of these patients. If this treatment is unsuccessful, surgery is necessary.

Investigational protocols are using chemotherapy, hyperfractionated radiotherapy, radiation sensitizers, and particle beam radiotherapy.

◆ *Glottis:* Surgery with postoperative radiotherapy, if necessary for the primary site and/or positive lymph nodes. Patients who refuse or cannot tolerate surgery are given radiation therapy.

Again, many centers are treating selected patients with radiotherapy as primary treatment. Careful follow-up is vital, since surgery is needed if the tumor recurs.

◆ *Subglottis:* Laryngectomy, including also thyroidectomy and tracheoesophageal lymph node dissection, all followed by radiotherapy. Some patients are not candidates for surgery and are treated with radiotherapy alone, but surgical treatment may still be needed if there is a recurrence. The Stage III investigational protocols described under supraglottic tumors should be considered.

Three-Year Survival 45 to 75 percent (supraglottis), 55 to 70 percent (glottis), no data for subglottis

STAGE IV
Standard Treatment

◆ *Supraglottis:* Total laryngectomy with pre- or postoperative radiotherapy. Patients who refuse surgery or who are inoperable are treated with radiotherapy. Investigational protocols as described earlier should be considered.

◆ *Glottis:* Same as for Stage III glottic cancer, except that radiation therapy is not an elective option initially, being used only in patients who refuse or cannot tolerate

surgery. Investigational protocols as described earlier should be considered.

◆ *Subglottis:* Same as Stage II subglottic tumors.

Three-Year Survival 15 to 35 percent (supraglottis), 10 to 25 percent (glottis), few data for subglottis

RECURRENT CANCER

Treatment includes further surgery or investigational protocols. If patients were treated initially with surgery alone or radiotherapy alone, further surgery and/or radiotherapy may be used. Some patients may respond to chemotherapy. Patients whose tumors recur after both radiotherapy and surgery are candidates for investigational palliative chemotherapy.

SUPPORTIVE THERAPY

Patients who have had their voice box (larynx) removed need supportive treatment to help them to learn to speak again. There are three methods.

◆ One involves the use of an esophageal voice, where a patient is taught to swallow air and bring it back up and speak.

◆ An electronic larynx—a buzzer-like battery-operated unit—may be pressed against the neck while the mouth and tongue form the words.

◆ A third method uses a unit that looks like a pipe. The sound is put into the mouth and the words are fashioned with the tongue and lips.

◆ There is also a method that requires a surgical procedure (tracheoesophageal puncture) to create a connection between the airway and the esophagus to insert a voice prosthesis ("button") and breathing valve.

METASTATIC SQUAMOUS NECK CANCER WITH A HIDDEN PRIMARY SOURCE

Enlarged neck lymph nodes containing squamous cell cancer may be the first sign of cancer elsewhere in the body. Since this type of cancer always begins elsewhere and never begins in these nodes, a search is made for the primary site. If a cancer has previously been diagnosed elsewhere, it naturally is the likely source, especially if the pattern under the microscope is similar.

Sometimes the biopsy of the lymph nodes will show adenocarcinoma or lymphoma. In these cases the primary site is less likely to be in the head and neck. For enlarged nodes containing squamous carcinoma in the lower half of the neck, the primary site may be the head and neck but may also be in the esophagus, lung or genitourinary tract.

Most epidermoid carcinomas found in lymph nodes in the upper half of the neck are a result of spread from primary head and neck cancers.

Evaluation A very careful history and physical examination is necessary to try to find the primary tumor. This frequently turns up cancer in the nasopharynx, oropharynx or larynx. If a cancer originating in the head and neck is found, other organs such as the lungs, liver and bones should be evaluated. If the cancer has already spread to one of these sites, then the treatment plan is directed towards metastatic disease and not to cure of the primary lesion (which would involve very aggressive local therapy).

Repeated examinations will sometimes find the primary tumor still at a treatable stage. A vital part of the solution to the puzzle is provided by pathologic examination of the biopsy specimen. Immunohistochemical and electron microscopic studies may be helpful. Special stains can be applied to the tissue slides to help in diagnosis. The problem is more significant in poorly differentiated tumors, since well-differentiated tumors tend to resemble the tissue of origin and the pathologist can often suggest the likely diagnosis. With poorly differentiated tumors the diagnosis is more uncertain.

Diagnosis and Staging If possible, biopsy is delayed until studies have tried to find the primary site. These studies include examination of head and neck areas directly and with mirrors and scopes. Suspicious areas are biopsied. If there are no suspicious areas, random biopsies are done of the nasopharynx, base of the tongue and the pyriform sinus on the same side as the neck lesion. If the tonsil is not present, a biopsy is done where the tonsil used to be. If the tonsil is present, it should be biopsied or removed. Sinus x-rays are often done and any abnormality is also biopsied. Other studies include MRI and CT scans.

Staging systems have been described, but of course the "T" classification has no relevance, since the primary tumor has not been found. Local control and survival rates for squamous cancers involving the lymph nodes of the neck, with unknown primary tumor, are:

N1 (single node smaller than 1 1/2 in./3 cm, one side) ....**40 to 50 percent**
N2 (nodes 1 1/4–2 1/2 in./3–6 cm, one side) ....**25 to 30 percent**
N3 (larger nodes, either or both sides) ....**10 to 15 percent**

Treatment If a head or neck primary is found with these studies, treatment is given as outlined. If the primary is not found, the treatment is a surgical neck dissection followed by radiation therapy.
♦ If the lymph nodes in the neck are enlarged or are on both sides, radiation

therapy is given first. If any lymph nodes persist after radiotherapy, then surgical lymph node dissection is done.

♦ Alternatively, many centers use radiotherapy as the first treatment for unknown primary cancer of the head and neck. External radiation may be about equally effective as neck dissection for control of neck metastases, although surgical neck dissection may be required for more well-differentiated tumors.

♦ Radiation fields to treat the likely primary sources are extensive and include the nasopharynx, the base of the tongue and the pyriform sinuses.

♦ Chemotherapy may also be appropriate for the most treatable likely primary site. Follow-up is extremely important.

♦ Options under clinical evaluation include neoadjuvant chemotherapy (cisplatin + 5-fluorouracil) followed by radiation therapy. Other investigational protocols are available.

RECURRENT CANCER

If the disease progresses, recurs or relapses, the prognosis is poor. Further treatment depends on the type of cancer, earlier treatment, site of recurrence and personal factors. Patients are candidates for investigational protocols.

THE MOST IMPORTANT QUESTIONS YOU CAN ASK

♦ What is the primary site or source of my cancer?

♦ What is the stage and what organs are involved?

♦ What tests are necessary to find this out? Are they uncomfortable?

♦ Is there a choice between surgery and radiation? Should you use both? In which order?

♦ Is there a role for chemotherapy? When?

♦ What kind of functional disability might I have? Will I have trouble eating, swallowing or speaking?

♦ How will I look after the treatments? Will I have a cosmetic disability?

♦ How much experience has the surgeon and radiation oncologist had with this type of tumor, and with what results?

♦ What complications can I expect from treatment?

♦ How long does it take to recover from the treatment?

♦ How often will you examine me afterwards?

♦ When will I know I am safe?

ISLET CELL
AND OTHER CARCINOMAS

Ernest H. Rosenbaum, MD, and Malin Dollinger, MD

◇

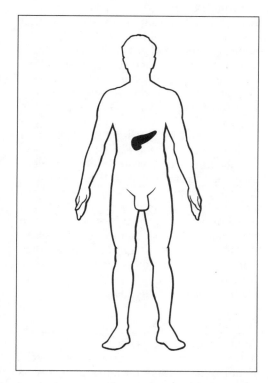

The pancreas is both an exocrine gland that produces enzymes to help digestion and an endocrine gland that produces insulin to regulate the body's metabolism of glucose. Cancer of the islet cells, or pancreatic endocrine gland, is a very uncommon tumor, making up about 5 percent of all pancreatic cancers (about 200 to 1,000 cases each year). Unlike the much more common exocrine pancreatic cancers, islet cell tumors are sometimes curable (*see* page 336).

These glandular tumors may be either functioning or non-functioning. What is meant by the term *functioning* is that the tumors secrete one or more hormones normally produced by the bowel endocrine cells and pancreatic islet cells. These hormones include insulin, gastrin, glucagon, vasoactive intestinal polypeptide (VIP), somatostatin, pancreatic polypeptide (PP), ACTH and others.

Most functioning tumors producing insulin are benign. But most islet cell cancers are non-functioning, and 90 percent of these non-functioning tumors are malignant.

Types The pancreatic islet cells have many different cell types, including alpha, beta and delta cells, each of which normally produces a specific hormone or polypeptide. Overproduction of the hormone or polypeptide by the tumor produces symptoms. Islet cell tumors, which are separate and distinct cancers, are named for the type of hormone or polypeptide they produce—those that produce gastrin are called gastrinomas, those that produce insulin are insulinomas and so on.

How It Spreads Spread may be by invasion of nearby tissues or metastases via the lymph system or bloodstream.

What Causes It Unknown.

RISK FACTORS

No special group is susceptible, but it is often found in those afflicted by the familial complex of tumors known as MEN (multiple endocrine neoplasia) type-I, a genetically transmitted group of endocrine abnormalities. These people develop several kinds of islet cell tumors—54 percent have multiple gastrinomas, 21 percent develop insulinomas, 3 percent glucagonomas and 1 percent VIPomas. They also have a tendency to develop pituitary gland tumors and parathyroid gland hyperplasia and hyperfunction.

SCREENING

When there is a family history of MEN-I, serum studies for gastrin, glucagon, insulin and VIP may be useful.

COMMON SIGNS AND SYMPTOMS

There is frequently a long delay between the initial symptoms and the diagnosis. The 90 percent of the non-functioning tumors that are malignant produce symptoms both by growing to a size where they put pressure on other tissues and by spreading to other organs.

The functioning, mainly benign islet cell tumors secrete active agents that have characteristic metabolic effects that create more symptoms than the tumor itself. When a functioning tumor becomes extremely large or metastatic, it will cause the same types of signs and symptoms as any other malignant tumor, as well as the hormonal symptoms.

♦ Gastrinomas produce an excess amount of gastrin (Zollinger-Ellison syndrome), leading to increased production of stomach acid, active peptic ulcer disease (with multiple and severe peptic ulcers) and often severe diarrhea. This accounts for less than 1 percent of peptic ulcers. The gastrin hypersecretion leads to diarrhea and fatty stools (steatorrhea). Other symptoms include abdominal pain and extreme weight loss.

♦ Insulinomas secrete increased insulin, leading to low blood sugar (hypoglycemia). Often, the symptoms of weight loss, fatigue, weakness and hunger are attributed to psychological or neurologic disorders. Symptoms may be worse during fasting.

♦ The overproduction of glucagon by glucagonomas causes a characteristic skin rash (necrolytic migratory erythema), painful tongue (glossitis) and decreased amino acids in the blood. Blood clots, which may travel elsewhere, have also been reported.

♦ An islet cell tumor producing VIP (vasoactive intestinal polypeptides) results in a syndrome with diarrhea, high serum calcium and low serum potassium, chloride and blood sugar (hypoglycemia). VIPomas are characterized by secretory diarrhea (pancreatic cholera), which persists even when fasting (this tumor is also referred to as WDHA—watery diarrhea, hypokalemic acidosis). With severe diarrhea, up to 1 1/2 gallons (6 L) of small bowel fluid can be lost each day. Persistent diarrhea over 48 hours is very suspicious for VIPomas. Weakness, low blood pressure, facial flushing and psychosis are common symptoms.

♦ Tumors that overproduce somatostatin cause electrolyte (mineral) abnormalities, diabetes mellitus, weight loss, malabsorption of food in the intestine (steatorrhea), loss of gastric acid (gastric achlorhydria) and occasionally gallstones.

DIAGNOSIS

Blood and Other Tests

♦ Diagnosis can be confirmed with specific hormonal assays measuring the levels of gastrin, glucagon, insulin, VIP, somatostatin or other hormones.

♦ An elevated serum gastrin level (often 10 times normal) and an elevated stomach basal acid output for those who have not had surgery should raise suspicions of the Zollinger-Ellison syndrome and its associated gastrinoma.

♦ Measurement of plasma proinsulin may be helpful for diagnosing an insulin-secreting carcinoma (insulinoma).

♦ Low serum potassium levels caused by secretory diarrhea may indicate a VIPoma.

♦ Elevated levels of serum somatostatin

and diabetes with severe malabsorption should suggest a somatostatin producing tumor.

Imaging
♦ Chest x-ray.
♦ Abdominal CT and MRI scans.
♦ Abdominal ultrasound, which may also be performed during surgery (intraoperative sonography).
♦ Pancreatic arteriography can diagnose about 50 percent of cases, for some tumors—insulinoma, for example—are rich in blood vessels and have a tumor "blush." This method is rarely used since the advent of ultrasound and CT.

Endoscopy and Biopsy
♦ Fine needle aspiration (FNA).

STAGING

There is no acceptable staging system for islet cell cancers. They can best be categorized as localized (in one site), regional (in several sites within the pancreas) and metastatic to regional lymph nodes or to distant sites.

TREATMENT OVERVIEW

Surgery and chemotherapy are the two treatment methods used, but only surgery can cure the disease. Careful observation may be an alternative approach for some islet cell tumors. Radiotherapy is not effective.

Surgery Surgical removal of the tumor may lead to a cure. Depending on the location of the tumor, part of the pancreas may be removed (partial pancreatectomy) or the tumor cells may be excised locally — or "shelled out"—of the head of the pancreas (enucleation). When the tumor can't be completely removed, reducing its size (debulking) may still be a helpful palliative measure, given that these tumors are slow growing.

Chemotherapy Several biological and chemotherapy agents appear to be active against islet cell tumors. These include interferon-alpha, a synthetic somatostatin analogue called Octeotride (Sandostatin), Adriamycin, Cytoxan, DTIC (dacarbazine), 5-fluorouracil (5-FU), streptozotocin and etoposide (VP-16) for advanced islet cell cancer.

TREATMENT BY TYPE
GASTRINOMA
Sixty to 75 percent of gastrinomas are malignant and metastatic at the time of diagnosis. In 90 percent of cases there are multiple tumors. Gastrinomas have also been reported in locations other than the pancreas.

Standard Treatment The tumor should be removed if it can be precisely located by preoperative imaging studies or during surgery. Usually, small lesions can be shelled out from the pancreas without the need for removing the organ.

The problem is that most of the time the lesion cannot be found. Either it is extremely small or there are several small lesions. When that is the case, most surgeons prefer not to give any additional treatment. The complete removal of the pancreas would create major problems and pose an unacceptable risk that would outweigh the benefits of removing the lesions.

Removal of half the pancreas has a success rate of only 50 percent, but any benefit of the operation is outweighed by the risks of the surgery and the potential for diabetes.

The main problem with this tumor is ulceration of the stomach from excess acid production. This can be adequately managed today with H-2 blockers such as Tagamet, Zantac and Pepcid. When they are no longer effective, a drug called Omeprazole (Losec) can be used to control gastric acid secretion effectively.

Cutting the acid secretion nerves to the stomach (vagotomy) and removing part of the stomach (partial gastrectomy) are not effective. If medical therapy fails to control acid secretion and ulcerations recur or diarrhea persists, a total gastrectomy is the treatment of choice.

In severe cases, primary management may include continuous stomach suction and intravenous replacement of sodium, potassium and chloride to maintain electrolyte balance. Surgery can then remove a functioning tumor when the patient is stable. Postoperative gastrin levels are used for monitoring.

Treatment for Metastatic Gastrinoma Occasionally active drugs include Adriamycin, streptozotocin, 5-FU, etoposide and Cytoxan. Chemotherapy is often reserved for patients who cannot tolerate surgery and cimetidine (Tagamet).
♦ Interferon-alpha has recently shown some effectiveness in controlling tumors and reducing symptoms.
♦ Blocking the blood supply to the liver (hepatic artery embolization) may successfully treat liver metastases.

 Palliation Octreotide (Sandostatin) is a synthetic, long-acting somatostatin analogue that significantly decreases hormone secretion by tumor cells. It is extremely useful for suppressing gastrin levels and inhibiting the hypersecretion of gastric acid on a sustained basis for managing the Zollinger-Ellison syndrome. This may be helpful when Omeprazole fails.

Five-Year Survival 65 percent

INSULINOMA

Insulinomas usually occur between ages 40 and 60. Eighty percent are benign and produce hormones (insulin).

Standard Treatment Removal of the pancreatic tumor is the basic approach, depending on the size and the site (in the head of the pancreas versus the body or tail). Most of these tumors can be excised locally without the risks of a major operation to remove part of the pancreas.

Metastases should be removed to help reduce symptoms of increased insulin and low blood sugar.

For pancreatic tumors that can't be removed or for metastatic tumors, combination chemotherapy (5-FU + streptozotocin) or diazoxide or somatostatin/octreotide (Sandostatin) can be given.

 Palliation Surgery may help reduce low blood sugar (hypoglycemia), as will dietary changes including frequent small meals and increased carbohydrates. Insulin-inhibiting drugs such as diazoxide may also help. Radiation therapy is not effective.

Five-Year Survival 60 percent

GLUCAGONOMAS

These tumors are often very large by the time they are discovered.

Standard Treatment The tumor should be removed, if possible.

Medical therapy can include Octreotide (Sandostatin) and the intravenous infusion of amino acids.

Chemotherapy with 5-FU and streptozotocin may also be given.

VIPomas

About 40 percent of these tumors are malignant. VIPomas have also been found in other parts of the body, usually of neurogenic origin.

Standard Treatment Single lesions can be removed or a partial pancreatectomy can be done for multiple lesions in the 50 percent of patients who do not have liver metastases. Debulking tumors that can't be removed may reduce diarrhea.

Prednisone may also help relieve diarrhea.

Combination chemotherapy with 5-FU + streptozotocin may be given if the tumors cannot be removed.

 Palliation Octreotide (Sandostatin) is effective in reducing VIPoma symptoms, but it is not curative and often works for only a limited time. Fluids and electrolytes have to be replenished.

SOMATOSTATIN-PRODUCING TUMORS

In this rare clinical entity, somatostatin is produced by the islet cell.

Standard Treatment Surgical removal of the tumor is the standard treatment for local and metastatic disease. Combined chemotherapy with 5-FU and streptozocin has also been used.

 Palliation Drugs used to relieve symptoms include the insulin-inhibiting drug diazoxide and phenoxybenzamine (Dibenzyline), an alpha-adrenergic blocking agent.

RECURRENT CANCER

Before deciding on further therapy for recurrences, the clinical situation will have to be re-evaluated. Surgery or medical therapy as indicated for metastatic disease could be considered depending on the stage, the site of recurrence, the presence of metastases and individual factors. Participation in clinical trials should also be considered.

THE MOST IMPORTANT QUESTIONS YOU CAN ASK

♦ Will the removal of my tumor reduce or eliminate my symptoms?
♦ Can medical treatment control my cancer and reduce my symptoms?
♦ Are there any cancer centers where I could go for a second opinion?

KAPOSI'S SARCOMA AND AIDS-RELATED LYMPHOSARCOMA

Ivan J. Silverberg, MD

◇

Kaposi's sarcoma (KS) consists of characteristic skin lesions that range from flat to raised purple plaques. These tumors have a rich network of small blood vessels, and red blood cells moving slowly through these channels lose their oxygen, changing from red to blue. The mixture of red and blue cells gives the KS lesion a characteristic purple color.

There are several forms of KS, based on cause rather than appearance. The "classic" Kaposi's sarcoma, found mainly in Mediterranean males and mid-European Jews, has always been rare. In the 1950s a large number of cases were found in Africa, and the incidence has dramatically increased since then. KS was later found to be a common result of an alteration of body immunity.

There are two circumstances under which this alteration takes place. The first is when depression of the immune system—the body's constant guard against outside threats—is part of some treatment, for example in kidney or other organ transplants. To prevent the foreign organ from being rejected, powerful drugs are given to shut down the immune system. KS may arise after such drugs are used and will sometimes disappear when the drugs are stopped. The second circumstance is associated with Acquired Immune Deficiency Syndrome (AIDS).

Types KS tumors are divided into three groups, based on appearance, with much overlap.

Nodular lesions are of varying size and thickness. They are purple and will at times have a halo of brown or yellow pigment around them.

Infiltrating lesions may be quite large, may be raised or grow downward beneath the skin.

Lymphatic lesions can mimic other causes of swollen lymph nodes and may require a biopsy to rule out infection.

Under the microscope, all three types of KS appear similar. But three sub-types have been identified, all of which are treated much the same. The spindle cell variety is the slowest growing, the anaplastic is the most aggressive, and the mixed cell has a somewhat intermediate growth rate.

How It Spreads Most malignancies develop from one cell or a small group of cells. As they grow, there comes a time when they spread either by direct invasion of other tissues or through the blood or lymphatic systems. But KS often appears simultaneously in many sites. This suggests that there is a causal agent, possibly in the blood, that triggers the formation of the lesions. In this, KS bears a strong resemblance to some viral "rash" diseases, like measles and chicken pox. As the lesions grow, they fuse together, thicken and may protrude from the skin or ulcerate.

What Causes It The cause of "classic" KS is unclear. KS as it originally occurred in Africa likewise has no clearly defined cause. But epidemic KS, occurring as a disease that accompanies AIDS, is thought to have a cause—the virus named HIV (human immunodeficiency virus). If given a blood test for HIV, nearly all patients with epidemic KS will show evidence of being infected.

Various ideas have been put forward to explain how this virus causes KS. One theory is that it causes a normal cell to become malignant either directly or by initiating a chain of events. Various agents that may be involved in such a change have been identified. Yet another idea has to do with the body's T cells, some of which hunt for malignant cells that have developed spontaneously and kill them off before they can become cancers. The T cell is known to be infected with the virus and cannot kill the malignant cells.

With AIDS-related KS there is also the continuing issue of whether HIV alone is responsible for the disease. Other factors have been suggested as coproducers of the illness, including drugs and other viruses. The agent most mentioned is CMV (cytomegalic inclusion virus), but this is by no means the only one.

Whatever the mechanism, KS in people who have taken drugs to depress the body's immune response is thought to occur in a fashion similar to that in patients with epidemic KS.

RISK FACTORS

Each form of this illness occurs in fairly specific groups. Classic KS is a disease of the elderly, with the average age of onset being over 70. The disease is more frequent in people of Mediterranean background and it is more common in Jews, with European (Ashkenazic) rather than the Spanish and Portuguese (Sephardic) Jews being affected. Men get classic KS 14 times more frequently than women.

The form that follows immune-suppressing drugs accounts for about 3 percent of all tumors that occur in people who have had kidney transplants, a very high rate of occurrence. Men get this form of the disease twice as frequently as women. The age of occurrence depends on the age when the medical treatment started.

African KS, which accounts for nearly 10 percent of all cancers in central Africa, attacks young adults, and about 10 males to every female. This ratio drops to three to one in children.

Epidemic, or AIDS-related, KS occurs in all age groups. Babies of infected mothers may develop the illness, and so may people who have contracted it from a blood transfusion received before 1985. (The risk of contracting HIV from a contaminated unit of blood with current blood screening methods is estimated to be once for every 153,000 units of blood. There is *no* risk of contracting HIV by donating blood.)

AIDS-related KS occurs through transmission of the virus from the body fluids of an infected person. There is no evidence of spread through casual contact. The rate of contagion with blood is high; lesser rates of spread are thought to occur with other body fluids including semen, urine, vaginal fluids and (very rarely) saliva.

Among the many unexplained observations in epidemic KS is that different rates of occurrence are found in each of the groups of people with AIDS. KS is nearly 10 times more frequent in gay men with AIDS than in people who have AIDS because of blood transfusions, IV drug use or hemophilia. The occurrence of AIDS-related KS is decreasing in all these groups at about an equal rate, again for unknown reasons.

At Significantly Higher Risk

♦ People who share or use HIV-contaminated needles. Spread can be eliminated in drug users by never sharing needles.
♦ People—both gay and straight—who have unprotected sexual contact with one or more partners infected with HIV. The risk increases with the number of partners. Convincing data from San Francisco shows that safe sexual practices can dra-

matically decrease the incidence of AIDS and, therefore, of KS.

SCREENING

There are no screening tests for KS. But because of the relationship of HIV to AIDS and KS, many health care workers now recommend routine blood testing for HIV in high-risk groups. Screening for HIV is now routinely done on all blood products in the United States.

COMMON SIGNS AND SYMPTOMS

There are no general symptoms of early Kaposi's sarcoma. In the epidemic form, KS may be the first sign of AIDS, or the first lesion may follow an illness of months or years. During this time the patient may have had non-specific symptoms such as fever, weight loss and sweating. Or there may have been other illnesses such as lymphoma or tuberculosis before the first KS lesion developed.

Once the disease occurs, symptoms relate to the site of involvement. Early and even more advanced skin lesions are usually only mildly uncomfortable, although painful ulcers may occur. Lesions in the gastrointestinal tract are very common but rarely cause significant symptoms. Early lesions in the lung have no symptoms either, but severe lung involvement produces a profound air hunger.

Physical findings also relate to the site of involvement. The most common sign of the illness is the appearance of the characteristic Kaposi's sarcoma lesion.

DIAGNOSIS

Careful physical examination of anyone suspected of having KS requires an evaluation of all organ systems. Lesions may be found in many locations, although the characteristic finding in classic KS is a single raised purple-red nodule or a cluster of lesions in a single area of the body, especially on the legs.

Physical Examination
♦ The skin must be carefully examined. Although the dominant lesion of classic KS is on the arms and legs, all forms of the disease can affect any area of the skin—on flat surfaces of the body, between fingers and toes, under nails, in the ear canal, on the penis and so on.
♦ Epidemic KS may have a peculiar appearance. Early lesions are usually flat to slightly thickened, round or slightly irregular purple spots. They are painless when they first appear and only infrequently during the course of the disease do they cause significant pain. As the disease progresses, the lesions grow, often reaching an inch or so in each direction. They also thicken.
♦ There may be different-sized spots at all stages, often growing at seemingly different rates. Many patients will have yellow-brown pigment around the purple lesions. This bruise-like appearance is due to a small amount of blood leaking into the tissue.
♦ In late stages of the disease, the plaques and nodules may grow together. They can occupy large areas of the skin and block drainage from an extremity, causing swelling and infection.
♦ Lymph nodes may be enlarged, but a biopsy is needed to distinguish KS in nodes from other causes of lymph node enlargement.
♦ Mucous membranes are often involved. In the mouth, the hard and soft palates are most frequently affected.
♦ The membrane covering the eye (conjunctiva) may be involved, or lesions may be seen beneath the white of the eye (sclera).
♦ There may be abnormal masses, including an enlarged liver or spleen. Although involvement of internal organs may be suspected by physical examination, it cannot be proven without further testing.

Blood and Other Tests
♦ Only the HIV-related form of KS has

associated abnormal blood tests. None of the tests, however—including HIV, P-24 antigen or beta-2 microglobulin—are predictive, meaning that they do not indicate that KS is about to occur, its rate of growth or the chances of its responding to treatment.

♦ Useful information can be obtained from the total lymphocyte count and the "helper/suppressor" ratio.

Imaging

♦ KS may appear on a chest x-ray but cannot be distinguished from infections or other tumors.

Endoscopy and Biopsy

♦ The only diagnostic test for KS is biopsy of a suspicious lesion.

♦ Examination with an anoscope or proctoscope may show rectal involvement.

♦ If KS is suspected on a chest x-ray, a direct view of the lung through a bronchoscope may be needed.

STAGING

There are several systems for staging KS, none entirely satisfactory or accepted by all physicians. Under a representative system designed at New York University, patients are divided into four groups:

1. Skin lesions, locally indolent (slow growing).

2. Skin lesions, locally aggressive, with or without local lymph node involvement.

3. Skin and mucous membrane involvement, generalized, with or without lymph node involvement.

4. Deep organ involvement.

All stages are then divided into either A (no symptoms) or B (with weight loss or fever).

TREATMENT OVERVIEW

KS is not considered curable. Neither surgical removal of the first-detected lesion nor obtaining a complete remission of multiple sites with chemotherapy or other techniques results in cure.

Long-term survival does occur both with and without treatment, however. Survival in classic KS is usually years and sometimes decades. Some patients with AIDS-related KS are still alive after 10 years, though most survive only a few years and treatment decisions are usually aimed at palliation.

New drugs are always being tried, however, and thought should be given to participation in clinical research programs in major medical centers and hospitals.

 Surgery A surgical biopsy of a suspicious lesion is needed to confirm the diagnosis of KS. Sometimes more than one biopsy is needed. But once the diagnosis is made, biopsy of other lesions is usually not needed except when a deep lesion—a lung tumor, for example—has to be evaluated.

Other than for a biopsy, surgery is not commonly used in KS treatment. Lesions in the gastrointestinal tract may uncommonly bleed or cause an obstruction and require surgical correction. Conventional surgery and lasers have been used to remove bulky lesions in the mouth. But removal of multiple skin lesions does little to provide any meaningful relief of symptoms.

 Radiation All forms of KS are sensitive to radiation therapy. Radiation is especially useful for lesions that are cosmetically disturbing, painful, involve the mouth extensively, block lymphatics, bleed or protrude from the skin. Response rates are quite high and treatment is usually well tolerated.

The mouth, however, is very sensitive to radiation in AIDS, resulting in a poor tolerance. The treatment itself is painless, but the surfaces of the mouth may become inflamed or ulcerated. The sore mouth can be quite uncomfortable during the time needed for healing, usually several days.

Mouthwashes can control pain and speed the healing.

Local radiation usually uses energy beams that do not penetrate deeply into the body. Various combinations of numbers of treatments and dose per individual treatment are used, ranging from one single high dose to small doses five days a week for four or five weeks. Response rates appear roughly similar with the different methods.

The use of small doses of radiation over half the body and very superficial electron beam radiation to the entire body over many weeks are being investigated.

 Chemotherapy Several problems are involved in treating KS with chemotherapy. One concern about using very aggressive therapy is that the treatment might further depress the immune system. Moreover, determining whether a lesion becomes smaller with treatment can be quite difficult. Many patients have multiple lesions that are hard to measure accurately and may not respond in the same way to therapy. Changes in a lesion's shape or color may indicate some effect of treatment but not a significant one.

The disease does respond to chemotherapy, however, both with single agents and combinations of drugs. Because of the rareness of the condition, there is no good information about how well patients with KS caused by immunosuppression respond. The response rates of classic KS to chemotherapy are not well known either, although this form is highly responsive to Velban, with response rates in the range of 90 percent. Little information is available on the response to other drugs. It would be logical, however, to assume response rates to the common drugs similar to those of epidemic KS. African KS appears to respond in a similar way to epidemic KS.

♦ Velban has been the most studied and used single agent. It is well tolerated when given intravenously weekly. In epidemic KS, response rates of about 25 percent are obtained, with rare complete responses.

♦ Oncovin, closely related to Velban, has very different side effects and a slightly lower response rate. Weekly treatment with both of these drugs combined, at a lower dosage or alternating full dosage on a weekly schedule, raises the response rate to 40 to 75 percent. Side effects are remarkably low, and some complete responses are seen.

♦ Etoposide (VP-16), given orally or intravenously, is an attractive drug because it is tolerated well. But it has the potential to depress blood counts in people who may already have marginal blood counts, making it sometimes unwise to use. Where it can be used, it has a high response rate. The same general comments apply to Adriamycin, which can be given only intravenously.

♦ Bleomycin is active against KS, although it appears to be more effective in combinations than as a single agent. Responses to it as a single agent appear to be short, although there is very little blood count depression.

♦ Methotrexate is similarly active, and ways can be found to give it with little blood count depression. Its use is limited, though, because it can cause rather marked blistering of the mouth.

Combination Chemotherapy In the early days of AIDS, combinations of chemotherapy drugs were nearly always used. They fell into disfavor because of the high death rate from drug toxicity, which often resulted in infections such as pneumocystis pneumonia. With newer drugs such as AZT, inhaled pentamidine and foscarnet now available to prevent, decrease or treat infections, combinations are being used again, with higher response rates. Many combinations are being studied, with either of the two Velban-Oncovin programs now standard therapy in some communities.

Whenever possible, patients should consider participating in a clinical trial with the hope of improved response and survival. Treatment should *always* be given by a physician experienced in using these agents.

Local Therapy KS is one of the few tumors that responds to local injections of chemotherapy. Many anticancer drugs cause intense local damage if they are accidentally injected into tissue. This undesirable side effect has been used in a positive way to treat skin lesions.

Diluted solutions of various drugs are injected with fine-gauge needles directly into the lesions. A small amount of inflammation may occur for a few days, but this is not usually painful. The lesions will often flatten and shrink so they look like freckles. They can stay this way for weeks or months before they recur.

Bleomycin, Oncovin and Velban have all been used in this way, with Velban the most commonly used because of its relative cheapness and ease of use.

Treatments are usually given weeks to months apart and are no more painful than any other injection. They will not permanently control the lesions, nor will they control lesions that have not been injected. There are no generalized side effects or bone marrow depression. These treatments are especially useful for cosmetically disturbing KS such as a lesion on the face.

 Biological Therapy Immunologic treatment of KS is primarily with the interferons, mainly alpha. Other agents, especially interleukin-2, are being studied but there is no clear data on their effects. Patients interested in these biologic response modifiers should ask their doctors for more information.

There is not much information available about the effects of interferon on classic KS, but it's not likely that it would respond because it does not involve an immunologic defect.

Drug-induced KS is often very responsive to removing whichever agent depressed the body's immune system in the first place. When this is done, frequent regressions of the disease, often complete, occur.

The most information on the effects of interferon is available with respect to HIV-associated KS. Treatment produces responses independent of the site of involvement or the amount of tumor present, which is a most unusual finding in cancer treatment.

The response rate drops if there are symptoms (fever, sweating, weight loss), opportunistic infections or low T4 cell counts. In one study, 45 percent of patients with T4 cell counts over 400 responded to immunotherapy, but only 2 percent of those with T4 cell counts less than 100 responded. There is some suggestion of an increase in survival if the amount of KS decreases, but final data are not yet available.

Responses are more frequent as larger doses are given, but higher doses cause unacceptable side effects much more often. Accordingly, some physicians start their patients at a low dosage of interferon and gradually increase it. This appears to result in fewer side effects when the higher dosage is eventually reached, but obviously the KS takes longer to respond.

Studies of interferon plus chemotherapy have failed to produce any consistent improvement over either agent used by itself.

AZT has been added to interferon with some suggestion of increased effect.

TREATMENT BY STAGE AND SITE

Treatment considerations for KS are different than for any other solid (non-blood origin) tumor. There are two major reasons.

The first is that there is *never* a stage or site of origin that can be cured.

The second is that there is no relationship between the stage of the tumor and the response to treatment. Starting therapy early in the disease does not appear to change either the prognosis or the overall length of survival.

Decisions on whether, when and how to treat patients are based on a number of factors such as the rate of growth, the site of involvement and the severity of symptoms.

Standard Treatment Many physicians will not treat early disease with systemic (drug) therapy. Patients with early localized disease may receive radiation to the lesions or local chemotherapy injections. Or their condition may be monitored without any treatment given until it is needed.

Lesions of the gastrointestinal tract (stomach, small and large bowel) are common but usually do not cause symptoms. When they do cause symptoms—such as pain, bleeding or an inability to eat a normal volume of food—either chemotherapy or local radiation may be useful.

Lung lesions have a poor prognosis. Patients find it harder and harder to get enough air. When this happens they may live only a few months. Radiation therapy to the lungs with chemotherapy given at the same time and then followed by so-called maintenance therapy has been used with a moderate degree of success.

A recent study of the combination of bleomycin and Velban (and in some patients Adriamycin) reported substantial improvement in lung symptoms.

SUPPORTIVE THERAPY

There are many common treatment-related problems with KS—hair loss and nerve damage from the medicines and especially depression of the bone marrow. This can lead to anemia, low white blood cell counts that make infections more likely and low platelet counts with the possibility of bleeding.

♦ Frequent checks of the blood counts help reduce the risk of serious bone marrow damage.

♦ Common as well as uncommon infections will often be seen and antibiotics may be needed.

♦ Nerve damage should regularly be checked for, with medications being changed as needed to minimize the problem.

♦ Fluid may build up in body tissues, especially the legs, because KS lesions can block drainage. Local radiation may relieve the obstruction. The use of diuretics (medicines that increase the flow of urine) under close supervision is also sometimes effective.

♦ Pain is not common, but if it does occur pain relievers may be needed.

♦ Poor nutrition is a common problem. Appetite stimulants such as Megace or Provera may be useful for those with poor appetites. Some patients who lose weight even with what appears to be good intake of food may benefit from nutritional counseling.

♦ Patients often need emotional and psychological support. Physical appearance is an important part of self-image, and cosmetics may be needed to cover lesions (*see* Chapter 22).

♦ Tourniquets or ice caps around the scalp can reduce blood flow to the scalp during treatment, which may reduce the amount of hair loss.

♦ Psychosocial aspects of the illness also have to be dealt with. Dealing with the fear of death is a continuing problem, and with the high incidence of AIDS-related KS in North America there are many other problems such as job loss and job discrimination, unwarranted public fear, treatment costs and death in young people.

Help may be found from a variety of organizations devoted to these problems. In some communities the spectrum of help ranges from psychiatry/counseling to the exceedingly valuable support given in one-to-one contact through such groups as Shanti.

TREATMENT FOLLOW-UP

To discover whether the treatment is working, the physician will often measure lesions in selected areas of the body. The physical examination will also try to detect areas of trouble such as internal organ involvement. Follow-up is primarily concerned with supportive care, however.

RECURRENT CANCER

Because KS is not now curable, the disappearance of detectable disease (clinical remission) means only that the disease's presence cannot be demonstrated at a particular time. The question really is how long treatment should be continued once remission has been obtained.

It is often the case that patients in either complete or partial remission who discontinue treatment relapse quite rapidly. So if the treatment program does not cause severe side effects and does not involve drugs that cause more damage the longer they are used, then treatment should continue indefinitely.

AIDS-RELATED LYMPHOSARCOMA

By the definition of the United States Center for Disease Control, only two malignancies establish an AIDS diagnosis when associated with a positive HIV test—Kaposi's sarcoma and high-grade, or aggressive, non-Hodgkin's lymphoma. It should be noted that most people with lymphomas—even those with high-grade lymphomas—do not have AIDS. There must be a positive HIV test in the patient with lymphoma to establish the diagnosis of AIDS as well.

Lymphomas are very rapidly growing tumors that may double in size in a few days. They have been found in every organ in the body.

Types The most common types of high-grade non-Hodgkin's lymphosarcoma are the Burkittoid lymphoma and immunoblastic lymphoma. For practical reasons, all AIDS-related high-grade non-Hodgkin's lymphomas are now treated identically.

How It Spreads Like KS, these tumors are believed to be widespread from their beginning. Although they may be first found in a single place—such as a lymph node—by then they probably involve many other parts of the body. What caus-

es the lymphoma probably initiates the change in multiple areas at the same time. These tumors also spread by direct extension and through the blood stream or lymphatic channels.

What Causes It The precise cause is not known, but it may involve the AIDS virus depressing the immune system's ability to guard against spontaneous malignancies.

Who Gets It Lymphomas occur in all the risk groups for AIDS. The number of new cases of lymphoma associated with positive HIV tests appears to be rising rapidly.

COMMON SIGNS AND SYMPTOMS

The most common sign of the illness is a lump, often an enlarged lymph node in the neck or under the arm.

Multiple symptoms can occur with internal masses. Lymphoma in the bowel may cause pain, loss of appetite or symptoms of obstruction. Lung involvement by lymphoma may produce a cough or blood in the sputum. Fever, weight loss and sweating are fairly common symptoms for all sites of origin.

DIAGNOSIS

♦ Besides the enlarged nodes, a physical examination may reveal an enlarged liver or spleen, fluid in the lungs, enlarged heart or evidence of brain abnormalities.

♦ A biopsy is always needed for a definitive diagnosis.

♦ Once the diagnosis is made, studies are then done to determine where the lymphoma is. These will include blood tests, a chest x-ray, whole-body gallium scan, bone marrow analysis, spinal tap and often various CT scans.

TREATMENT OVERVIEW

Lymphosarcoma can be cured in some patients even though the HIV virus does not disappear and other AIDS-related diseases can and do occur. Because this tumor will often respond dramatically to chemotherapy—sometimes in hours—chemotherapy is usually the initial treatment of choice.

 Chemotherapy There is no clear consensus on standard chemotherapy, but multiple drug programs are generally

used by physicians who see many of these patients.

Drug dosages have to be reduced, however, because people with AIDS cannot tolerate conventional doses. For the same reason, the duration of treatment is often shorter than usual and meticulous care has to be taken to prevent the infections that people with AIDS are more likely to get, especially those such as pneumocystis pneumonia.

 Radiation Some patients may receive local radiation to specific areas in addition to chemotherapy.

THE MOST IMPORTANT QUESTIONS YOU CAN ASK

♦ When should treatment begin?

♦ When in the disease is interferon helpful?

♦ What types of drug treatment are available?

♦ When is radiation useful?

♦ How long will treatment last?

♦ Are there any new treatments available?

♦ What supportive services and treatments are available?

KIDNEY

Alan Yagoda, MD

◇

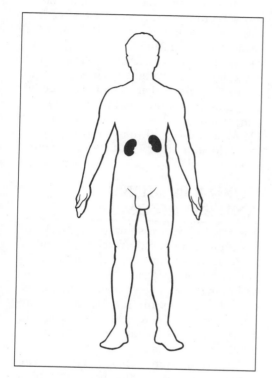

Cancer of the kidney—also called renal cell cancer, kidney adenocarcinoma or hypernephroma—accounts for about 2 percent of new cancers in the United States, 24,000 cases a year. It ranks as the eleventh most common cancer. Unfortunately, five-year survival rates have not changed for the past 30 years, partly because two-thirds of these cancers are not localized in the kidney when they are diagnosed. About 10,700 persons will die of kidney cancer in 1991.

The kidneys, which lie between the lining of the body cavity (peritoneum) and the back muscles at the level of the last two ribs, do not lend themselves to early diagnosis. By the time symptoms such as back pain and bloody urine are noted, the tumor is large (average size is 3 in. or 7.5 cm), has invaded lymph nodes and/or surrounding structures and is very vascular because of its ability to attract blood vessels. This increased vascularity soon leads to spread to the lungs, liver and bone. Five-year survival ranges between 30 to 80 percent for small tumors within the kidney that can be completely removed by surgery, whereas high-grade advanced disease has a cure rate of only 5 to 15 percent.

Renal cancer arises from the outer portion of the kidney called the parenchyma (as opposed to the renal pelvis, which briefly collects the urine, which is then carried by a tube, the ureter, to the bladder for storage before it is expelled). The parenchyma is made up of many single units called nephrons that filter water and toxic products from the blood.

Types More than 85 percent of renal cancers develop in glandular tissue (adenocarcinoma). The clear cell variety is the most common, followed by granular or clear cell mixed with other more aggressive components such as granular and sarcomatous elements. Studies using a test called flow cytometry suggest that the number of chromosomes in the tumor cells may help predict the chance for recurrence and disease-free survival. The normal two chromosomes (diploid) is favorable, while any other number (aneuploid) is less favorable.

Another renal cancer, Wilms' tumor, is found exclusively in children.

How It Spreads Kidney cancer cells frequently spread through the bloodstream by penetrating blood vessels within the tumor, then entering the renal vein and/or the inferior vena cava, the largest abdominal vein. Once cells have entered the bloodstream, they can lodge in the lungs, liver, brain or bone.

Cells also can directly invade the abdominal lymph nodes that drain the kidney and extend into structures surrounding the kidney (perinephric) such as fat, adrenal gland and liver. This kind of invasion is found at diagnosis in about 45 percent of cases. Invasion of the inferior vena cava is found in 10 to 15 percent of cases and of local lymph nodes in 10 to 30 percent. In over half the cases with lymph node involvement, distant metastases are found.

In over 40 percent of patients, the symptoms that cause them to seek medical attention are due to metastases.

What Causes It Risk factors are poorly defined, although the incidence is twice as high for those using tobacco (cigars, chewing tobacco, cigarettes). In fact, it has been estimated that one-quarter of renal cancers may be caused by cigarette smoking.

RISK FACTORS

At Significantly Higher Risk
♦ This tumor is twice as frequent in men than in women, occurring mostly between the ages of 30 and 70.
♦ Those who smoke tobacco.
♦ Patients on long-term dialysis with acquired polycystic kidneys have an increased risk, as do those with the inherited disease von Hippel-Lindau syndrome.
♦ Other (but weak) risk factors include obesity in women and a high animal-fat diet, both of which suggest a hormonal imbalance.
♦ A new finding is the frequent abnormality in chromosome 3, which may relate to onset of these tumors.

SCREENING

Examination of the urine for blood (hematuria) is used for detecting early lesions that can be surgically removed. Ultrasound screening of the kidney, which is used in some countries, would be more accurate but is not cost-effective. Intravenous pyelography (IVP) and CT scans are used in the diagnostic work-up to discover the cause of persistent and unexplained symptoms such as abdominal or flank pain, anemia and fever. Better screening procedures will have to await a simplified and less expensive urine or blood test using kidney cancer specific monoclonal antibodies. Such tests should soon be available.

COMMON SIGNS AND SYMPTOMS

The most common symptom is blood in the urine (hematuria), which is present in up to 65 percent of cases. Abdominal pain is found in 40 percent of patients and an abdominal mass in 35 percent. Other common symptoms include anemia, bone pain, unexplained weight loss, low-grade fever, general weakness or loss of energy and loss of appetite.

Unusual symptoms may include hypercalcemia (high blood calcium), high blood pressure, abnormal liver tests or too many red cells in the blood (polycythemia). These symptoms develop because renal tumors can produce substances that indirectly affect other organs, producing conditions called paraneoplastic syndromes.

DIAGNOSIS

Physical Examination
♦ Abdominal mass.
♦ Neck mass due to enlarged lymph node.
♦ Abdominal bruit (sound over renal artery).

Blood and Other Tests
♦ Liver function tests.
♦ Complete blood count.
♦ Blood calcium determination.
♦ Urinalysis.

Imaging
♦ Intravenous pyelogram (IVP).
♦ Ultrasound is the most sensitive test, being able to find masses as small as 3/4 in. (2 cm) in over 90 percent of cases. Sonograms can readily distinguish between the more commonly occurring benign or non-cancerous cyst and a solid tumor. When this test is combined with the intravenous pyelogram (IVP), the accuracy of a tumor diagnosis is over 90 percent. The sonogram can also be very helpful in determining whether the tumor has induced a clot in or invaded the renal vein or the inferior vena cava.

♦ CT with intravenous dye (the same dye used for intravenous pyelograms) will accurately diagnose renal tumors in 95 percent of cases and be falsely positive in fewer than 2 percent. This test may also show the tumor extension outside the kidney and can determine the extent of lymph node, liver and blood vessel involvement.

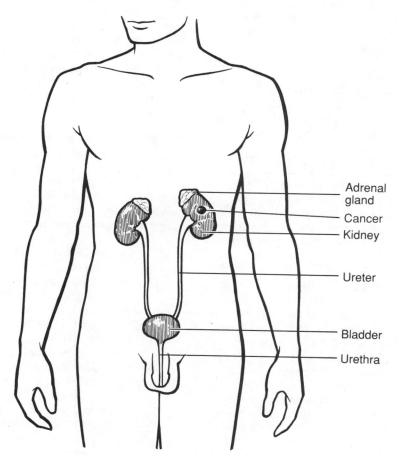

Kidneys and adrenal glands

♦ MRI has replaced the inferior vena cavagram for determining more clearly the extent of blood vessel involvement and involvement of adjacent structures.

♦ Selective renal arteriography is helpful in finding small tumors and providing information that sometimes may be needed at the time of surgery about uncommon blood vessel patterns and, in selected cases, determining the possibility of a partial nephrectomy (removal of only a portion of the kidney) for small localized tumors.

♦ Other tests before surgery simply assure that there are no distant metastases. These include chest x-rays (if abnormal it may be followed by a chest CT scan), bone scans or skeletal x-rays and a liver scan (unnecessary when an abdominal CT scan is performed).

Endoscopy and Biopsy
♦ Ultimately, the diagnosis is made either by removing the kidney (nephrectomy) or by a thin needle aspiration through the skin for cytologic slide examination.

TREATMENT OVERVIEW

Surgical removal of the kidney (simple nephrectomy) and the surrounding fat, adrenal gland and lymph nodes (radical nephrectomy) can lead to a cure for Stages I and II and can even cure Stage III in a few cases.

Surgery Partial nephrectomy can be performed in selected cases, such as for a tumor in patients with only one kidney or with tumors in both kidneys and for small, low-grade tumors. If both kidneys have to be removed, long-term renal dialysis may be required.

Renal transplantation can play a role for cancers in both kidneys. However, there is a risk of metastases being increased because the immune system has to be suppressed by drugs to prevent rejection of a transplanted kidney.

While there is renewed debate about the effectiveness of radical compared to simple nephrectomy in prolonging survival, no evidence exists that preoperative or postoperative radiation therapy, radiation therapy alone without surgery or renal artery embolization—clotting the arterial supply, thereby destroying both the tumor and the kidney—are beneficial in preventing metastases.

Adjuvant Therapy Without any effective treatment for advanced disease, there is no role for preoperative (neoadjuvant) or postoperative (adjuvant) therapy. Nor is there any role for immunotherapy with interferon, interleukin-2 (alone or combined with lymphokine-activated killer cells), monoclonal antibodies or vaccines. Similarly, there is no role for hormone manipulation (female hormone progesterone) or chemotherapy (vinblastine), except when given as part of an investigational study.

Radiation Although radiation therapy can control bone and brain lesions, it has not successfully prevented local tumor recurrence, nor has improvement in survival been definitely shown with radiation given before or after surgery.

Chemotherapy The most effective standard chemotherapy drugs for metastatic disease are vinblastine and nitrosoureas—lomustine (CCNU) and carmustine (BCNU)—which produce tumor regression in 5 to 10 percent of cases. Combination chemotherapy regimens have not yet demonstrated any superiority to single-drug therapy.

Biological Therapy Interferon-alpha reduces tumors in 10 to 20 percent of patients, mostly those with lymph node and lung metastases. The usual dose of 6 million units—self-administered under the skin in the thigh three times weekly—should be continued for about three months before a decision is made about its effectiveness. There may shortly be a test using a monoclonal antibody (uro-II) that can predict tumor responsiveness to interferon.

Investigational programs include interleukin-2—with and without lymphokine-activated killer (LAK) cells or tumor-infiltrating lymphocytes (TIL)—and autolymphocyte therapy. In some studies, these have been combined with interferon and/or low-dose chemotherapy with cyclophosphamide.

Vaccines are being explored but are as yet of unproven benefit.

Monoclonal antibodies, either given alone or with drugs attached to the antibody, are now being used in clinical trials and may well be a more promising treatment method. The use of these monoclonal antibodies is being investigated for both diagnosis and treatment.

TREATMENT BY STAGE

STAGE I
TNM T1, N0, M0
T2, N0, M0
In Robson's staging system, Stage I means the tumor is confined within the renal capsule and is either less than 3/4 in. (2 cm) (T1) or more than 3/4 in. (2 cm) (T2) and with no lymph node or distant metastases.

About one-third of cases present with Stage I disease, many of which are Grade I (very well-differentiated) to Grade II (moderately well-differentiated). Almost one-third of Stage I cases are found to have micrometastases or microscopic disease after surgery.

Standard Treatment Simple or radical nephrectomy. It can be partial in selected cases, for low-grade small masses less than 1 1/4 in. (3 cm) in the cortex or outer

area of the kidney, for tumors within one kidney and for tumors in both kidneys.

As long as tumor-free surgical margins are obtained, partial nephrectomy can be performed either with the kidney in place but isolated from the normal blood supply or by using an *ex vivo* technique, in which the kidney is removed from the body (so-called bench surgery). After excision of the tumor, the remaining normal kidney is autotransplanted back into an appropriate area.

Radical nephrectomy involves tying the renal artery and vein, removing the surrounding fibrous layer (called Gerota's fascia) and thereby completely excising the kidney, the surrounding fat, the adrenal gland, regional lymph nodes and the ureter.

Five-Year Survival 60 to 80 percent

Investigational
♦ Postoperative interferon, as well as autolymphocyte therapy, is being evaluated in clinical trials.

STAGE II
TNM T3a, N0, M0
The tumor invades the surrounding fat or adrenal gland.

About 10 percent of cases are diagnosed in Stage II, and one-third of those patients will have micrometastases found at the time of surgery.

Standard Treatment Radical nephrectomy or, in selected cases, a simple nephrectomy.

Five-Year Survival 50 to 65 percent

Investigational Same as for Stage I.

STAGE III
TNM T3b, N1–3, M0
The tumor invades the renal vein (T3b, N0, M0), the inferior vena cava (T3b) or regional lymph nodes (T3b, N1–3, M0).

Approximately 25 to 35 percent of cases

are found in Stage III, 60 percent of whom will have micrometastases found at the time of surgery.

Standard Treatment Radical nephrectomy.

Five-Year Survival 30 to 45 percent

Investigational Same as for Stage I.

STAGE IV
TNM T4, N3–4, M1
The tumor invades adjacent organs (T4), nearby lymph nodes (N4) or has distant metastases (M1).
   Approximately 30 percent of cases are diagnosed in Stage IV, with 10 percent having a low-grade and more than 60 percent a high-grade tumor.

Standard Treatment The role for radical nephrectomy is debatable, since most patients die from metastatic disease. In the past it was thought that removing the primary cancerous kidney would cause the metastases to shrink. But spontaneous shrinkage of tumors has been documented in only 2 to 10 percent of cases at best, so the era of radical nephrectomy following embolization is over.
   Nephrectomy is again being considered, however, to debulk the tumor volume in order to make immunological treatment more effective for remaining disease. Nephrectomy for Stage IV cases should only be considered when part of an investigational study or for severe hemorrhage.

Five-Year Survival 5 percent

Investigational
♦ Participation in an experimental protocol, as outlined for Stage I, would be very appropriate.

TREATMENT FOLLOW-UP
♦ Regular physical examinations.
♦ Blood chemistry panel (includes alkaline phosphatase, which may signify bone or liver metastases if elevated).
♦ Chest x-rays (every 3 months) and abdominal CT scan (every 3-6 months).
♦ Bone scan (and specific bone x-rays) if bone pain is present or serum alkaline phosphatase is elevated.
♦ Selected x-rays or imaging studies for specific areas (brain CT or MRI for persistent headaches; spine MRI for back pain with leg weakness or nerve symptoms).

RECURRENT CANCER
New investigational treatments should be explored before starting standard therapy. The results with currently used standard cytotoxic agents—vinblastine and a nitrosourea such as lomustine or carmustine—as well as immunological agents (interferon) are very limited.

THE MOST IMPORTANT QUESTIONS YOU CAN ASK
♦ Has my cancer spread?
♦ What is the chance for cure with surgery?
♦ What are the complications of surgery?
♦ Is there any role for other treatments such as chemotherapy?
♦ Is there a role for biological therapy with interferon, IL-2 or other agents?

LEUKEMIA

Timothy S. Gee, MD

◇

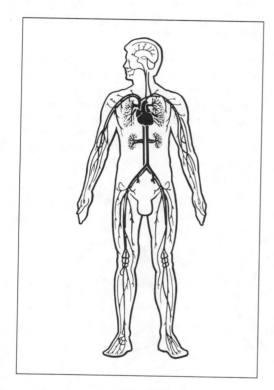

Leukemia is a cancer of the cells in the blood. It usually involves the various forms and stages of the white blood cells, although on rare occasions it may involve red blood cells and platelets.

Leukemia is often thought of as primarily a childhood disease, but it strikes many more adults than children. Adults account for 25,000 of the estimated 29,000 new cases expected in the United States in 1991. Acute leukemia is the most common childhood malignancy. The incidence of leukemia has not changed dramatically over the past 50 years, but survival rates

for some forms of the disease have improved, especially in children, with the development of new types of treatment and chemotherapy agents. With acute lymphocytic leukemia in adults, for example, the five-year survival has increased from 4 percent in the early 1960s to about 50 percent today. More than half of the children who develop acute lymphocytic leukemia are alive five years after diagnosis, the majority being considered cured.

Types The many different forms of leukemia are generally divided into acute or chronic and then classified according to the cell type involved. There are two major types of white blood cells—granulocytic (myeloid) and non-granulocytic (lymphoid). Under a microscope, myeloid cells contain particles (granules), lymphoid cells generally do not. The diagnosis may be confirmed by new techniques for identifying certain biological markers and chromosomal characteristics.

♦ *Acute* An acute leukemia is associated with early (precursor) white blood cells called blast forms that do not become mature. These abnormal cells interfere with the production of the more mature cells normally seen in the bone marrow and blood, with the result that the normal cells are generally diminished or not seen at all. Because of the decreased number of normal cells, symptoms may include anemia, easy bruising, bleeding and sometimes infections. Without treatment, people with acute leukemia have an average survival of three to five months after diagnosis.

♦ *Chronic* Chronic leukemia usually involves the white blood cells, although the red blood cells may rarely be involved. Unlike acute leukemia, the leukemic cell clone involved in chronic leukemia does show all stages of maturation, with only a few blast forms. But even though they appear normal, the cells are abnormal. They do not function like normal cells. The white cells, for example, are not able to help fight infection. Because the bone marrow shows normal-appearing maturing cells, the diagnosis is made on the basis of the clinical picture, blood counts, the predominance of a particular cell line, genetic characteristics and the presence of certain proteins on the cell surface (cell surface markers).

The disease is controlled easily with medication or may not even need medication in its early stages. Average survival is measured in years rather than months.

How It Spreads Because it is a cancer of the blood, leukemia is found wherever blood travels. It is most commonly found in the bone marrow, spleen, liver and lymph nodes. In extremely rare cases, leukemia may first appear as a single localized mass of leukemia cells (chloroma) in the breasts, ovaries, testicles or brain. There may also be skin involvement by leukemic cells.

What Causes It There is no known cause. There are, however, known oncogenes in leukemia cells that may be associated with some types of the disease. Some forms of leukemia are associated with exposure to a retroviral infection such as HTLV-1. Certain abnormalities in the chromosomes are also associated with specific types of leukemia.

Two Types of Leukemic Cells

RISK FACTORS

At Slightly Higher Risk

♦ Men are slightly more likely than women to develop leukemia, and whites are more likely than blacks.

♦ People who have been exposed to prolonged or significant doses of radiation have a higher risk of developing leukemia.

♦ Prolonged exposure to toxic organic chemical compounds may be associated with increased risk.

COMMON SIGNS AND SYMPTOMS

A significant proportion of people with leukemia are completely free of symptoms and are diagnosed on a routine physical examination. The doctor may find an enlarged lymph node or an enlarged liver or spleen. Then again, the physical examination may be completely normal, but the routine blood test is abnormal.

People who do have symptoms commonly complain about generalized weakness, fevers, frequent infections, anemia or easy bruising or bleeding. Bleeding may be from the gums or nose or there may be blood in the stool or urine. Some people may have enlarged lymph glands, abdominal fullness or pain from enlargement of the liver or spleen. Less commonly, there may be complaints of headaches, fevers, skin rash or breast masses.

DIAGNOSIS

The initial diagnostic work-up—and treatment—of adults with acute leukemia can be carried out in many community medical centers, but children with acute leukemia should usually be evaluated in a pediatric cancer center because of the sophisticated testing required.

Physical Examination

♦ Enlarged lymph nodes.

♦ Swollen gums.

♦ Enlarged liver and spleen.

♦ Bruises or a small pinpoint red rash (petechiae) on the skin.

Blood and Other Tests

♦ A complete blood count (CBC) usually is abnormal, but on rare occasions may be normal.

Endoscopy and Biopsy

♦ The definitive test is a bone marrow aspiration and biopsy. The aspiration is performed by putting a needle into the breastbone (sternum) or pelvic bone under local anesthesia.

♦ A marrow biopsy may also be required. It is performed in the same fashion as an aspirate but with a larger, specialized needle.

♦ Additional amounts of marrow may be withdrawn for more specialized tests, such as chromosomal or DNA analysis.

STAGING

There is no staging system for leukemias, except for the chronic lymphocytic form (CLL). With CLL there are several staging classifications, the most frequently used being the RAI and the International. Both systems are based on the presence or absence of enlarged lymph nodes, liver or spleen and, most important, on the degree of anemia or low platelet counts.

Staging in the RAI system varies from Stage 0 to Stage IV, with average survivals ranging from over 12 years in the early stage to about a year in the late. Average survivals are comparable in the International classifications of A, B and C.

TREATMENT OVERVIEW

Leukemia is treated mainly with chemotherapy, although radiotherapy and biological therapy can play a part with some forms of the disease. Surgery has no role. The goals of therapy are to relieve symptoms and obtain a remission. Remission is the condition in which leukemia is no longer detected and the marrow is normal again.

Bone Marrow Transplantation This is still an investigative procedure (*see* Chapter 12). There are two forms of marrow transplantation.

♦ Autologous transplantation uses the patient's own marrow. The marrow is collected while the patient is in remission, and it is often treated with chemotherapy agents or monoclonal antibodies before being given back. This is an effort to eliminate the few leukemic cells that might still be present but are undetectable.

♦ An allogeneic bone marrow transplant uses marrow from a normal donor, preferably a brother or sister who has the same tissue types. If a sibling is not available, a search of national and international tissue banks could be made for a non-related normal donor.

A bone marrow transplant requires four to six weeks in a hospital and the cost is currently about $150,000 to $175,000. Not all hospitals are able to perform the procedure.

The risk of dying is higher for an allogeneic marrow transplant than for an autologous one. Comparison studies are now evaluating this situation. Early results of mortality and long-term results between patients with first remission and second remission transplants show no significant difference. Because the long-term results between first remission patients treated with chemotherapy alone rather than bone marrow transplant are similar, bone marrow transplants are generally used for patients in their second remission—that is, patients who went into remission at the beginning of their illness, later relapsed, then again went into remission with chemotherapy.

PRELEUKEMIA (MYELODYSPLASTIC SYNDROME)

Preleukemia is a form of early leukemia that in most if not all cases will progress into an acute leukemia in a few months to a year.

A significant number of people with this syndrome will have a chromosomal abnormality associated with the disease. The syndrome is often found in patients who have had chemotherapy or radiation therapy for some other malignancy. Exposure to toxic organic chemicals or radiation may also be possible causative agents associated with myelodysplasia.

Like other types of leukemias, a definitive diagnosis is generally made by evaluating a bone marrow sample. Treatment is often not urgently necessary—not within hours or days of a diagnosis. Some patients with preleukemia may be followed closely by their physicians without treatment for weeks or months, with blood transfusions given at two- to four-week intervals if necessary.

In almost all cases, however, the disease will eventually progress to a point where treatment with chemotherapeutic agents should be started. The progression will be signaled by physical deterioration, an increase in the white blood cell counts, lowering of platelet counts and/or progressive anemia.

It is not yet known whether there is any significant difference in survival between people treated immediately after diagnosis and those who defer their treatment until there is a clinical indication.

Standard Treatment Treatment depends on the overall goal at a given point in the course of the disease. Approaches include:

♦ *Palliative* Treatment is intended to control the disease, not necessarily to eradicate it or bring about a remission. This is particularly true when the white blood count rises. At that point, in addition to palliative blood transfusions, the white blood count may be controlled by Hydrea (hydroxyurea), an oral chemotherapy agent. Other agents such as Thioguanine (6-thioguanine) and Myleran (busulfan) may also be used. Eventually, in spite of these palliative attempts, the disease will break through. There is no remission or cure for patients on palliative treatment.

♦ *Chemo-modulation* This concept of therapy involves an attempt to "differenti-ate" the leukemia cells to a more normal stage of development in the hopes that they may behave more like normal cells in growth pattern and function.

The treatment commonly involves the use of a standard chemotherapy agent—Cytosar (cytosine arabinoside)—in low doses given by a 24-hour intravenous infusion or daily injections for 10 to 14 days. This has been temporarily helpful in 20 to 30 percent of cases, but the disease eventually progresses.

♦ *Investigational* Treatment with other, more experimental, agents can also try to "push" the leukemic cells in the direction of normal cells in appearance and func-tion. Investigative agents now being eval-uated include growth factors or cytokines such as G-CSF (granulocyte colony stimu-lating factor), a new synthetic chemical agent called HMBA (hexamethylene bisac-etamide), IL-3 (interleukin-3) or vitamin A analogues (retinoic acid). It is too soon to know how effective these innovative treat-ments are.

♦ *Intensive chemotherapy* When the preleukemic stage becomes similar to an acute leukemia—in other words, it becomes a more aggressive form with sur-vival a matter of months—standard thera-py is similar to that described for acute leukemia.

♦ *Bone Marrow Transplantation* Even though bone marrow transplantation has been available for the past 15 years, it is still a new type of management. In a few patients with myelodysplasia, transplants from matched donors (a family member) have been performed before chemotherapy although results have not been encouraging.

ACUTE LEUKEMIAS

There are two major subdivisions in adult acute leukemias, with the identification of the various forms based on the appear-ance of the cells and on studies of various biological and cell surface markers. Chromosome analysis often helps to iden-tify the type of leukemia involved.

♦ Eighty percent of adult patients have an acute myeloid (AML) form. AML is divid-ed into many subtypes such as acute myelogenous or myeloblastic, acute monocytic or monoblastic (AMOL), acute myelomonocytic (AMML), acute promyelocytic (APL) or, less commonly, erythroleukemia. There are slight differ-ences in the prognosis and treatment response for each of these subtypes, but for practical purposes therapy is similar for all of them.

♦ Twenty percent of patients have acute lymphoblastic leukemia (ALL), which is similar to the childhood form of leukemia. The treatment for ALL is generally differ-ent than for AML, because the lym-phoblasts respond to a larger variety of chemical agents and also because ALL occurs in a younger population.

The probability of a long-term remis-sion is better for ALL, with one exception. People with ALL cells that have a specific chromosome abnormality (the "Philadel-phia chromosome") have a prognosis sim-ilar to patients with AML.

Adult patients with ALL, like children with ALL, are at risk of their leukemia eventually involving the central nervous system—the brain and spinal cord. Both treatment and prognosis are influenced by this potential complication.

AML and ALL patients are susceptible to the development of localized areas of leukemia involvement. These may show up as skin rashes or lumps in the breasts, testicles or ovaries. The prognosis is worse when these localized areas of leukemia appear.

Treatment Overview The goal of treatment is to obtain a complete and long-term remission. Anything short of that offers no substantial survival benefit. Treatment is divided into two phases:
♦ Induction. This is the attempt to attain a remission, meaning that the bone marrow appears normal.
♦ Consolidation. This involves giving the same or different treatment, even when someone appears to be in remission, because of the suspected or assumed presence of residual disease that cannot be detected.

Some patients may receive a third phase called maintenance treatment to prolong the remission. Maintenance treatment is more commonly associated with the treatment of ALL than AML.

Survival Remission rates are inversely related to age. The response rate decreases as the patient's age increases, and age is directly related to increased risk for complications and death during the induction phase of treatment. On average:
♦ Patients with AML have a 60 to 70 percent probability of having a remission. Twenty percent of those who do attain a remission can expect to survive three years or more with a possibility of being cured.
♦ Patients with ALL have an 80 to 90 percent probability of achieving a remission, with 35 to 45 percent surviving five or more years, again with a possibility of being cured.

ACUTE MYELOID LEUKEMIA (AML)
Standard Treatment Standard treatment includes two drugs, Daunomycin (daunorubicin) and Cytosar (cytosine arabinoside). These are commonly given intravenously, Daunomycin for three days and Cytosar for five to seven days.

These drugs may cause significant nausea and vomiting, so patients are also given drugs such as Benadryl, Compazine, Vistaril, Reglan and Ativan.

The chemotherapy drugs will kill normal and leukemic cells equally, so the most significant side effect besides nausea and vomiting is a temporary reduction of normal white blood cells and platelets. The deficiency of white cells means a loss of normal defenses against bacterial and fungal organisms, leaving the patient open for infections. Low platelets mean that the patient may bruise or bleed easily. All patients should be closely watched in the hospital until this effect is over.

Supportive treatment during this period includes blood and platelet transfusions and intravenous antibiotic treatment. Because of the intensive supportive treatment required, therapy for AML is given in the hospital, with the duration of hospitalization ranging from four to six weeks.

Investigational
♦ Different combinations of chemotherapy agents such as mitoxantrone and etoposide, amsacrine (AMSA) and higher doses of Cytosar alone or carboplatinum and Cytosar are being evaluated. All combinations have the common side effects of bone marrow suppression with resulting low white blood cell and platelet counts. The benefits of treatment with these newer combinations are not yet clear.
♦ Treatment with growth factors such as GM-CSF (granulocyte/macrophage colony stimulating factor) or G-CSF (granulocyte colony stimulating factor), or differentiation agents such as HMBA, or cisor trans-retinoic acid are also being evaluated. It is hoped that treatment with these agents will be less toxic and more

effective than current chemotherapy programs.

♦ Another new concept in therapy involves using specific antibodies. These are proteins that bind to leukemia cells and not to normal cells. The antibodies can carry some cell killing agent such as ricin or radioactive isotopes directly to the leukemia cells, letting the agent kill the leukemia cells while sparing the normal white blood cells and platelets. In this way, complications such as infection and bleeding may be avoided. Results on this type of treatment will be available in the next few years.

ACUTE LYMPHOBLASTIC LEUKEMIA (ALL)

Standard Treatment ALL patients have a higher response rate to chemotherapy than do patients with AML and more drugs are available to treat this form of the disease. Drugs commonly used for induction treatment include vincristine (Oncovin), prednisone, daunomycin (Daunorubicin) or doxorubicin (Adriamycin), L-asparaginase, Cytoxan and Cytosar.

Again, treatment includes an induction and consolidation phase, and generally a maintenance phase for one to two years. Because of the known risk of central nervous system leukemia (leukemic meningitis), patients are also treated with chemotherapy (usually methotrexate) via a spinal tap or an Ommaya reservoir surgically implanted under the scalp or by radiation therapy to the head in an effort to prevent this complication. As with AML treatment, most patients will be in the hospital when treatment is started.

Investigational

♦ New combinations of chemotherapy agents or different ways of administering the drugs are being evaluated, along with monoclonal antibodies.
♦ Bone marrow transplantation.

CHRONIC LEUKEMIA

Like acute leukemia, there are two major categories based on cell appearance, histochemical stains and biological markers. Because chronic leukemias involve cells that are either mature or become mature, these cells may have a normal appearance.

The two major types of chronic leukemia are chronic myelogenous leukemia (CML) and chronic lymphocytic leukemia (CLL). They are easily distinguished under the microscope.

♦ CLL involves mature lymphocytes, cells that differ from the cells in CML in size, nuclear pattern and generally by the absence of cellular particles. The diagnosis of CLL can be confirmed by cell surface marker studies. These studies can be particularly helpful because sometimes appearance alone may not distinguish between CLL and lymphoma.

♦ The CML cells are larger and appear normal. Chromosome studies on CML cells are sometimes needed to tell the difference between a person with CML or preleukemia (myelodysplastic syndrome) or even someone with a normal elevation in peripheral blood counts because of an infection. The more sensitive DNA analysis of the CML cells may be used to confirm a diagnosis. In 80 to 90 percent of CML patients, the chromosomal and DNA abnormality will confirm the presence of the (abnormal) Philadelphia chromosome.

Most people with CML and CLL have a high white blood cell count but may have few or no symptoms. A good number of these cases are diagnosed on a routine blood test performed as part of a routine or pre-employment physical examination. A doctor may find an enlarged spleen in someone with CML, and enlarged lymph nodes, with or without an enlarged spleen, in those with CLL.

CHRONIC LYMPHOCYTIC LEUKEMIA (CLL)

The decision on whether or when to treat

patients with CLL depends on many factors, including the stage of disease. Because CLL is not curable and because it generally occurs in older people without symptoms and often progresses slowly, it is usually treated in a conservative fashion.

Standard Treatment In the early stages, most patients do not require any treatment. In a typical case, the white blood cell count is very high but there are no symptoms. Management ranges from periodic observation by the physician (with treatment of infection, bleeding or immunologic complications as they occur) to standard chemotherapy.

In moderate to advanced disease—RAI Stage II, III, IV or International B and C—observation without treatment may still be the plan if there are no symptoms and the CLL does not progress.

If therapy is indicated because of symptoms or signs—enlarging lymph nodes or spleen or adversely changing blood counts—the conventional treatment is chemotherapy with medications taken by mouth such as Leukeran and Cytoxan, singly or in combination with a steroid preparation like prednisone.

On uncommon occasions when there is one single site of lymph node enlargement, radiation to the site is appropriate. The use of total lymph node irradiation for CLL is no longer used as conventional treatment.

Investigational Patients with newly diagnosed CLL or early stage CLL are generally not candidates for investigational treatments.

♦ Chemotherapy agents are constantly being developed. Fludarabine is now being tried as a single agent or in combination with conventional drugs. Results show some activity, but it is too soon to know the full effectiveness of this drug. It has recently become available to practicing medical oncologists for use with people who are resistant to standard therapy.

♦ Cytokines and biologic response modifiers such as monoclonal antibodies, interferon-alpha and 2'-deoxycoformycin are being evaluated.

CHRONIC MYELOGENOUS LEUKEMIA (CML)

This chronic leukemia affects the myeloid cell line rather than the lymphocytes. The disease usually affects people in their fifth and sixth decades of life, but may occur even in infants.

The average survival for people with CML is 42 to 45 months with current therapies. About 60 to 70 percent of CML patients with the Philadelphia chromosome abnormality will progress into an acute or blastic phase. Without change in treatment at this stage, the average survival is four or five months.

The only possible chance for a longer survival or possible cure is the use of an allogeneic bone marrow transplant while the disease is in the chronic phase. With such a transplant soon after diagnosis, there will perhaps be a 25 to 40 percent chance for a longer survival. Once the disease is in the blastic phase, even with intensive treatment similar to the treatment for acute leukemia there is only about a 20 percent response rate at best, with the duration of the response generally less than a year.

Since no standard treatment offers a cure, prevents the blastic phase from occurring or prolongs the average survival, all newly diagnosed patients should be considered for an allogeneic marrow transplant and for clinical trials of new therapeutic approaches.

Standard Treatment Most CML patients have unusually high white blood cell counts, so the initial standard therapy tries to lower the counts toward more normal levels. There are two ways of doing this:

♦ Chemotherapy is the most common method, with either Hydrea or Myleran taken as an oral medication. Both are effective and offer excellent control over a prolonged period. Myleran is longer acting and has the potential of over-dosage unless the blood counts are followed closely. It also has the potential long-term side effect of causing lung complications. Hydrea also has to be monitored closely by the physician. It is a much shorter acting drug so the problem of overdosage is less. Hydrea has no known complications after long-term use, so it is now more in favor as the chemotherapy agent for CML.

Along with these drugs, patients with CML who have unusually high counts will be placed on Zyloprim (allopurinol). This drug prevents high levels of uric acid that can be caused by the rapid killing of the leukemia cells. A high level of uric acid may cause problems such as kidney stones or impaired kidney function.

♦ The other method is called leukopheresis. This is effective, but generally only as a short-term means of control.

Leukopheresis involves using a mechanical centrifuge machine to remove the white blood cells. To perform this procedure, a large needle is placed in a vein in each arm. The needles are attached to a catheter, which allows the blood from one arm to run into the centrifuge. There the white cells are separated out and the remaining blood cells and plasma are returned through the other arm. The procedure takes two to three hours.

The white blood count will stay lowered for a few days to a few weeks before the procedure has to be repeated. Obviously, this is not an acceptable method for controlling the disease over a long time. But it may be useful over a brief period, especially if the white blood count is very high, which is associated with risks of brain complications (strokes) as well as respiratory and vascular complications.

Further therapy may involve the removal of the spleen if it is enlarged, causing symptoms and not responding to chemotherapy. In rare cases, the spleen may be removed to improve the abnormally low counts of normal blood cells caused by the removal of these cells by the spleen.

Investigational

♦ Interferon-alpha, a biologic protein given by injection first daily then several times a week, has been shown in CML patients to effectively control white blood counts and decrease the size of the spleen. It has also been effective in reducing the number of leukemia cells with the Philadelphia chromosome in the marrow for a short period (months to one or two years). Early results indicate an improved survival in patients who respond to interferon.

Bone Marrow Transplantation All patients under 50 should be tissue-typed along with their immediate family members to determine if there is a relative who could be a marrow donor. If there is, then an allogeneic marrow transplant should be considered.

The current consensus is that a marrow transplant should be performed within two years of diagnosis. Transplants further from diagnosis have been performed, but preliminary results have not been as good as when transplants were performed earlier in the course of the disease.

Again, marrow transplantation is the only treatment that offers the chance of a cure to CML patients. There is a 20 percent probability that a transplant patient may die during or shortly after the transplant from a variety of problems—infections, graft rejection, graft-versus-host (GVH) problems, lung complications and bleeding. Patients who survive the procedure are also susceptible to a recurrence of the disease.

MISCELLANEOUS LEUKEMIAS

This is a group of leukemias rarely seen in adults. They either do not belong to the usual classification of acute and chronic leukemias or are unusual variations of the forms already described.

HAIRY CELL LEUKEMIA

This is a moderately rare leukemia that is more like a chronic than an acute leukemia.

The diagnosis is usually made by reviewing the bone marrow and blood smear and finding a lymphoid cell, a cell that uniquely describes this leukemia. Some special blood stains and antibodies help confirm the diagnosis made on the marrow. The tartrate resistant acid phosphatase (TRAP) stain, for example, is diagnostic for hairy cell leukemia.

People who get this leukemia are usually elderly and go to their doctor with symptoms of weakness and/or after finding a lump in their abdomen, which is an enlarged spleen. Blood counts are abnormal. Usually the white count is low and in some cases the counts of red cells and platelets are also low.

This disease is rarely cured and about 10 percent of patients may not need treatment for years. Patients may have prolonged survival with treatment.

Standard Treatment Before 1985, the recommended standard treatment was quite limited. The surgical removal of the spleen relieved symptoms and improved the blood counts in over 60 percent of the patients. But about half of those who did show improvement from the splenectomy would again get the same symptoms. The best long-term response to a splenectomy is found in patients with a very enlarged spleen.

Now there is an effective form of treatment in addition to or instead of removing the spleen. Interferon-alpha treatment without a splenectomy began in 1985 and is effective in 70 to 80 percent of patients. Interferon-alpha is given by injection, daily at first, then usually three times a week. Patients are taught how to give themselves interferon just as diabetics are taught how to inject insulin.

Most patients continue the treatment for two years. When the interferon is discontinued, about a quarter to a third of patients will develop the disease again. At that time, retreatment with interferon, removal of the spleen or treatment with newer forms of treatment might be used.

Investigational
♦ Preliminary results with a new drug— 2'-deoxycoformycin (pentostatin)—seem to show that this compound is just as effective or more effective than interferon. More important, it has been found to be effective in cases where interferon-alpha is not.
♦ Another new agent, 2-chlorodeoxy-adenosine, is showing great promise, but its final role has yet to be determined.

PROLYMPHOCYTIC LEUKEMIA

It is difficult to distinguish this rare leukemia from chronic lymphocytic leukemia and some types of lymphoma.

Like hairy cell leukemia, the diagnosis is made by examining the cells in blood and bone marrow samples. Even the most current technologic methods find it difficult to specifically identify lymphocytic cells as to their placement in the diagnosis of CLL or lymphoma.

The clinical course is moderately aggressive with enlarging spleens, lymph nodes and progressive blood count change.

Standard Treatment Chemotherapy with the drugs used in the treatment of CLL or lymphoma.

MEGAKARYOCYTIC, BASOPHILIC AND EOSINOPHILIC LEUKEMIA

These extremely rare leukemias are probably associated with the blastic phase of chronic myelogenous leukemia.

Because they are so rare, there is no standard treatment. People with these forms of the disease are managed like those who have acute non-lymphoblastic leukemia.

The prognosis and survival rates with these leukemias are very poor.

THE MOST IMPORTANT QUESTIONS YOU CAN ASK

♦ What is the prognosis for my type of leukemia?

♦ Is treatment necessary immediately? If not, when will it be necessary and how do you decide when to start?

♦ What type of treatment is needed and what are the chances of a response?

♦ How long will the treatment continue?

♦ What are the risks and complications?

♦ Are any investigational treatments available?

♦ Should the treatment be done at the local community hospital or should it be directed or done at a major specialty institution?

LIVER
Alan P. Venook, MD

◇

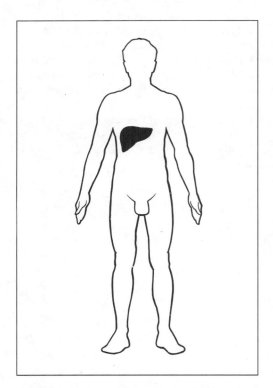

Primary liver cancer—also called hepato-cellular carcinoma or hepatoma—may be the most common cancer worldwide. It occurs with great frequency in Asia and Africa, but is relatively uncommon in the United States. About 4,000 cases are diagnosed yearly in the U.S., although immigration patterns are changing the rates at which primary liver cancer is seen in this country.

Partly because it is so uncommon here, liver cancer is generally not suspected and is at an advanced stage by the time it is diagnosed. Because the liver plays a vital role in removing toxins from the blood,

cancer within it causes major metabolic problems. The treatment now available for advanced liver cancer is not particularly effective, and the principal goal of therapy is to relieve the symptoms related to the disease.

Types The most common type of cancer originating in the liver itself—referred to as primary liver cancer—develops in liver cells and is called hepatocellular carcinoma. Rarely, tumors arise from blood vessels in the liver (hemangioendothelioma), other glands in the liver (adenocarcinoma) or connective tissue in the liver (sarcoma, angiosarcoma). An unusual type of hepatocellular carcinoma called fibrolamellar tends to occur in young women. Tumors that develop in the bile ducts are called cholangiocarcinomas (*see* "Bile Duct").

Most commonly, cancer in the liver has spread there from another organ and is therefore a type of metastatic cancer (*see* "Metastatic Cancer").

How It Spreads Liver cancers can spread to other areas through either the lymph system or the blood. Most often the cancer first moves into the lymph nodes in the region of the liver (porta hepatis), then goes to other lymph nodes or into the lung or bones. Tumor cells can also spread into the abdominal cavity, causing the accumulation of fluid (ascites) or masses elsewhere in the abdomen (*see* Gall Bladder, page 334).

What Causes It Hepatocellular carcinoma most often develops in damaged livers. Long-standing infection with either the hepatitis B or hepatitis C virus often precedes it and is therefore seen as a significant risk factor.

Cirrhosis of the liver (from, for example, a viral infection, alcohol, toxin exposure or a genetic defect of metabolism) also increases the likelihood of hepatocellular carcinoma, presumably because of chronic inflammation in the liver. In fact, an estimated 5 percent of all people with cirrhosis of the liver will eventually develop liver cancer. Fifty to 80 percent of all people with liver cancer have cirrhosis.

Certain chemicals are associated with increased liver cancer, and a link has been established with a plant fungus (aflatoxin) that is ingested with the normal diet in a region in Africa. Oral steroid use may also increase the risk.

RISK FACTORS

At Significantly Higher Risk

♦ Worldwide, men are twice as likely as women to develop liver cancer.

♦ Chronic hepatitis B and/or hepatitis C virus infection, with or without cirrhosis of the liver. The usual route of transmission of hepatitis B and C is through blood transfusions or drug needles. Because hepatitis B virus may also be transmitted by a mother to her offspring during pregnancy or childbirth or may be transmitted between partners during sexual intercourse, it is not unusual for members of the same family to develop liver cancer after becoming infected with hepatitis B.

♦ Cirrhosis of the liver from any cause—alcohol damage or inborn errors of metabolism such as hemochromatosis or enzyme deficiencies.

♦ Exposure to aflatoxin, a fungus contaminant found in the soil in Africa.

♦ Exposure to the fumes of vinyl chloride or to Thorotrast (a contrast material no longer used for radiologic procedures) is associated with an increased risk of angiosarcoma of the liver but not hepatocellular carcinoma.

At Slightly Higher Risk

♦ Anabolic steroid use, as by weightlifters and other athletes, is known to increase the risk of benign liver tumors and may cause an increase in liver cancer.

♦ Estrogen therapy, such as oral contraceptives, may increase the risk, although this has not been proven.

SCREENING

People with known chronic hepatitis and/or cirrhosis of the liver may benefit from the use of screening tests to try to find the cancer before it has spread beyond the liver. Thorough screening includes frequent monitoring of serum alpha-fetoprotein (a product found in the blood of 50 to 70 percent of all hepatocellular carcinoma patients in the U.S. and more commonly worldwide) and ultrasound of the liver. These tests are not useful for identifying primary liver tumors other than hepatocellular carcinoma.

Although these screening methods may be useful in Asia and Africa, where liver cancer is very common, they are not routinely used in North America because of this cancer's rarity. Screening of hepatitis B virus-infected Asian and African immigrants to the U.S. may be beneficial.

COMMON SIGNS AND SYMPTOMS

Common symptoms include bloating, abdominal pain, fever, weight loss, decreased appetite and nausea. But because liver cancer is so rare, its symptoms are usually attributed to more common, benign conditions. Frequently, the diagnosis of cancer is not considered until these symptoms persist or until a person develops an enlarging abdominal mass or fluid in the abdomen. Jaundice (the skin turning yellow) and swelling in the legs are usually associated with more advanced tumors. Sometimes, people with liver cancer feel entirely well.

DIAGNOSIS

Physical Examination

There are no findings specific only to liver cancer on physical examination. Findings may include the following, all of which may have other explanations:

♦ Fever.
♦ Enlarged liver and spleen.
♦ Enlarged, hard lymph nodes.
♦ Swelling of the abdomen from fluid (ascites).
♦ Jaundice (the skin turning yellow).
♦ Swelling of the legs (edema).

Blood and Other Tests

♦ A complete blood count may be normal or may show a decrease (anemia) or increase in red blood cells.

♦ Routine liver function studies—blood tests measuring serum bilirubin and liver enzymes—may be abnormal, but can be entirely normal even in advanced stages of primary liver cancer.

♦ Prothrombin Time and Partial Thromboplastin Time (PT and PTT) tests of clotting—usually done if a liver problem is suspected—may be abnormal.

♦ The serum alpha-fetoprotein (AFP) is elevated in 50 to 70 percent of people in the U.S. with primary liver cancer. It may also be elevated in people with germ cell cancer, gastric cancer or cirrhosis of the liver or in pregnant women.

Imaging

♦ Abdominal ultrasound can evaluate the density of the liver if there is a suspicion of a mass. It can reveal the presence of fluid in the abdomen and is particularly useful for distinguishing a solid mass from a non-cancerous accumulation of fluid within the liver (benign cyst).

♦ A CT scan is useful for determining the extent of a tumor within the liver and evaluating the possible extension of tumorous tissue into lymph nodes or to other structures within the abdomen.

♦ Magnetic resonance imaging (MRI) may be helpful in determining if the liver cancer can be surgically removed by revealing whether the tumor involves both lobes of the liver or is invading blood vessels. Usually, MRI is not necessary because the CT scan provides essentially the same information.

♦ An x-ray involving the injection of dye into the artery going to the liver (arteriography) is necessary before any attempts are made to remove the tumor, since the surgeon needs to know exactly what the blood supply of the tumor is in order to remove it.

♦ If surgery is being considered, a chest x-ray should be done. If the cancer has spread to the lungs or any other organ, surgery should be reconsidered.

Endoscopy and Biopsy

♦ Biopsy, either by fine needle aspiration (FNA) or with a regular needle, is almost always necessary. This procedure can be done through the skin without significant danger. Because of the variation in the tumor cells of different types of cancer, the biopsy sample can be used to distinguish between a primary liver cancer or a cancer that has spread from another organ. Occasionally, if the AFP is extremely high and the tumor very large, a biopsy may not be necessary.

STAGING

Although a TNM staging system exists for hepatocellular carcinoma, for purposes of deciding about therapeutic options, there are only three stages—localized resectable, localized unresectable and advanced disease.

TREATMENT OVERVIEW

Surgery is the only way to cure primary liver cancer, so the goal of the diagnostic work-up is to discover if all the cancerous tissue can be removed. This is often not possible, either because the tumor has already spread beyond the liver or because the liver is too damaged and removal of liver tissue would leave a person without enough liver function to survive.

Chemotherapy and radiation therapy are occasionally helpful in relieving symptoms. Primary liver cancer may progress rapidly, but these and other measures can be taken to maintain the quality of life. Newer treatments, such as more effective chemotherapy or liver transplantation, may someday allow the surgical removal of cancers now felt to be inoperable.

Surgery Surgery can cure liver cancer if the entire tumor can be removed. The liver has two distinct lobes—right and left— and a tumor confined to one lobe can often be removed even if the patient has cirrhosis of the liver. If cirrhosis is only minimally or not at all present, a tumor involving parts of both lobes of the liver can be removed with an extensive operation (trisegmentectomy). This surgery is potentially dangerous, however, and people with poor liver function may not survive it.

Liver transplantation may be considered for someone whose cancer has not yet spread and who cannot tolerate the removal of part of the liver because of underlying liver disease or the size of the tumor. So far, this approach has been beneficial only in people with the fibrolamellar variant. Even if patients with hepatocellular carcinoma have no evidence of metastases, the tumor almost always redevelops after transplantation, perhaps because of the suppression of the immune system that allows the transplanted liver to function. Rarely, cancer is not found in the liver until after a person has had a transplant for another reason. Such patients may be cured because the cancer is in an earlier stage.

The presence of tumor anywhere else in the body—lung, bone or lymph nodes, for example—means that removal of the liver tumor alone will not bring about a cure. If the disease has already metasta-sized, removing part of a liver tumor is not considered beneficial because of the side effects of surgery, including a long recuperative period.

♦ **Investigational** A new surgical technique called cryosurgery involves freezing the tumor tissue by placing a cold probe directly into it. A tumor that cannot be removed because it is too close to blood vessels or because of extensive underlying liver disease may be "killed" by this technique. The effectiveness of this therapy is being evaluated.

Chemotherapy Chemotherapy may result in tumor shrinkage, but this does not necessarily prolong survival. The standard drug, Adriamycin, may shrink tumors in 15 to 20 percent of patients and seems to help some. But the side effects of this drug, including nausea, vomiting and hair loss, may leave patients in a worse condition even if the tumor shrinks. Other drugs that may decrease the tumor size are 5-fluorouracil, mitomycin-C, etoposide and mitoxantrone, although these have similar side effects to Adriamycin.

These drugs seem to shrink tumors more successfully when administered directly into the liver via the hepatic artery. Although tumors within the liver regress in about 50 percent of patients, the therapy is difficult to give and is extremely toxic to an already damaged liver. Because few patients feel better after such therapy and because distant metastases nearly always develop, it is generally not advisable to surgically implant an infusion device into the hepatic artery.

♦ **Investigational** There is substantial experience in Asia and at some institutions in the U.S. with a process called chemoembolization. This involves administering a combination of chemotherapy and colloid particles directly into the liver tumor via its main (hepatic) artery.

Generally, it is performed as a single treatment and does not require surgery or prolonged bed rest. Preliminary results show that tumors will shrink in about 50 percent of patients, although prolonged survival has not been proven.

There may also be a role for chemoembolization before the surgical removal of the liver tumor, since significant shrinkage may enable the removal of a previously unresectable tumor. This has not yet been proven, however.

Radiation The usefulness of radiation is limited in liver cancer because it is extremely damaging to non-cancerous liver tissue. It is sometimes used to treat the liver area after a tumor has been removed, although this has not been shown to be of definite benefit. The principal role for radiation is the management of painful liver masses or metastases.

♦ **Investigational** The combination of external beam radiation, chemotherapy and a unique antitumor monoclonal antibody has been shown recently to benefit some patients with otherwise unresectable cancer. The effectiveness of this combination is still not certain. Institutions studying this therapy are best equipped to perform it.

TREATMENT BY STAGE

LOCALIZED RESECTABLE

The tumor is confined to a portion of the liver that allows for its complete surgical removal. The tumor may be localized to either the right or the left lobe of the liver or possibly involve the right lobe and only a portion of the left lobe.

Standard Treatment Surgery is the standard therapy but depends on the relative health of the remaining underlying liver, since a person with cirrhosis of the liver may not be able to tolerate the removal of one-half or two-thirds of the liver tissue. Surgery also depends on the presence of a clear zone between the tumor and the neighboring blood vessels. Only a small percentage of people are candidates for surgery and, unfortunately, the majority experience a tumor recurrence.

Five-Year Survival 10 to 30 percent

Investigational
♦ The role for chemotherapy after surgery is unknown. Although Adriamycin is often recommended, no systematic studies have been done to see if it increases the chances of cure.
♦ Similarly, radiation is often applied to the liver area after surgery but has never been proven to be beneficial in such patients.

LOCALIZED UNRESECTABLE
Despite being a localized mass, the tumor may be unresectable because crucial blood vessel structures are involved or because the liver is impaired.

Standard Treatment There is no standard therapy, so patients should be considered for clinical trials.

Two-Year Survival Less than 5 percent

Investigational
♦ Liver transplantation may be attempted in patients who are deemed unresectable because of poor liver function and whose tumors are not intertwined with blood vessels in the abdomen. This has been shown to be beneficial in patients with the fibrolamellar variety of liver cancer, but people with a more typical cancer invariably develop tumor metastases shortly after transplantation.
♦ Cryosurgery holds some promise to allow the removal of otherwise unresectable tumors, but the technique is done only by a few specialized physicians.

♦ Radiation and an antibody that identifies and attacks liver tumor cells (the polyclonal antiferritin antibody) may allow some patients to be treated surgically, as might chemoembolization.

ADVANCED DISEASE
The tumor involves all lobes of the liver and/or has spread to involve other organs such as the lungs, intra-abdominal lymph nodes or bone.

Standard Treatment No standard therapy is known to prolong survival. The usual approach is a trial of single-agent chemotherapy such as Adriamycin or 5-fluorouracil. Radiation to the tumor along with intravenous chemotherapy may relieve the pain of large liver masses, and radiation to painful bone or other metastases may also be appropriate.

Two-Year Survival Less than 5 percent

Investigational
♦ Combination chemotherapy or new drugs may prove to be better treatment than those currently available. These would best be administered in a clinical trial, rather than using random combinations.
♦ Chemoembolization may improve symptoms even if there is metastatic disease.
♦ Newer drugs, including interleukin-2 and interferon, are being studied.

TREATING OTHER PRIMARY LIVER TUMORS
The approach taken with other primary liver tumors is generally the same as for hepatocellular carcinoma. Patients with these other tumors are more likely to be candidates for surgery because they usually do not have underlying liver disease.

ANGIOSARCOMA AND HEMANGIOENDOTHELIOMA
These diseases are less predictable than hepatocellular carcinoma and survival is variable.

♦ They may not have spread at the time of diagnosis and surgery should be considered.
♦ As in hepatocellular carcinoma, no systematic study of adjuvant chemotherapy or radiotherapy has been done.
♦ Localized unresectable disease may respond to the same intravenous chemotherapy used for sarcomas and the tumors may occasionally shrink enough to allow the surgeon to remove them completely.
♦ Advanced disease is approached in the same way as a sarcoma.

ADENOCARCINOMA
This type of tumor is approached in the same way as hepatocellular carcinoma. Its prognosis is similar.

SUPPORTIVE THERAPY
♦ Pain relievers are sometimes called for in liberal doses. Narcotics may have excessive side effects because they are metabolized by the liver, which may not be functioning properly.
♦ Non-steroidal anti-inflammatory drugs may be surprisingly effective even against the severe pain associated with liver cancer.
♦ Frequent small meals may be necessary to provide enough nutrition, since an enlarged liver might reduce the capacity of the stomach.
♦ The loss of appetite that frequently accompanies liver cancer may be relieved with a medication called Megace.
♦ The use of water pills to relieve fluid in the abdomen or legs may cause significant imbalance in kidney function and can create major problems if not carefully monitored.
♦ Nausea should be adequately treated with standard medications, including suppositories.
♦ Sleep disturbances are common. Most sleeping pills are metabolized by the liver, however, so they should be used carefully.

TREATMENT FOLLOW-UP

Careful follow-up is important after the removal of localized liver cancer because patients are at risk for a second occurrence as well as tumor metastases. Such follow-up should include:

♦ Serum alpha-fetoprotein (AFP) every two to three months. A rising AFP suggests tumor recurrence, which might still be curable with further surgery.

♦ CT scans should be done every two to three months for the first year after surgery. Tumors are most likely to grow again within the first year and they may still be curable if caught in the early stages.

♦ The liver function of patients with underlying cirrhosis or hepatitis has to be closely monitored, since it may deteriorate after surgery.

THE MOST IMPORTANT QUESTIONS YOU CAN ASK

♦ Should I see another physician to confirm that this tumor can or cannot be removed for cure?

♦ Could I benefit from an investigational therapy available at another institution?

♦ How sick will the proposed chemotherapy or radiation treatment make me relative to the potential benefit?

♦ Should any tests be done on my spouse or children to see if they are at risk for developing this cancer?

♦ Is a liver transplant an option for me?

LUNG: SMALL CELL

Alan B. Glassberg, MD

◇

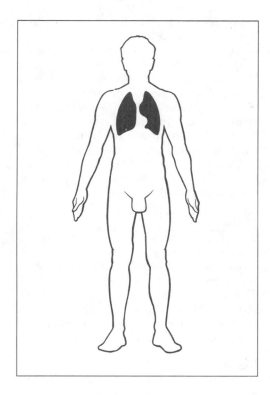

In 1991, there will be 161,000 new cases of lung cancer in the United States. Small cell lung cancer accounts for about a quarter of all lung cancer cases. Also called oat cell carcinoma of the lung, it has the most rapid clinical course of any type of lung cancer, with average survival from diagnosis of only several months without treatment. Compared with other types of lung cancer, small cell carcinoma has a greater tendency to have spread widely by the time of diagnosis, but is more responsive to treatment with chemotherapy and radiation than are the other types of lung cancer.

Seventy percent of patients with small cell carcinoma of the lung have distant metastases at the time of diagnosis. With modern staging procedures, the areas of spread can be discovered in two-thirds of these patients.

Small cell cancer is not confined to the lung. It may occur in other organs such as the esophagus or cervix and sometimes without one primary site of origin being able to be defined. The management of these tumors will be addressed in chapters concerning those organs; chemotherapy remains the fundamental basic treatment.

Types There are several kinds of small cell cancer, including oat cell, intermediate and combined. It is unclear, however, whether these are real differences or if the apparent differences are due to various methods of staining the slides during biopsies.

This tumor arises from what are called neuroendocrine cells and is known as an APUD (amine precursor uptake decarboxylation) tumor. Under the electron microscope, hormone-producing (neurosecretory) granules can be seen. These tumors, therefore, can abnormally produce hormones and cause what have been known as paraneoplastic syndromes. For example, if the tumor produces too much cortisone, the condition is called Cushing's syndrome. If antidiuretic hormone (ADH) is produced, water is retained in the body and the apparent salt (sodium) level decreases. Each of these paraneoplastic syndromes produces its own signs and symptoms.

How It Spreads Small cell lung cancer can spread via lymphatic vessels to the lymph nodes in the center of the lung (hilar nodes), the center of the chest (mediastinal nodes), in the neck and above the collarbone (supraclavicular nodes), and in the abdominal cavity. It is likely to spread through the bloodstream to the liver, lungs, brain and bone.

What Causes It Cigarette smoking has been a major factor in the development of both small cell and non-small cell lung cancers. The increase in cigarette smoking by men in the 1920s, apparently related to increased cigarette advertising about that time, was followed in the 1940s by a dramatic increase in the incidence of lung cancer in men. The marked increase in cigarette smoking by women in the 1940s, perhaps because it became more socially acceptable during the war, was unfortunately followed 20 years later by a similar increase in the incidence of lung cancer among women. It has been estimated that if all tobacco disappeared from the earth, 17 percent of all cancers would also disappear. The attempt to discontinue cigarette smoking remains one of the most crucial medical issues in our society.

Lung cancer may predispose a person to a higher risk of developing another lung cancer later.

RISK FACTORS

There are no specific environmental or genetic factors known except those discussed in the section on non-small cell lung cancer.

At Significantly Higher Risk
♦ Cigarette smokers.
♦ Workers exposed to industrial substances such as asbestos, nickel, chromium compounds and chloromethyl ether and/or air pollutants.

SCREENING

There is no good screening test for this kind of cancer.

COMMON SIGNS AND SYMPTOMS

As with non-small cell cancer, a new or changing cough, sometimes containing blood, is a common symptom, along with hoarseness and shortness of breath or increased shortness of breath on exertion. There may also be an increase in the amount of sputum, recurrent episodes of lung infection (sometimes in the same lobe of the lung as the cancer), weight loss and swelling of the face or arms.

✳ If the tumor has metastasized, the symptoms can include severe headaches, double vision, and pain in the bones, chest, abdomen, neck and down the arms.

One point that needs to be emphasized is that this disease is usually widespread at the time of diagnosis.

DIAGNOSIS

Electron microscopy can detect the neuroendocrine granules that will help differentiate between small cell and non-small cell cancers. Newer techniques of diagnosis such as oncogene analysis may show specific oncogenes. Patients with the specific oncogene of the *myc* family may experience a more aggressive course.

Blood and Other Tests
♦ Chemistry profile.
♦ Sputum (phlegm) examination.
♦ Removal of fluid from the chest and examination of it for malignant cells.

Imaging
♦ Chest x-ray.
♦ CT scan of the chest and abdomen.
♦ MRI or CT scan of the brain.
♦ Bone scan.

Endoscopy and Biopsy
♦ Fiber-optic bronchoscopy with brushings or biopsy.
♦ Mediastinoscopy with biopsies. In this safe and easy procedure, a small incision is made at the base of the neck and a long

thin tube called a mediastinoscope is inserted down to the lymph nodes in the middle of the chest. Tissue can be removed through this instrument for analysis.

♦ Needle biopsy through the chest wall, under local anesthetic and often under CT guidance.

♦ Biopsies of the chest lining, lymph nodes, bone and liver.

STAGING

The staging techniques and classifications used for non-small cell lung cancer apply as well to small cell cancer. All patients with small cell cancer initially receive the same treatment—chemotherapy—so it is not necessary to stage in the same fashion. Determining the stage by non-surgical means, however, allows a better evaluation and assessment of prognosis. Therefore, a staging evaluation is carried out.

When stage affects the choice of treatment, especially the use of chest radiation or surgical excision of the primary cancer, results of staging have therapeutic implications.

The staging procedures commonly used to document distant metastases include bone marrow examination, CT scans of the brain and liver and radionuclide bone scans. MRI scans are also used to evaluate the brain and bones.

Limited-stage means that tumor is confined to the side of the chest where it originated, the mediastinum and the supraclavicular nodes. This area can be encompassed within a tolerable radiotherapy port. There is no universally accepted definition of "limited-stage." Patients with fluid around the lung (pleural effusion), massive or multiple pulmonary tumor masses on the same side and enlarged supraclavicular nodes on the opposite side have been both included in and excluded from "limited-stage" by various treatment centers.

Extensive-stage disease means that tumor is too widespread to be included within the definition of limited-stage disease. (*See* page 409)

TREATMENT OVERVIEW

At the time of diagnosis, about one-third of patients with small cell lung carcinoma will have limited-stage disease. Most people who survive at least two years without a recurrence of the cancer come from this group. In limited disease, average survival of 10 to 16 months is a reasonable expectation with current treatments. The small proportion of patients with limited disease who can undergo surgery have an even better prognosis.

With extensive-stage disease, the prognosis is worse. Average survival is 6 to 12 months with current treatments. There is long-term disease-free survival in some patients, so treatment is certainly recommended. Patients who achieve a complete response to treatment (the tumor appears to go away completely) have the best overall survival.

In small cell lung cancer, 10 to 20 percent of patients may achieve long-term remissions with aggressive combined radiation and chemotherapy. Most of the improvement in survival has been the result of treatments dicovered by clinical trials.

 Surgery Removing the primary tumor produces little benefit with this type of cancer, although a very small number of patients might possibly benefit from surgery followed by adjuvant chemotherapy. This is an option only for those whose lung function is adequate and whose tumor is confined to the lung where it started or to the lung and the hilar lymph nodes on the same side.

 Chemotherapy Because of the frequent presence of hidden and undetectable spread to other parts of the body, chemotherapy is the cornerstone of treatment for small cell lung cancer, since it also treats tumors too small to detect. Once remission is achieved, there is no evidence that maintenance therapy is beneficial. There is little evidence that more than six months of treatment is of value.

 Radiation Doses in the range of 5,000 cGy or more are needed to control chest tumors effectively. If radiation therapy is given with combination chemotherapy, there are higher response rates and better survival than when radiation therapy is given alone. Radiation therapy plus combination chemotherapy is also superior to chemotherapy alone for controlling the primary chest tumor, but there is no evidence that this provides better control for metastatic disease.

Studies have shown some survival benefit when combined therapy is given so long as radiation therapy does not result in a delay of the administration of proper doses of chemotherapy. There are increased side effects with combined programs, and some treatment-related mortality because of lung and bone marrow toxicities.

Some patients have a tumor mass in the center of the chest that presses on the large vein draining blood from the head and arms (the superior vena cava). This pressure causes a fluid backup, resulting in swelling of the face and arms and sometimes even the brain. If this superior vena cava syndrome is present, combination chemotherapy alone can be given or radiation therapy given with it.

Because of the high frequency of brain metastases in small cell lung cancer, especially in patients with prolonged survival, prophylactic radiation of the head has been used by many physicians. This reduces the frequency of clinically detected brain metastases, especially in patients with complete responses to therapy, but has not been shown to influence survival. There may be late complications of this type of treatment, with significant neurologic, mental and thinking deficits in some long-term survivors who were given high daily dose fractionation. It may be preferable to give smaller doses each day.

It must also be emphasized that many treatment centers do not recommend the use of prophylactic brain irradiation because there has not been ample proof of a survival benefit and there is a valid concern about the neurologic side effects of the treatment. If necessary, radiation therapy can be given when the brain metastases are demonstrated to occur.

TREATMENT BY STAGE

LIMITED STAGE
Standard Treatment Limited-stage small cell lung cancer is highly responsive to treatment with combination chemotherapy. Multiple drugs are clearly superior to single-agent treatment. Current programs give objective response rates (the tumor gets smaller) of 80 to 90 percent, with complete response rates (the tumor disappears) of 45 to 75 percent.

As noted, a small minority of limited-stage patients without evidence of tumor in the mediastinum might benefit from surgery followed by adjuvant chemotherapy.

Two-Year Survival 15 percent

EXTENSIVE STAGE
Standard Treatment Extensive-stage small cell lung cancer patients are given chemotherapy in much the same fashion as those with limited-stage disease. Current programs result in response rates of 70 to 85 percent and complete response rates of 20 to 30 percent.

Combination chemotherapy regimens include CAV (cyclophosphamide + Adriamycin + vincristine), cyclophosphamide + Adriamycin + etoposide and cisplatin + etoposide. Other protocols include agents such as methotrexate, lomustine and ifosfamide.

There is no pressing need to include chest irradiation with combination chemotherapy, but radiotherapy may relieve symptoms caused by the primary tumor or metastatic disease. For example, symptoms from brain metastases and pain from bone metastases can be promptly relieved with radiation.

If the superior vena cava syndrome is present, chest irradiation may result in very rapid initial response.

Two-Year Survival 2 percent

TREATMENT FOLLOW-UP

After treatment is completed, patients should be seen every one or two months for at least two years. Visits can then be spread out, perhaps every four months for two years and every six months for another two years.

During the first two years, follow-up should include:

♦ Physical examination of the lungs, chest wall, lymph nodes and abdomen.
♦ Chest x-ray every three to four months, or more frequently if indicated.
♦ Blood chemistry tests every three to four months.
♦ Neurologic examination.

RECURRENT CANCER

If small cell lung cancer recurs, the prognosis is very poor regardless of stage or treatment. The expected average survival is two to three months, so a patient should be considered for either palliative therapy or participation in clinical trials.

♦ Palliative therapy could include chemotherapy agents that have not yet been used or radiation therapy for bone metastases or when otherwise appropriate.
♦ Other palliative treatments include measures for pain relief and orthopedic aids.

THE MOST IMPORTANT QUESTIONS YOU CAN ASK

♦ What is the stage of my disease and what is my prognosis?
♦ How sick will I be on chemotherapy and what can be done to control the side effects?
♦ If chemotherapy cannot cure my cancer, why should I expose myself to its side effects and toxicities?
♦ What is the chance that I will die from this tumor? How much time am I likely to have?

LUNG: NON-SMALL CELL

Alan B. Glassberg, MD

◇

Lung cancer is the second most common cancer. Although there has always been a higher incidence in men, the incidence in women has risen rapidly in recent years. In fact, lung cancer has now surpassed breast cancer as the number-one cancer killer of women. It has long been the number-one cancer killer of men.

An estimated 161,000 people will develop lung cancer in the U.S. in 1991, and about 143,000 people will die of it. This is especially unfortunate because it is one of the most preventable cancers. The cause is well known. It has been estimated that if all tobacco were removed from the earth, the number of cancers would fall by 17 percent.

There are two general types of lung cancer—small cell and non-small cell. The non-small cell variety is much more common, accounting for 75 percent of all lung cancer cases. Although some of these tumors can be cured by surgery, the overall five-year survival for people with this kind of cancer is only 10 percent. There has been no improvement in the survival rate in decades, which is a reflection of both the lack of a satisfactory screening test that could detect it in the early stages and, up to the present time, the lack of truly effective treatment with clear survival benefits.

Types Non-small cell cancer contains at least three distinct types—squamous cell, large cell and adenocarcinoma—but the treatment of all three is generally similar. Squamous cell carcinoma is the most common type, but for reasons not understood adenocarcinoma is increasing in frequency.

Squamous cell (epidermoid) carcinoma of the lung is the microscopic type most frequently related to smoking. This type is also more commonly associated with spread of the tumor to distant sites (metastasis), but surgical removal of the tumor along with the nearby lymph nodes more often produces a cure than in other types.

Adenocarcinoma of the lung accounts for 30 percent of all lung cancer cases. It is more common in women and is the most frequent type seen in non-smokers, although it occurs in smokers as well. It is more likely than other types to be in the peripheral portions of the lung (near the edge) and therefore may invade the lining of the chest and produce fluid in the chest cavity more commonly than in other types.

Large cell carcinoma of the lung is more commonly associated with spread of the tumor to the brain.

How It Spreads Non-small cell cancer can spread by the lymphatic route and through the blood. It can also directly invade to involve the center of the chest (mediastinum), the lining of the chest, the ribs or, if it is in the top part of the lung, the nerves and blood vessels leading into the arm. When this kind of cancer enters the bloodstream, it can spread to distant sites such as the liver, bones, the brain and other places in the lung.

What Causes It Cigarette smoking has been a major factor in the development of both small cell and non-small cell lung cancers. The increase in cigarette smoking by men in the 1920s, apparently related to increased cigarette advertising about that time, was followed in the 1940s by a dramatic increase in the incidence of lung cancer in men. The marked increase in cigarette smoking by women in the 1940s, perhaps because it became more socially acceptable during the war, was unfortunately followed 20 years later by a similar increase in the incidence of lung cancer among women.

Lung tissue affected by the connective tissue disease scleroderma may be associated with bronchoalveolar carcinoma. Lung cancer may predispose a person to a higher incidence of developing another lung cancer later. Lung cancer may also occur at sites of old scars in the lung resulting from an infection (tuberculosis, for example) or injury (scar carcinoma).

RISK FACTORS

At Significantly Higher Risk

♦ Cigarette smokers.

♦ The male to female ratio remains 4 to 1. Peak incidence occurs between ages 50 and 60, with less than a 1 percent incidence under the age of 30 and about a 10 percent incidence in people over 70.

♦ Workers exposed to industrial substances such as asbestos, nickel, chromium compounds and chloromethyl ether, especially those who smoke.

At Slightly Higher Risk

♦ Patients with previous or pre-existing lung disease.

♦ Former smokers.

♦ People exposed to second-hand smoke over many years.

♦ People exposed to Radon.

SCREENING

Lung cancer is very difficult to detect at an early stage. Tests such as the examination of sputum (phlegm) for malignant cells and regular chest x-rays have not proved to be beneficial. Cancer may be detected earlier in cigarette smokers, however, by regular chest x-rays.

COMMON SIGNS AND SYMPTOMS

A new or changing cough, sometimes containing blood, is a common symptom, along with hoarseness and shortness of breath or increased shortness of breath during exertion. There may also be an increase in the amount of sputum, recurrent episodes of lung infection (sometimes in the same lobe of the lung as the cancer), weight loss and swelling of the face or arms.

If the tumor has spread or metastasized, the symptoms can include severe headaches, double vision, and pain in bones, the chest, abdomen, neck and down the arms.

DIAGNOSIS

Physical Examination

♦ Lymph node enlargement in the neck or in the region above the collarbones.

♦ Enlarged liver or another mass in the abdomen.

♦ Signs of a mass in one lung such as decreased breath sounds, noises in the lung that are not usually present, or areas of dullness when the chest is tapped with the fingers.

Blood and Other Tests

♦ Sputum examination for malignant cells.

Imaging

♦ If a chest x-ray shows an abnormality, this does not establish a diagnosis until some tissue is obtained and examined under the microscope.

♦ CT scans of the chest and often the liver and adrenal glands.

♦ Sometimes CT or MRI scans of the brain.

Endoscopy and Biopsy

♦ Fiber-optic bronchoscopy with brushing or biopsy.

♦ Mediastinoscopy with biopsies. In this

procedure, a small incision is made at the base of the neck and a long thin tube called a mediastinoscope is inserted down to the lymph nodes in the middle of the chest. Tissue can be obtained through this instrument, and the procedure is safe and easy.

♦ Needle aspiration of a mass in the chest, often with CT guidance.

♦ Removal and analysis of fluid in the chest to detect tumor cells.

♦ Pleural (chest lining) biopsy.

♦ Lymph node biopsy.

♦ Bone biopsy.

♦ Liver biopsy.

♦ Biopsy of a nodule during surgery.

♦ DNA analysis. With the advent of genetic probe studies, certain genes appear to be more frequent in patients who develop lung cancer. Patients with amplification of the k-*ras* oncogene, for example, have a much worse prognosis. There may come a time when we can have our genes analyzed and be made aware of our risks, not only for lung cancer but for other cancers as well.

STAGING

Once a diagnosis of a malignant tumor is made, further staging studies are carried out because the stage of disease determines prognosis and the selection of treatment.

Stage is based on a combination of clinical findings (physical examination, chest x-ray and lab studies) and pathologic findings (biopsy). The stages are now commonly defined according to the TNM classification.

TREATMENT OVERVIEW

 Surgery Surgical treatment—removal of the tumor—remains the mainstay of curative treatment for non-small cell lung cancer. This will involve removing a lobe of the lung or, if appropriate, a wedge resection of the tumor. Sometimes the entire lung has to be removed.

 Radiation If surgery is not considered feasible either because of the patient's condition or because the lymph nodes are so involved that surgery could not remove all the cancer, then radiation therapy can be used as the primary treatment.

 Chemotherapy The role of chemotherapy has not yet been completely defined, although it has been found to be more successful since the advent of platinum compounds. Up through Stage II disease, the response rate has been reported to be in excess of 50 percent. In Stage IV disease, the response rate is lower.

When a platinum drug is combined with drugs such as vinblastine, vindesine or etoposide, response rates of about 30 percent have been observed in Stage IV cancer. Although there is no evidence of major survival improvement by the use of these agents in Stage IV disease, they may give palliative benefit by reducing the size of the tumors and relieving the symptoms. Recent trials using a cisplatin-based regimen showed a four- to five-month improvement in average survival. This exciting work has suggested that chemotherapy might be used earlier in treatment in hopes of improving survival.

Neoadjuvant Chemotherapy and Radiation New protocols to explore curative strategies in lung cancer include using chemotherapy, radiation therapy or both before surgery to try to convert some patients from an inoperable stage to one where the tumor can be removed. Examples are the use of cancer chemotherapy initially in Stage IIIB lung cancer patients. Several studies have indicated that this approach may be beneficial, although it is too early to make any definite claims about this technique.

In view of the poor survival rate in Stage IIIA lung cancer, similar studies have been carried out using chemotherapy and radiation therapy before surgery in patients who are potentially operable. Again, preliminary results are providing optimism about the future management of locally advanced lung cancer.

 Laser Therapy Laser bronchoscopy with light-sensitizers has been an interesting experimental technique to try to open the airways when they are blocked by a tumor (*see* Chapter 9).

Bone Marrow Transplantation A general principle of chemotherapy has been to increase the dose to increase the destruction of tumor cells. Generally, the amount of chemotherapy that can be given is limited by the effect of the drugs on the bone marrow. If these effects could be overcome, higher dosages could be given.

Accordingly, autologous bone marrow transplantation is being investigated. In this technique, bone marrow is removed from the patient and stored while very high doses of chemotherapy are administered. This could be lethal but the patient is "rescued" by reinfusion of his or her own bone marrow, which then grows back. It is not yet known whether this will result in longer survival.

TREATMENT BY STAGE

STAGE I
TNM T1–2, N0, M0
The tumor can be removed surgically and has not spread to involve the lymph nodes.

Standard Treatment If possible, the tumor is removed along with the nearby lymph nodes. At times, such as with a T1 tumor, only the tumor rather than the entire lobe of the lung has to be removed.

Some patients are unable to withstand surgery because of severe lung or heart disease. In those cases, radiation therapy is sometimes used. Patients who have impaired lung function may be consid-

ered for a lesser operation such as a wedge resection of the primary tumor.

Five-Year Survival 30 to 80 percent

STAGE II
TNM T1–2, N1, M0
The tumor has spread to the hilar nodes.

Standard Treatment This stage is likewise treated with surgery. Once again, patients unable to withstand this kind of rigorous surgery may be candidates for radiation therapy with intent to cure.

Five-Year Survival 10 to 35 percent

Investigational
♦ Trials are exploring the use of radiation therapy and/or chemotherapy before surgery to see if the cure rate can be improved.

STAGE IIIA
TNM T1–2, N2, M0 or T3, N0–2, M0
Stage III is divided into IIIA and IIIB. Both show involvement of nodes in the center of the chest, but Stage IIIA tumors may be removed under certain circumstances.

Standard Treatment These tumors are treated mainly with radiation therapy, surgery or both, depending on the clinical circumstances.

Although most patients do not completely respond to radiation therapy alone, 5 to 10 percent do experience long-term survival benefit.

Radiation therapy is frequently given after surgery. Although there is no evidence that this improves survival, there can be a decrease in recurrences at the original tumor site.

Patients whose tumors invade the chest wall can sometimes be treated with surgery, which may involve the removal of some of the chest wall, including ribs. Radiation therapy is often used along with surgery.

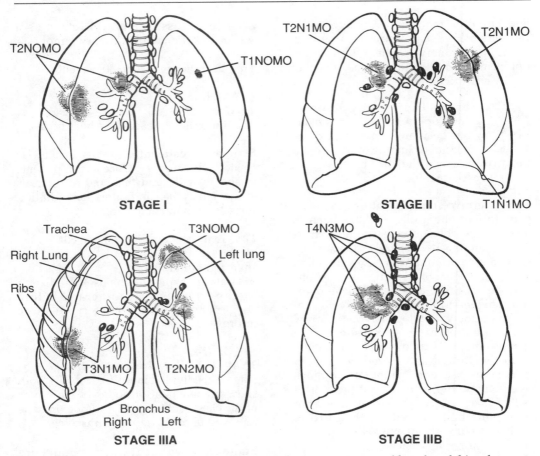

Stages of Lung Cancer, showing size and location of primary cancer, and lymph nodal involvement
Credit: Based on drawings in *Contemporary Internal Medicine* Sept. 1990.

Some patents with extensive metastatic disease in the center of the chest may develop what is called the superior vena cava syndrome, in which the great vessels in the chest are compressed by the tumor. When this involves the large vein that returns blood to the heart, the blood gets backed up into the tissues of the neck, head and arms. This is an urgent situation and patients should be given prompt radiation therapy.

A special situation under Stage III is called a superior sulcus tumor, which involves cancers in the top of the lung that invade local nerves and cause pain in the arm. These tumors seem to have a reduced potential for distant metastases, so local radiation therapy is possible for cure. Surgery is frequently used after radiation.

Five-Year Survival 10 to 15 percent

Investigational
♦ Adjuvant chemotherapy must still be considered investigational, but it can provide a slight increase in disease-free survival and a trend toward improved overall survival.

♦ Treatment with radiation or chemotherapy or both before surgery has been used on an investigational basis.

Preliminary results suggest that there may be benefit by combining all three treatments in selected cases. Newer trials are giving cisplatin + etoposide together with radiation, followed by surgery.

STAGE IIIB
TNM Any T, N3, M0 or T4, any N, M0
The tumor cannot be removed because of technical reasons or because there would be no benefit to the patient.

Standard Treatment These tumors are best managed with radiation therapy. Surgery usually has no benefit at this stage.

Five-Year Survival Less than 5 percent

Investigational
♦ Trials are examining the effectiveness of chemotherapy and/or radiation therapy before surgery. These treatments have occasionally converted some patients to an operable stage, but it is too soon to know if using this aggressive approach will increase the rate of cure.

STAGE IV
TNM Any T, any N, M1
The cancer has spread to distant sites.

Standard Treatment Metastatic disease cannot be cured by surgery, so treatment for this stage is directed toward relieving symptoms with either radiation therapy or chemotherapy.

Radiation may relieve local symptoms such as tracheal, esophageal or bronchial compression, bone or brain metastases, pain, vocal cord paralysis, coughing blood (hemoptysis) or superior vena cava syndrome. Patients without symptoms should be kept under close observation. Sometimes treatment may appropriately be deferred until symptoms or signs of a progressive tumor develop.

Chemotherapy with, for example, a platinum compound combined with drugs such as vinblastine, vindesine, etoposide or mitomycin-C has response rates of about 30 percent in Stage IV cases. Although there has been no evidence of major survival improvement with these agents, they may give palliative benefit by reducing the size of the tumors and relieving symptoms.

Recent trials using a cisplatin-based regimen of chemotherapy showed some survival benefit and give hope for more benefit in the future. Combinations currently in use include: cisplatin + etoposide, carboplatin + etoposide, cisplatin + mitomycin-C + vinblastine and cisplatin + etoposide + ifosfamide.

Other useful adjuncts to the treatment of advanced lung cancer include feeding gastrostomies when the esophagus is obstructed by the cancer and the use of lasers to open up an airway obstructed by a tumor mass.

Adjuvant or neoadjuvant protocols may be useful.

Five-Year Survival Less than 5 percent

SUPPORTIVE THERAPY
The importance of supportive therapy in the treatment of lung cancer cannot be overemphasized.
♦ Quite clearly, malnutrition results in a bad outcome in patients with lung cancer. Patients must be served a palatable meal and attempts must be made to work with patients to determine food likes and dislikes.
♦ Pain control is of critical importance, and the tools to achieve control are available even for the most advanced cases. These include the use of pain-relieving (analgesic) drugs such as non-steroidal anti-inflammatory agents, mild narcotics, strong narcotics, continuous narcotics and narcotics delivered into the spinal canal (epidural). This can control pain without interfering with mental competence.
♦ Nausea can be controlled with a variety of drugs (*see* Chapter 17).

♦ Physical therapy will help maintain muscle strength to keep life as normal as possible.

Maintaining the Quality of Life In the management of lung cancer (as well as all other malignancies), it is critical that the patient maintain as high a quality of life as possible. Patients must feel that they are contributing members of society. Certainly, this keeps them in a happier mental frame.

Being with family and friends, going out to meals and movies and participating in enjoyable recreational events are all important parts of maintaining lifestyle. Family members and physicians should try to provide as much of this as possible. With the services now available, it is usually possible to maintain these goals.

However, when the time comes that patients are no longer able to participate in such activities, we must all be sensible enough to ensure comfort by whatever methods we can. Even if mental ability has been compromised in order to relieve the pain, pain control should come first and remain all-important. Comfort care is the key phrase at that stage of life.

TREATMENT FOLLOW-UP

People who have lung cancer have to be followed carefully by their physicians, generally being examined every one to three months during the first two years, for that is when the risk of relapse is greatest.

♦ Chest x-ray every three to four months in the absence of symptoms.

♦ Chest x-rays more often should symptoms occur.

♦ Blood chemistry tests every three to four months.

♦ Physical examination of the chest, lymph nodes and abdomen.

♦ Neurologic examination.

♦ After two years, follow-up every six months with x-rays and blood surveillance.

Patients should, of course, see their physician if any unusual symptoms occur.

RECURRENT CANCER

See treatment for Stage IV disease.

THE MOST IMPORTANT QUESTIONS YOU CAN ASK

♦ What is the stage of my disease and what is my prognosis?

♦ What is the role of surgery and what is the chance of it curing me?

♦ What is the role of radiation therapy?

♦ How sick will I be on chemotherapy and can we control the sickness?

♦ If chemotherapy cannot cure my cancer, why should I expose myself to its side effects and toxicities?

♦ What is the chance that I will die from this tumor? How much time am I likely to have?

LYMPHOMA: HODGKIN'S DISEASE

Russell Hardy, MD, and Sandra J. Horning, MD

◇

Hodgkin's disease—also called Hodgkin's lymphoma—is a cancer of the lymphoid system. It has special historical interest because it was the first malignancy of the lymphoid system to be described. The first cases were reported in 1832 by British physician Thomas Hodgkin, who recognized that this disorder was distinct from other causes of enlarged lymph nodes such as tuberculosis or other infectious diseases. Hodgkin's lymphoma has characteristic features that distinguish it from all the other cancers of the lymphoid system, and so these other cancers have come to be collectively referred to as non-Hodgkin's lymphomas.

Hodgkin's disease (HD) is an uncommon malignancy. Hodgkin's and non-Hodgkin's lymphomas combined account for 6 percent of newly diagnosed cancers each year, with HD accounting for only 20 percent of all lymphomas. In 1991, about 7,400 new cases of HD will be diagnosed in the U.S. out of a total of 1 million new cases of cancer. Despite the relatively low incidence, it is an important disease because it afflicts adolescents and young adults and because it has a substantial cure rate. Treatment is approached with much optimism.

The systematic approach to the pathologic diagnosis, staging, treatment strategies and clinical trials that have been developed for Hodgkin's disease over the past 30 years serves as a model for all modern cancer therapy. These methods transformed an almost always fatal disease into one of the most curable cancers. With so many cases being cured, attention has recently turned toward the complications of therapy and issues of "survivorship." Here again, HD is leading the way in treatment design and evaluation.

Types The malignant cell characteristic of Hodgkin's disease is known as the Reed-Sternberg cell, named after the two pathologists who first described it. One feature unique to Hodgkin's disease among all cancers is that the "tumors" contain very few cancer cells. In most cases, the affected lymph nodes contain mixtures of mostly normal and less frequent malignant cells. It is believed that the collections of normal cells and scar tissue within affected lymph nodes represent a host response to the tumor cells. Occasionally it can be very difficult or impossible to locate a single diagnostic Reed-Sternberg cell, but Reed-Sternberg "variants" or atypical large cells are regularly identified in HD tissues.

Like the non-Hodgkin's lymphomas, Hodgkin's is divided into sub-types according to the appearance of the affected lymph nodes under the microscope. In the commonly used scheme called the Rye classification, there are four major categories based on the types and arrangements of malignant and non-malignant cells and on associated pathologic features. Each sub-type is associated with characteristic age groups, sex and stages of the disease, but because of the overall success of therapy, sub-type generally has less prognostic importance in HD than in the non-Hodgkin's lymphomas.

RYE CLASSIFICATION

Nodular sclerosis (NS) The affected lymph node has nodules of normal lymphocytes and other "reactive" cells, together with Reed-Sternberg cells, separated by bands of scar-like tissue. This is the most common type of HD and is the only type more common in women than in men. It is usually found as a limited-stage disease involving the lymph nodes of the lower neck, above the collarbones and within the chest in adolescents and young adults. This type is unusual in people over age 50.

Lymphocyte predominant (LP) The affected lymph nodes are composed largely of reactive lymphocytes. The malignant cells have a "popcorn" appearance, distinct from Reed-Sternberg cells (which are rare in this sub-type). The cells may be arrayed in a nodular or diffuse pattern. This type is most common in people under 35 and affects men more frequently than women. The disease is

most often in limited stage when it is discovered and patients rarely have symptoms at the time of diagnosis. Recent information has linked the nodular variety to the B cell of the immune system, similar to most non-Hodgkin's lymphomas.

Mixed cellularity (MC) The affected lymph node contains a mixture of inflammatory cells in addition to abundant Reed-Sternberg cells. Adults with this type are often older and have widespread disease at the time of diagnosis.

Lymphocyte depletion (LD) This is the least common variant and is usually discovered in an advanced stage. Two forms have been described. One has abundant scar-like tissue (fibrosis) with sparse lymphocytes and Reed-Sternberg cells. The other has sheets of malignant cells of different sizes and shapes. It is important to distinguish this sub-type from non-Hodgkin's lymphoma.

How It Spreads One of the unique features of Hodgkin's disease is its pattern of spread. As a rule, HD progresses in an orderly fashion from one lymph node group to the next group on the same side (ipsilateral) or the opposite side (contralateral). Non-Hodgkin's lymphomas, by contrast, are often widespread at diagnosis.

The most characteristic pattern of HD spread is extension of the disease from the lymph nodes in the neck (cervical) to the nodes above the collarbones (supraclavicular), then to the nodes under the arms (axillary) and within the chest (mediastinal and hilar). Although there are different patterns, it is unusual to find areas that have been "skipped," meaning that no apparent disease is found at a site where it would be expected by the rule of orderly progression.

Hodgkin's disease often involves the spleen and may spread to the liver, bone and bone marrow. Involvement of the central nervous system is extremely rare.

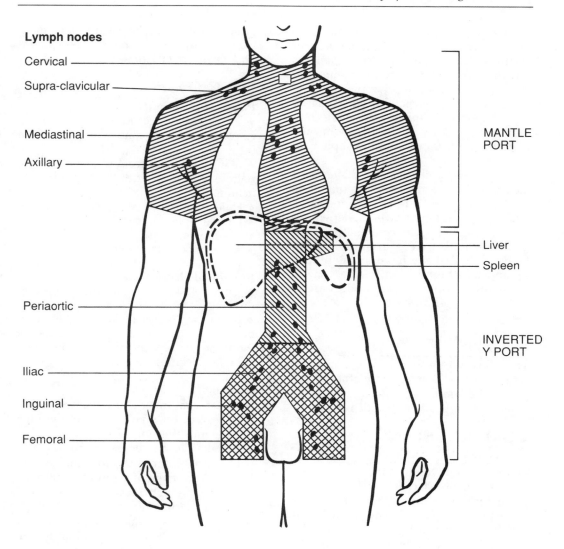

Lymph nodes

- Cervical
- Supra-clavicular
- Mediastinal
- Axillary
- Periaortic
- Iliac
- Inguinal
- Femoral

MANTLE PORT

Liver
Spleen

INVERTED Y PORT

Lymph nodes potentially involved in Hodgkin's disease and non-Hodgkin's lymphomas, and radiotherapy fields

What Causes It Unknown. There is a theory that HD is the rare result, possibly determined by genetics, of an infection acquired in late adolescence or early adulthood. Family clusters have been reported and several viruses have been suggested as the cause, but no genetic or infectious basis for the disease has been proved.

RISK FACTORS

In developed countries there are two peaks of incidence of Hodgkin's disease, the first in young adults (ages 15 to 35) and the second after age 50. Men are affected slightly more commonly than women.

The frequency of the various sub-types depends on age. At the National Cancer Institute, where the majority of patients are young, nodular sclerosis accounts for 70 percent of cases and lymphocyte predominant for 15 percent. Mixed cellularity and lymphocyte depletion are more common in the elderly, in socioeconomically underdeveloped areas and in people with AIDS.

There are no clearly established risk factors for Hodgkin's disease, although in the United States there is some increased risk with small family size, higher education and higher socioeconomic position. Brothers and sisters of people with Hodgkin's disease have an incidence seven times higher than in the general population. Sophisticated studies are in progress to explore the genetics of Hodgkin's disease.

SCREENING

There are no known effective ways to screen for Hodgkin's disease other than a physical examination and a chest x-ray when an enlarged lymph node is found.

COMMON SIGNS AND SYMPTOMS

People who develop Hodgkin's disease often see their physicians because of the persistent swelling of painless lymph nodes in the neck or underarms. The swollen nodes may be the only sign of disease or they may be accompanied by unexplained fevers, chills, night sweats, weight loss or itching.

Young people with limited disease usually feel entirely well, but occasionally have symptoms such as itching. Cough, shortness of breath or chest discomfort can be the first symptoms of HD in the chest, although it is not unusual for a mass to be detected on a chest x-ray done for totally unrelated reasons. Less commonly, Hodgkin's disease in the abdomen may be signaled by an enlarged spleen or enlarged groin lymph nodes. These are much more likely to be signs of non-Hodgkin's lymphoma than of HD, however.

DIAGNOSIS

Physical Examination
♦ Enlarged lymph nodes in the neck, above the clavicles, under the arms or in the groin.
♦ Skin breakdown from scratching (excoriation) over most of the body because of itching.
♦ Fluid around the lungs (pleural effusion).
♦ Liver or spleen enlargement.
♦ Abdominal mass.
♦ Areas of bony tenderness.

Blood and Other Tests
♦ Complete blood count, including erythrocyte (red cell) sedimentation rate.
♦ Blood chemistries, including serum copper. These may be abnormal because of the tumor or because of the involvement of bone, the kidneys or liver.

Imaging
♦ Chest x-ray may show masses within the chest, direct involvement of the lung or a pleural effusion.
♦ CT scan of the chest, abdomen and pelvis to look for enlarged lymph nodes or the involvement of the liver or spleen.
♦ Lymphangiogram, which uses a contrast dye injected into the feet to highlight the lymphatic system. The dye will stay within the pelvic and abdominal lymph nodes for many months or years, during which the disease can be followed by simple x-rays of the abdomen.
♦ Bone x-rays and/or bone scan if there are tender bony areas.
♦ After injection of the isotope gallium, scanning may reveal "hot spots" indicating areas of HD.

Endoscopy and Biopsy
♦ Bone marrow biopsy to look for the presence of Hodgkin's disease.

♦ Biopsy of an enlarged lymph node.
♦ Surgical exploration of the abdomen (laparotomy) with removal of the spleen (splenectomy) may be needed to evaluate any hidden disease that could influence the choice of treatment.

STAGING

The stage is identified through a careful history, physical exam and laboratory and x-ray studies including a lymphangiogram. For those patients whose treatment decision requires it, exploratory abdominal surgery (staging laparotomy) may also be done.

The classification used for staging Hodgkin's disease is known as the Ann Arbor Staging System.

Stage I Involvement of a single lymph node region (Stage I) or localized involvement of a single organ or site other than lymph nodes (IE).

Stage II Involvement of two or more lymph node regions on the same side of the diaphragm (either above or below the breathing muscle separating the chest from the abdomen) (Stage II) or localized involvement of a single associated organ or site other than lymph nodes (extralymphatic) and its nearby lymph nodes, with or without other lymph node regions on the same side of the diaphragm (IIE).

Stage III Involvement of lymph node regions on both sides of the diaphragm (Stage III) that may also be accompanied by localized involvement of an extralymphatic organ or site (IIIE), involvement of the spleen (IIIS) or both (IIIS+E).

Stage IV Widespread involvement of one or more sites other than lymph nodes, with or without associated lymph node involvement, or isolated extralymphatic organ involvement with distant lymph node involvement.

Each stage may be further sub-divided into A or B according to the presence or absence of general symptoms. "A" means the absence of "B" symptoms, which include any of: unexplained fevers over 38°C (100.4°F), drenching night sweats or the unexplained loss of at least 10 percent of body weight.

TREATMENT OVERVIEW

About 75 percent of all newly diagnosed people with Hodgkin's disease can be cured with current radiotherapy and combination chemotherapy.

The most important factors for determining the prognosis and outlining treatment plans are the stage of disease, the presence or absence of symptoms and the presence of large masses. Other factors include the patient's age, the extent of splenic disease found during a laparotomy, the extent of abdominal lymph node involvement and the results of a laboratory test measuring the erythrocyte (red cell) sedimentation rate.

 Radiation Radiation therapy is considered the treatment of choice for those with favorable localized disease—Stage I and Stage II, with no large masses and no symptoms.

 Chemotherapy For all other patients, chemotherapy is required. Combined radiation and chemotherapy is commonly used for large individual tumor masses, so-called bulky disease. Even patients who have recurrent disease after initial treatment with radiation have an excellent chance for a prolonged disease-free survival with combination chemotherapy. Patients with recurrent disease after chemotherapy have a less favorable prognosis, but long remissions have been reported after more chemotherapy or intensive chemotherapy and radiation therapy followed by bone marrow transplantation.

Investigational The leading clinical investigations in early-stage Hodgkin's disease are designed to decrease the toxicity of treatment without reducing the overall excellent results.

More effective therapy is needed for patients with very extensive disease and better chemotherapy programs are needed for the elderly. The use of hematopoietic growth factors is likely to improve treatment for both (*see* Chapter 8). Current studies will eventually define the best use of intensive chemotherapy, radiation therapy and bone marrow transplantation.

TREATMENT BY STAGE

STAGE IA and IIA "FAVORABLE"
The disease is classified as favorable if there are no large masses.

Standard Treatment Patients will usually have exploratory abdominal surgery (a staging laparotomy), but this might be avoided when there is little likelihood of disease below the diaphragm. This may be the case with disease that appears only in the chest (no lymph nodes), with high neck disease of the nodular sclerosis or lymphocyte predominant sub-types and with young women with Stage I disease.

The standard treatment is radiation to the chest and the deep abdominal lymph nodes.

Alternatives include involved field radiation plus mild chemotherapy and combination chemotherapy alone.

Five-Year Survival About 90 percent

STAGE IB and IIB "FAVORABLE"
Standard Treatment If radiotherapy alone is to be considered, a staging laparotomy is essential. Sub-total or total lymphoid irradiation is favored in some centers, particularly those with modern radiotherapy equipment and extensive experience.

Combination chemotherapy programs commonly used include:

MOPP (mechlorethamine [nitrogen mustard] + vincristine + procarbazine + prednisone), ABVD (Adriamycin + bleomycin + vinblastine + dacarbazine [DTIC]), a MOPP-ABV hybrid (without dacarbazine) and alternating cycles of MOPP and ABVD.

An alternative therapy in laparotomy-staged patients is involved field radiation plus mild chemotherapy.

Five-Year Survival 75 to 90 percent

STAGE IA or IB and IIA or IIB "UNFAVORABLE"
The disease is classified as unfavorable if there is a large mass.

Standard Treatment Staging laparotomy is not indicated.

Combination chemotherapy such as those mentioned before in combination with radiation therapy to the involved field is the standard treatment.

Five-Year Survival 75-90 percent

Investigational
♦ New chemotherapy combinations are being investigated, either alone or together with radiotherapy.

STAGE IIIA
Standard Treatment The treatment for Stage IIIA patients is controversial. For laparotomy-staged IIIA patients with limited splenic disease (fewer than five nodules), total lymphoid irradiation alone may be considered in centers specializing in radiotherapy.

For patients staged clinically (on the basis of physical examination, x-rays and laboratory tests) or patients pathologically staged with more than five splenic nodules, combination chemotherapy such as MOPP, ABVD or the MOPP-ABV hybrid should be used.

For patients with Stage IIIA disease with bulky masses, both chemotherapy and irradiation are recommended.

Five-Year Survival 65 to 85 percent

Investigational
♦ New chemotherapy combinations, alone or together with radiotherapy.

STAGE IIIB and STAGE IV
Standard Treatment Combination chemotherapy with MOPP, ABVD, the MOPP-ABV hybrid and MOPP alternated with ABVD.

Radiation therapy may be added to sites of bulky disease.

Five-Year Survival 60 to 80 percent

Investigational
♦ Chemotherapy alternated with total lymphoid irradiation.

TREATMENT FOLLOW-UP

All patients must be followed up at regular intervals with a physical examination, blood counts and radiological studies. This is particularly important because of the young age of the population and the ability to cure patients with secondary therapy.
♦ For patients treated with limited radiation after clinical staging alone, annual abdominal CT scans are recommended. Sites of previous bulky disease should receive particular attention.
♦ All patients receiving radiation therapy to the thyroid should have annual thyroid function tests. In a significant percentage of patients, thyroid function may become low (hypothyroid) because of radiation treatments, requiring the taking of thyroid hormone.
♦ Surveillance is needed to be on the lookout for secondary malignancy, solid tumors in patients treated with irradiation and acute leukemia in patients treated with MOPP (*see* "Complications of Therapy").

Complications of Therapy These may be divided into acute and chronic. Acute toxicities for the various chemotherapy drugs are well described and should be discussed before treatment. Acute toxicities of radiation therapy depend on which area of the body is irradiated.

Now that the cure rate for Hodgkin's disease is so high and so many patients are alive many years after treatment, the late complications of therapy are receiving more attention. These include:
♦ Nearly universal sterility in males and infertility and premature menopause in women over age 25 who receive the equivalent of six cycles of MOPP. These effects appear to be largely irreversible. But children born to parents treated for Hodgkin's disease by any of the standard treatments have had normal birth weights and no increased incidence of birth defects.
♦ MOPP is also associated with an increased risk—between 1 and 5 percent—of acute leukemia, which is most common about four years after treatment and is no longer appreciated by 10 years. The risk of leukemia may be increased by the combined use of MOPP with radiotherapy or after splenectomy.
♦ Non-Hodgkin's lymphomas are increased in HD patients treated by any method.
♦ Patients receiving radiotherapy are at increased risk of developing a second malignancy in the irradiated tissues, particularly skin cancer, breast cancer, stomach cancer, soft tissue and bone cancer and lung cancer. Any patient who is irradiated would be very wise to stop smoking, since the incidence of lung cancer is strongly related to tobacco use.
♦ There are theoretical concerns with the use of ABVD in that bleomycin may be toxic to the lungs and doxorubicin is associated with cardiac toxicity. Both of these effects depend on the dose used and are also affected by the combined use of radiotherapy.

RECURRENT CANCER

Combination chemotherapy with the outlined programs is used for patients who were initially treated with radiotherapy alone.

Cancer that recurs more than one year after chemotherapy has been given as the initial treatment may be treated with either the same chemotherapy program or an alternative combination.

Relapse during the first year after chemotherapy may be treated with intensive chemotherapy or chemotherapy and radiation therapy (depending on the earlier treatment) followed by bone marrow transplantation.

THE MOST IMPORTANT QUESTIONS YOU CAN ASK

♦ What is my stage? Is it favorable or unfavorable?

♦ Do I need to have a laparotomy for staging?

♦ Should I have treatment with radiation only, chemotherapy only or both? Why?

♦ What side effects can I expect from the treatment and how can they be minimized?

♦ Will this treatment make me sterile (or infertile)?

♦ What is my risk of future malignancy?

♦ If the Hodgkin's disease recurs, what therapy will be required and what are my chances for cure? Should bone marrow transplantation be considered?

LYMPHOMAS: NON-HODGKIN'S

Russell Hardy, MD, and Sandra J. Horning, MD

◇

Malignant lymphomas are cancers that arise from the lymphoid system, the complex network of cells and channels that runs throughout the body as a basic part of the immune system. Normally, the cells of the lymphoid system, lymphocytes, are either arranged in clusters—called lymph nodes or lymph glands—or they circulate through the bloodstream and the lymphatic channels to all the tissues of the body except the brain.

Cancers that develop within the lymphoid system—malignant lymphomas—may be found wherever normal lymphocytes go. They may occur in an isolated lymph node, a group of lymph nodes, in organs such as the stomach or intestine, the sinuses, bone, skin or any combination of these sites.

About 37,200 new cases of malignant lymphoma and lymphocytic leukemia (a lymphoid cancer that primarily involves the blood and bone marrow) will occur in 1991 in the United States. They are the seventh most common cause of cancer deaths. The increase in the incidence of non-Hodgkin's lymphoma between 1973 and 1987 was larger than the increase during that period for any other major cancer except melanoma and lung cancer.

Although lymphoma refers to any cancer of the lymphoid system, malignant lymphomas actually represent a variety of cancers ranging from slow-growing chronic diseases to rapidly progressive, acute diseases that may be life-threatening if appropriate therapy is not begun quickly. The first cancer of the lymphoid system was described by British physician Thomas Hodgkin, in 1832. The form he described behaves in a very predictable way and has come to be called Hodgkin's disease. Despite their diversity, all of the other malignant lymphomas are referred to as non-Hodgkin's lymphomas (NHL).

Types There are two main types of cells in the lymphoid system—B cells, which make antibodies in response to infection, and T cells, which are responsible for the regulation of the immune system. Both B cell and T cell lymphomas occur, but the vast majority of lymphomas in the U.S. are of B cell origin.

Whatever the origin, the features that best predict the prognosis and guide decisions about therapy are the size, shape and pattern of the lymphocytes as seen under the microscope. Malignant lymphocytes may be small and round or angulated (cleaved). Others may be large. Combinations of small and large cells may also be seen. Intermediate-sized lymphocytes with rapidly dividing cells are characteristic of aggressive (high-grade) lymphomas.

Within normal lymph nodes there are microscopic clusters (follicles) of specialized lymphocytes. In some malignant lymphomas, the lymphocytes arrange themselves in a similar pattern that is called follicular or nodular. Small cell and follicular lymphomas typically have a chronic course with an average survival of 6 to 12 years. In the more aggressive lymphomas, the normal appearance of the lymph node is lost by diffuse involvement of tumor cells, which are usually moderate-sized or large.

Follicular small cleaved cell lymphoma, which is a favorable low-grade lymphoma, is the most common sub-type seen in the United States and Canada. The other major sub-type is diffuse large cell lymphoma, which is an aggressive intermediate- or high-grade lymphoma.

A variety of systems have been used to classify NHL sub-types according to their microscopic appearance and the behavior of the disease. The Rappaport classification is an older scheme still commonly used. More recently, an international group of pathologists and clinicians developed a Working Formulation to establish a common terminology. This defined 10 major sub-types categorized as low-, intermediate- or high-grade. These terms relate to the relative malignant potential and the growth rate—low (slow), high (rapid) or intermediate (moderately rapid).

International Working Formulation	*Rappaport Classification*
Low-Grade	
Small lymphocytic, consistent with chronic lymphocytic leukemia	Diffuse lymphocytic, well-differentiated
Follicular, predominantly small cleaved cell	Nodular lymphocytic, poorly differentiated
Follicular mixed, small cleaved and large cell	Nodular mixed, lymphocytic and histiocytic
Intermediate-Grade	
Follicular, predominantly large cell	Nodular histiocytic
Diffuse, small cleaved cell	Diffuse lymphocytic, poorly differentiated
Diffuse mixed, small and large cell	Diffuse mixed, lymphocytic and histiocytic
Diffuse large cell (cleaved or non-cleaved)	Diffuse histiocytic

International Working Formulation	Rappaport Classification
High-Grade	
Immunoblastic, diffuse large cell	Diffuse histiocytic
Lymphoblastic (convoluted or non-convoluted)	Diffuse lymphoblastic
Small non-cleaved cell, Burkitt's or non-Burkitt's	Diffuse undifferentiated, Burkitt's or non-Burkitt's

How It Spreads Since lymphocytes normally travel throughout the body via the blood and the lymphatic system, malignant lymphomas can either start in or spread to virtually any organ.

A lymphoma may arise in a single lymph node or organ and stay there even when a large mass is present, or many different sites may be involved at the time of diagnosis. Low-grade lymphomas most often involve lymph nodes, bone marrow and the spleen when they are diagnosed. Intermediate- and high-grade lymphomas are most commonly found in lymph nodes, but about one-third of cases primarily involve organs separate from lymph nodes and are called extranodal.

What Causes It The immune system is so complex and dynamic that there are many opportunities for errors in regulation. Many lymphomas are thought to result from such errors or "accidents," which are statistically more probable when the immune system is continually stimulated.

Chronic disorders of the immune system or the chronic administration of drugs to suppress the immune system (such as those used after an organ transplant) predispose a person to lymphoma. Exposure to radiation increases the risk too.

Several types of viruses have been linked. The Epstein-Barr virus, which causes infectious mononucleosis, is associated with African Burkitt's lymphoma. A T cell virus related to the HIV virus associated with AIDS has been linked to an aggressive T cell lymphoma found in Japan, the Caribbean and the southeastern United States.

The mechanism common to each of these appears to be a significant alteration in the normal regulation of the immune system.

RISK FACTORS

At Significantly Higher Risk
♦ The incidence of lymphoma increases with age and is more common in men that in women. Most occur in people who were previously healthy.
♦ Occupational exposure in the flour and agricultural industries has been reported to increase the risk of developing certain types of intermediate- and high-grade lymphoma.
♦ People with congenital or acquired abnormalities of their immune systems or who take medicine to suppress their immune systems have a higher incidence of lymphoma.
♦ Recent National Cancer Institute statistics indicate that the incidence of intermediate and high-grade lymphomas in people infected with the HIV virus for four or more years is markedly increasing.
♦ Exposure to radiation or chemotherapy.

SCREENING

There are no known effective ways to screen for lymphoma.

COMMON SIGNS AND SYMPTOMS

People with lymphoma most often seek medical attention because of one or more enlarged lymph nodes. Sometimes these have developed in association with a variety of non-specific symptoms such as fatigue, fevers, chills, night sweats, decreased appetite and weight loss.

But many people are found to have lymphoma when they see their doctors about a variety of symptoms related to the site and extent of tumor involvement. People may develop shortness of breath or cough because of chest disease; abdominal pain or fullness because of an abdominal mass; ulcers, or bleeding or a change in bowel habits because of stomach or intestinal involvement. There can also be nasal stuffiness or sore throat or difficulty swallowing because of a lymphoma involving the sinus, upper airway or throat. If the brain is involved, there may be headaches, changes in vision or seizures. If the bone marrow is involved, there may be recurrent or persistent infections, bleeding or profound fatigue.

Disease outside the lymphatic system is more common in intermediate- and high-grade lymphomas.

DIAGNOSIS

Physical Examination
◆ Enlarged lymph nodes in the neck, under the arms or in the groin.
◆ Swelling in the area of the tonsils, throat or upper airway.
◆ Fluid around the lungs (pleural effusion).
◆ Liver or spleen enlargement.
◆ Abdominal mass.
◆ Soft tissue swelling.
◆ Tenderness when pressure is applied to areas of the skeleton.
◆ Neurologic findings such as numbness or muscle weakness.

Blood and Other Tests
◆ Complete blood count may show circulating lymphoma cells or other blood abnormalities because of lymphoma in the bone marrow.
◆ Blood chemistries may be abnormal because of the tumor or because of the involvement of bone, the liver or the kidneys.
◆ HIV test.

Imaging
◆ Chest x-ray may show masses within the center of the chest (mediastinum or hilum), involvement of the lungs or fluid around the heart or lungs.
◆ CT scan of the chest, abdomen and pelvis may show enlargement of lymph nodes, spleen or liver or the involvement of the lungs or other organs.

There are also several optional imaging methods, including:
◆ Lymphangiogram, which uses a contrast dye injected into the feet to highlight the lymphatic system. The dye will stay within the pelvic and abdominal lymph nodes for many months or years, during which the disease can be followed by a simple x-ray of the abdomen.
◆ A spinal tap or CT or MRI scans of the brain may be done if central nervous system involvement is suspected. MRI may allow more accurate assessment of the tumor, particularly in the spinal cord and vertebrae.
◆ An imaging scan using the radioactive isotope gallium may show "hot spots" in areas of lymphoma.

Endoscopy and Biopsy
◆ Bone marrow biopsy may detect the presence of lymphoma, in which case further studies will be done to identify the type.

STAGING

The staging system used for non-Hodgkin's lymphomas is the Ann Arbor convention developed for the staging and treatment (primarily with radiation) of Hodgkin's disease.

Several proposals for a revised staging system for NHL have been made, but none is universally recognized. Sometimes a distinction has been made between "clinical" and "pathologic" staging. Clinical staging describes the apparent stage of the disease as determined by physical examination, x-rays and blood tests. Pathologic staging has generally involved exploratory abdominal surgery (laparotomy) to assess lymph nodes, the liver and spleen for lymphoma. Laparotomy cannot now be recommended for staging of NHL. Strictly speaking, biopsy of the bone marrow is pathologic staging, but the procedure is commonly included as part of clinical staging.

Stage I Involvement of a single lymph node region (Stage I) or localized involvement of a single organ or site other than lymph nodes (IE).

Stage II Involvement of two or more lymph node regions on the same side of the diaphragm (either above or below the breathing muscle separating the chest from the abdomen) (Stage II) or localized involvement of a single associated organ or site other than lymph nodes (extralymphatic) and its regional lymph nodes, with or without other lymph node regions on the same side of the diaphragm (IIE).

Stage III Involvement of lymph node regions on both sides of the diaphragm (Stage III) that may also be accompanied by localized involvement of an extralymphatic organ or site (IIIE), involvement of the spleen (IIIS) or both (IIIS+E).

Stage IV Widespread involvement of one or more extralymphatic sites, with or without associated lymph node involvement, or isolated extralymphatic organ involvement with distant lymph node involvement.

Each stage may be further sub-divided into A or B according to the presence or absence of general symptoms. "A" means the absence of "B" symptoms, which include any of: unexplained fevers over 38°C (100.4°F), drenching night sweats or the unexplained loss of more than 10 percent of body weight.

TREATMENT OVERVIEW BY GRADE

The microscopic appearance and the stage of the lymphoma are the most important factors in determining both the prognosis and the appropriate therapy. Other factors affecting the prognosis for a particular person include age, the presence of "B" symptoms, abnormal laboratory tests, the presence of large masses and general physical condition.

With greater understanding of the biology of NHL, other factors have recently been recognized—biologic parameters such as determination of growth fraction or chromosomal analysis—that can be related to the clinical outcome of the disease. It is expected that these will play a greater role in deciding on treatment in the future.

Low-Grade Although low-grade lymphomas grow slowly and respond readily to chemotherapy, they almost invariably return and are generally regarded as incurable cancers.

It is usual for the low-grade lymphomas to be widespread at the time of diagnosis, including involvement in the bone marrow. Despite this, the average survival of people with these lymphomas is 6 to 12 years.

The long-term outcome of the disease has not been favorably affected by the use of immediate chemotherapy in patients who have no symptoms, so close observation alone may be the initial therapy of choice, particularly in patients over age 60. Chemotherapy or radiation therapy may be required when the disease progresses or begins to cause symptoms.

Because of the apparent inability to cure low-grade lymphoma patients, it is important that patients with this diagnosis are presented with the opportunity to participate in clinical trials designed to test new strategies or new agents with the goal of improving the prognosis for low-grade lymphoma.

Patients with limited (Stages I and II) disease provide the exception. They may have prolonged responses to radiation therapy. It is well known that low-grade lymphomas may transform into more aggressive lymphomas. Therapy appropriate for the more aggressive cancer is required at that time.

Intermediate- and High-Grade These lymphomas are curable. Combination chemotherapy is almost always necessary for successful treatment.

Chemotherapy alone or abbreviated chemotherapy and radiation cure 70 to 80 percent of patients with limited (Stages I and II) intermediate-grade lymphoma. Advanced (Stages III and IV) disease can be eradicated in about 50 percent of patients. As noted, elderly patients and those with a high tumor burden have the least favorable prognosis, while patients with no adverse factors enjoy a cure rate that approaches 80 percent.

♦ Patients with B cell immunoblastic lymphoma respond in a manner similar to those with intermediate-grade large cell lymphoma. Several recent reports indicate that T cell lymphomas may be somewhat less favorable for cure.

♦ The intermediate sub-types follicular large cell and diffuse small cleaved cell lymphoma are less common and less well characterized. Some physicians suggest that they should be treated more like the low-grade lymphomas, but others favor an aggressive approach.

♦ Lymphoblastic lymphoma is a high-grade malignancy treated with an inten-sive drug program similar to that used for acute leukemia, including treatment of the central nervous system.

♦ The small non-cleaved cell lymphomas, including Burkitt's lymphoma, are rapidly progressive neoplasms that are exquisitely sensitive to chemotherapy.

For each of these high-grade malignancies there is a 40 to 50 percent cure rate with conventional therapy. Some limited stage high-grade lymphomas have a high rate of cure, but more effective treatment approaches are needed for patients with the greatest tumor burden.

Because of medical problems that may occur when treatment is started, patients with extensive lymphoblastic lymphoma or Burkitt's lymphoma should receive their initial chemotherapy treatment in the hospital.

TREATMENT BY GRADE AND STAGE

LOW-GRADE LYMPHOMA
STAGE I and STAGE II
Standard Treatment Radiation therapy is the standard treatment, particularly for patients under the age of 40. While total lymphoid irradiation has been associated with longer disease-free survival, there is no overall survival benefit over regional or limited irradiation.

STAGE III and STAGE IV
Standard Treatment The best treatment for advanced-stage disease remains controversial. Options include:
♦ No initial treatment, with close observation for patients who have no symptoms.
♦ Single-drug therapy, most often oral chlorambucil or Cytoxan.
♦ Combination chemotherapy with CVP (Cytoxan + Oncovin + prednisone), C(M)OPP (Cytoxan + Oncovin + procarbazine + prednisone) or CHOP (Cytoxan + Adriamycin + Oncovin + prednisone).

Five-Year Survival 90 percent for Stages I and II, 80 percent for Stages III and IV

Investigational
♦ A variety of biologic agents have been used, most notably interferon-alpha. This is a modest antitumor agent when used alone and is being studied in combination with chemotherapy or as an adjuvant to chemotherapy in an attempt to prolong remission.
♦ Monoclonal antibodies directed against specific surface markers or more general B cell markers have been used alone, tagged with a radioisotope, combined with a toxin or used in a combined approach with chemotherapy and interferon.

Therapy for Relapsed Disease The treatment used initially is often successful when used again after a relapse in the low-grade lymphomas. Radiotherapy may be useful to reduce bulky or painful disease sites. Any of the investigational treatments may also be used.

INTERMEDIATE-GRADE LYMPHOMAS

FAVORABLE STAGES I AND II
Limited-stage lymphomas are generally considered favorable if the disease is not bulky (usually less than 4 in./10 cm in diameter) and there are no "B" symptoms.

Standard Treatment Treatment options for favorable Stages I and II include:
♦ Chemotherapy alone with CHOP (Cytoxan + Adriamycin + Oncovin + prednisone).
♦ Abbreviated combination chemotherapy plus limited radiation therapy.
♦ Primary radiation therapy to the site of disease in selected Stage I cases, particularly in patients with minimal disease who cannot tolerate chemotherapy.

Five-Year Survival 80 to 90 percent for Stage I, 70 to 80 percent for Stage II

Investigational Because initial therapy is so successful, the goals of investigational

efforts are reducing the toxicity of treatment and trying to predict which patients are most likely to fail primary therapy and therefore need other treatment approaches.

UNFAVORABLE STAGES I AND II, STAGE III AND STAGE IV
Standard Treatment Combination chemotherapy, with programs such as:
♦ CHOP (Cytoxan + Adriamycin + Oncovin + prednisone).
♦ m-BACOD (methotrexate + bleomycin + Adriamycin + Cytoxan + Oncovin + dexamethasone).
♦ ProMACE-CYTABOM (prednisone + high-dose methotrexate + Adriamycin + Cytoxan + etoposide [VP-16] + cytosine arabinoside + bleomycin + Oncovin).
♦ MACOP-B (methotrexate with leucovorin rescue + Adriamycin + Cytoxan + Oncovin + prednisone + bleomycin).
♦ COP-BLAM (Cytoxan + Oncovin + procarbazine + bleomycin + Adriamycin + methotrexate).

Radiation therapy may be given to the sites of bulky disease to boost the effect of chemotherapy. Central nervous system therapy is required for patients with tumor involvement in the area adjacent to the spinal cord (epidural), the testes, paranasal sinuses and bone marrow.

Five-Year Survival About 40 to 50 percent, although the prognosis for patients over 60 is not as good.

Investigational Most investigational efforts have the goal of increasing the intensity of treatment by using hematopoietic growth factors or bone marrow transplantation.
♦ A major challenge is the proper separation of patients who have a high likelihood of cure with the standard treatments from those who require more intensive or innovative therapy.
♦ Combination chemotherapy regimens

which use newer drugs with activity against lymphoma such as etoposide (VP-16), mitoxantrone, ifosfamide and epirubicin are being actively investigated. These regimens include:

♦ CEPP (Cytoxan + etoposide [VP-16] + procarbazine + prednisone)

♦ VACOP-B (etoposide [VP-16] + Adriamycin + Cytoxan + Oncovin + prednisone + bleomycin)

♦ MINE (mesna + ifosfamide + mitoxantrone + etoposide [VP-16])

Therapy for Relapsed Disease A number of chemotherapy combinations have demonstrated antitumor activity, but secondary chemotherapy has generally failed to provide a cure.

♦ Many patients under age 55 have been been given high-dose chemotherapy and radiation followed by a bone marrow transplant with moderate success. An international clinical trial is testing the benefit of autologous marrow transplant compared with secondary chemotherapy.

HIGH-GRADE LYMPHOMAS
LYMPHOBLASTIC LYMPHOMA
Standard Treatment Multi-agent chemotherapy, primarily with Cytoxan, Adriamycin, Oncovin and prednisone, is given together with central nervous system prophylactic therapy.

Patients with extensive disease—usually Stage IV on the basis of bone marrow and/or central nervous system involvement—and a high serum lactate dehydrogenase (LDH) have generally done poorly with conventional therapy. Early use of intensive chemotherapy and radiation followed by bone marrow transplantation has been reported to improve the outlook for these patients markedly.

Five-Year Survival 80 percent for limited disease, 20 percent for extensive disease with bone marrow and central nervous system involvement

Investigational
♦ Intensified treatment for high-risk patients is being investigated. One strategy is early use of bone marrow transplantation.

Therapy for Relapsed Disease Secondary chemotherapy and bone marrow transplantation at relapse have some antitumor activity but have most often failed to cure this rapidly fatal condition.

SMALL NON-CLEAVED CELL LYMPHOMA (BURKITT'S/ NON-BURKITT'S)
Standard Treatment The management of this lymphoma is similar to that of lymphoblastic lymphoma. Multi-agent chemotherapy, based upon high-dose Cytoxan, frequently incorporates metho-trexate, Oncovin, prednisone and Adria-mycin together with central nervous system prophylactic therapy.

Patients with extensive disease—usually Stage IV on the basis of bone marrow and/or central nervous system involvement—and a high serum lactate dehydrogenase (LDH) have generally fared poorly with chemotherapy.

More intensive treatment programs similar to those used for acute leukemia, with or without bone marrow transplantation, are under investigation.

Survival data, investigational approaches and therapy for relapsed disease are essentially the same as for lymphoblastic lymphoma.

TREATMENT FOLLOW-UP
Follow-up varies considerably, depending on the initial grade of lymphoma and the treatment.

♦ Patients with low-grade lymphoma require follow-up because of the strong likelihood that the disease will recur and/or will transform into a higher-grade malignancy.

♦ Some forms of intermediate-grade lymphoma, particularly diffuse small cleaved cell and follicular large cell lymphoma, may also relapse over long periods.

♦ Recurrence of intermediate-grade diffuse large cell and mixed lymphomas or high-grade lymphomas usually occurs within three years after treatment. Relapse is rarely hard to find, given the rapid growth characteristics of these lymphomas. All patients should be seen at regular intervals for physical examination, complete blood counts and radiologic studies. Newer biologic markers of minimal disease may be used in the future.

THE MOST IMPORTANT QUESTIONS YOU CAN ASK

♦ What is my prognosis? What is the likelihood of cure?

♦ If the standard treatment won't cure me, are there any investigational treatments I should consider?

♦ What side effects can I expect from the treatment and how can they be minimized?

♦ If I have a low-grade lymphoma, what are the risks and benefits of immediate treatment as opposed to no initial therapy?

♦ If I have recurrent (relapsed) lymphoma, should bone marrow transplantation be considered?

MELANOMA
Malcolm S. Mitchell, MD

◇

Most skin cancers are not generally considered very dangerous, since they are easily cured by surgery or medicines applied to the skin. The malignant mole called melanoma—which means black tumor—is a notable exception. Not only is melanoma the most malignant of all skin cancers, it is among the most malignant of *all* cancers.

Melanoma can spread to nearly every organ and tissue in the body and can lead to death within a year after it recurs in distant sites. Although it is very rare for a mother's tumor to spread to her fetus, melanomas lead the list among those tumors that do spread in this way.

Melanoma is also one of the most common tumors to spread to the brain and spinal cord.

While by no means a common cancer, the incidence of melanoma is increasing yearly, with about 29,000 cases expected in the U.S. during 1991.

Yet amidst all these bleak aspects there are some very encouraging ones. When melanoma first appears as a malignant mole of the skin or eye—and occasionally on the gums, in the vagina or in the anus—it is often curable by limited surgery. This points up the importance of recognizing the early signs of melanoma and bringing them to the attention of a physician so that an experienced dermatologist, surgeon or oncologist can become involved.

Once the melanoma has penetrated deeply into the skin and has reached the lymphatic and blood vessels in the second level of the skin (the dermis), it is often impossible to cure, although a long period of quiescence may still be achieved by surgery.

Types There is only one type of malignant cell composing all melanomas—the malignant pigment-producing cell called a melanocyte—but there are a few variants distinguished by their shapes, such as cuboidal or spindle-shaped. The behavior of each is generally similar in skin melanomas, although in eye melanomas the shape determines the behavior to a significant degree.

All melanocytes have pigment granules in them even when the cells are not black or dark brown. In all cases, they have the enzymes necessary to produce melanin, the black pigment. When melanomas spread, they often do not produce pigment and are said to be amelanotic, but the degree of malignancy of both amelanotic or melanotic melanomas seems to be the same.

Melanomas are most commonly found on the skin, but 10 percent arise in the eye. The most common variants in the skin are called the superficial spreading melanoma and the nodular melanoma, terms that describe the pattern of enlargement.

Melanomas can arise in somewhat unusual locations, such as under the nail of a finger or toe or on the mucosa lining the inside of the mouth, vagina or anus. Primary melanomas have also been found on the pigmented tissue covering the brain (the meninges). It is important not to confuse melanomas under the nail with fungal infections, although that mistake is sometimes made at the beginning of the disease.

Melanomas of the eye occur in the colored regions at the front (the iris), just behind the iris in the structure controlling the shape of the lens (the ciliary body) and in the pigmented layer (the choroid) covering the eyeball behind the retina.

How It Spreads There are two phases of growth of melanomas—the radial (outward on the surface of the skin) and the vertical (deeply into the layers of the skin). Sometimes, superficial spreading melanomas can remain in a radial growth phase for over a year. Nodular melanomas grow vertically soon after their appearance. Detection in a biologically early phase is, therefore, more likely with superficial spreading melanomas, but these tumors do eventually enter a vertical growth phase. When they do, they are as dangerous as nodular melanomas.

Most eye melanomas grow very slowly. They may be observed by ophthalmologists for 5 to 10 years with little increase in size. The eye melanomas composed of spindle-shaped cells (called spindle A and spindle B) are almost non-malignant in

their behavior, with almost all patients surviving more than 10 years after the tumor is detected. Other varieties, composed of cells shaped more like skin cells (epithelioid) are much more malignant.

Melanomas can also spread through the lymphatic system and the blood to just about every organ in the body, with the lungs and liver being the most common sites.

What Causes It Intermittent episodes of intense sun exposure causing sunburns rather than tanning is more commonly associated with melanoma than the sort of chronic exposure to sunlight associated with more benign skin cancers. Typically, office workers or schoolchildren who spend hours on the beach on weekends, rather than farmers, dockworkers or sailors who work in the sun daily, are liable to develop melanomas.

There is no conclusive evidence to support an association with hormones, although anecdotes continue to surface that suggest at least some women are highly susceptible to developing melanoma or recurrent melanoma when they are pregnant or have taken oral contraceptives. Individual patients have had a striking history of recurrences and rapid progression of disease related to pregnancy. Taking oral contraceptives, which contain mostly progestational agents, has also been associated with an increased incidence of superficial spreading melanomas.

RISK FACTORS

Caucasians living in tropical or sub-tropical climates, such as the American Southwest, equatorial Africa, Hawaii or Australia, have the highest incidence. Obviously, exposure to ultraviolet light, particularly that leading to sunburn, is strongly suspected as a cause.

There are about 15 cases among each 100,000 Caucasians in California or Arizona, while 30 cases are found per

100,000 Caucasians in Hawaii and Australia. Blacks, brown-skinned people and Orientals in the same regions have a much lower incidence.

Even in the Northeast, the incidence is more than 10 per 100,000, up from 8 per 100,000 10 to 15 years ago. Melanoma is becoming a major concern in countries of the Northern hemisphere such as Sweden, Finland and England, where the incidence is increasing for reasons that are not entirely clear.

Melanoma is most common in people in their forties to sixties and is rare before puberty. An increasing number of young adults with primary melanomas are being seen, however; many of them had episodes of intense sun-burn in their childhood. A tumor known as clear cell sarcoma, arising in the soft tissues such as muscle or the tissue under the skin, is made up of the same type of malignant melanocytes as adult melanomas. Children and adults can have this form.

Eye melanomas are most common in fair-skinned people living in sunny climates, suggesting that dark glasses completely blocking ultraviolet rays should be worn by blue-eyed people when out in bright sunlight.

Levels of Invasion
1. 0.75 mm (L1)
2. 0.76-1.5 mm (L2)
3. 1.6-4.0 mm (L3)
4. 4.0 mm (L4)
5. over 4.0 mm (L5)

Layers of skin, showing a malignant melanoma and a basal cell carcinoma

♦ Among Caucasians, red-haired people with very fair complexions are at the highest risk, followed by blond, blue-eyed people.

♦ Primary melanomas can occur even in dark-skinned people on the palms and soles, under the skin and in the membranes lining the mouth, rectum and anus.

♦ White people with a large number of moles are at increased risk. Those with sporadic dysplastic nevi—unusual moles that under the microscope have features resembling melanoma—are probably not at increased risk of developing melanoma from those nevi. People with a strong family history, however (familial dysplastic nevus syndrome), have an increased tendency to develop melanoma.

SCREENING

There is no effective screening procedure, but because melanoma arises on the skin or in the eye its presence is usually obvious to anyone aware of its features.

COMMON SIGNS AND SYMPTOMS

Cure requires early diagnosis and appropriate surgery. Family practitioners, internists and patients themselves must recognize the early-warning signs that ordinarily occur in sequence: *darkening* of an existing mole, an *increase* in its size, *irregularity* of margins and *elevation* of the lesion. The American Cancer Society's often quoted sign of bleeding is one of the later signs of the disease.

Further changes in the color of the mole, such as depigmentation of a portion of it or a reddish or bluish tinge, may also occur. Bleeding usually occurs after some minor injury sometime after these changes become apparent. Itching is common, as is scaling or crusting of the lesion. Occasionally, an entirely new pigmented spot appears.

It should be emphasized that most pigmented spots are not melanomas. Chronic inflammatory conditions, benign fibrous tumors (fibromas) and basal cell carcinomas—one of the most common low-malignancy skin tumors—are sometimes pigmented. Benign tumors can also bleed after being irritated by underwear or after shaving. It is nevertheless better to bring any suspicious changes to the attention of a doctor. It is far better to risk being thought a hypochondriac than to run the risk of letting a melanoma get out of hand.

DIAGNOSIS
Blood and Other Tests
♦ There are no blood tests available for screening or confirming the diagnosis of primary melanomas.

♦ Tumor-associated antigens shed by the tumor are now being looked at as possible markers in the bloodstream, but results are inconclusive. Carcino-embryonic antigen (CEA), which is found in several cancers, is not found in melanomas.

Endoscopy and Biopsy
♦ An adequate—in other words, an excisional—biopsy is necessary for diagnosis. Examination of the tumor under the microscope reveals characteristic melanoma cells, which are typically plump and usually contain dustlike grains of melanin pigment. The malignant melanocytes are seen to migrate into the dermis to various depths, where they are found singly, in small groups or in large aggregations. Immunological staining procedures with special antibody-carrying dyes are now available to confirm the diagnosis in cases that do not appear typical.

♦ Shave biopsies are not recommended. They do not allow the depth of invasion into the skin to be determined, and this needs to be known to help predict whether the patient will be cured or has a risk of recurrence.

♦ Cauterization or freezing should never be done. These procedures destroy the superficial part of the melanoma, making diagnosis and staging impossible. They also leave tumor cells in deeper locations at the site, which could later give rise to seeding of other parts of the body.

♦ Eye melanomas are not biopsied to avoid damage to sight. The appearance of eye melanomas is so characteristic that experienced ophthalmologists have no difficulty in making an accurate diagnosis in almost all cases.

STAGING

Several systems are used to stage skin melanomas. The depth of invasion is the best predictor of outcome. One classification categorizes primary melanomas into five levels of invasion that a pathologist can easily recognize under the microscope.

♦ Level 1 is melanoma at the place of origin, in the basal layer of the epidermis at the epidermal-dermal junction, where the outer and underlying layers of the skin meet.

♦ Level 2 is extension to the upper third of the dermis, the papillary dermis.

♦ Level 3 melanoma extends to the border of the papillary and reticular dermis.

♦ Level 4 involves the reticular dermis.

♦ Level 5 invades subcutaneous tissue, such as fat.

Level 1 melanomas are almost always curable by surgical removal of the lesion. Levels 4 and 5 recur in over 85 percent of cases. Level 3 melanomas recur in perhaps 60 percent of patients.

Another classification system using the exact measurement of the thickness of the tumor under the microscope has recently been introduced and is used together with the other system.

Melanomas less than 0.75 mm are usually considered highly curable by surgery alone, although some people with such "thin" lesions have had recurrences. Tumors 0.76 mm to 1.5 mm are considered to have a moderately deep invasion and have a worse prognosis than thin lesions. Melanomas 1.6 mm or more are very deep, particularly those over 4 mm.

While no exact relationship exists between the two classification schemes, an approximate correlation can be made between levels and thicknesses.

It is prudent to consider any lesion deeper than 0.75 mm potentially recurrent and, therefore, dangerous. Close contact with the surgeon or a medical oncologist for follow-up examinations and scans is required in these circumstances.

The presence of the tumor in regional lymph nodes draining the site of the primary tumor—such as the lymph nodes in the armpit draining a melanoma of the forearm—is another sign of a poor prognosis. Lymph nodes usually provide an immunological barrier against the tumor. When they are filled with tumor, they have obviously lost the battle and cancer cells have usually passed beyond them into the blood and traveled to distant organs. Over 80 percent of patients with involved nodes have a recurrence elsewhere.

Melanomas of the eye are classified by direct observation and ultrasound measurements into small, medium and large tumors, based on their diameter and elevation.

♦ Small tumors have a better prognosis and are often followed without removal to see how fast they are growing.

♦ Medium tumors are often followed, but there is some debate about whether this is the best course of action.

♦ Large melanomas are usually treated early, but if they are not significantly impairing vision they can also be watched for a time.

If the rules that govern skin melanomas are correct, any size of eye tumor carries a significant hazard of permitting the tumor to reach the bloodstream (the eye has few lymph vessels). Since the ocular melanoma appears to be much more slow growing than skin melanoma and usually occurs in elderly people, however, it does not have the same degree of risk.

The appearance of eye melanoma cells under the microscope is also an indicator of outcome. Spindle-shaped cells are less malignant and patients almost always live 15 years. Melanoma cells resembling skin cells (epithelioid) are more malignant, with 34 percent of patients living 5 years and 28 percent 15 years. Survival is a little better for melanomas in which spindle cells are mixed with epithelioid cells (46 percent and 41 percent, 5- and 15-year survivals respectively).

In general, small melanomas of the spindle cell type are almost entirely benign and the patient may never have widespread disease or require treatment of any kind.

♦ Melanomas arising from the colored portion at the front of the eye (the iris) are usually noted very early and frequently contain spindle cells.

♦ Large melanomas of the epithelioid variety require treatment soon after discovery. Despite treatment, there is spread to a different part of the body—often the liver—in 65 percent of all patients.

TREATMENT OVERVIEW

Surgery The removal of the tumor, along with sufficient margins of normal skin, is the only curative treatment for all but the most advanced stages of disease. Nearby lymph nodes may also be removed if they are involved.

Chemotherapy Single-drug chemotherapy is effective in no more than 20 percent of patients with advanced disease. Recent reports suggest that drug combinations can cause responses—more than 50 percent shrinkage of all tumor masses for at least four weeks—in 40 to 64 percent of cases. The percentage of complete remissions is low and the duration of response is still fairly short, but the increased percentage of responses is encouraging.

High-dose chemotherapy with drugs such as Thiotepa or melphalan, followed by replacement of the patient's own stored bone marrow—autologous bone marrow transplantation—has similar high response rates, but the short duration of remission (four months) does not yet justify the considerable risk of mortality (15 to 25 percent).

Radiation Radiation therapy can help shrink isolated large lesions, particularly nodules under the skin, or relieve pain, but high doses of at least 500 cGy are usually required to overcome the resistance of melanoma cells to radiation. Somewhat lower radiation doses (300 to 400 cGy) are used for brain metastases.

Hyperthermia in conjunction with radiation may improve local control of large lesions.

Biological Therapy Stimulating the immune system with biological response modifiers to reject the tumor has already shown some degree of success, sometimes with less severe side effects than chemotherapy.

Giving moderate doses of interferon-alpha three times a week under the skin (subcutaneously) has resulted in about a 20 percent response rate. Major advantages include self-administration by the patient or family members, minor side effects (controllable fever, chills and fatigue) and availability. The high cost of interferon-alpha is a drawback, but the two major companies that manufacture it both offer cost-assistance programs for those suffering financially because of the treatment.

Various doses of a new biological substance called interleukin-2 (IL-2) has had responses in approximately 25 percent of patients. Remarkable degrees of shrinkage have been observed in the liver (usually a very difficult site to treat), as well as in the lungs, lymph nodes, skin, bone and adrenal glands.

It is not necessary to receive so-called

LAK cells (IL-2 or lymphokine-activated killer cells) or very high dose IL-2 to achieve this response rate. IL-2 can also be given subcutaneously, which allows patients to administer it to themselves.

Active specific immunotherapy (melanoma vaccines) has also shown considerable promise in treating advanced melanoma and theoretically should be even more effective in early stages of the disease. About 20 to 25 percent of patients have had partial or complete remissions with the most successful of the melanoma vaccines.

There are no side effects from the vaccine except for some short-term soreness at the site of injections and, possibly, painful lumps after a long series of treatments. This makes it one of the easiest cancer treatments to tolerate. Melanoma and kidney cancer appear to be unusually sensitive to biological therapy, and a great variety of emerging biological agents and approaches will be tried first in these two diseases.

Adjuvant Therapy The removal of lymph nodes as a preventive (prophylactic) measure in patients without clinically enlarged lymph nodes has not been proved to improve the cure rate but still has its advocates among surgeons. The issue is being studied by university surgeons in an international trial nearing completion.

Several trials are addressing the issue of whether biological response modifiers such as tumor vaccines, interferons or interleukins that have proved useful in Stage IV disease can help prevent recurrence when used after surgery for Stage II and III disease.

There is suggestive evidence that some tumor vaccines can prolong disease-free survival, and more definite results should be forthcoming from several trials within the next few years.

Investigational Several new treatment methods have shown some promise in treating melanoma.

♦ Highly specific antibodies engineered in the test tube (monoclonal antibodies) to act against surface components of melanoma cells are being evaluated. Antibodies by themselves have not been too effective, but when used as carriers for killer molecules—radioactive isotopes, strong chemotherapeutic drugs, enzymes or toxins—good effects have been achieved in animals. Trials in humans have already shown that antibodies have "homed" to the tumor and can show its location accurately on radioisotope scanning (*see* Chapter 8).

♦ There are at least seven interleukins. IL-1 and IL-4 are ready for testing in humans. Both help IL-2 stimulate killer T lymphocytes (white blood cells that kill tumors) and the helper T cells that help educate the killer T cells. Both should be useful either alone or in combination with IL-2 in treatment protocols. Other combinations include interferons and interleukins together or in sequence.

♦ High-dose chemotherapy, with single drugs or in combinations, followed by autologous bone marrow transfusion, has had too many dangerous side effects associated with the drugs in current trials and too short a duration of response. The general approach, however, is very promising. Even now the rate of response is in the order of 60 percent.

♦ Several groups, including one at the National Cancer Institute, have begun investigating immunotherapy with tumor-infiltrating lymphocytes (TIL) or cloned killer and helper T cells. This form of "adoptive" immunotherapy involves removing blood cells from the patient, stimulating and multiplying them, then returning them, usually with IL-2. Initial results are very promising, with response rates in the 50 to 60 percent range.

SKIN MELANOMAS
STAGE I
Standard Treatment Surgery with a wide excision of normal tissue and a skin graft, if necessary, is preferred except when the

lesion is on the face. A margin of at least 1/2 in. (1 cm) and preferably 1 1/4 in. (3 cm) away from the edges of the tumor is usually maintained on cosmetically less important areas such as the back.

Five-Year Survival 80 to 100 percent

STAGE II
Standard Treatment Surgery, as for Stage I.

Five-Year Survival Up to 65 percent

STAGE III
Standard Treatment For deep melanomas without palpable lymph nodes, surgery as for Stage I is the standard procedure. If the melanoma was called Stage III because of an enlarged lymph node, that node should be removed. The radical removal of all lymph nodes at the site is highly controversial and cannot be routinely recommended. Such radical surgery has not brought about cure.

Five-Year Survival 20 to 50 percent

STAGE IV
Standard Treatment Systemic therapy using immunological or chemotherapy agents or regional therapy with radiation (*see* "Treatment Overview").

Five-Year Survival Less than 10 percent

EYE MELANOMAS
Standard Treatment Small tumors are usually followed closely by direct observation by an ophthalmologist, who uses a slit lamp and ultrasound or CT scanning to chart the exact diameter and height of the lesions. If they become large, they can be treated in the same way as medium and large melanomas.

Such medium and large melanomas are treated either by removing the eye (enucleation) or by applying radioactive plaques.

If the melanoma extends outside the eye to the surrounding bone, the prognosis is very poor. Surgical treatment combined with radiation therapy is usually given, but there is no solid evidence that this intensive therapy alters the bad outcome.

If the eye melanoma spreads to other parts of the body, it is usually handled in the same way as widespread skin melanoma, even though the tumors arising in the two locations may not be completely similar.

Investigational
♦ Immunological treatment found to be effective against skin melanomas will be studied against medium and large primary eye melanomas within the next few years. It would be a major advance if at least partial sight could be preserved by arresting tumor growth (if not outright regression) by immunological means.

TREATMENT FOLLOW-UP
Melanoma can involve so many parts of the body that any new symptom should be reported to the doctor.
♦ Since the liver and the lung are common sites for tumor cells to lodge and grow after traveling through the bloodstream, these organs should be watched carefully at three-month intervals after removal of the primary melanoma and more often during treatment of disseminated disease.
♦ Liver function tests (especially LDH and alkaline phosphatase) should be done.
♦ CT scans of the abdomen with contrast material injected to show the liver should be done every six months. MRI or ultrasound examinations of the abdomen are good alternatives. MRI is better than CT for evaluating the pelvis.
♦ A chest CT scan is preferable to a chest x-ray and can be performed at the same time as an abdominal scan, but a chest x-ray can suffice as a screening tool in

patients with no known lung metastases. Expense and exposure to radiation are major problems with frequent CT scans, even though the scans' ability to detect lesions is far better than with routine x-rays.

♦ Lumps under the skin, usually colorless or reddish-purple and occasionally black if *in* the skin, can be felt and seen by patients, often during a bath. Lymph nodes under the arms or in the groin can also be felt and/or seen.

♦ Brain involvement causing neurologic symptoms is becoming more common as therapy improves for disease elsewhere in the body and patients live long enough to allow the slow-growing brain metastases to enlarge. Therefore MRI scans (or, less desirably, a CT scan) of the brain should be performed at least semi-annually or at the first sign of headaches or changes in mental ability, vision, muscle strength, sensation or balance.

RECURRENT CANCER
Similar to Stage IV.

SUPPORTIVE TREATMENT
Melanoma usually has remarkably few debilitating effects on the system. Patients feel and look good through most of their disease.

Unless the tumor is in a place where it can cause symptoms because of its size—such as pressing on a nerve and causing pain, or causing headaches if it is in the brain—melanoma is not generally associated with severe symptoms. This is in sharp contrast to cancers such as those of the head and neck or the bowel, where patients may lose their appetite and become thin fairly early in the course of their disease. Patients should do everything they feel like doing, without fear of adversely affecting their disease. Modern treatments are designed to permit and encourage a full and active life.

♦ Low-or non-impact aerobic exercise, such as swimming or walking, can be pursued by all patients who feel good. More active exertion is often possible so long as there are no bad results, such as damage to the bones.

♦ Good, balanced nutrition is helpful, which means whole grains, lean meats and complex carbohydrates. Fad diets should be avoided, as they often lack essential nutrients. Many patients who are doing well are convinced that their use of high doses of some vitamin or extract is causing their response, although most are also receiving conventional treatments such as immunotherapy or chemotherapy.

♦ As in any cancer, psychological support is essential to a good outcome. An upbeat attitude is an important element. Support groups emphasizing psychological adjustment and channeling of mental strength into overcoming the tumor, often with visualization techniques, are increasing in popularity and perform a valuable function. While no one can yet explain it, there is little doubt that people who believe they will do well in fact do better than those who give up hope when they learn they have cancer. Mental attitude alone cannot do everything, but without a positive outlook even an objective remission of disease cannot make a patient truly better.

OTHER ISSUES
Melanoma is such a variable disease that someone who is diagnosed should not feel totally disheartened. Long disease-free intervals are often achieved after the deep primary tumors are removed, and early melanomas are usually curable. If the disease comes back in a lymph node, it can be removed surgically. If it comes back elsewhere, such as in the lungs or liver, a variety of treatments are available. Some of the most exciting developments

in immunotherapy are occurring in the treatment of melanoma.

It is important for all patients to know that there is now good news to replace the old bad news, when there was very little anyone could do about widespread disease.

Check any information you may gain from reading about the disease with an oncologist who knows about melanoma. Above all, don't let your relatives, neighbors or friends tell you all they "know" about melanoma.

THE MOST IMPORTANT QUESTIONS YOU CAN ASK

♦ What are the alternatives to the plan you are suggesting?
♦ Can you arrange a second opinion about the surgery you are proposing?
♦ What is the response rate and duration of response of the therapy you are proposing, and do you think they justify the side effects I may have?
♦ Are there investigational treatments available anywhere in the country? Can you help me find out about them?

MESOTHELIOMA

Malin Dollinger, MD and Ernest H. Rosenbaum, MD

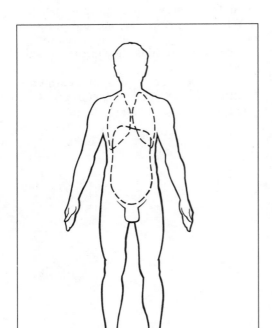

Mesothelioma is a malignant tumor in the lining of the chest and abdominal cavities. It is a rare form of cancer, with about 2,000 cases diagnosed in the United States each year. Most people who develop this cancer have a history of exposure to the widely found carcinogen asbestos.

Malignant mesothelioma is usually not curable, although some surgical cures have been reported in a very few patients with very localized tumors. Most patients, however, have widespread disease at the time of diagnosis, with chest pain and a buildup of fluid within the cavity involved that causes shortness of breath. Treatment at this stage, which may involve removing the fluid and the tumor, is usually directed toward relieving these symptoms.

Types Malignant mesothelioma is a sarcoma that can have both fibrous and epithelial elements. Epithelial cancers that develop in the tissues that cover the surface or line internal organs are carcinomas, so the epithelial form of mesothelioma is sometimes confused with adenocarcinomas of the lung or metastatic carcinomas. Epithelial mesotheliomas seem to have a better prognosis than other types.

How It Spreads Mesotheliomas start in the membranes lining the chest (pleural cavity) or the membranes of the abdominal cavity (the peritoneum). They can extend within and beyond the cavity of origin and metastasize to other organs such as the lungs, the chest wall and abdominal organs such as the bowel.

What Causes It Inhalation of asbestos fibers is a primary cause. About 70,000 tons of asbestos are used in the United States each year, in cement, brake linings, roof shingles, insulation, flooring products and packing materials. Asbestos has also been found as a contaminant in talc, which is also associated with ovarian cancer. Many urban water reservoirs contain asbestos-like fibers and most public and private buildings contain asbestos. Only recently has the strong association between asbestos exposure and malignancy been recognized and appropriate industrial and health standards for exposure been put into effect.

It is sometimes difficult to prove the relationship between asbestos exposure and the development of mesothelioma.

The increase in the disease is first detectable about 15 years after the first exposure and increases each year up to 40 to 45 years after the first exposure. It is estimated that about 8 million people living in the United States have been occupationally exposed to asbestos over the last half century during the mining and milling of the mineral and during various manufacturing processes.

RISK FACTORS

At Significantly Higher Risk
Anyone exposed to asbestos fibers, even for a few months, particularly:
♦ Miners and millers in contact with asbestos.
♦ Producers of asbestos products.
♦ Laborers who install plumbing, boilers and heating equipment in ships, factories and homes.
♦ Workers who are near the material but do not handle it directly (carpenters, electricians and shipyard welders, for example).
♦ Heating and construction tradespeople.
♦ People living near asbestos mines have an increased chance of developing asbestosis, the associated scarring of the lung, as well as mesothelioma.
♦ Inhabitants of the Anatoli region of Turkey, where zeolite is found in the soil and in homes.

At Somewhat Higher Risk
♦ Spouses and children of asbestos workers presumably because of asbestos fibers brought home in the hair and on clothing.
♦ Demolition workers and workers who repair structures that contain asbestos.
♦ Although smoking greatly increases the risk of lung cancer in asbestos workers, it does not increase the risk of mesothelioma.

SCREENING

Regular chest x-rays are essential to follow the course of people with any significant asbestos exposure, although the scar tissue and shadows related to asbestosis that are seen on the x-rays will be chronic and may progress slowly over the years even without the development of malignant mesothelioma. The tumor may not appear on a chest x-ray as a single mass with sharp edges, so rather than depend on x-rays as a screening method, the best procedure is to biopsy any suspicious area for a possible malignancy.

COMMON SIGNS AND SYMPTOMS

Patients with mesothelioma may have shadows on their chest x-rays related to asbestosis, though the development of chest pain, significant shortness of breath and especially fluid around one lung or in the abdomen should suggest a diagnosis of mesothelioma. People with peritoneal mesothelioma usually have signs of advanced disease, including an abdominal mass, pain, fluid in the abdomen (ascites) and weight loss.

If the tumor has extended to the ribs, bones, nerves and the superior vena cava, common symptoms include pain, trouble swallowing, nerve compression syn-dromes or swelling of the neck or face.

Involvement of the the membrane around the heart (pericardium) may cause heart rhythm disturbances. Tumors in the lining of the abdominal cavity (peritoneum) may extend to produce bowel obstruction. Fever, clotting abnormalities, thrombophlebitis and anemia have also been seen in a large number of patients with peritoneal mesothelioma.

DIAGNOSIS

Careful questioning about the history of asbestos exposure should focus on the period 20 to 50 years before diagnosis and include possible exposure to years of household contacts. Because asbestos is so widespread, a brief exposure may have been forgotten.

Chest membranes that may be involved with mesothelioma

Physical Examination
♦ Swelling of the neck and face.
♦ Abdominal mass.

Blood and Other Tests
♦ Lung function tests usually show a smaller amount of normal lung tissue available for breathing.
♦ A test for elevated levels of the carcinoembryonic antigen (CEA) in the blood may help distinguish an adenocarcinoma from mesothelioma, with a markedly elevated level suggesting an adenocarcinoma. This distinction may be important, for adenocarcinoma of the lung can be much more treatable than mesothelioma.
♦ Patients with peritoneal mesothelioma may have elevated platelet counts and clotting abnormalities.

♦ Laboratory studies are not particularly helpful.

Imaging
♦ CT scan to assess the extent of disease and to assist decision-making on therapy.
♦ Chest x-rays will often reveal thickening of the pleural membranes in half the patients with peritoneal mesothelioma.

Endoscopy and Biopsy
♦ If mesothelioma is suspected, attempts at a diagnostic biopsy should be made. Sometimes fluid removed during a chest "tap" (thoracentesis) may be examined for tumor cells in a way similar to a Pap test. A needle biopsy may also be done.
♦ Most cases require an open surgical biopsy, since needle biopsies seldom

produce enough diagnostic material. Since a simple biopsy done with a surgical incision into the chest under general anesthesia (thoracotomy) may make it technically difficult to remove the tumor later, the surgeon doing the biopsy should be prepared to do the definitive surgical treatment if that seems appropriate.

♦ The usual examination of the biopsied tissue under the microscope will often prove that the tissue is malignant but may not distinguish adenocarcinoma of the lung from mesothelioma. So a specimen is often processed by special methods—electron microscopy and special stains—to help document the type of tumor.

♦ Cytology of the sputum either coughed up by the patient or obtained through a bronchoscopy may document a bronchogenic adenocarcinoma, which may not be visible on routine chest x-rays.

♦ Patients with peritoneal mesothelioma eventually have exploratory surgery of the abdomen (laparotomy), with an open directed biopsy. Sometimes a simpler procedure, peritonoscopy, may yield enough tissue for diagnosis. An adequate biopsy is essential, since peritoneal mesothelioma can be confused with adenocarcinomas arising in other tissues, especially the ovary.

STAGING

There are a number of different staging systems for malignant mesothelioma, including a TNM system. All list four stages of tumor from very localized to metastatic, but no one system is universally agreed upon. The PDQ classification into localized and advanced disease seems most appropriate for decision-making.

There is no satisfactory staging system for peritoneal mesothelioma, although the tumor is usually confined to the abdomen. Since metastasis is rare, extensive staging studies outside the abdomen may not be necessary. CT scans will usually adequately define the extent of tumor.

TREATMENT OVERVIEW

Surgery is the only treatment method that can lead to a cure, but only people with very early stage disease—a small minority of patients—have long-term survival. Mesothelioma is usually incurable, so treatment efforts are designed to control the accumulation of fluids (effusion) as well as pain and other symptoms.

There is a large number of clinical trials investigating aggressive radiation therapy and chemotherapy programs.

 Chemotherapy Extensive attempts have been made to discover chemotherapeutic agents that have some effectiveness against this tumor. Many drugs have been tested, but only a few appear to have any activity. Doxorubicin, cyclophophamide and cisplatin are active, and so are 5-azacytidine, 5-fluorouracil and high-dose methotrexate with leucovorin rescue.

Response rates to combinations of chemotherapy drugs may be higher. Recent studies evaluating combinations containing doxorubicin indicate that this drug should be a part of all combinations.

 Radiation The usefulness of radiation therapy is difficult to define. The natural history of these tumors varies and interpretation of the effects after treatment is difficult, both because of chronic shadows on the chest x-ray before and after treatment and because so few patients have been treated with this method. Early research did suggest some benefit from radiation therapy.

One problem is that usually one entire side of the chest is at risk for tumor and has to be treated. It may be difficult to administer a dose of radiation high enough to control tumor growth without risking toxic effects to the stomach, intestines, liver and kidneys.

The radiation therapy physician must

also be careful in giving radiation to the area of the heart. This is even more of a problem after surgery to remove the left lung, with the resulting shift of the heart toward the left side of the chest. Sophisticated radiation methods have to be used with this cancer, which may involve electron beam treatments as well as the usual external radiation therapy.

Combined Therapy There has been a lot of interest in combined treatments, especially with radiation therapy being used as an adjuvant to surgery. This has also included the use of adjuvant intraoperative radiotherapy (IORT). New cooperative studies are evaluating various chemotherapeutic agents such as radiation sensitizers, especially doxorubicin.

Very recent research has also involved the preliminary use of chemotherapy, followed by surgery if the disease responded.

TREATMENT BY STAGE

LOCALIZED MALIGNANT MESOTHELIOMA
Localized mesotheliomas are either solitary tumors or tumors that have spread within the cavity involved (intracavitary) but are confined to the serosal sufaces where they started.

Standard Treatment Occasional patients with this stage of disease can be cured by aggressive surgery. A solitary tumor can be completely removed along with adjacent structures to ensure wide margins of cancer-free tissue.

Standard surgery for intracavitary mesothelioma will also involve the removal of portions of the lung and diaphragm in selected patients. Some surgeons favor more extensive operations to include whatever tissue is necessary to remove all visible tumor as long as this doesn't interfere with the functioning of the remaining organs.

To relieve the symptoms of disease, collections of fluid in the cavity (effusions)

are drained. A chemical irritant can then be introduced into the chest to make the layers of the membranes adhere to one another. This may prevent further fluid accumulations.

Radiotherapy is also sometimes given to the lung involved to eliminate blood flow in the area and improve breathing.

Five-Year Survival Not determined since cases are rare.

Investigational
♦ Chemotherapy within the chest cavity (intracavitary) after aggressive surgery.
♦ Clinical trials of new chemotherapeutic agents and radiotherapy techniques.

ADVANCED MALIGNANT MESOTHELIOMA
In this stage, the tumor has spread beyond the cavity of origin, with metastasis outside the serosal surface. This extension can include the lung, the chest wall, as well as abdominal organs such as the bowel.

Standard Treatment In some patients, surgical removal of the tumor may be done as a palliative measure. Radiation therapy may also be given in an attempt to control the growth of the malignancy and reduce symptoms in the lung.

As for localized disease, chemical irritants are used to control collections of fluid caused by irritation from the tumor. The fluid is drained beforehand and the chemical irritants introduced through a chest tube.

Five-Year Survival Less than 10 percent

Investigational Same as for localized disease.

PERITONEAL MESOTHELIOMA
Standard Treatment Therapy for peritoneal mesothelioma is difficult, especially as it is usually widespread by the time it is diagnosed. Removal of the tumors for

cure is rarely possible and the role of surgery is generally confined to relief of bowel obstruction, relief of ascites by placing shunts for drainage or the palliative removal of large tumors.

Radiation therapy has often been used, but its role has not yet been defined. Since the entire abdomen is at risk, all of the abdominal organs will also be affected by radiation. To protect the liver, kidney, bowel and spinal cord, the dose has to be lower than would be desirable for tumor control.

Although radiation may not be effective in most patients with large, bulky tumors because of the problems posed by an adequate dose, there may be some benefit from lower doses—in the range of 3,000 cGy—if most of the tumor has been successfully removed and only small amounts remain.

The use of chemotherapy for peritoneal mesothelioma has lately focused on the use of chemotherapy given via a catheter directly into the abdominal cavity (intraperitoneal). This permits a much higher concentration of drug to be delivered to the area of the tumor. Intraperitoneal cisplatin, with special measures to neutralize the drug's toxic effects in the body, resulted in a significant complete response rate in one study, but unfortunately many of these patients relapsed after treatment.

Survival Beyond one year is unusual

Investigational

♦ Important studies are currently underway with combined treatment therapy, using, for example, surgery and chemotherapy (cyclophosphamide + doxorubicin + dacarbazine) in combination with abdominal radiotherapy.

♦ Another current trial involves the removal of larger tumor nodules, followed by intraperitoneal chemotherapy with cisplatin and doxorubicin and a "second-look" operation to determine response. Radiotherapy is given if there has been complete control of the tumor and more chemotherapy is given before the radiation treatment if there is any residual disease left. The preliminary results of this combined program did produce a very significant response rate with acceptable toxicity.

TREATMENT FOLLOW-UP

Mesotheliomas usually progress rapidly and frequent follow-up evaluations are needed.

♦ A physical examination every six to twelve weeks.

♦ Chest or abdominal x-rays or CT scans every three to six months.

♦ Blood counts and chemistry panel every three to six months.

♦ Lung function tests, depending on symptoms.

THE MOST IMPORTANT QUESTIONS YOU CAN ASK

♦ Should I stop smoking?
♦ What can surgery accomplish?
♦ Should radiation be used?
♦ Is there any role for chemotherapy?
♦ How long can I live with this tumor?

METASTATIC CANCER

Alan P. Venook, MD

When a cancer spreads (metastasizes) from its original site to another area of the body, it is termed metastatic cancer. Virtually all cancers have the potential to spread this way. Whether metastases do develop depends on the complex interaction of many tumor cell factors, most of which are not completely understood.

The treatment of metastatic cancer depends on where the cancer started. When breast cancer spreads to the lungs, for example, it remains a breast cancer and the treatment is determined by the tumor's origin within the breast, not by the fact that it is now in the lung. About 5 percent of the time, metastases are discovered but the primary tumor cannot be identified. The treatment of these metastases is dictated by their location rather than their origin (*see* "Cancer of an Unknown Primary Site").

Although the presence of metastases generally implies a poor prognosis, some metastatic cancers can be cured with conventional therapy.

Types Virtually all cancers can develop metastases.

How It Spreads Metastases spread in three ways—by local extension from the tumor to the surrounding tissues, through the bloodstream to distant sites or through the lymphatic system to neighboring or distant lymph nodes. Each kind of cancer may have a typical route of spread. The most likely sites of metastases for each tumor are listed in the individual tumor chapters.

What Causes It The characteristics of each tumor are different, and it is not known what factors make the metastasis develop in particular places.

COMMON SIGNS AND SYMPTOMS

Many patients have no or minimal symptoms related to the tumor, and their metastases are found during a routine medical evaluation. If there are symptoms, they depend on the site involved.

♦ Brain metastases may cause headaches, dizziness, blurred vision, nausea or other symptoms related to the nervous system.

♦ Bone metastases may be evident because of pain, although they frequently cause no symptoms. The first sign of a bone metastasis may be when the affected bone breaks, often after a minor injury or no injury at all.

♦ Lung metastases may cause a non-productive cough, or a cough producing bloody sputum, chest pain or shortness of breath.

♦ Liver metastases may cause weight loss, fevers, nausea, loss of appetite, abdominal pain, fluid in the abdomen or jaundice (the skin turning yellow).

DIAGNOSIS

Physical Examination

There are no specific findings for metastatic cancer on physical examination. But there may be:

♦ fever
♦ tenderness of the bones
♦ tumors under the skin
♦ enlarged liver and spleen
♦ enlarged, hard lymph nodes
♦ fluid in the abdomen (ascites)
♦ jaundice (the skin turning yellow)
♦ swelling of the legs (edema)

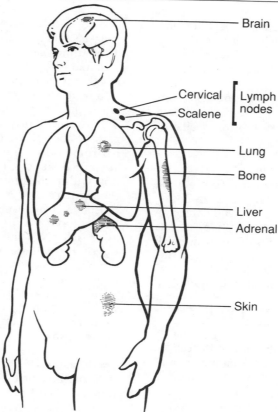

Brain

Cervical ⎤ Lymph
Scalene ⎦ nodes

Lung
Bone
Liver
Adrenal

Skin

Areas of Potential Cancer Metastases

Blood and Other Tests

♦ Routine liver function studies—blood tests looking at serum bilirubin and liver enzymes—may be abnormal. They can, however, be completely normal even in advanced stages of metastatic cancer.

♦ There may be serum blood tests that are abnormal. Metastatic colon cancer, for example, may be associated with an elevated carcinoembryonic antigen (CEA), testicular cancer with a high alpha-feto-protein (AFP) and/or elevated HCG and ovarian cancer with an elevated CA-125. But not all tumors have specific serum markers.

Imaging

♦ Abdominal ultrasound is one way to evaluate the abdomen if a mass is suspect-

ed. It can reveal the presence of fluid in the abdomen and is particularly useful for distinguishing a solid mass from a non-cancerous accumulation of fluid within the pelvis or liver (benign cyst).

♦ A bone scan will identify most tumor spread to the bones. It involves the injection of a special contrast agent into a vein, followed by whole-body imaging by a special camera. The image produced is a miniaturized skeleton that may show abnormal areas. But abnormal findings on a bone scan almost always have to be evaluated further with plain x-rays of the suspicious area.

♦ A CT scan is useful for determining the extent of a tumor within the head, chest or abdomen and for evaluating the possible spread of tumorous tissue into lymph

nodes or other structures in the abdomen.
♦ Magnetic resonance imaging (MRI) may help determine if the cancer can be surgically removed, but it is usually not necessary.
♦ If metastases have been found on biopsy, a chest x-ray should be done because the lungs are a very common site of metastases.

Endoscopy and Biopsy
♦ A biopsy, either with a fine needle (FNA) or regular needle, is often necessary. This procedure can be done through the skin without significant danger. The biopsy sample can be used to distinguish between types of malignancy because the tumor cells of different cancers have characteristic features under the microscope.

TREATMENT BY TYPE
Treatment of metastatic cancer primarily depends on the original site of the cancer, so for specific treatment recommendations refer to the chapters dealing with the primary cancers. In some clinical situations, however, metastases may be treated in specific ways.

BRAIN METASTASES
The treatment of brain metastases depends on many factors such as the tumor of origin, the number and location of lesions within the brain and the extent of cancer in places other than the brain.

Standard Treatment Most patients are placed on steroids (Decadron) to relieve significant brain swelling that can cause severe symptoms. Many patients will also take an antiseizure medicine (Dilantin), since seizures are a common complication.

Patients with brain metastases from lymphoma, leukemia or small cell cancer should generally be given radiation therapy to the entire brain, although these tumors may also be treated with systemic chemotherapy.

The standard approach with brain metastases of any other origin is to decide if the tumor can be removed. Both a CT scan and MRI should be done to discover whether there is more than one tumor and to define the specific site in the brain where the tumor or tumors are located.
♦ If there is only one tumor and the patient's overall condition is good, surgical removal of the metastasis may be attempted, although factors such as location within the brain, the duration since the primary cancer was treated and the presence of metastases elsewhere in the body have to be considered. This approach gives the best short-term and long-term palliation. After the tumor is removed, radiation therapy is given to the entire brain.
♦ In patients with more than one brain metastasis, surgery is not usually an option and radiation is delivered to the entire brain.

Investigational
♦ A method of biopsying or removing tumors called stereotaxic surgery is being studied. This allows for access to the brain tissue without causing extensive side effects (*see* "Brain Tumor").

LUNG METASTASES
Metastases to the lung are common for many types of cancer. Patients may have no symptoms or they may have symptoms such as shortness of breath or coughing up blood.

Standard Treatment Lung metastases are generally treated with chemotherapy directed against the primary tumor type. But occasionally tumors metastasize to form a single deposit in the lungs. The likeliest primary tumor to do this is a sarcoma, although it may occur with almost any primary cancer.

If the CT scan and MRI suggest that the tumor is isolated, it may be surgically removed without causing significant loss of lung function. In fact, sarcomas may metastasize slowly enough that as many as three or four discrete tumors can be removed. This aggressive approach should be considered in any patient with a solitary lung metastasis, although most of the time the presence of other systemic tumors is likely to limit any gains from surgery.

One problem caused by metastases to the lung and the tissue lining the lung (pleura) is the accumulation of fluid within the chest. This may make the lung collapse, creating breathing difficulties. The fluid can be removed through a needle or through a larger tube inserted through the skin into the chest cavity. After the fluid is removed, an irritant such as tetracycline or bleomycin may be injected into the cavity to cause scarring of the tissues and prevent the reaccumulation of fluid.

If a metastatic tumor causes bleeding into the lungs, a patient may begin coughing up blood. Radiation therapy directed precisely at the tumor may alleviate the problem. If that cannot be done, it may be possible to stop the bleeding by injecting a special material into a blood vessel in the lung. This requires a specific radiologic technique but occasionally is very effective.

BONE METASTASES
Bone metastases may be discovered on a routine x-ray or bone scan or may be found because of pain, swelling or a fracture of the weakened bone.

Standard Treatment Bone metastases that don't produce symptoms and involve bones that are not weight-bearing (weight-bearing bones include the hip, upper leg, and shoulder) may be treated with the chemotherapy appropriate for the primary tumor.

Bone metastases that cause symptoms can also be treated with systemic therapy, although to take this approach depends on the type of cancer and the likelihood of

getting much benefit from the treatment. If the tumor is not likely to respond to chemotherapy or if the bone involved is a weight-bearing one, the best option is to give radiation focused only on the involved area. The symptomatic relief is usually rapid and complete. Each bone can tolerate only a limited amount of radiation, although radiation can often be used to treat many different sites of tumor involvement.

If the bone metastases become apparent because of a fracture, the management issues are complicated. Surgery may be required to repair the bone and should be done if it is a weight-bearing bone. Fractured ribs, on the other hand, are not treated with a cast or immobilization. All such fractures should be treated with radiation therapy as well.

Bone metastases to the spine are a particular concern because a fractured vertebra can result in the loss of function of the limbs or bowel and bladder. Tumors in these bones, therefore, may need to be treated even though they are not weight-bearing bones and even when there are no symptoms.

LIVER METASTASES
Treatment of liver metastases depends on the organ where the cancer originated.

Standard Treatment For most metastatic tumors to the liver, systemic chemotherapy directed at the tumor type should be offered. But metastases from some cancers may be approached in a different way.

Occasionally, metastases to the liver are localized in one part of the liver or exist as solitary masses. Such tumors may be surgically removed with a possibility of achieving a cure, particularly with metastases from colon and kidney cancers or sarcoma. Generally, no more than four tumors should be removed from the liver, however. Removing more than four metastases rarely results in a cure and exposes the patient to significant surgical risks.

Liver metastases from colon cancer may be treated with combination chemotherapy, but because of the particular biological properties of some colon cancers, patients may develop liver metastases without ever having other sites of tumor involvement. Patients with such limited cancer may benefit from chemotherapy infused directly into the liver. Delivered by an implanted pump connected to the hepatic artery, this therapy takes advantage of the liver's ability to metabolize some drugs, meaning that the tumor may be exposed to high concentrations of chemotherapy while the rest of the body is spared the side effects.

This approach initially requires surgery for the implantation of the pump and the removal of the gall bladder, but the rest of the therapy can be done on an outpatient basis. The treatment causes tumor regression more often than standard chemotherapy.

Investigational

♦ New combinations of chemotherapy drugs may improve results for patients with colon cancer metastases, both to the liver and elsewhere. Such treatments are being studied for systemic treatment as well as for treatment to the liver.

♦ A treatment called chemoembolization involves administering a combination of chemotherapy and colloid particles directly into the liver tumor via its main (hepatic) artery. The procedure is performed by a radiologist and does not require surgery or prolonged bedrest. It is very effective for primary tumors, but it is much less effective for metastases.

♦ Cryosurgery—cold surgery—holds out some promise of allowing the removal of some otherwise unresectable tumors. So far, this technique is performed only by a few specialized physicians.

♦ Liver transplantation can be performed. But it should almost never be done for patients with metastatic tumors in the liver, for it can be assumed that the cancer will spread to other organs.

SUPPORTIVE THERAPY

♦ Pain relievers are sometimes called for in liberal doses. Narcotics may have excessive side effects, however, because they are metabolized by the liver, which may not be functioning properly.

♦ Non-steroidal anti-inflammatory drugs may be effective even against the severe pain associated with metastatic cancer.

♦ The loss of appetite that often accompanies metastatic cancer may be relieved with a medication called Megace.

♦ The use of water pills to alleviate fluid in the abdomen or legs may cause a significant imbalance in kidney function, creating major problems if their use is not carefully monitored.

♦ Nausea can be adequately treated with standard medications, including suppositories.

♦ Sleep disturbances are common, but sleeping pills (sedatives) should be used carefully, since most are metabolized by the liver.

TREATMENT FOLLOW-UP

Careful follow-up is necessary after treatment of metastases. Depending upon the organs involved, diagnostic tests will be done to identify new areas of tumor involvement that may cause problems and to look for tumor recurrences.

THE MOST IMPORTANT QUESTIONS YOU CAN ASK

♦ Should I see another physician to confirm that my metastatic tumor is being treated in the right way?

♦ Could I benefit from an investigational therapy available at another institution?

♦ How sick will the proposed chemotherapy make me relative to its potential benefit?

♦ How sure are you that you know the primary source of my cancer?

MULTIPLE MYELOMA

Robert A. Kyle, MD

Multiple myeloma is a cancer of the plasma cell, a type of B lymphocyte responsible for producing antibodies that take part in the immune response. A treatable but rarely curable disease, multiple myeloma—also called plasma cell myeloma, myelomatosis or Kahler's disease—is characterized by the overgrowth of malignant plasma cells, mostly in the bone marrow. Although multiple myeloma usually involves the bones, it must be distinguished from cancers that begin in another organ such as the breast or lung and then spread to the bones.

Multiple myeloma is an uncommon malignancy, making up only 1 percent of all cases of cancer. In a population of 1 million people, only 30 to 40 cases would be found each year. There have been reports that the incidence of myeloma has increased two- to threefold during the past 40 years, but careful studies from the United States and Europe suggest that the incidence has not truly changed. The apparent increase is most likely due to more and better medical facilities and diagnostic techniques.

Types Ninety percent of multiple myeloma cases involve the bone marrow. There are several types, each with its distinctive features and each producing a variety of diagnostic findings and symptoms:

♦ Patients with smoldering multiple myeloma (SMM) have enough myeloma cells in the bone marrow and a large amount of an abnormal protein (monoclonal or M-protein) in the blood to indicate multiple myeloma, but they do not have the anemia, kidney failure or skeletal lesions that are also characteristic of the disease. There are no symptoms.

♦ Patients with plasma cell leukemia have large numbers of plasma cells circulating in the blood. Plasma cell leukemia may be the first feature of multiple myeloma leading to a diagnosis or it may occur late in its course after a resistance to chemotherapy has developed.

♦ With non-secretory myeloma, patients have abnormal plasma cells in the bone marrow and frequently have holes (lytic lesions) in the skeleton, but no abnormal protein is detectable in the blood or urine.

♦ Osteosclerotic myeloma patients usually have pain, burning, numbness and weakness produced by the involvement of nerves by the disease (polyneuropathy). The liver and spleen are often enlarged, there may be a darkening of the skin and increased growth of body hair. The breasts may become enlarged and the testicles smaller. Bone x-rays usually reveal dense (sclerotic) areas in the bone. Anemia, kidney failure and fractures are rare with this type.

♦ Solitary plasmacytoma (solitary myeloma of bone) means there is a single plasma cell tumor in the bone. X-rays of the bones show no other lytic lesions and the bone marrow is normal. Characteristically, the patients have no abnormal M-protein in the blood or urine. This tumor can be treated with high doses of radiation to the lesion, but about 60 percent of patients will develop multiple myeloma within 10 years.

♦ Extramedullary plasmacytoma is a tumor consisting of myeloma cells but occurs *outside* the bone marrow. The most commonly involved area is the back of the nose and throat (nasopharynx), and the sinuses or larynx (voice box) may also be involved. Eighty percent of cases involve the upper respiratory area.

Extramedullary plasmacytomas may also involve the stomach, small bowel, colon, urinary bladder, thyroid, breast or the brain. Examination of the bone marrow is normal, and the patients have no lytic bone lesions or M-protein in the blood or urine. If the abnormal protein is present, it should disappear after treatment. Diagnosis of plasmacytomas is made after a biopsy of the tumor. It is treated with large doses of radiation therapy. Most patients are cured, but the disease may recur in a nearby area. The development of typical multiple myeloma is uncommon.

What Causes It The cause is not known, although exposure to radiation may be a factor in some cases. Survivors of the atomic bomb explosions in Japan had an increased incidence of multiple myeloma.

There is little evidence that chemicals cause myeloma in humans, although some reports have linked multiple myeloma with benzene or asbestos. An increased risk of multiple myeloma has been recognized in farmers in several countries and has been noted in rubber workers, furniture workers and those exposed to pesticides. The number of cases is small, however, and more information is needed to confirm this association.

There have been reports of two or more family members with multiple myeloma, but if a genetic factor exists it is of little importance. There is no evidence that allergies, chronic infections or other immune-stimulating conditions play a role.

RISK FACTORS

At Significantly Higher Risk
♦ Multiple myeloma occurs in older people. The average age is approximately 60 years; 2 percent are under 40.
♦ Its incidence in blacks is twice that in caucasians.

SCREENING

Screening is of no value in a healthy person because anyone with multiple myeloma should not be treated unless there are symptoms or serious laboratory abnormalities. Many patients are found to have an M-protein in their blood during a routine examination, but if there is no other evidence of multiple myeloma these patients are considered to have a benign condition called monoclonal gammopathy of undetermined significance (MGUS).

Bone with lytic myeloma lesion and stabilizing rod

COMMON SIGNS AND SYMPTOMS

At the time of diagnosis, more than two-thirds of people with multiple myeloma have bone pain, typically in the back or chest and less often in the arms and legs. The pain is usually made worse by movement and does not occur at night except after a change in position. Patients may lose several inches in height because of the collapse of vertebrae.

Weakness and fatigue are common and are often associated with anemia. Fever is rare, and when it occurs it is usually from an infection. Occasionally, there may be bleeding from the nose and gums or easy bruising. The initial symptoms may result from an acute infection, most often pneumonia, though meningitis or bloodstream infections may also occur. There may also be symptoms of elevated serum calcium (*see* "Supportive Therapy").

DIAGNOSIS

There are strict minimal criteria for the diagnosis of multiple myeloma. There must be at least 10 percent abnormal plasma cells in the bone marrow or proof of an extramedullary plasmacytoma *plus* the usual clinical features of multiple myeloma *and* at least one of the following abnormalities:
♦ an M-protein in the blood (usually greater than 3 gm/dL)
♦ an M-protein in the urine (Bence Jones protein)
♦ osteolytic lesions.

Connective tissue diseases (such as rheumatoid arthritis, polymyositis or scleroderma), chronic infections, metastatic cancer, lymphoma and leukemia may resemble some of the characteristics of multiple myeloma.

The diagnosis must differentiate those with true multiple myeloma from those with monoclonal gammopathy of undetermined significance (MGUS) and smoldering multiple myeloma (SMM), since people with these conditions should be observed indefinitely and not given therapy unless they develop features of multiple myeloma.

Physical Examination
♦ Physical findings are often general and non-specific. Pallor (paleness) is the most common physical finding.
♦ The liver can be felt in about one-fifth of patients; the spleen is rarely felt.
♦ There may be tumors outside the bone marrow (extramedullary plasmacytomas).

Blood and Other Tests
♦ A complete blood count (CBC) reveals anemia in two-thirds of patients.
♦ A serum chemistry profile includes measures from about 15 chemistry tests. An elevated serum calcium occurs in about 30 percent of patients. The level of serum creatinine (a measure of kidney function) is abnormal in one-fourth of patients at diagnosis. An increased total serum protein may be one of the first clues to the presence of an M-protein. The serum beta-2 microglobulin level is helpful in prognosis.
♦ Serum protein electrophoresis shows an M-protein "spike" in 75 percent of patients. Immunoelectrophoresis or immunofixation is necessary to determine the type of M-protein. The amount of M-protein is measured by serum protein electrophoresis or by the measurement of IgG or IgA, the two major types of M-protein found in multiple myeloma.
♦ Ninety-nine percent of patients with multiple myeloma will have an M-protein in the blood or in the urine. If the level of M-protein in the blood is high or if the patient has blurred vision or bleeding, determining the viscosity (thickness) of the serum is necessary. Measuring of the M-protein in the serum and urine is a good way to determine whether the disease is getting worse or is responding to chemotherapy. The level of the M-protein is a direct measure of the tumor mass.
♦ A 24-hour urine specimen is essential. The total protein is determined and elec-

trophoresis is performed, making it possible to measure the amount of monoclonal light chain (of kappa or lambda origin). This is often called Bence Jones protein and should be detected by immunologic techniques.

♦ Bone marrow examination is essential for diagnosis, allowing the physician to determine the number of plasma cells (myeloma cells) in the marrow and their appearance. It also provides a measure of normal red cell, white cell and platelet production.

Serum protein electrophoresis (SPEP) patterns in multiple myeloma.
Note the M protein spike

Imaging

♦ X-rays of the skull, the entire spine, pelvis, upper legs and upper arms are necessary to detect lytic lesions, bone thinning (osteoporosis) or fractures. Skeletal abnormalities occur in 80 percent of patients.

♦ Bone scans with technetium-99 can be done but are not as effective as conventional x-rays for detecting lesions.

♦ CT or MRI scans may be helpful when the patient has skeletal lesions and negative x-rays.

Monoclonal spike
(M protein)

Normal

Albumin α_1 α_2 β γ
          Alpha$_1$ Alpha$_2$ Beta   Gamma

GLOBULINS

STAGING

A clinical staging system based on a combination of laboratory findings that correlate with the myeloma cell mass has often been used. Patients are generally separated into those with low-cell mass (Stage I), high-cell mass (Stage III) and those whose cell mass is between Stages I and III (Stage II). A further classification divides patients according to whether they are "A" (kidney function test is normal or only slightly elevated, with a creatinine less than 2.0 mg/dL) or "B" (the serum creatinine is equal to or greater than 2.0 mg/dL).

All patients in Stage III and almost all in Stage II should be treated, but many Stage I patients will have no symptoms and need no treatment.

TREATMENT OVERVIEW

Multiple myeloma involves all of the red bone marrow and is widespread when the diagnosis is made. Consequently, there is no adjuvant or neoadjuvant treatment and no therapy for metastatic disease. Treatment is not given only on the basis of the stage of disease.

Not all patients who meet the minimal

criteria for diagnosis of multiple myeloma should be treated. Because the disease is not curable and therapy involves cost and potential side effects, treatment should be delayed until there is evidence of progression, symptoms appear or treatment is needed to prevent complications.

When symptoms do develop, chemotherapy is the preferred treatment.

Chemotherapy The major controversy in chemotherapy is whether treatment should be with a single alkylating agent such as melphalan (Alkeran) together with prednisone or a combination of alkylating agents.

Melphalan + prednisone is given daily by mouth for four to seven days every four to six weeks. This produces an objective response in 50 to 60 percent of patients. The dosage of melphalan must be changed depending upon the white count and platelet count, with the dosage increased to the point that some decrease in the white count or platelets occurs three weeks after the start of each cycle of therapy.

Many combinations of chemotherapy drugs—including melphalan, cyclophosphamide, carmustine (BCNU), vincristine, doxorubicin (Adriamycin) and prednisone—produce an objective response in about 75 percent of patients. But the average survival of those treated with the single alkylating agent (melphalan) and those receiving multiple alkylating agents is about the same—two to three years.

How long chemotherapy should be continued is unknown. Stopping treatment after one or two years usually results in relapse, but patients receiving chemotherapy may also relapse or develop bone marrow damage resulting in a myelodysplastic syndrome or acute leukemia. So it is advisable to continue treatment for one to two years, then discontinue therapy if there has been a response and the patient is in a stable (plateau) state. Patients must be followed closely, however, and chemotherapy must be started again when there is a relapse.

Radiation The use of radiation therapy should be limited to those patients with disabling pain who have a local process that has not responded to chemotherapy. The use of Tylenol with codeine or other narcotics can usually control the pain. This approach is preferred to local radiation because pain frequently recurs in another site anyway and local radiation does not benefit anyone with generalized disease.

Five-Year Survival 25 to 40 percent for Stage I, 15 to 30 percent for Stage II, and 10 to 25 percent for Stage III

Investigational Chemotherapy
♦ Interferon-alpha appears to be beneficial in prolonging the plateau state (remission) of patients with multiple myeloma. This preliminary observation must be confirmed by more extensive studies.
♦ The combination of alkylating agents and interferon shows promise. VBMCP (vincristine + BCNU + melphalan + cyclophosphamide + prednisone) in alternating cycles with interferon-alpha produces an objective response in 80 percent of patients. Complete responses—disappearance of the M-protein from blood and urine and a normal bone marrow—or near-complete responses were found in 46 percent of patients in a pilot study. This exceeds the 19 percent with similar responses in those treated with VBMCP alone. The average survival is about three years with a combination of interferon-alpha and VBMCP.

Bone Marrow Transplantation This procedure, while investigational, is promising in the treatment of multiple myeloma. There are three methods of bone marrow transplantation, but not all are useful for this disease.

◆ With allogenic transplantation, bone marrow is given from a matched donor following high-dose chemotherapy and total body irradiation. The mortality is high (25 percent within the first three months) and the patient often suffers from a peculiar form of rejection called graft-versus-host disease, in which the transplanted marrow attacks the host tissue. This procedure is also possible only for people under 45, which greatly limits its use in multiple myeloma.

◆ Autologous transplantation—in which marrow is removed from a patient before high-dose radiation or chemotherapy, then returned—is applicable to far more people because it can be used in older patients and there is no problem with graft-versus-host disease.

◆ With autologous bone marrow transplantation with peripheral blood stem cell rescue, normal stem cells are obtained from the patient's blood and then stored. The patient is then given a high dose of chemotherapy plus total body irradiation, and the stem cells from the blood are returned. The advantage to this procedure is that blood contains fewer myeloma cells than the bone marrow.

But there are two major problems for patients with multiple myeloma. First, it is difficult to destroy all the myeloma cells from the bone marrow even with high doses of chemotherapy and radiation. Second, it is difficult to remove the malignant myeloma cells from the bone marrow or blood before reinfusion. Using chemotherapy or monoclonal antibodies directed against myeloma cells (or both monoclonal antibodies and chemotherapy) may be helpful.

SUPPORTIVE CARE

Multiple myeloma produces many complications that require close medical attention and management.

◆ *Hypercalcemia* (elevated blood calcium level) This occurs in almost one-third of all patients and should be suspected if symptoms such as loss of appetite, nausea, vomiting, excessive thirst, increased urine, constipation, weakness, change in mental alertness or confusion develop. Treatment is urgent because kidney failure is common. Therapy with intravenous fluids and prednisone is usually effective, but if it isn't there are a variety of other effective agents such as mithramycin, calcitonin or diphosphonates.

◆ *Infections* Bacterial infections may occur and must be diagnosed and treated promptly with appropriate antibiotics. All patients should receive pneumococcal vaccine and influenza immunization. Prophylactic penicillin or intravenous gamma globulin should be considered for those with serious recurrent bacterial infections.

◆ *Pain* Bone pain should be treated with analgesics or narcotics. People with multiple myeloma have to be as active as possible because confinement to bed increases the bone loss. Patients should do all they can to avoid falling because a fall can result in multiple fractures. The use of an intramedullary rod in the long bones of the arm or leg should be considered when a large hole (lytic lesion) is seen on x-ray. The rod will stabilize the bone and prevent fractures. Radiation therapy to relieve pain may not be necessary for someone who is beginning chemotherapy but is sometimes used.

◆ *Fluid Balance* Increased fluid intake is necessary for patients with Bence Jones protein in the urine. They should drink enough fluids so that they produce 3 quarts (3 L) of urine daily. Patients with acute kidney failure must be treated promptly with maintenance of fluid and electrolyte balance. An artificial kidney (hemodialysis) may be necessary. In some cases, removing large amounts of plasma from the blood (plasmapheresis) may be helpful.

♦ *Hyperviscosity* This condition of "thick blood" is characterized by bleeding from the nose or gums, blurred vision, dizziness, shortness of breath or mental confusion. It can be treated effectively with plasmapheresis.

♦ *Muscle Weakness* People with multiple myeloma may develop weakness or paralysis of their legs and have difficulty urinating or controlling their bowels. If this happens, a myeloma tumor pressing on the spinal cord is a possibility and can be diagnosed with a CT or MRI scan or myelography. The tumor can be treated effectively with radiation therapy.

♦ *Emotional Support* Anyone with multiple myeloma needs substantial and continuing emotional support. The approach must be positive, emphasizing the potential benefits of therapy. It is reassuring to know that some patients survive for 10 years or more while receiving treatment. It is vital that the physician caring for patients with multiple myeloma has the interest and capacity to deal with an incurable disease over a span of years with assurance, sympathy and resourcefulness and that patients can sense the doctor's confidence.

TREATMENT FOLLOW-UP

♦ Complete blood count (CBC) every three weeks after each cycle of therapy and before each treatment course.
♦ Calcium and creatinine measured every 6 to 12 weeks.
♦ Serum protein electrophoresis every 6 to 12 weeks.
♦ Electrophoresis of a 24-hour urine specimen every 6 to 12 weeks if an M-protein was found at the time of diagnosis.
♦ Metastatic bone survey every six months or x-rays of bones in the event of new pain.
♦ Bone marrow examination to confirm remission or relapse.

RECURRENT (AND RESISTANT) CANCER

About one-third of all patients treated initially with chemotherapy will not obtain an objective response. And almost all patients with multiple myeloma who do respond to chemotherapy will eventually relapse if they do not die of some other disease in the meantime.

The decision about further treatment after a relapse has to take a number of factors into account, including prior treatment, where the recurrence occurs and personal considerations.
♦ If the relapse occurs after the initial therapy has been stopped, therapy with the same melphalan-prednisone or multiple alkylating agent treatments may be effective.
♦ If the relapse occurs while melphalan and prednisone therapy is being used, a combination called VBAP (vincristine + BCNU + Adriamycin + prednisone) will be of some benefit to 40 percent of patients.
♦ If a patient has already received these agents or does not respond to VBAP, a combination of vincristine + Adriamycin + dexamethasone (VAD) can be given.
♦ If a patient is resistant to all of these agents, a trial of high-dose prednisone or methylprednisolone may be beneficial.

THE MOST IMPORTANT QUESTIONS YOU CAN ASK

♦ Should I be treated now or should therapy be delayed until I have symptoms?
♦ Should I receive single or multiple alkylating agents?
♦ Should I get a second opinion?
♦ When should chemotherapy be discontinued?
♦ Should I receive an autologous bone marrow transplant?

OVARY

Jeffrey L. Stern, MD

◇

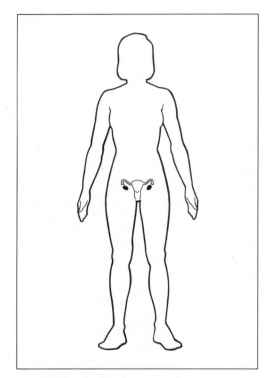

Carcinoma of the ovary is one of the most common gynecologic malignancies. In many cases, it is curable when found early, but because it does not cause any symptoms in its early stages most women have widespread disease at the time of diagnosis. Partly because of this, the mortality rate from ovarian cancer exceeds that for all other gynecologic malignancies combined. It is the fourth most frequent cause of cancer death in women in the United States. About one in every 70 women will develop cancer of the ovary and one in every 100 women will die from it. The American Cancer Society estimates that there will be 20,700 cases of ovarian cancer diagnosed in 1991 with approximately 12,500 deaths.

Types The most common form of ovarian cancer arises from the cells covering the surface of the ovary and is known as epithelial carcinoma. There are five major types of this carcinoma—serous, mucinous, endometrioid, clear cell and undifferentiated. Epithelial carcinomas are further divided into grades, according to how virulent they appear on microscopic examination.

Tumors of low malignant potential, also known as borderline tumors, are the most well-differentiated malignancy (Grade 0) and account for 15 percent of all epithelial carcinomas of the ovary. The other three grades are well-differentiated (Grade 1), moderately differentiated (Grade 2) and poorly differentiated (Grade 3). Well-differentiated tumors have a better prognosis than poorly differentiated tumors. Clear cell carcinoma and especially undifferentiated carcinoma have a poorer prognosis than the other cell types.

The two other major kinds of ovarian cancer—germ cell tumors, which arise from the eggs, and ovarian stromal tumors, which arise from supportive tissue—are relatively uncommon and account for less than 10 percent of all ovarian malignancies (*see* "Ovarian Germ Cell Tumors").

How It Spreads Ovarian cancer spreads early by shedding malignant cells into the abdominal cavity. The cells implant on the lining of the abdominal cavity (peritoneum) and can grow on the surface of the liver, the fatty tissue attached to the stomach and large intestine (omentum), the small and large intestines, the bladder and the diaphragm.

Disease on the diaphragm may at times result in impaired drainage of fluid from the abdominal cavity, resulting, for some women, in a large collection of abdominal fluid known as ascites. The cancer cells can occasionally cross the diaphragm and spread to the surface of the lungs and chest cavity, resulting in a collection of fluid around the lungs known as a pleural effusion.

Ovarian cancer may also spread to the pelvic, aortic, groin and neck lymph nodes (*see* page 278).

What Causes It Unknown.

RISK FACTORS

There is a much higher incidence of ovarian cancer in industrialized countries. Some researchers have implicated talcum powders, which until recently contained asbestos, as a possible cause. Ovarian cancer can occur in any age group, but it is most common in postmenopausal women. Not ovulating—by having children, using birth control pills or having a medical condition that interferes with ovulation—may offer some protection against developing ovarian cancer.

There may also be a genetic predisposition to this cancer. There are rare families in which several members of the same or different generation develop ovarian cancer.

SCREENING

There is no diagnostic method accurate enough to be used for routine screening of women who have no symptoms. Nonetheless, the American College of Obstetricians and Gynecologists recommends that all women have an annual pelvic and rectal examination, since an ovarian mass can occasionally be detected.

A Pap smear will detect ovarian cancer in only 15 percent of women with the disease.

Recent studies have shown that a serum tumor marker known as CA-125 is elevated in 80 percent of women with epithelial ovarian cancer. Unfortunately, this is not accurate enough for screening all women for ovarian cancer. There is a great deal of research now exploring it and other tumor markers for screening, however, and it is useful for assessing response to treatment.

A pelvic ultrasound examination may become part of the routine annual gynecological exam in the future.

COMMON SIGNS AND SYMPTOMS

Many women with early stages of ovarian carcinoma have no symptoms. The unfortunate result is that two-thirds of all women with ovarian carcinoma have advanced disease at the time of diagnosis.

Many women have vague, non-specific abdominal symptoms including pain, pelvic pressure, low back discomfort, mild nausea, feeling full early when eating, constipation and gas. Some women have abnormal uterine bleeding. Although some cases are diagnosed during a routine gynecologic examination, many women are diagnosed only when they have developed abdominal distension because of ascites.

Advanced ovarian cancer often results in blockage of the intestines, causing severe nausea, vomiting, pain and weight loss.

DIAGNOSIS

Physical Examination
♦ A careful pelvic exam is performed with attention to the ovaries, uterus, bladder and rectum.
♦ The neck, groin and underarms (axilla) are examined for enlarged lymph nodes.
♦ The lungs are carefully examined for excess fluid.
♦ The abdomen is examined for the presence of an enlarged liver, a mass or ascites.

Blood and Other Tests
♦ Complete blood count (CBC).
♦ Serum liver and kidney function tests.
♦ Serum CA-125.

Imaging
♦ Abdominal and pelvic CT or MRI scans.
♦ X-rays of the upper gastrointestinal tract (UGI series) may occasionally be done.
♦ Intravenous pyelogram (occasionally).
♦ Barium enema.

Endoscopy and Biopsy
♦ A definitive diagnosis requires microscopic examination of part or all of the involved ovary or any other suspicious abdominal mass. Cystic ovarian tumors that are less than 2 1/2 in. (6 cm) in diameter occurring in premenopausal woman are usually benign cysts.

Surgical evaluation should be performed for any mass in a postmenopausal woman, masses that are larger than 2 1/2 in. (6 cm) in diameter, masses persisting longer than one menstrual cycle and masses that are suspicious on imaging of the pelvis.

STAGING

Ovarian carcinoma is staged at surgery. Stages are usually defined according to the classification system devised by FIGO (International Federation of Gynecology and Obstetrics). The TNM system corresponds to the stages accepted by FIGO.

Stage I Cancer is confined to one or both ovaries.

♦ **Ia** Cancer is limited to one ovary. There is no ascites and no tumor on the surface of the ovary and the surface of the tumor is unruptured.

♦ **Ib** The cancer is limited to both ovaries. There is no ascites and no tumor on the

surface of either ovary and the surfaces of the tumors are unruptured.

♦ **Ic** The cancer is either Stage Ia or Ib and one or more of the following applies: there is tumor on the surface of one or both ovaries, at least one of the tumors has ruptured, ascites is present or the abdominal washings contain malignant cells.

Five-Year Survival 60 to 100 percent, depending on the histologic type, grade and sub-stage.

Stage II The tumor involves one or both ovaries with extension to other pelvic structures.

♦ **IIa** There is extension of the cancer or metastases to the uterus and/or fallopian tubes.

♦ **IIb** There is extension to the bladder or rectum.

♦ **IIc** The cancer is either stage IIa or IIb and one or more of the following applies: there is tumor on the surface of one or both ovaries, at least one of the tumors has ruptured, the ascites contains malignant cells or the washings from the abdominal cavity contain malignant cells.

Five-Year Survival About 60 percent

Stage III The tumor involves one or both ovaries with tumor implants confined to the abdominal cavity but outside the pelvis, or there is cancer in the pelvic, para-aortic or groin lymph nodes (*see* figure page 278).

♦ **IIIa** The tumor is grossly limited to the pelvis and the lymph nodes are negative, but there is biopsy-proven microscopic cancer on the intra-abdominal (peritoneal) surfaces.

♦ **IIIb** The tumor involves one or both

ovaries and there are tumor implants on the peritoneal surfaces less than 3/4 in. (2 cm) in diameter. The lymph nodes are negative.

♦ **IIIc** The tumor involves one or both ovaries, there are tumor implants on the surface of the abdominal cavity greater than 3/4 in. (2 cm) in diameter or there is cancer in the pelvic, para-aortic or groin lymph nodes.

Five-Year Survival About 20 percent

Stage IV Growth involves one or both ovaries. There are distant metastases to the liver or lungs, or there are malignant cells in the excess fluid accumulated around the lungs.

Five-Year Survival 10 percent

TREATMENT OVERVIEW

 Surgery In women with early-stage cancer, one or both ovaries are usually removed (with or without removal of the uterus) and meticulous surgical staging is performed. This involves washings from the abdominal cavity to detect malignant cells, selective sampling of pelvic and aortic lymph nodes and meticulous inspection of the abdominal cavity surfaces with biopsy of any suspicious lesion and removal of the fatty tissue attached to the stomach and large intestines (omentectomy).

In women with advanced cancer, surgical removal of as much tumor as possible, also called tumor debulking, is standard therapy. If possible, the uterus, both fallopian tubes, both ovaries, the omentum and as much of the grossly visible cancer as possible is removed.

Recent studies have shown that 25 to 35 percent of women with ovarian carcinoma will require intestinal or urologic surgery to obtain optimal tumor debulking

(defined as leaving behind no tumor implant greater than 3/4 in. (2 cm) in diameter). A permanent colostomy may occasionally be necessary but is rare in women who have had a preoperative bowel prep—a cleansing of the intestines with enemas and laxatives and administration of oral antibiotics.

To decide if further treatment is required, second-look abdominal surgery is often performed after six cycles of chemotherapy in women without evidence of persistent cancer (*see* "Treatment Follow-up"). In advanced recurrent cancer, surgery is sometimes required to relieve intestinal obstruction.

Complications of surgery can include infection, bleeding and injury to the bladder, rectum or ureter causing a leak, although this is rare. There may be blood clots in the legs, which can occasionally dislodge and travel to the lungs (pulmonary embolism).

 Chemotherapy In most cases chemotherapy is begun one to two weeks after surgery. The standard regimen includes cisplatin or carboplatin + Cytoxan, given intravenously every three to four weeks as tolerated for at least six cycles. Forty to 80 percent of patients can be expected to respond. The response rate depends to a large degree on the amount of cancer remaining after surgery, with those who have an optimal tumor debulking having a better response rate.

Carboplatin is now being used more often than cisplatin because it can sometimes be given on an outpatient basis. It causes less kidney damage, hearing loss, nausea and vomiting and peripheral nerve damage (manifested by muscle weakness and numbness or tingling). Unfortunately, it does have more bone marrow toxicity than cisplatin. Cisplatin + Cytoxan and carboplatin + Cytoxan appear to have equal response rates.

Over the past several years, a technique

known as intraperitoneal (intra-abdominal) chemotherapy has been developed to deliver the chemotherapy directly into the abdominal cavity. This procedure requires surgery to place a port and its attached catheter beneath the skin. The catheter is brought through the abdominal wall and placed directly into the abdominal cavity. The cancer drugs are then given via a needle directly into the subcutaneous port. Complications can include infection, malfunction of the catheter and occasionally intestinal blockage.

Intraperitoneal chemotherapy is generally given monthly for six months. Although preliminary results are encouraging, it has been tested in a small number of women who have been followed only for a short time, so it is still considered investigational. Large trials are now under way to compare the effectiveness of intraperitoneal versus intravenous chemotherapy.

Chemotherapy can cause hair loss, nausea and vomiting, infection or bleeding because of bone marrow toxicity, and damage to the heart, kidneys, nerves and liver.

Intraperitoneal Chemotherapy for Ovarian Cancer

 Radiation There is some evidence that external beam radiation therapy is as effective as chemotherapy for patients with early stages of ovarian carcinoma who have no visible cancer remaining after their operation.

Sometimes radiation therapy is used for microscopic recurrent ovarian cancer or cancer that has not responded well to chemotherapy. Radiation may be given only to the pelvis or, more typically, to the entire abdomen (usually five days each week for four to five weeks), which results in a better survival rate. Complications and side effects can be considerable and can include diarrhea, nausea and vomiting, bleeding from the bladder or rectum, vaginal scarring, intestinal obstruction, or leaks (fistulas) in the urinary or intestinal tracts.

Radioactive phosphorus inserted directly into the abdominal cavity is sometimes given to women who have no visible cancer or less than 1 mm of residual disease after surgery.

TREATMENT BY STAGE

STAGE Ia

Standard Treatment Therapy depends primarily on the age of the patient and the grade of the cancer.

For borderline, well-differentiated tumors (Grade 1) in women who want to preserve their reproductive function, standard therapy includes removal of the cancerous ovary and the adjacent fallopian tube (the other, apparently healthy ovary should be biopsied, however), partial removal of the omentum and biopsies of the pelvic and para-aortic lymph nodes.

For postmenopausal women and those who do not want to preserve their reproductive function, standard therapy includes a total hysterectomy, removal of both fallopian tubes and ovaries and careful surgical staging. Women with Stage Ia borderline or Grade 1 carcinoma are usually cured with surgery alone.

Standard therapy for Grade 2 or 3 tumors is total hysterectomy, removal of both tubes and both ovaries, meticulous surgical staging and six monthly cycles of combination chemotherapy, usually with cisplatin or carboplatin + Cytoxan. Other therapies that are sometimes recommended are total abdominal and pelvic radiation or intra-abdominal administration of radioactive phosphorus (P32).

Investigational

♦ A Gynecologic Oncology Group trial is comparing giving intra-abdominal radioactive phosphorus given once with giving six cycles (once every three weeks) of intravenous cisplatin + Cytoxan for women with poorly differentiated (Grades 2–3) tumors.

♦ Intra-abdominal chemotherapy with agents such as cisplatin or carboplatin.

STAGE Ib

Standard Treatment A total hysterectomy, removal of both tubes and ovaries and meticulous surgical staging is performed. Women with tumors of low malignant potential or Grade 1 carcinomas may not require further treatment.

Women with Grade 2 or 3 cancers usually receive postoperative combination chemotherapy (usually carboplatin or cisplatin + Cytoxan given every three weeks as tolerated for a total of six cycles), whole abdominal and pelvic radiation therapy or intra-abdominal radioactive phosphorus.

Investigational Same as Stage Ia.

STAGE Ic

Standard Treatment Hysterectomy, removal of both fallopian tubes and ovaries, partial omentectomy and biopsy of the pelvic and para-aortic lymph nodes is done. Careful inspection of the remaining intra-abdominal surfaces is vital. Suspicious lesions should be biopsied, and washings of the abdominal cavity should be taken to check for malignant cells.

In the absence of progressive disease, standard therapy after surgery includes six courses of cisplatin or carboplatin + Cytoxan.

Investigational

♦ Intra-abdominal cisplatin or carboplatin with or without other anticancer drugs.

♦ Intra-abdominal radioactive phosphorus.

♦ Whole-abdomen and pelvic radiation therapy.

STAGE IIa

Standard Treatment The surgical procedure is the same as for Stage Ic, again with biopsy of any suspicious lesions and washings of the abdominal cavity to check for malignant cells.

If all tumor implants are less than 3/4 in. (2 cm) in diameter after surgery, combination chemotherapy including cisplatin or carboplatin + Cytoxan is given to the majority of patients for six cycles (one course every three weeks).

Whole-abdomen and pelvic radiation may be given if the residual disease is less than 1/4 in. (0.5 cm) in diameter. Intra-abdominal radioactive phosphorus can be given if the residual disease is less than 1 mm in diameter.

If there is residual cancer greater than 3/4 in. (2 cm) in diameter, intravenous chemotherapy is used exclusively. There are several commonly used combinations—CP (Cytoxan + cisplatin or Cytoxan + carboplatin), CAP (Cytoxan + Adriamycin + cisplatin), AP (Adriamycin + cisplatin) and CHAD (Cytoxan + hexamethylmelamine + Adriamycin + cisplatin).

Investigational
♦ One-time intra-abdominal administration of radioactive phosphorus versus six cycles of intravenous cisplatin + Cytoxan.
♦ Intra-abdominal carboplatin or cisplatin with or without other anticancer drugs.

STAGES IIb, IIc, IIIa, IIIb, IIIc, IV
Standard Treatment In women with advanced ovarian carcinoma, standard therapy involves removing as much of the tumor as possible as well as the uterus, both fallopian tubes and ovaries and the omentum. Biopsies from the pelvic and para-aortic nodes are also performed.

If there is optimal residual disease after surgery—no tumor implant greater than 3/4 in. (2 cm) in diameter—combination chemotherapy including cisplatin or carboplatin + Cytoxan is given for six cycles (one course every three weeks).

Total abdominal and pelvic radiation may be given, but only if the residual disease is less than 1/4 in. (0.5 cm) in diameter. Intra-abdominal radioactive phosphorus may be given only if the residual disease is less than 1 mm in diameter.

If there is residual cancer larger than 3/4 in. (2 cm) in diameter or metastases outside the abdominal cavity, intravenous chemotherapy is used exclusively. The commonly used combinations are the same as used for Stage IIa, namely CP, CAP, AP and CHAD.

Investigational Many investigational protocols are being used in the treatment of ovarian cancer:
♦ Intra-abdominal administration of single agents such as interferon-alpha, cisplatin, carboplatin, ARA-C, bleomycin, mitoxantrone, 5-fluorouracil (5-FU) and etoposide.
♦ Intra-abdominal melphalan + ARA-C, carboplatin + etoposide (VP-16), monoclonal antibodies to ovarian carcinoma cells and cisplatin + etoposide with thiosulfate.
♦ Continuous infusion of intravenous 5-FU.
♦ Intravenous fludarabine, hexamethylmelamine or cisplatin + 5-FU + VP-16.
♦ Intravenous carboplatin + ifosfamide.
♦ Intravenous taxol.
♦ Intravenous cisplatin + Cytoxan + hyperfractionated (twice daily) abdominal radiotherapy.
♦ Sodium thiosulfate, which has been shown to protect kidney function as well as lessen the bone marrow complications of cisplatin chemotherapy.
♦ High-dose intravenous carboplatin + etoposide with autologous (self-donated) bone marrow transplant.
♦ High-dosage Cytoxan + cisplatin plus chest and abdominal radiation followed by autologous bone marrow transplant.
♦ High-dose carboplatin + ifosfamide + Mesna with autologous bone marrow transplant.
♦ Intravenous Thiotepa with autologous bone marrow transplant.
♦ Immunotherapy with interleukin-2 or interleukin-2–activated mononuclear cells.
♦ Leuprolide acetate (Lupron) in women with low malignant potential tumors.
♦ Tamoxifen.
♦ Megace.

◆ Taxol, a plant product with significant activity in ovarian cancer, is being actively studied.

TREATMENT FOLLOW-UP

Follow-up is generally performed every three months for the first two years after treatment.

◆ The neck, lungs, abdomen and pelvis are carefully examined at each visit.

◆ The serum CA-125 level is followed closely and is sometimes the first indication of recurrent cancer.

◆ Abdominal and pelvic CT or MRI scans may be done, but their routine use has not been shown to be effective in the absence of symptoms.

Second-Look Surgery If after six cycles of chemotherapy there is no evidence of progressive disease—as determined by physical examination, the serum CA-125 level and pelvic and abdominal CT scans—then second-look exploratory abdominal surgery may be performed. Although it is sometimes considered the standard of care, there has been no proven survival benefit of this procedure. It is, however, the most reliable way of determining whether any cancer is left after treatment. Any residual cancer can also be removed.

If there is no cancer found during the second-look operation, a thorough procedure requires taking peritoneal washings and biopsies from any adhesions or 20 to 30 random biopsies from the surfaces within the abdomen. These include the surfaces of the bladder, pelvis, pelvic sidewalls, diaphragm and the pelvic and aortic lymph nodes if not sampled previously. If any of the omentum is still present, it is also removed. Traditionally, if the second-look operation and microscopic examination of all the biopsies reveal no cancer, no further treatment is required.

In the hands of a gynecologic oncologist, approximately 25 to 30 percent of the women who have sub-optimal disease at the second-look surgery (any tumor nodule greater than 3/4 in./2 cm in diameter) will undergo an optimal surgical debulking. An intra-abdominal catheter for intraperitoneal chemotherapy can also be placed during the operation.

Prognosis The prognosis primarily depends on the stage, grade and type of carcinoma as well as on the amount of residual disease after the initial surgery.

Women who have Stage II, III or IV Grade 1 carcinoma and a negative second-look procedure have an excellent prognosis. Women with Grade 2 or 3 cancers and a negative second-look also have a good prognosis, but have a significant risk for developing recurrent disease. It is estimated that 30 to 50 percent of women with Grade 3 cancer will develop a recurrence within five years even after a negative second-look. As a result, many gynecologic oncologists recommend giving additional treatment—intravenous or intraperitoneal chemotherapy, radioactive phosphorus or whole-abdomen radiation—after the second look.

For women who have microscopic disease at their second-look procedure, the prognosis is not as good and is partially dependent upon the grade of the cancer. These women are excellent candidates for intra-abdominal chemotherapy or whole-abdomen radiation.

Women with bulky residual cancer (implants greater than 3/4 in./2 cm) after a second-look procedure have a poor prognosis despite treatment with second-line chemotherapy.

RECURRENT CANCER

Women whose cancer returns are sometimes candidates for exploratory surgery for further aggressive tumor debulking.

Postoperative therapy varies and may include intra-abdominal chemotherapy, intravenous chemotherapy or pelvic and whole-abdomen radiation therapy. In most cases treatment is only palliative.

Numerous combinations of chemotherapy have been used with some benefit, including various combinations and doses of Cytoxan, hexamethylmelamine, 5-fluorouracil, ifosfamide and Cytoxan, Adriamycin, carboplatin and Alkeran (melphalan).

THE MOST IMPORTANT QUESTIONS YOU CAN ASK

♦ What is the cell type, grade and stage of my cancer?

♦ How much cancer remained after surgery?
♦ What is the benefit of second-look surgery?
♦ What is the reason for the type of therapy you recommended after surgery?
♦ Is there a medical oncologist and radiation oncologist available for consultation?
♦ What qualifications do you have for treating cancer? Will a gynecologic oncologist be involved in my care?

OVARIAN GERM CELL TUMORS

Jeffrey L. Stern, MD

◇

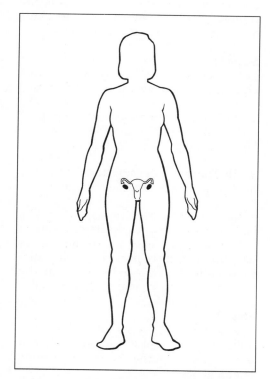

Germ cell tumors account for approximately 5 percent of all ovarian malignancies. They almost always occur in women of reproductive age and are frequently found in women in their teens or twenties. Many types of germ cell tumors are extremely aggressive, fast-growing malignancies. In the past they were often fatal within one or two years even though frequently confined to one ovary at the time of diagnosis. With surgery and modern multi-agent chemotherapy, the cure rate is higher.

Types There are six main cell types: dysgerminoma, endodermal sinus tumor, embryonal carcinoma, choriocarcinoma, immature teratoma and mixed germ cell tumors.

There are also rare cell types such as struma ovarii, carcinoid and malignant transformation of a benign dermoid.

How It Spreads Ovarian germ cell tumors can spread directly to the adjacent pelvic organs and through the lymph system to the pelvic, aortic, chest (mediastinal), groin and neck lymph nodes. They may also spread to the surfaces of the abdominal cavity and to distant organs such as the liver, lungs and brain. (*See* page 278)

What Causes It The cause is not clear.

RISK FACTORS

At Significantly Higher Risk
♦ Premenopausal women.

At Slightly Higher Risk
♦ Women with abnormal (dysgenetic) ovaries usually containing male chromosomes.

SCREENING

No definitive screening method is available, except for a routine annual pelvic, abdominal and rectal examination.

COMMON SIGNS AND SYMPTOMS

These tumors often do not cause any symptoms. Some women, however, will have a rapidly enlarging pelvic or abdominal mass and vague pain in the lower abdomen. Other women can experience acute abdominal symptoms, including pain and shock.

DIAGNOSIS

Physical Examination
♦ In addition to a careful pelvic exam, a general physical examination should pay particular attention to the lymph nodes above the collarbone, the axillae and the groin.
♦ An abdominal examination may find an enlarged liver, a mass or masses or excessive fluid (ascites).

Blood and Other Tests
♦ Serum beta human chorionic gonadotropin (βHCG) is elevated in choriocarcinoma.
♦ Serum alpha-fetoprotein (AFP) is elevated in endodermal sinus tumors.
♦ Serum lactate dehydrogenase (LDH) is elevated in dysgerminoma.
♦ One or more of the tumor markers—serum βHCG, AFP and LDH—may be elevated in mixed germ cell tumors.

Imaging
♦ Abdominal and pelvic CT scan.
♦ Chest x-ray.

Endoscopy and Biopsy
♦ The definitive diagnosis is made on histologic evaluation of the removed ovary.

STAGING

The International Federation of Gynecology and Obstetrics (FIGO) staging classification for malignant epithelial carcinomas of the ovaries is also used for staging malignant germ cell tumors of the ovary. Germ cell tumors of the ovary are surgically staged.

Stage I
Cancer is confined to one or both ovaries.

♦ **Ia** Cancer is limited to one ovary. There is no tumor on the surface of the ovary, the surface of the tumor is unruptured and there is no ascites.

♦ **Ib** Growth is limited to both ovaries.

There is no tumor on the surface of either ovary, the surfaces of the tumors are unruptured and there is no ascites.

♦ **Ic** The tumor is either Stage Ia or Ib, but there is tumor on the surface of one or both ovaries, at least one of the tumors has ruptured, ascites is present or the abdominal washings contain malignant cells.

Stage II
The cancer involves one or both ovaries with extension to other pelvic structures.

♦ **IIa** There is extension of the tumor or metastases to the uterus and/or the fallopian tubes.

♦ **IIb** There is extension to other pelvic organs such as the bladder or rectum.

♦ **IIc** The cancer is either stage IIa or IIb, but there is tumor on the surface of one or both ovaries, at least one of the tumors has ruptured, there is ascites with malignant cells or the washings from the abdominal cavity contain malignant cells.

Stage III
The tumor involves one or both ovaries with tumor present outside the pelvis or there is cancer in the abdominal or groin lymph nodes.

♦ **IIIa** The tumor is grossly limited to the pelvis, but there is microscopic cancer involving the abdominal cavity (peritoneal) surfaces. The lymph nodes are negative.

♦ **IIIb** The tumor involves one or both ovaries, there are tumor implants on the peritoneal surfaces less than 3/4 in. (2 cm) in diameter. The lymph nodes are negative.

♦ **IIIc** The tumor involves one or both ovaries, there are tumor implants on the surface of the abdominal cavity greater than 3/4 in. (2 cm) in diameter or there is cancer in the pelvic, para-aortic or groin lymph nodes.

Stage IV
There are distant metastases to the liver or lungs or there are malignant cells present in the fluid accumulated in the chest cavity.

TREATMENT OVERVIEW

 Surgery Surgical removal of the involved ovary or ovaries and removal of as much of the grossly visible tumor as possible is performed in all cases. If there is no spread beyond the ovaries, treatment will involve meticulous surgical staging, including sampling of the pelvic and para-aortic lymph nodes, washings of the abdominal cavity to look for malignant cells and careful inspection of the abdominal surfaces.

The cell type of the tumor is an extremely important factor in determining the prognosis and the appropriate therapy after surgery.

 Chemotherapy Women with a tumor confined to one ovary (Stage I) or with a well-differentiated (Grade 1) immature teratoma or dysgerminoma do not require postoperative chemotherapy. All others are usually treated with multi-drug chemotherapy.

Until recently, external radiation therapy to the abdomen and pelvis (1,500 to 3,000 cGy with a 1,500 cGy boost to the para-aortic region given in divided doses daily over five to six weeks) was standard therapy for dysgerminomas, but chemotherapy is now used more often to preserve fertility.

Women with other malignant germ cell tumors are treated with chemotherapy after surgery because radiation therapy is ineffective. The most commonly used chemotherapeutic drug regimen includes cisplatin, bleomycin and etoposide given monthly for three courses.

Second-Look Surgery In those women with Stage II, III or occasionally IV disease who have no evidence of persistent cancer after chemotherapy, "second-look" exploratory abdominal surgery is performed to see if they are truly disease-free.

Second-look surgery is not usually performed on correctly staged women with well-differentiated immature teratomas, Stage Ia and Ib dysgerminomas or other Stage I germ cell tumors who had elevated alpha-fetoprotein, βHCG or LDH levels before treatment that returned to normal with chemotherapy.

Women who have bulky disease after chemotherapy may occasionally benefit from a tumor debulking at a second surgery.

TREATMENT BY STAGE AND CELL TYPE

DYSGERMINOMAS
STAGE Ia
Standard Treatment The involved ovary and fallopian tube and a wedge biopsy of the opposite, normal-appearing ovary and meticulous surgical staging is performed in women who want to preserve their fertility. Women with Stage Ia disease require no further treatment.

About 20 percent of women will have microscopic disease in the opposite, apparently normal ovary (Stage Ib). For women who do not desire more children or who are approaching menopause, a hysterectomy and removal of both tubes and both ovaries is performed.

Investigational None.

STAGE Ib
Standard Treatment Women with this stage of disease are usually treated with three courses of cisplatin, bleomycin and etoposide or whole-abdominal radiation

therapy after hysterectomy, removal of both fallopian tubes and ovaries and meticulous surgical staging.

Investigational
♦ Combinations of chemotherapy including carboplatin and ifosfamide.

STAGE Ic
Standard Treatment After surgery most gynecologic oncologists recommend three courses of cisplatin, bleomycin and etoposide or whole-abdomen radiation.

Investigational Same as Stage Ib.

STAGES II, III and IV
Standard Treatment Depending on the extent and location of disease, standard therapy includes a hysterectomy, removal of both tubes and both ovaries, aggressive tumor debulking and three courses of cisplatin, bleomycin and etoposide.

If the opposite ovary and the uterus are normal, they can be preserved in women who want to maintain their reproductive capacity. Whole-abdomen radiation may be given to those women who fail to respond to chemotherapy or who are not interested in preserving their reproductive function.

Investigational Same as Stage Ib.

NON-DYSGERMINOMATOUS GERM CELL TUMORS
These include endodermal sinus tumors, embryonal carcinoma, immature teratoma, choriocarcinoma and mixed germ cell tumors.

STAGE I
Standard Treatment Removal of the affected tube and ovary is generally all that is required since these tumors rarely occur in both ovaries.

Postoperative chemotherapy including cisplatin, bleomycin and etoposide is given to all patients for four courses with the exception of Grade 1 (well-differentiated) immature teratomas.

Vincristine, actinomycin-D and Cytoxan may be used in women who develop progressive disease.

Investigational
♦ Other combinations of chemotherapy, including carboplatin and ifosfamide, are currently under investigation.

STAGES II, III and IV
Standard Treatment Depending on the extent and location of disease, a hysterectomy, bilateral removal of the tubes and ovaries, and aggressive tumor debulking. If the opposite ovary and uterus are normal, they can be preserved in women who want to maintain their reproductive function. Four courses of chemotherapy including cisplatin, bleomycin and etoposide are given after surgery.

Investigational
♦ Experimental therapy for advanced non-dysgerminomatous germ cell tumors include combinations of other chemotherapeutic drugs such as carboplatin and ifosfamide.

FIVE-YEAR SURVIVAL RATES

The five-year survival rate for Stages Ia and Ib dysgerminomas and Grade 1 immature teratomas is over 95 percent. Even Stage III dysgerminomas have approximately an 80 percent survival rate.

The survival rate for the other stages of dysgerminomas and other histologic types of germ cell tumors are not as well established. But over the past 10 years there has been a marked improvement in prognosis since the advent of cisplatin-based chemotherapy regimens.

Survival rates for women with Stages I and II non-dysgerminomatous germ cell tumors are greater than 90 percent. Even women with Stage III and IV disease have survival rates estimated to be greater than 75 percent.

TREATMENT FOLLOW-UP

All women with germ cell tumors need careful follow-up every three months for the first two years after treatment.

♦ Follow-up should include a careful physical examination and serum βHCG, alpha-fetoprotein and LDH levels (depending on which was elevated before therapy).

♦ Occasionally, radiologic studies such as an abdominal and pelvic CT or MRI scan are performed as required.

RECURRENT CANCER

Germ cell tumors may recur in the pelvis, the abdominal cavity, liver, lungs and lymph nodes. Symptoms may include pelvic or abdominal pain, nausea, vomiting, abdominal swelling, weight loss and chronic cough.

♦ Women with recurrent cancer usually undergo an exploratory laparotomy with aggressive surgical debulking of the tumor.

♦ Women with recurrent dysgerminoma who did not receive radiation therapy previously can be treated with pelvic radiation up to a dose of 3,000 to 5,000 cGy over four to five weeks and whole-abdomen radiation therapy, up to 1,500 cGy, with a boost of up to 1,500 cGy to the para-aortic area over several weeks.

♦ Women with recurrent dysgerminoma who were initially treated with radiation therapy are treated with combination chemotherapy such as cisplatin + etoposide + bleomycin, vincristine + actinomycin-D + Cytoxan or carboplatin + ifosfamide.

♦ Women with non-dysgerminomatous tumors are generally treated with chemotherapy after surgery, as radiation is not effective for these tumors. The chemotherapeutic drugs of choice are cisplatin + etoposide + bleomycin or ifosfamide, vinblastine or vincristine + actinomycin-D + Cytoxan, or carboplatin + ifosfamide.

THE MOST IMPORTANT QUESTIONS YOU CAN ASK

♦ What qualifications do you have for treating cancer? Will a specialist in gynecologic oncology be involved in my care?

♦ What kind of germ cell tumor do I have?

♦ What stage is it?

♦ Will I still be able to have children?

♦ Will I need chemotherapy?

♦ Do I need a second-look operation?

PANCREAS

Ernest H. Rosenbaum, MD and Malin Dollinger, MD

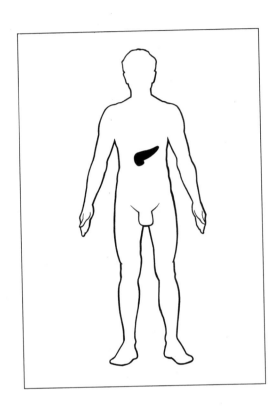

Pancreatic cancer is a common malignancy that is treatable if diagnosed early but is rarely curable. Diagnosis is usually not possible until symptoms appear and by that time the cancer is often well advanced. Because the pancreas is a deep organ resting close to the backbone and involving vital structures, and because tumors often produce few early symptoms, this cancer is not easily diagnosed at a possibly curable stage. Ninety percent of pancreatic cancers cannot be removed surgically.

Pancreatic cancer is the fifth most common cause of cancer deaths in the United States, with about 28,000 cases and 25,000 deaths projected for 1991. For unknown reasons, the number of cases is increasing every year, especially in industrialized countries.

Types Ninety percent of pancreatic cancers are adenocarcinomas. These develop in the exocrine glands that produce enzymes that travel through the pancreatic duct to the small intestine to aid digestion. Adenosquamous, undifferentiated, small cell carcinomas, cystadenocarcinomas, and lymphomas are rare. The other cancers of the pancreas develop in the pancreatic endocrine or islet glands, which produce hormones such as insulin that are released directly into the bloodstream (*see* "Islet Cell Carcinoma").

How It Spreads Two-thirds of pancreatic cancers are located in the head of the organ (right side), one-third in the body and tail (left side). (*See* page 336.) Tumor cells may spread to adjacent structures by direct extension and/or lymphatic metastasis to the small intestine (duodenum), bile duct, stomach, spleen, colon and lymph nodes (regional, celiac and supraclavicular). The most common sites for distant metastases are the liver, peritoneum (by lymphatic spread) and lungs (by spread through the bloodstream).

What Causes It It is not definitely known what causes pancreatic cancer, although age is a factor. There also may be racial or dietary factors. Smoking increases the risk of developing pancreatic cancer threefold. Concerns have been raised about the role of coffee, but there is no proof of an association.

RISK FACTORS

At Significantly Higher Risk

♦ Men outnumber women by a ratio of three-to-one.

♦ Rare before age 40, the incidence peaks around age 60.

♦ Smokers of over two packs a day.

♦ Over 10 years' exposure to chemicals, particularly petroleum compounds and solvents.

♦ Sufferers of chronic inflammation of the pancreas (chronic pancreatitis).

At Slightly Higher Risk

♦ Some association with alcohol consumption.

♦ History of diabetes, particularly in women.

SCREENING

No effective screening methods are available.

COMMON SIGNS AND SYMPTOMS

The most common symptom is pain in the upper abdomen, indicating celiac lymph node involvement (in more than 90 percent of cases). There may also be loss of appetite, nausea and vomiting, constipation (50 percent of patients), weight loss (early feeling of fullness is usual in 50 percent of cases), diarrhea, bloating, belching and hiccups. Other symptoms include itching skin, swollen legs, sleeping problems and fatigue.

Other symptoms vary according to the location of the cancer:

♦ Progressive jaundice, often painless (66 per cent), can be a sign of cancer in the head of the pancreas.

♦ Itching (pruritis) due to bile duct obstruction.

♦ Diarrhea and swollen legs or mild diabetes may also develop.

There are few symptoms of cancer in the tail of the pancreas until the tumor is a large, often baseball-sized, mass.

DIAGNOSIS

Physical Examination

♦ Jaundice.

♦ Abdominal masses.

♦ Enlarged gallbladder—50 percent of cases (carcinoma of head of pancreas).

♦ Enlarged liver (hepatomegaly).

♦ Abdominal fluid (ascites).

♦ Enlarged lymph nodes.

♦ Phlebitis (swollen legs).

Blood and Other Tests

♦ Complete blood count (CBC) and platelet count.

♦ The carcinoembryonic antigen (CEA) is elevated in 50 percent of cases.

♦ CA 19-9 is elevated in 70 to 80 percent of pancreatic cancer cases and is a better test than the CEA because it is 87 percent specific. (In many cases of pancreatic cancer, both the CEA and the CA 19-9 are elevated.)

♦ Serum bilirubin is elevated in patients with bile duct obstruction.

♦ Serum alkaline phosphatase will be elevated if there are liver or bone metastases or if there is bile duct obstruction.

♦ Stools should be examined for hidden blood. The color may be abnormal. If they are white or clay-colored, the bile duct is obstructed.

Imaging

♦ Abdominal ultrasound. Ultrasound is also used at surgery to locate the exact borders of the tumor.

♦ CT scans may not detect small tumors but may identify pancreatic masses, liver metastases, enlarged lymph nodes and fluid in the abdomen (ascites).

♦ MRI may complement the CT scan.

♦ PET (Positron Emission Tomography) imaging is an experimental method for diagnosis and evaluation for liver metastases.

Endoscopy and Biopsy

♦ ERCP (endoscopic retrograde cholangiopancreatography) involves placing a gastroscope into the stomach and inserting a tube into the opening of the pancreatic duct.

♦ For a definite diagnosis, a biopsy is essential. Tissue can be drawn out with a fine needle (FNA) inserted into the tumor using CT guidance (80 percent diagnostic). This will be necessary to differentiate pancreatic cancer from benign pancreatitis or pseudocyst, islet cell carcinoma or lymphoma.

Tests to Surrounding Organs

♦ Upper gastrointestinal tract x-rays (UGI series) may be done to examine the duodenum (the portion of the small intestine that surrounds the pancreas) to look for abnormalities.

♦ A needle may be inserted into the liver to discover obstructions in the bile duct (percutaneous transhepatic cholangiogram).

♦ Liver biopsy to confirm metastases, if indicated.

Ninety percent of cases can be diagnosed with abdominal ultrasound, CT scans, ERCP and a positive CA 19-9.

STAGING

The staging system for pancreatic cancer is still evolving. However, staging has limited value because treatment, regardless of stage, has had little influence on survival. Knowing the location of the cancer in the head, body or tail of the pancreas will help determine if surgery is feasible.

TREATMENT OVERVIEW

Surgery Surgery is rarely curative but can be used for palliation, improving survival and the quality of life. The radical surgical approach (pancreaticoduodenal resection) depends on whether the tumor is in the head, body or tail of the pancreas.

Cure may be achieved when the tumor is truly localized, but this stage is diagnosed in fewer than 20 percent of cases. Radical surgery (the Whipple procedure) is more feasible when the tumor is small (less than 3/4 in./2 cm), no lymph nodes are involved and there is no extension of the cancer beyond the "capsule" of the pancreas (a rare situation).

Surgery may also be advantageously used to bypass any obstruction of the biliary or gastrointestinal tract. In addition, before surgery pancreatic cancer cannot be differentiated from other cancers involving bile ducts. Overall, surgery results in only about 5 percent survival after five years, although about 22 percent are alive five years after radical surgery (Whipple procedure).

Radiation When the tumor cannot be removed surgically, radiation can play a palliative role after surgery. The risks of radiotherapy can be reduced with proper treatment planning.

The risks of damage to the kidneys, spleen, liver, spinal cord and the bowel surrounding the pancreas can be minimized by careful treatment planning. Combination radiotherapy and chemotherapy (5-fluorouracil) may offer a survival advantage (22 weeks of radiotherapy alone to 40 weeks with combination therapy) and palliation with decreased pain.

Intraoperative radiotherapy (IORT) and interstitial I-125 radioactive implants have helped local tumor control but have not increased survival.

Chemotherapy No major palliative role for chemotherapy has been proven. The most commonly used drugs are 5-fluorouracil (5-FU), Adriamycin, mitomycin-C and streptozotocin. 5-fluorouracil has had the best response but in no more than 20 percent of patients.

Various combinations such as FAM (5-FU + Adriamycin + mitomycin-C) and SMF (streptozotocin + mitomycin-C + 5-FU) may increase survival a few months and have had a good response in selected cases, but there is little proof that combination therapy is superior to 5-FU alone.

 Palliation Although surgery and radiation therapy will not improve survival, both may improve the quality of life. A biliary tract obstructed by a tumor at the head of the pancreas can by bypassed (with surgery or a stent), an obstruction of the stomach outlet can be relieved, and pain control can be improved dramatically.

Other palliative measures include pain control using analgesics, celiac and splanchnic nerve blocks, spinal morphine, antiemetics to control nausea or vomiting, and nutritional support with diets and replacement of pancreatic enzymes. (*See* Chapter 18.)

TREATMENT BY STAGE

STAGE I
TNM T1 or T2, N0, M0
The cancer is confined to the pancreas or has directly spread to involve the adjacent small intestine, the bile duct or tissues surrounding the pancreas.

Standard Treatment Stage I cancer is treatable by surgery and is occasionally curable. Radical surgery—the Whipple procedure (pancreaticoduodenal resection)—is the standard treatment for cancer of the head of the pancreas or the opening of the pancreatic duct, although only about 20 percent of patients are eligible for total resection (80 to 90 percent have lymph node involvement at the time of diagnosis, and 70 percent have liver metastases).

A radical pancreatic resection, removing the head or all of the pancreas is very difficult surgery. Five to 30 percent of patients may not survive the operation. Fluid leaks at the connection to the small bowel (jejunum) and bleeding are the major postoperative problems.

Postsurgical local radiotherapy and 5-FU may improve survival. About 40 percent of patients treated with such combined therapy may be alive at two years, representing a twofold increase in survival. (Metallic clips are inserted during surgery to help localize the tumor for radiotherapy.)

Removing cancer involving the tail of the pancreas is uncommon because tumors in the tail are usually large and far advanced before diagnosis.

Three-Year Survival 15 percent

Investigational
♦ Radiation given during the operation—intraoperative radiotherapy (IORT)—is being evaluated.
♦ Some trials of split course radiotherapy of 4,000 to 6,000 cGy over six to eight weeks have shown one-year survival of 34 percent and five-year survival of 20 percent
♦ Brachytherapy—implanting irradiating seeds of radon or boron—is under clinical evaluation at a few centers. Results so far have not been promising.
♦ Postoperative large-field radiation with 5-FU chemotherapy is also being evaluated and it appears that this combination improves survival. Side effects include diarrhea, inflammation of the mucosa and toxicity in the liver.

 Palliation Eighty percent of pancreatic cancer patients have jaundice caused by an obstruction. A bypass from the gall bladder or the common bile duct to the intestine may be helpful.

STAGE II
TNM T3, N0, M0
The cancer has directly spread to involve adjacent organs such as the stomach, spleen or colon.

Standard Treatment Surgical bypass procedures can be carried out as a palliative measure (*see* Stage I) and neurosurgical procedures such as blocking the nerves from the stomach and pancreas (celiac ganglion nerve blocks) may relieve much of the pain.

Combined radiation and chemotherapy may be helpful. Radiation therapy alone may relieve symptoms, but clinical trials should be considered, since survival is not significantly increased with radiotherapy alone.

If the patient is jaundiced, the bile ducts can be drained through the skin (transhepatic percutaneous biliary bypass). Alternatively, a drainage tube can be placed inside the small bowel by means of a gastroscope (endoscopic stent placement).

Investigational

♦ Radiation therapy with radiosensitizers.
♦ Intraoperative radiotherapy (IORT) and implantation of radioactive seeds (brachytherapy) are sometimes combined, with and without chemotherapy for resectable or unresectable tumors.
♦ Postoperative radiation therapy plus 5-FU in resected patients.

Three-Year Survival 2 percent

STAGE III
TNM Any T, N1, M0
The cancer has spread to the regional lymph nodes.

Standard Treatment There is no reliably curative treatment and no proven adjuvant therapy. The standard palliative treatment options for Stage II and/or clinical trials should be considered.

Three-Year Survival 2 percent

Investigational
♦ Surgery plus radiation therapy with radiosensitizers.
♦ Intraoperative radiotherapy with and without resection.

♦ Particle beam radiation therapy if a special research facility is available.

STAGE IV
TNM Any T, any N, M1
The cancer has spread to distant sites, most commonly the liver or lungs.

Standard Treatment Palliative surgical bypass, bile drainage procedures (see Stage II description).
♦ Chemotherapy (*see* Stages II and III) and pain-relieving procedures are standard treatments. Clinical chemotherapy trials should be considered.
♦ Combination chemotherapy with SMF (streptozotocin + mitomycin-C + 5-fluorouracil), which has a 30 to 45 percent response rate, FAM (5-fluorouracil + Adriamycin + mitomycin-C) or 5-fluorouracil + leucovorin.

Three-Year Survival 2 percent

SUPPORTIVE THERAPY

Nutrition Malnutrition is a common problem because of loss of appetite, diarrhea, poor fat absorption and the loss of bile salts because of bile drainage diversions or bile duct obstruction. Fat-soluble vitamin deficiencies (A, D, E, K) may also occur.
♦ Frequent feedings, use of digestive replacement enzymes (pancreatin, Viokase) and antinausea drugs will be needed.
♦ Low-fat food or supplements (medium-chain triglycerides) may help provide proteins and calories.
♦ Gastric and jejunal tube feeding or intravenous hyperalimentation can help reduce malnutrition.

Pain Control This often becomes a major problem, but morphine or narcotics can help. If these are not effective, celiac nerve blocks or the infusion of morphine by vein or the spinal canal can help control pain in a majority of patients.

RECURRENT CANCER

The three major signs of recurrent pancreatic cancer are increased pain, jaundice and fluid in the abdomen (ascites).

Recurrent cancer can be treated with palliative surgical or radiation therapy.

♦ Chemotherapy may produce tumor regression. Treatment options are the same as for Stages II, III and IV—5-FU, FAM, SMF, 5-FU + leucovorin and PALA + 5-FU. (PALA is an investigational drug that increases the antitumor activity of 5-FU.)

THE MOST IMPORTANT QUESTIONS YOU CAN ASK

♦ Will diet help my treatments?
♦ What are the limiting factors for a surgical cure of pancreatic cancer?
♦ Are there any new chemotherapy treatments?
♦ How can using chemotherapy and radiation together help improve the chance for cure?

PARATHYROID

Malin Dollinger, MD

◇

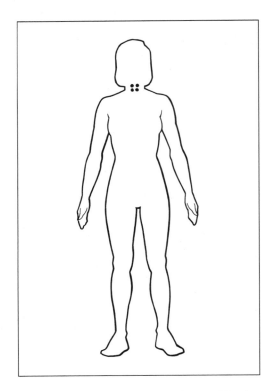

The parathyroid glands are located in the neck, two on each side of the thyroid gland (*see* page 538).

Parathyroid cancer is a rare and sometimes curable endocrine gland cancer. Though not all these tumors are functioning, those that are produce increased amounts of parathyroid hormone (parathormone), which leads to a marked elevation in blood calcium level. It is usually the signs and symptoms of elevated calcium that lead to the diagnosis.

Benign tumors of the parathyroid (adenomas) and an overgrowth of parathyroid tissue (hyperplasia) are much more common than malignant tumors. These also produce parathyroid hormone and elevated blood calcium levels, so it is sometimes difficult to know at surgery if the tumor is benign or malignant. This distinction is extremely important because the treatment of a malignant parathyroid tumor requires not only removal of the tumor but removal of the thyroid gland on that side. Adjacent muscles and tissues are also removed if they are affected by cancer.

Recognition by the surgeon that the tumor is malignant rather than benign and performing the appropriate surgery, including removal of the lymph nodes, is important for good results. Malignancy is more likely if there is a very high serum calcium, a palpable or hard mass in the neck or hoarseness due to paralysis of the vocal cords on the same side.

Because this tumor usually grows slowly and because the main clinical problem is usually the effects of the elevated calcium levels, palliative reduction or debulking of the primary tumor or metastases is recommended. This may lower the blood calcium level, which is difficult to treat any other way.

Types Parathyroid tumors are carcinomas, with pure cell, chief cell, transitional clear cell and mixed cell types.

How It Spreads Parathyroid tumors can spread directly to adjacent tissues, as well as through the lymphatic system to nearby lymph nodes and distant sites, usually the lung, bones and liver.

What Causes It Unknown.

RISK FACTORS

There are no known risk factors for

parathyroid carcinoma, although benign tumors of the parathyroids (adenoma) occur more often if there has been previous radiation to the head and neck. Parathyroid tumors also occur in association with tumors of the adrenal and thyroid glands (multiple endocrine neoplasia—MEN).

SCREENING

Specific screening for this type of cancer is generally not done, because it is so rare. But appropriate methods to search for parathyroid tumors, whether benign or malignant, include measuring the serum calcium levels—commonly performed as part of a chemistry panel—as well as examining the thyroid region for suspicious masses during routine physical examinations.

COMMON SIGNS AND SYMPTOMS

Symptoms are due to mass in the neck, and also to the elevated calcium.

Symptoms usually include fatigue, muscle weakness, nausea and vomiting, kidney stones or other kidney disease, peptic ulcer and inflamation of the pancreas (pancreatitis).

DIAGNOSIS

The diagnosis of overactive parathyroids is characterized by a combination of an elevated level of serum calcium plus an elevated level of serum parathyroid hormone.

Diagnosis may be complicated because, very rarely, some other cancers can produce parathyroid hormone and so are also associated with high calcium levels. More frequently a similar substance called parathyroid hormone-related peptide is responsible for elevated calcium levels in patients with cancer.

Physical Examination
♦ Mass in the neck. Benign tumors rarely have a mass in the neck.

♦ Vocal cords may be paralyzed on one side, causing hoarseness.

Blood and Other Tests
♦ Urinary cyclic AMP levels are elevated in almost all patients.
♦ The normal serum calcium level is about 10 mg/dl and the levels in benign tumors average 12 mg/dl, but most parathyroid cancers have levels over 14 mg/dl.
♦ Sometimes the presence and location of a primary parathyroid tumor can be confirmed by placing a plastic catheter into the veins draining the parathyroids or metastatic deposits. Blood samples are then taken from each of the parathyroid areas to measure the level of the serum parathyroid hormone.

Imaging
♦ Reabsorption of bone on x-ray.
♦ Confirmatory tests can be done before surgery, especially if a mass is not present. These include ultrasound examination of the parathyroid region of the neck as well as CT or MRI scans.
♦ An isotope scan using radioactive thallium or technetium.

STAGING

There are only two stages for parathyroid cancer. One stage is localized, meaning that the disease is confined to the parathyroid with or without invasion of adjacent tissues. The other is metastatic, in which the cancer may have spread to regional lymph nodes and may or may not involve other distant sites such as the lung, bones and liver.

TREATMENT OVERVIEW

The major problem with these tumors is not predominantly the tumor itself, which grows rather slowly, but the severe elevation in calcium levels, which produces a condition (hypercalcemia) that is difficult to control medically and may eventually be fatal.

For this reason, aggressive surgical removal of bulk disease or even metastatic disease has been favored. But this type of surgery is not always possible, either because of widespread metastasis or because the area that has to be operated on is not accessible or involves vital structures.

A variety of medical means can inhibit the the action of parathyroid hormone and to improve the hypercalcemia, including the use of calcitonin. The use of mithramycin or diphosphonates has not been remarkably successful.

TREATMENT BY STAGE

LOCALIZED
Standard Treatment Localized parathyroid cancer is treated with removal of the tumor and the thyroid gland on the same side. Adjacent muscles and other tissues are included if they appear to be involved. Local recurrence is common, however, and may require repeat surgery.

Five-Year Survival About 50 percent

Investigational
♦ Clinical trials are evaluating combinations of surgery and radiation therapy, as well as radiation therapy alone.

METASTATIC
Standard Treatment For metastatic parathyroid cancer, an operation is performed similar to that for localized parathyroid cancer, with removal of adjacent neck muscles and regional lymph nodes if they are involved.

An attempt is made to remove as much tumor as possible to help eliminate the source of parathyroid hormone and in turn to reduce the problems of elevated serum calcium.

Five-Year Survival 20 percent

Investigational
♦ As for localized cancer, clinical protocols are studying combinations of surgery and radiation therapy, as well as radiation therapy alone for metastatic parathyroid cancer.
♦ A few patients with metastatic parathyroid cancer have been treated with chemotherapy combinations, including the active agent dacarbazine (DTIC), as well as that agent combined with 5-fluorouracil and cyclophosphamide. There are no current adjuvant treatment protocols for this tumor.

TREATMENT FOLLOW-UP

♦ Physical examination of the neck and determinations of blood calcium and parathyroid hormone levels are the most appropriate methods of follow-up.
♦ Appropriate x-ray studies and scans will be useful for patients with metastases.

RECURRENT CANCER

The treatment of recurrent parathyroid cancer is generally surgical removal of the primary tumor—with or without removing the lymph nodes—or debulking the tumor to reduce the production of parathormone. Under investigation are the combinations of surgery with radiation therapy, radiation therapy alone, as well as chemotherapy.

THE MOST IMPORTANT QUESTIONS YOU CAN ASK

♦ If you are not sure at surgery whether this is benign or malignant, how will you decide what kind of surgery to do?
♦ Is a frozen section reliable in helping to decide if the tumor is benign or malignant?
♦ Would radiation therapy be helpful along with surgery?

PENIS

Norman R. Zinner, MD, MS

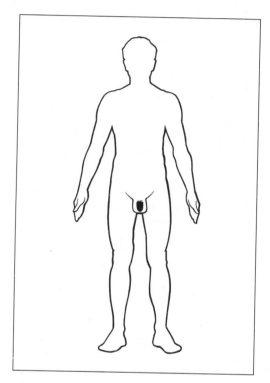

Cancer of the penis is rare in the United States, affecting only one or two men in 100,000. It is almost never seen in those who have been circumcised as babies, which is a major argument in favor of newborn circumcision. It can occur anywhere along the penile shaft, but most are on the foreskin or head (glans). It is usually a slow-growing cancer and is curable if discovered early. Unfortunately, some men do not seek medical attention until after it has spread.

Types Nearly all penile malignancies are cancers of the skin, the most common being squamous cell carcinoma similar to squamous cell carcinomas on other parts of the skin such as the face or hands. Some penile cancers are melanomas, which appear as blue-brown flat growths and tend to spread more rapidly and more widely. Occasionally, the deep tissues of the penis develop cancer, typically sarcomas.

How It Spreads The tumor spreads gradually, becoming larger in the area of the skin where it first develops. Ultimately, it spreads to deep tissues inside the body of the penis and to lymph nodes in the groin (inguinal area) or pelvis. When the cancer is in the penis itself (local) and involves no more than a few nearby inguinal lymph nodes, it can be cured, but cure rates fall rapidly once it spreads to the pelvic lymph nodes.

What Causes It This is one of the few cancers where the cause is fairly well known. Men who are circumcised at birth (a common practice among whites in the United States) almost never get cancer of the penis. If circumcision is performed at puberty, the incidence of cancer is slightly higher, and men who are circumcised as adults are not protected and experience the same incidence of penile cancer as men who are never circumcised at all.

Cancer of the penis is, in a sense, a disease of poor hygiene. It is believed that the decaying cells of the undersurface of the foreskin (smegma) produce irritation leading to cancer. Cancer of the uterine cervix may be higher in the female sexual partners of men who are not circumcised. Penile warts (condylomata) are also associated with penile cancer. This is of special importance to female sexual partners of these men because the women often develop cancer of the cervix when exposed to the viruses that produce penile warts, even if the men do not have cancerous change in their warts.

RISK FACTORS

The cancer is one of later years, being rare before age 25 and typically occurring after age 50. The highest incidence is among uncircumcised men, especially those who cannot pull back their foreskins and clean them. In the United States, the highest incidence is among Afro-Americans.

SCREENING

There are no blood tests to screen for cancer of the penis. All uncircumsised men should examine the foreskin and head of the penis monthly. It is essential that they be able to retract the foreskin to be able to see all the tissue on its undersurface.

COMMON SIGNS AND SYMPTOMS

The most common finding is a painless sore on the foreskin or glans that won't heal. If the man cannot retract the foreskin the cancer may not be discovered until it grows large and appears as a cauliflower-like mass growing from beneath the pouch of the foreskin. If left alone, it will usually become inflamed and often infected. This may produce a foul odor and discomfort. It can also lead to enlargement of inguinal lymph nodes. Penile cancer rarely interferes with urination.

DIAGNOSIS

Physical Examination
♦ The main physical finding is a sore or rash on the penis that may be inflamed. It will erode and destroy the penis if not treated early.
♦ There may be swelling in the groin from inflamed lymph nodes or from nodes involved with cancer.

Imaging
♦ CT scan, chest x-ray and bone, liver and lymph node scans (lymphangiogram) are used to discover if there is spread once a cancer is confirmed on biopsy.

Endoscopy and Biopsy
♦ A biopsy is the main diagnostic test.

TREATMENT OVERVIEW

The tumor size and degree of spread locally and to other sites (stage) determines treatment options.
♦ If the tumor is small and local, it can be treated surgically, chemically or with radiation or laser without major damage to the appearance or function of the penis.
♦ If it has penetrated the deeper penile tissues or if it is large, surgery is the preferred treatment for most men. Radiation is an option, but results are less certain.
♦ If the tumor has spread to lymph nodes, surgery or radiation are used.
♦ Chemotherapy is of little value in extensive carcinoma of the penis.

TREATMENT BY STAGE: SQUAMOUS CELL CARCINOMA

CARCINOMA IN SITU
This tumor appears either as a reddish, velvety rash (erythroplasia of Queyrat) or as small, crusty bumps (Bowen's disease).

Standard Treatment These tumors are best treated with 5-fluorouracil cream applied locally twice daily for four to five weeks. If this is not successful, the local lesions can be treated with laser or removed surgically. Usually, there is little or no disfigurement, but this depends upon the size and location of the growth.

Five-Year Survival 100 percent

STAGE I
The cancer is limited to the foreskin or head of the penis and does not invade the deep layers beneath the skin.

Standard Treatment An extensive circumcision may be all that is necessary if the cancer is small and limited to the foreskin. If it is large or on the glans, surgical removal of the tumor with a wide margin may be acceptable, but partial amputation is usually needed. The remaining penile stump can be remarkably serviceable for urination and sexual intercourse, but partial amputation is disfiguring and most younger men find the emotional trauma hard to take. The main advantage of surgery is that it usually results in a cure. Because of the high incidence of microscopic metastases to inguinal lymph nodes, surgery to remove these nodes is under evaluation.

Radiation therapy, administered by external beam or with radiation implants, may preserve the entire penis. But recurrence rates are high and the urine canal often becomes very narrow. If this happens, surgical amputation can then be done.

Five-Year Survival 100 percent

STAGE II
The cancer is locally invasive but has not spread to the groin (inguinal) lymph nodes.

Standard Treatment Partial or complete amputation of the penis (penectomy) depending upon the location of the cancer. If the tumor is at the tip of the penis, a partial penectomy can be done. If it develops closer to the root of the penile shaft or has spread, a total penectomy is usually needed. Cure rates are excellent for Stage II penile cancers treated surgically.

The decision to remove all of the penis depends on whether enough of a stump can be left to allow the man to have sexual intercourse and to urinate while standing without voiding in uncontrolled directions. Penile reconstruction or the construction of a new penis is possible with plastic surgery.

Radiation therapy can be tried in younger men and those who refuse surgery, but rates of recurrence and urethral strictures are high. If radiation fails, surgery can usually be accomplished with excellent results.

Five-Year Survival 88 percent

STAGE III
These cancers have spread to inguinal or pelvic lymph nodes, and cure rates are poor.

Standard Treatment Stage III disease is suspected when there is swelling of the inguinal lymph nodes, but this swelling can be misleading. Sometimes the lymph nodes are enlarged not because of cancer but because of an infection or inflammation. To find out if this is the case, the tumor is first treated in the same way as Stage II tumors.

If the nodes are involved with infection or inflammation, the swelling will usually subside four to six weeks after the cancer is surgically removed from the penis. The lymph nodes will no longer be felt through the skin.

If the lymph nodes can still be felt through the skin four to six weeks after surgery, some of the inguinal lymph nodes can be biopsied and examined. If they are found to contain cancer, all of the nodes of the groin and pelvis are removed.

If the patient is treated with radiation therapy rather than by surgery, the swollen inguinal lymph nodes will usually not disappear within the four-to-six-week period of observation.

Five-Year Survival 75 percent

STAGE IV
The cancer has spread to distant sites.

Standard Treatment There is no standard treatment for cure. Treatment is directed at the control of symptoms by selected radiation, surgery or experimental chemotherapy protocols.

Five-Year Survival Less than 5 percent

TREATING VENEREAL WARTS

Occasionally, venereal warts (malignant transformation of condyloma acuminata) become cancerous. Since they are also known to cause cancer in the female partners of men with some types of these warts even if the men do not have cancer themselves, all venereal warts should be treated. Treatment methods include:

♦ applying a liquid chemical (podophyllin) directly to the area,
♦ applying supercooled liquid gases (cryotherapy),
♦ charring (fulguration),
♦ vaporization by a laser, or surgical removal,
♦ intradermal interferon-alpha.

If there is any suspicion of malignancy, warts should be removed surgically and examined under the microscope.

THE MOST IMPORTANT QUESTIONS YOU CAN ASK

♦ Is surgery necessary, and how extensive must it be?
♦ Are you going to remove my lymph nodes? Which ones and when?
♦ Is this tumor transmitted sexually?
♦ What is the relationship of this cancer to venereal warts?
♦ What is the relationship to circumcision?

PITUITARY

Malin Dollinger, MD, and Ernest H. Rosenbaum, MD

◇

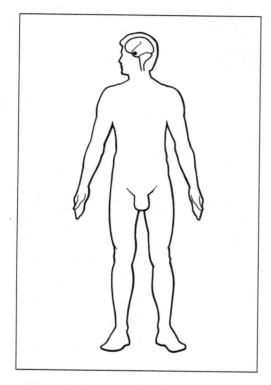

Tumors in the pituitary gland, which is located at the base of the brain (*see* page 232), are benign (adenomas) and curable over 90 percent of the time. But these tumors can become large enough to damage nearby nerves and brain tissue, sometimes permanently. By pressing on the nerves to the eyes, a pituitary tumor can cause a progressive loss of vision and even blindness. In some cases, the tumor compresses the pituitary gland, preventing it from producing the normal amount of hormones. Hypothyroidism, adrenal insufficiency and a deficiency in growth hormone can result.

Types In some cases, pituitary adenomas produce excess hormones, causing significant symptoms. The increased production of growth hormone can produce a disease called acromegaly. Excess prolactin can cause impotence in men and the loss of menstrual periods and breast secretion in women. Excess ACTH (adrenocorticotropic hormone) can result in Cushing's disease. Some tumors, chromophobe adenomas, are non-functional.

How It Spreads Since most pituitary tumors are benign, they do not spread like cancerous tumors. But they do become larger and may grow outside the bony cavity surrounding the pituitary (sella turcica).

What Causes It There is no known cause, although the use of birth control pills may be a contributing factor in some cases.

COMMON SIGNS AND SYMPTOMS

Early symptoms depend on which hormone is involved. As the tumor grows, sight may deteriorate, starting with loss on the edges of the field of vision. Sometimes there may also be headaches.

DIAGNOSIS

Blood and Other Tests
♦ Sensitive radioimmunoassays for any hormone suspected of overproduction.

Imaging
♦ CT and MRI scans of the brain. MRI is the more sensitive study.
♦ X-rays of the skull may show destruction of the sella turcica.

TREATMENT OVERVIEW

Treatment depends on the type of tumor and whether it has grown beyond the area of the pituitary gland.

Tumors that produce hormones are treated with surgery or radiation, with the surgical approach—a transsphenoidal hypophysectomy—usually the treatment chosen for tumors that have not grown outside the bony cavity. Larger tumors, usually non-functioning adenomas, need additional treatment with radiation.

Prolactin-secreting tumors may stabilize and improve with time. People with these tumors may be given bromocriptine to help control symptoms.

Tumors that produce growth hor-mone and ACTH usually grow slowly. With any of the pituitary tumors, however, surgery is called for immediately if vision starts to deteriorate rapidly.

TREATMENT BY TYPE

ACTH-PRODUCING TUMORS

Standard Treatment Surgery, radiation therapy, a combination of both or Mitotane plus radiation.

Investigational
♦ Heavy-particle radiation.

PROLACTIN-PRODUCING TUMORS

Standard Treatment Surgical removal of the tumor, radiation, bromocriptine or combinations of these treatments. Bromocriptine has been of considerable benefit in reducing symptoms. A new drug, CV205-502, has been successful in patients who have failed to respond to bromocriptine.

Investigational
♦ Heavy-particle radiation.

GROWTH HORMONE–PRODUCING TUMORS

Standard Treatment Surgery, radiation therapy, bromocriptine or somatostatin. Which treatment is chosen depends on the size and extent of the tumor and on how urgent it is to eliminate the excess hormone production.

NON-FUNCTIONING TUMORS

Standard Treatment These tumors, usually chromophobe adenomas, are treated with surgery and radiation. The choice depends on how big the tumor is, how fast it's growing and its effect on adjacent body structures.

The surgical and radiotherapy techniques used to treat these tumors are very complex and sophisticated. Neuro-surgeons and radiation oncologists experienced in treating them are best able to judge which method is the most appropriate.

TREATMENT FOLLOW-UP

The intensity and schedule of follow-up depends on the amount of damage done to adjacent tissues before treatment and on whether the tumor was completely removed during surgery.

♦ An internist or endocrinologist will often be involved in following up after surgery, since replacement hormones may be needed.

♦ Follow-up CT or MRI scans may be useful.

♦ Hormone levels may be measured periodically if a hormone-producing tumor was treated.

THE MOST IMPORTANT QUESTIONS YOU CAN ASK

♦ Is my tumor producing extra hormones?

♦ Is surgery or radiation the best treatment for my type of tumor?

♦ What is the probability that the treatment will eliminate the tumor?

♦ What are the risks, complications and side effects of treatment?

♦ Will I have to take hormones after surgery and, if so, for how long?

♦ What are the chances that my vision will improve?

PROSTATE

Norman R. Zinner, MD, MS

◇

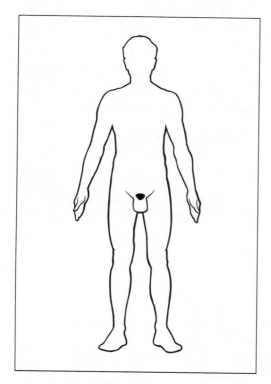

Cancer of the prostate is the most common cancer in American men, overtaking both lung cancer and cancer of the colon and rectum during the 1980s. Since this is usually a disease of men over 65, the increase appears to be due to the aging of the population. The American Cancer Society estimates that over 100,000 men will contract the disease in 1991 and about 29,000 will die from it. It is the third leading cause of cancer death in men. Prostate cancer is not related to the problem of an enlarged prostate in most older men, a condition called benign prostatic hyperplasia (BPH).

If the disease is to be cured it has to be discovered before it spreads beyond the prostate gland. Unfortunately, only about one-half of newly diagnosed patients fall into this category. Advances in ultrasound and increased public awareness of the importance of early discovery through annual rectal examinations may lead to earlier detection. Even then, the benefit to the public is uncertain. Most men with prostate cancer will die from other illnesses never knowing they had the problem.

Types Nearly all prostate cancer arises from the glands of the prostate. Glandular cancer (adenocarcinoma) accounts for 95 percent of all prostate cancer cases. Over half of these cancers develop from the rear (posterior) portion of the prostate that lies closest to the rectum, which is why rectal examination is useful to detect the tumor.

Other types are rare. Most, including leiomyosarcoma and rhabdomyosarcoma, arise from supporting or connective tissues within or around the prostate. Others develop in the ducts within the prostate. Tumors can also spread to the prostate from other locations such as the bladder or adrenal gland.

Some types are not actually cancer but have characteristics that appear precancerous. These are called prostatic intraepithelial neoplasia (PIN), a term referring to cell growths that are almost active cancers or may soon become cancer. Men with PIN have to be observed closely and have periodic biopsies.

How It Spreads Prostatic cancers spread through the lymphatic system to pelvic lymph nodes and through the bloodstream to bones and other tissues. The earliest spread is usually detected in lymph nodes in the pelvis near the prostate. Other areas of spread are to lymph nodes around the arteries and veins leading to the legs and pelvic organs and to bones in the spine, legs, arms and hips. Ultimately, it can reach almost any organ in the body. The tumor may also spread directly through the prostate to surrounding tissues or may grow inward, blocking the flow of urine.

What Causes It The exact cause isn't known, but hormones play a role. Any man who had his testicles removed before he reached puberty—and so did not get to produce the male hormone testosterone— will rarely develop prostate cancer. The use of hormones such as steroids by athletes or cortisone for certain diseases, however, will not cause the problem.

Some people have recently speculated that foods high in fat may play a role, but this is far from certain. Genetic factors are suspected, since prostate cancer patients with relatives who also have prostate cancer are up to three times more likely to die of their disease than those patients who do not have relatives with prostate cancer.

We know a great deal more about what does not cause it. There is no conclusive evidence that one can get cancer of the prostate from "too much sex," masturbation, infection of the prostate or benign prostatic hyperplasia (BPH). Prostatic stones or infection have no proven influence.

RISK FACTORS

There is speculation about a relationship between prostatic cancer and industrial cancer-causing agents such as cadmium. No relationship has been shown between prostate cancer and smoking, use of alco-

Bladder

Seminal vesicle

Prostate

Cancer

Urethra

Testicle

The prostate gland and associated pelvic organs

hol, disease patterns, circumcision, weight, height, blood group, hair distribution, sexual activity or benign prostatic hyperplasia.

There are no known ways to protect against the development of prostatic cancer.

At Significantly Higher Risk

♦ The probability of having the disease increases with age. Men under 50 have less than one chance in a hundred of getting prostate cancer while about half of all men over 80 will have it.

♦ The risk is twice as high in blacks than in whites and is lowest for Asians. Jews have the lowest mortality rate from prostatic cancer, blacks the highest.

♦ The United States death rate is high compared with other countries. The urban rate is slightly higher than the rural rate.

SCREENING

A digital rectal examination remains the best way to detect cancer of the prostate early, for the gland's location within the rectum makes it easy to feel. The cancer often produces a lump or an irregularity that can be felt, and about one suspicious area in three will prove to be malignant.

Half the cancers will have spread by the time they are discovered, which has led to a search for more sensitive methods to detect the tumor early. Ultrasound is one method now being tested. It is painless and does not involve radiation. Although its value as a screening tool is not yet proved, early results suggest that ultrasound is especially helpful in confirming results of a digital exam and in guiding needle biopsy.

Prostate-specific antigen (PSA) is a blood antigen specific to the prostate and is often elevated when cancer is present. But it is also elevated in benign disease, so efforts to use PSA as a screening test have not been fruitful. Since PSA will usually rise as tumors grow, its measurement is a good way to monitor the course of cancer once it is found.

COMMON SIGNS AND SYMPTOMS

When symptoms occur, they can be local or generalized. Local symptoms include painful or frequent urination, a sudden decrease in the size and force of the urinary stream or blood in the urine. Generalized symptoms relate to spread to bone and include pain in the back, hips, thighs or shoulders. There is weight loss and fatigue as the tumor progresses. Prostate cancer is seldom curable once symptoms develop, which is the best argument for early detection through screening.

DIAGNOSIS

Physical Examination

♦ The main finding is a lump or irregularity in the prostate, which can be felt with the examining finger. The prostate may seem enlarged but can also be normal size.

Blood and Other Tests

♦ Blood chemistry tests to measure prostate-specific antigen and prostatic acid phosphatase, which can become elevated in prostatic cancer.

♦ Urinalysis to detect evidence of bleeding or infection in the urine.

♦ A complete blood count may show anemia if the tumor has invaded the bone marrow.

♦ A serum chemistry profile looks at 15 to 20 chemistry tests measuring liver and bone enzymes, kidney function and other studies.

Imaging

♦ Transrectal ultrasound to view the prostate and direct a biopsy needle into the tumor.

♦ X-rays of the abdomen, pelvis, kidneys and bladder to see if the tumor has spread to these structures.

♦ Intravenous pyelogram (IVP) of the urinary system (kidneys, ureters and bladder).

♦ Chest x-ray.

♦ Abdominal and pelvic CT or MRI scans.

Endoscopy and Biopsy
♦ A transrectal needle biopsy is the removal of a small piece of the tumor for examination by a pathologist. Its accuracy can often be increased by guiding the needle with ultrasound.

♦ Cystoscopy (passage of a small tube through the urinary canal) will provide a different view of the prostate and allow the doctor to move the prostate while it is being examined with a finger in the rectum. In this way, the lump can be felt from a variety of angles and it can be discovered whether the lump has become attached to adjacent tissues.

♦ Flow cytometry and nuclear shape analysis are tests to evaluate the characteristics of the prostate cells removed by biopsy. Cancer cells are less uniform than normal ones.

STAGING/GRADING
Stages of prostate cancer are divided into A, B, C and D according to the degree of spread. Slower-growing cancer cells take longer to spread, and the grade of the tumor cells—how aggressive they are—is described by the Gleason grading system, which categorizes prostate cell growth and behavior. The Gleason rating, which is between 1 and 10, represents a total score of two parts. One part is given to the predominant cell type and the second part is given to the most aggressive cell type. These two scores are added to become the Gleason rating. Tumors rated 2 to 4 are generally slow growing and are less likely to be life-threatening. Tumors rated 8 to 10 are the more dangerous ones.

TREATMENT OVERVIEW
Treatment options depend on the tumor's stage (its size and degree of spread to other sites) and grade (the aggressiveness of the particular tumor cells). If the cancer can be caught while still confined to the prostate it can be cured. If it has spread, it

Stages of prostate cancer

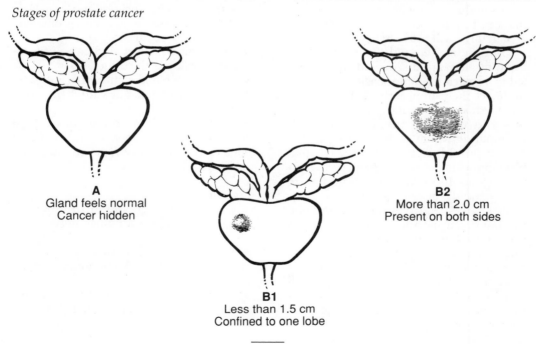

A
Gland feels normal
Cancer hidden

B1
Less than 1.5 cm
Confined to one lobe

B2
More than 2.0 cm
Present on both sides

can be treated but not cured. If it is low grade it is less likely to have spread than if it is high grade.

Surgery and radiation therapy are the treatments of choice if the tumor is going to be cured. The decision depends on the patient's age, medical condition and personal desires. Therapy with hormones, removal of the testicles (orchiectomy) and chemotherapy may relieve symptoms of advanced disease but will not produce a cure.

Surgery Surgical removal of the prostate and the seminal vesicles—a radical prostatectomy—is the only certain way to remove all of the cancerous gland. This will lead to a cure if the cancer is confined to the prostate.

The surgeon will often sample lymph nodes—in a procedure called a pelvic lymphadenectomy—during the operation but before the prostate is removed. If the lymph nodes are positive for cancer, the prostate will not be removed, for there will be little benefit for the patient.

The newest procedure for lymph node sampling is called laparoscopic lymphadenectomy. A long telescope (laparoscope) is inserted through a tiny opening in the abdomen and is used to observe and guide the sampling of pelvic lymph nodes to see if they contain cancer. This will simplify and shorten the testing process and may eliminate a major surgical procedure without sacrificing the result. It also creates the option for other definitive surgical procedures that are easier on the patient and that may have fewer side effects. In time, it may also be used in conjunction with radiation therapy.

The removal of the prostate will produce intermittent loss of urine in about half the patients and complete incontinence (leaking of urine) in 5 to 10 percent of patients. Newer techniques permit the majority of younger men to preserve their sexual ability, but it is lost in most men

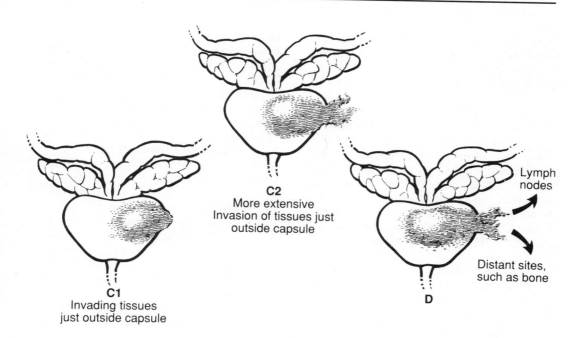

C2
More extensive
Invasion of tissues just
outside capsule

C1
Invading tissues
just outside capsule

Lymph
nodes

Distant sites,
such as bone

D

over 70. However, urine loss and impotence can be treated.

The operation is complex and as with any major surgical procedure there can be wound breakdown and infection. Nearly everyone survives the operation.

 Radiation Radiation therapy can be given by external beam or implantation of radioactive seeds into the tumor. External beam radiation usually takes about six weeks. It has the advantage of avoiding an incision, but sometimes it may not kill all the cancer cells. If so, the tumor may grow back, although it can take ten to fifteen years to return. The risks and complications of external beam radiation therapy are equivalent in number to those of surgery, but there are differences in the nature of specific problems. Six weeks of radiation can cause moderate and sometimes considerable fatigue. Severe rectal pains with diarrhea and spasms (radiation proctitis) and severe bladder urgency, frequency and pain on urination (radiation cystitis) can also occur. These can be permanent. Loss of urine (incontinence) and impotence occur nearly as often as they do with a radical prostatectomy. As well, external beam radiation may not kill all the cancer cells.

Interstitial radiation is administered by inserting pellets or ribbons of radiation-emitting material directly into the prostate. This can be done by open surgery or via needles inserted through the skin. The main advantage of this therapy is that the radiation dosage is concentrated to the tumor and does not harm normal tissues. There is also less radiation cystitis and proctitis. If the pellets or ribbons are inserted at open surgery, the surgeon can at the same time sample the lymph nodes to see if the tumor has spread (although the use of laparoscopic sampling may make open surgery less common).

The disadvantages of interstitial radiation are that the pellets or ribbons may not be placed evenly in the tumor and areas can be missed. Also, all the cancer cells may not be killed and the tumor may recur. Interstitial radiation can also produce erosion into the rectum causing urine to pass into the rectum, and stool into the bladder.

Radiation therapy is also used to relieve symptoms. Radiation to bone for local control of pain, for example, can often produce dramatic relief.

Surgery vs Radiation There is controversy about the relative benefits of surgical treatment versus radiation therapy. Most data suggest that surgery produces the greater likelihood of avoiding tumor recurrence, since radiation may not kill all the cancer cells and injured ones may recover and grow back. Not all experts agree.

If life expectancy is the sole issue, surgery and radiation therapy produce about the same results for the first 5 to 10 years. After that time, surgery is somewhat better.

Hormonal Therapy When the prostate cancer can no longer be cured with surgery or radiation or when the patient is not a candidate for these methods perhaps because of other illness, hormonal therapy is used to slow the growth of the tumor and reduce symptoms. It is not a cure, but results can be very good. The idea behind this treatment is that the male hormone testosterone helps prostate tumor cells thrive. Depriving the tumor cells of this hormone will often retard the tumor's growth.

Hormonal therapy can be given by removing the testicles (the body's main source of male hormone) or by giving other hormones or chemicals to shut down the body's production of testosterone or counteract its effects. Patients receiving hormonal therapy often experience dramatic relief of symptoms, which can sometimes last for years. But ultimately, the tumor returns.

All the methods used to manipulate the male hormone system will cause men to lose their desire for sex. They may also produce hot flashes.

♦ Removing the testicles (orchiectomy) is a simple surgical procedure that can be done under local or general anesthesia in an outpatient department. Once this is done there is no need for further hormonal therapy. Some men find this procedure undesirable, but the effect is the same as for other hormonal treatments.

♦ Giving men the female hormone estrogen will shut down the gland in the brain (pituitary) that stimulates the testicles to make testosterone. The effect of estrogens on prostate cancer is similar to the effect of orchiectomy, but the female hormone can cause breast development and breast tenderness, although this can usually be prevented by first giving a small dose of radiotherapy to the breast area. Estrogens can also be associated with an increased incidence of heart disease. The pills must be taken daily for life.

♦ Newer hormones such as leuprolide have much the same effect as orchiectomy or estrogen therapy but are less likely to produce the breast enlargement or heart problems experienced with estrogens. These hormones are expensive and are administered by daily or monthly injections for life.

♦ There are hormonal agents (progestins) that bind to the prostate cell and prevent testosterone from helping it thrive. And there are non-hormonal chemical agents such as ketoconazole that reduce male hormone levels and mimic the effect of orchiectomy.

 Chemotherapy When orchiectomy or hormonal therapy fail, chemotherapy may be used in advanced stages, but results are poor.

TREATMENT BY STAGE

STAGE A

These tumors are hidden from usual clinical observation. They cannot be felt and are typically found in tissue samples taken after the prostate has been removed because of a benign obstructive disease or when biopsies are taken after ultrasound shows something suspicious.

STAGE A-1

The tumor is limited to less than 5 percent of the prostate tissue removed at surgery and is low grade.

Standard Treatment Most men do not require treatment for this stage of tumor. It is slow growing and will rarely cause symptoms. Fewer than 2 percent will have unsuspected spread to lymph nodes when the tumor is discovered.

Men under 60 may consider radical prostatectomy or external beam radiation therapy because their longer life expectancy will give the slow-growing tumor a greater time to produce symptoms.

STAGE A-2

The tumor extends to more than 5 percent of the tissue removed at surgery and is usually medium to high grade. It is a dangerous tumor, and 34 percent of patients have unexpected spread to lymph nodes when the tumor is found.

Standard Treatment Removal of the pelvic lymph nodes, followed by radical prostatectomy during the same operation if the lymph nodes are found to be negative. If the tumor location and tissue conditions permit, nerve-sparing methods may be used to preserve sexual ability.

Postoperative radiation therapy should be considered if the tumor is found to invade or penetrate the prostate capsule or if serum PSA levels remain elevated three weeks after surgery.

♦ External beam radiation therapy using the linear accelerator.

♦ Careful observation or hormonal therapy may be acceptable in patients with other serious medical problems that might indicate a short life expectancy or an inability to withstand the stress of surgery or radiation.

Five-Year Survival 60 percent

Investigational
♦ Interstitial radiation with I-125 inserted at open surgery, often with removal of the pelvic lymph nodes. With ultrasound guidance, the isotope can also be inserted without an open incision.
♦ Lymph node sampling without open surgery (laparoscopic lymphadenectomy).
♦ Therapeutic trials using newer isotopes such as iridium-191 and palladium are under way.

STAGE B
Stage B tumors are palpable lumps that are confined to the prostate and do not penetrate the prostate capsule. The size and grade of the tumor determine the possibility for cure.

STAGE B-1
The tumor is less than 5/8 in. (1.5 cm), does not invade the capsule and is limited to one lobe of the prostate. Approximately 15 to 20 percent of patients have unsuspected lymph nodes with cancer when the lump is discovered, which is why pelvic lymph node sampling is required before the prostate is removed.

Standard Treatment Same as Stage A-2.

Five-Year Survival 75 percent

Investigational Same as Stage A-2.

STAGE B-2
The tumor is larger than 3/4 in. (2 cm) and involves more than one lobe of the prostate. It does not invade the capsule. Thirty-four percent of patients have unex-

pected spread to lymph nodes at the time the tumor is found.

Standard Treatment Same as Stage A-2.

Five-Year Survival 60 percent

Investigational Same as Stage A-2.

STAGE C
These tumors have penetrated the prostate capsule and spread to nearby structures such as the seminal vesicles or fat next to the prostate gland.
    This stage is further divided into:
♦ C-1, indicating spread just beyond the prostate;
♦ C-2, indicating spread still in the local area but involving more of the immediately surrounding tissues. Stage C-2 will often obstruct the flow of urine, producing voiding difficulties.
    About half of Stage C-1 patients and 80 percent of Stage C-2 patients have unsuspected lymph node metastases when the tumor is detected.

Standard Treatment The approach to Stage C cancer depends on the extent of the tumor and the patient's medical condition.
    Treatment can be directed toward curing the cancer if the tumor can be removed or seems able to be treated successfully and if the patient's medical condition permits.
    If the tumor seems too large or if the patient is too old or not in good health, palliative therapy can be provided to slow tumor growth and reduce symptoms.

♦ *Treatment for Cure* External beam radiation therapy using the linear accelerator is the treatment of choice. Some experts, however, believe that a radical retropubic prostatectomy can be done successfully in certain cases of Stage C-1 cancers where the tumor is confined closely to the prostate and the surgeon can get well around the tumor. In these cases, as always, the lymph nodes are first sampled to be certain they have no cancer. If nodes are positive, the prostatectomy is not done. Interstitial implants using radioactive palladium have also been used.

◆ *Treatment for Palliation* Radiation therapy to the prostate can reduce the size of the tumor, but long-term effects in prolonging life are not well documented. This therapy can reduce obstructions and make urination easier.

A transurethral prostatectomy (TURP) will also help urination and is less burdensome than radiation therapy. But incontinence is more likely afterwards when cancer spreads to the urinary control zone, the urethral sphincter.

Hormonal therapy is the mainstay of palliative therapy for prostate cancer.

Five-Year Survival 50 to 55 percent for C-1, 40 to 45 percent for C-2

Investigational Same as Stage A-2.

STAGE D
The tumor has spread to lymph nodes and distant locations and is rarely curable. There are often symptoms of urinary obstruction or pain from metastases to bone.

This stage is further divided into:
◆ D-0. The tumor appears localized to the prostate as if it were Stage B, but the blood test tumor marker prostatic acid phosphatase is elevated, indicating that the tumor has spread to distant sites.
◆ D-1. Spread to lymph nodes in the pelvis.
◆ D-2. Spread to bone or distant organs.
◆ D-3. Patients with Stage D-2 disease who have relapsed after adequate hormonal therapy.

Standard Treatment Most treatment aims to control symptoms—relieving obstruction or pain—and tries to prolong life. Radical surgery is generally not useful.

The standard treatment is hormonal manipulation through hormonal therapy or removal of the testicles. Hormonal therapy includes giving estrogens (diethylstilbestrol), antiandrogens (flutamide), luteinizing hormone-releasing hormone (LH-RH) agonists such as leuprolide, and progestational agents (Megace).

Impressive improvement often follows hormonal treatment, with reduction in pain and improvement in overall well-being. Voiding symptoms sometimes disappear, although this effect may take several months to occur. Relief of pain is often dramatic after the testicles are removed. This procedure produces the quickest results and does not require the use of any further medication for tumor control.

◆ A chemotherapeutic-hormonal agent called estramustine phosphate concentrates in the prostate cancer tissue and is believed to have some direct action against the tumor. Whether this effect is because of the hormonal activity or antitumor activity is not well understood. The agent is still unproven and is used mainly for patients who fail traditional hormone therapy measures.

◆ When voiding problems are severe and there is no time to wait, a transurethral prostatectomy (TURP) will produce immediate relief of urinary obstruction. Incontinence (leakage of urine) is a risk in TURP because the tumor may extend to the urethral sphincter muscle and prevent the canal from closing properly.

◆ Pain in areas of bone involved by tumor and that does not respond to hormonal therapy is best treated by external beam radiation to the area of pain. Relief is often felt within days.

◆ Observation without further immediate treatment may be suitable for selected patients who have no symptoms.

◆ External beam irradiation for possible cure in highly selected Stage D-1 patients, since patients with this limited Stage D disease will occasionally respond to external beam radiation to the prostate and pelvic area. Cure is rare.

Five-Year Survival 55 percent for D-0, 40 percent for D-1, 35 percent for D-2 and D-3

Investigational
♦ Combination hormonal manipulation with LH-RH agonists and progestational agents.
♦ Chemotherapy protocols.
♦ Alternative forms of radiotherapy with neutron beams. New devices producing more powerful forms of external radiation using proton and neutron beams have been developed, and patients are being treated in clinical trials.

TREATING OTHER PROSTATE TUMORS
DUCTAL CARCINOMAS
These arise within the prostatic ducts and comprise less than 5 percent of prostate cancers. There are four types:
♦ transitional cell carcinoma;
♦ intraductal adenocarcinoma;
♦ mixed ductal carcinoma; and
♦ endometroid carcinoma.

Transitional cell and mixed ductal carcinomas are aggressive cancers that require complete removal of the prostate and bladder (cystoprostatectomy) if found while the tumor is still confined to the prostate. The outlook is not good for patients with these cancers.

Intraductal adenocarcinomas are treated by radical prostatectomy.

Endometroid carcinomas arise near a structure called the verumontanum and are similar to certain types of uterine cancers in women. If the tumors are confined to the prostate, the treatment of choice is the removal of the prostate and bladder. Some patients with advanced disease respond to external beam radiation therapy, hormonal treatment or chemotherapy with 5-fluorouracil and doxorubicin.

CARCINOSARCOMAS, RHABDOMYOSARCOMAS, CHONDROSARCOMA AND OSTEOSARCOMA
These make up the rest of the prostate tumor types. If found early, complete removal of the prostate, bladder and adjacent pelvic structures offers the best chance for cure.

Radiation, hormonal therapy and chemotherapy are not effective.

TREATMENT FOLLOW-UP
Prostate-specific antigen (PSA) is monitored shortly after prostate surgery and at regular intervals following all therapy for prostate cancer. Cured patients will have no measurable PSA in their blood.

Regular examination, chest x-rays, bone scans and various blood tests are performed at frequent intervals to detect recurrence or spread as early as possible.

TREATING IMPOTENCE AND INCONTINENCE
Impotence is nearly always treatable. There are a variety of external appliances, surgical implants or penile injection techniques that function quite well. Over 85 percent of patients and their mates are satisfied with the results of these methods.

Patients who become incontinent after the surgical removal of the prostate or radiation therapy have a wide selection of incontinence aids—diapers, condom catheters and penile clamps, for example—to collect urine, protect the skin and maintain hygiene. Exercises to try to strengthen the urethral sphincter muscle are usually not helpful but are worth the try.

The leaking will often subside after 6 to 12 months. If not, surgically inserted sphincter implants are successful in about three-quarters of patients. Recent experiments with collagen and Teflon injections seem encouraging. Drugs such as Pro-Banthine or oxybutinine reduce bladder contraction and may control the wetness.

RECURRENT AND METASTATIC CANCER

The cure rate is low or non-existent for patients with metastatic disease, but hormonal therapy, external beam radiation, experimental chemotherapy and supportive measures can often extend life and well-being for years.

♦ Locally recurrent tumors in the pelvis are best treated by external beam or interstitial radiation therapy if radical prostatectomy was the initial form of treatment.

♦ Patients originally receiving external beam radiation therapy usually cannot be given additional external beam treatments, but selected patients can undergo interstitial radiotherapy.

♦ As is the case for most cancer of the prostate, hormonal therapy is the mainstay for metastatic disease.

♦ Chemotherapy protocols are continuing, but there are no truly promising developments.

THE MOST IMPORTANT QUESTIONS YOU CAN ASK

♦ Is my cancer confined to the prostate and how can you tell?
♦ Do I need a radical prostatectomy?
♦ What is the difference in results between surgery and radiation? Are they the same?
♦ What are the advantages and disadvantages of various hormone treatments?
♦ What are the chances that I'll become incontinent or impotent?
♦ How can I decide which treatment is best for me?
♦ Is my surgeon a Board-certified urologist experienced in this kind of operation?

SARCOMAS OF BONE AND SOFT TISSUE

Frederick Eilber, MD, and Malin Dollinger, MD

◇

Sarcomas are uncommon malignant tumors that begin either in bones or in soft tissues such as muscles, cartilage, fat or connective tissue. There are about 7,000 cases of soft tissue sarcoma and 3,000 cases of bone sarcomas in the United States each year, making up about 1 percent of cancers in adults and 15 percent in children (*see also* "Childhood Cancer: Bone and Soft Tissue Sarcomas," "Kaposi's Sarcoma," "Mesothelioma" and "Uterus: Uterine Sarcoma").

Malignant bone tumors tend to affect certain age groups. Osteosarcoma primarily affects teenagers. Ewing's sarcoma tends to affect children (ages 5 to 9) and young adults (ages 20 to 30). Chondrosarcomas tend to affect the older age groups (50 to 60 years). For childhood soft tissue sarcomas (specifically rhabdomyosarcoma) the age group most affected is children aged 1 to 3 years. Most adults with soft tissue sarcoma are 40 to 60 years old.

Over the past 15 years there has been a major advance in the early diagnosis of these tumors with CT scanning, as well as a dramatic improvement in overall survival, mainly because of effective chemotherapy. The overall survival for people with soft tissue sarcomas rose from about 40 percent in 1968 to about 70 percent in 1989. In the same years, survival for sarcomas of bone rose from less than 20 percent to over 70 percent.

In 1968, the usual treatment for tumors that began in an arm or leg was amputation of the limb. Now it is possible to preserve the limb in more than 90 percent of sarcomas in an arm or leg by using limb-sparing surgery followed by radiotherapy (although for osteosarcomas, the possibility of sparing the limb is not as high).

Types There are at least 56 different types of soft tissue sarcomas named according to the normal tissue from which the tumor is derived. Many have characteristic patterns of growth and spread. Specialists use the specific type to help plan work-up, tests and treatment, but the likely behavior of the tumor is more often related to its grade. There are three tumor categories related to the tumor's grade or activity as defined by the percentage of dividing cells (mitotic rate)—low grade, intermediate grade and high grade. The last is the most highly malignant.

The four common types of bone sarcomas are osteosarcoma, Ewing's sarcoma, chondrosarcoma and fibrosarcoma. All are usually high grade.

How It Spreads Sarcomas may spread early to adjacent tissues without being confined by a shell or capsule, as is common with other types of tumors. If this capsule were present, it would tend to delay local spread and also make surgery easier. They also spread to nearby lymph nodes and distant sites.

What Causes It In most cases the cause is unknown, although some sarcomas are related to certain diseases or exposure to specific agents. Soft tissue sarcomas do not arise from benign tumors, but some apparently benign bone tumors—cartilage or benign giant cell tumors, for example—can become malignant. Malignant bone tumors are more common in adolescence, supporting the theory that these tumors may occur because of rapid growth.

RISK FACTORS

♦ About 10 percent of people with von Recklinghausen's disease, a rare genetic abnormality affecting nerves, will develop neurofibrosarcoma. Malignant schwannomas may also develop as part of the condition.

♦ Other genetically linked diseases that have a slightly increased incidence of associated sarcomas include Werner's syndrome, tuberous sclerosis, intestinal polyposis, basal cell nevus syndrome and Gardner's syndrome.

♦ Lymphangiosarcoma is associated with people who have chronic swelling of an arm or leg and rarely may develop after many years in a swollen arm after mastectomy.

♦ Fibrosarcomas may develop after high-dose radiation given for benign conditions, such as tuberculosis of the joints or thyroid disease.

♦ The risk of angiosarcoma of liver increases with exposure to thorotrast (no longer in use), arsenic, vinyl chloride or in association with cirrhosis or hemochromatosis.

♦ The risk of osteosarcoma increases with radiation exposure, and sarcomas of both bone and soft tissue can occur many years after radiotherapy, especially if it was given in childhood. Radiation exposure causes less than 5 percent of osteosarcomas and fibrosarcomas, however. (Many years ago, exposure to radium caused osteosarcomas in painters of glow-in-the-dark watch faces.)

♦ Various causes of chronic irritation or stimulation to bones, including chronic bone infection, fractures and Paget's disease increase the risk.

♦ Sarcomas have developed in old scars or areas of trauma, but any definite cause has not been proved. There may be an associa-

TYPES OF SARCOMAS

Tumor Type	Tissue of Origin
Bone	
Chondrosarcoma	Cartilage
Osteosarcoma	Bone
Ewing's sarcoma	Probably neural crest (primitive nerve)
Fibrosarcoma	Connective (fibrous) tissue
Soft Tissue	
Liposarcoma	Fat
Rhabdomyosarcoma	Skeletal muscle
Synovial sarcoma	Membranes lining joints
Neurofibrosarcoma	Nerve structures
Angiosarcoma	Blood vessels
Leiomyosarcoma	Smooth muscle, such as found in the wall of the bowel
Mesenchymoma	Primitive connective tissue
Malignant fibrous histiocytoma	Primitive connective tissue
Epithelioid sarcoma	Unknown
Clear cell sarcoma	Unknown
Dermatofibrosarcoma protuberans	Connective tissue
Parosteal sarcoma	Bone surface
Malignant schwannoma	Nerve structures
Hemangiosarcoma	Blood vessels
Primitive neuroectodermal tumor	Nerve tissues
Lymphangiosarcoma	Lymph vessels
Alveolar soft part sarcoma	Unknown
Granular cell myoblastoma	Skeletal muscle
Hemangiopericytoma	Blood vessels

tion with certain viruses (RNA type C).

♦ Many types of bone and soft tissue sarcoma have been found to have associated characteristic chromosome abnormalities. Some families appear to have an increased incidence of sarcomas. Another inherited genetic abnormality—deletion of the retinoblastoma gene—also increases risk.

♦ Some chemotherapeutic agents, particularly "alkylating" agents, increase risk.

SCREENING

Because these are rare tumors that can arise virtually anywhere in the body, there are no standard screening measures. Both bone and soft tissue sarcomas may appear silently with an enlarging mass or swelling that may not be apparent until it causes pain or pressure symptoms.

Early detection requires that all unexplained masses or lumps in the soft tissues be assessed clinically and with CT and MRI scans and that they be biopsied or removed. Early detection is often difficult, however, not only because these cancers grow without producing symptoms but also because they arise in inaccessible places.

COMMON SIGNS AND SYMPTOMS

The most common complaints are a swelling or mass, most often painless, or pain in an affected bone or joint, especially at night. There may rarely be general symptoms such as fever, malaise, weight loss or bleeding. Some sarcomas cause a low blood sugar, with symptoms of hypoglycemia. Malignant bone sarcomas cause pain as they become larger.

DIAGNOSIS

Blood and Other Tests

♦ Blood tests—including serum chemistry panel, LDH, serum protein electrophoresis, calcium, and acid and alkaline phosphatase levels—to aid in differential diagnosis.

Imaging

♦ X-rays will suggest a diagnosis and the most probable type of bone sarcomas, but soft tissue sarcomas do not show up well on regular x-rays.

♦ For soft tissue tumors, CT or MRI scans are useful for finding masses and determining their size and relationships to surrounding structures.

♦ Bone scans may add additional information about the tumor type and extent.

♦ Arteriography (x-rays of the tumor blood vessels) can outline tumor margins and help select a perfusion vessel for chemotherapy.

♦ Chest x-ray or CT to determine spread to lungs.

Endoscopy and Biopsy

♦ Biopsy of the suspected lesion is essential. The type of biopsy procedure used has to take the possible surgical treatment into account. Definitive surgery may be done at the same time as the biopsy or later.

STAGING

Stage is determined by the tumor's size and grade and whether it has spread to nearby lymph nodes or distant sites. Several staging systems are used for adult soft tissue sarcomas, pediatric sarcomas and bone sarcomas.

The TNM system is useful to specialists, but a simplified staging system uses the grade of the tumor—the primary factor determining survival—to divide adult soft tissue sarcomas into four stages. Stages I, II and III, none of which involve spread to nearby lymph nodes or distant sites, are also divided into sub-stages A (tumors less than 2 in./5 cm in diameter) and B (tumors larger than that). Stage IV tumors have spread to regional lymph nodes (IVA) or to distant sites (IVB).

Grade is determined primarily by the percentage of dividing cells in the tumor. Grade 1 tumors are well-differentiated and have only a small chance of spreading to another site. Grade 2 tumors are moderately differentiated and have a less than 20 percent chance of spreading. Grade 3 tumors are poorly differentiated, meaning that they contain immature cells that divide rapidly. They have a greater than 50 percent chance of metastasizing.

Five-year survival is usually better than 75 percent for low-grade tumors and less than 25 percent for high-grade tumors.

ADULT SOFT TISSUE SARCOMAS: TREATMENT OVERVIEW

Sarcomas are best treated by an experienced team of specialists in surgical oncology (often orthopedic oncologists in the case of bone tumors), radiation oncology, medical oncology and often physical medicine and rehabilitation.

The initial biopsy must be carefully planned to ensure that enough tissue is available for diagnosis, but also to allow for subsequent surgery. This is especially important with sarcomas involving arms or legs, where the appropriate biopsy can make limb-sparing surgery more effective.

Prognosis is affected by a patient's age, the size of the primary tumor, grade and stage, degree of lymphatic and blood vessel invasion, the duration of symptoms and the location of the tumor on the arm, leg or trunk. Unfavorable prognostic signs include age over 58, a tumor larger than 2 in. (5 cm), a high-grade tumor, spread to lymph nodes or distant sites, a deep rather than a superficial malignancy, and symptoms lasting less than one year.

Low-grade tumors can usually be cured by surgery alone. Higher grade sarcomas have more tendency to recur in the same area or metastasize and so are often treated with surgery, radiotherapy and/or regional chemotherapy.

Many of these tumors are often treated by a combination of surgery, radiation therapy and chemotherapy to improve the possibility of cure.

 Surgery Surgery for these tumors often has to be extensive, with a wide margin of tissue around the tumor being removed. Sarcomas involving muscles require removal of the entire affected muscle group.

Bone sarcomas must be removed with a wide margin of apparently normal bone. Amputation can be avoided most of the time, as limb-salvage surgery is now often possible in selected patients.

After primary malignant tumors of bone are partially or completely removed, the bone may be reconstructed. This procedure may include bone grafts, but these are not always satisfactory. A more reliable method is custom-made metal bones with artificial joint replacement. Remarkable achievements have made it possible to avoid amputation by substituting a prosthetic bone tailored to the patient. In children, an arm or leg prosthetic bone can be lengthened as the child grows.

 Radiation Radiation therapy is used to prevent local recurrences of radiosensitive tumors and may be given either before or after surgery.

 Chemotherapy Several drugs have proven to be effective in treating bone and soft tissue sarcomas. The dosages required to provide a good chance for cure often produce significant side effects, though.

Effective single agents include doxorubicin (Adriamycin), cyclophosphamide, high-dose methotrexate (with leucovorin rescue), ifosfamide, dacarbazine (DTIC), vincristine, dactinomycin (Actinomycin D), etoposide and investigational agents.

Commonly used combinations include doxorubicin + cyclosphosphamide + methotrexate, CyVADIC (cyclophosphamide + vincristine + doxorubicin + dacarbazine), ifosfamide + etoposide, doxorubicin + cyclophosphamide and doxorubicin + dacarbazine + cyclophosphamide. Other combinations have been used, chiefly of these drugs but also of others available for investigational use.

Chemotherapy is part of the standard and optimal initial treatment for Ewing's sarcoma and osteosarcoma. For Ewing's sarcoma, radiation therapy of approximately 4,500 cGy is added. Surgery then follows for all patients with osteosarcoma and most patients with Ewing's sarcoma. Additional chemotherapy is mandatory for both Ewing's sarcoma and osteosarcoma after surgery. To see if the same chemotherapeutic agent should be given again, another tumor specimen is examined for significant tumor destruction.

Adjuvant Chemotherapy Even if a bone or soft tissue sarcoma is apparently localized and could apparently be completely removed, there is a significant risk that tumor cells too small to detect have already spread to other places in the body. Additional treatment with chemotherapy (adjuvant) attempts to eliminate these tumor deposits.

Adjuvant chemotherapy is commonly used for certain sarcomas, especially childhood sarcomas (rhabdomyosarcoma and Ewing's sarcoma) and osteosarcoma. The use of adjuvant chemotherapy for other sarcomas is under clinical investigation.

The role of adjuvant chemotherapy for soft tissue sarcomas is not fully established. The combination of doxorubicin, high-dose cyclophosphamide and high-dose methotrexate may be of value. Several trials have shown an advantage to giving chemotherapy combined with radiation or radiation therapy combined with surgery for the treatment of the primary tumor.

♦ **In Metastatic Disease** The treatment of metastatic disease in both bone and soft tissue sarcomas involves the use of chemotherapy first. If there is a response with tumor shrinkage, an attempt is made to surgically remove the metastatic deposits, since the majority are in the lungs. Removal of only a small wedge or triangular-shaped portion of the lung may be needed, rather than the entire lung or a major portion of it.

Investigational
♦ Current investigational protocols for soft tissue sarcoma include an adjuvant trial that divides patients (after adequate primary therapy with either surgery or surgery plus radiation) into two groups. One receives no chemotherapy, the other receives an adjuvant combination of doxorubicin + dacarbazine (DTIC) + ifosfamide.
♦ There are investigational protocols for patients with high-risk Ewing's sarcoma (large tumors in the pelvis) that don't respond well to preoperative treatment. As well as the standard chemotherapy, radiation and surgery, patients are now being entered into trials of high-dose chemotherapy and autologous bone marrow transplantation.

ADULT SOFT TISSUE SARCOMAS: TREATMENT BY STAGE

(For treatment of soft tissue tumors and sarcomas of bone in children, *see* "Childhood Cancer: Sarcomas of Soft Tissue and Bone.")

STAGE I
These are well-differentiated (low-grade) tumors that have not spread to nearby lymph nodes or other sites.

Standard Treatment The primary treatment is surgery, with wide (3/4 in./2 cm) margins free of tumor being essential. Radiotherapy is used for tumors that cannot be removed, when the tumor-free margins are uncertain and residual tumor cells are likely, or when wider resection would mean amputation or removal of a vital organ. Adjuvant therapy is generally used only in clinical trials.

Five-Year Survival Over 90 percent

STAGE II
These are moderately well-differentiated tumors (medium grade) that have not

spread to nearby lymph nodes or to other sites. They are highly treatable and curable, but are more likely to spread than Stage I tumors.

Standard Treatment For sarcomas involving the arms or legs, limb-sparing surgery is often combined with preoperative or postoperative radiotherapy. In some centers, intra-arterial chemotherapy is also given. Research is continuing on the best way to combine these treatments.

In some cases involving limbs, amputation may still be necessary if conservative surgery combined with radiotherapy is not possible. The use of adjuvant chemotherapy in this stage is still under investigation, but studies so far seem to show benefit.

Sarcomas of the trunk, head and neck, and abdomen are treated with surgery, often followed by high-dose radiotherapy. Preoperative radiotherapy sometimes permits more conservative surgery, with radiotherapy also given postoperatively. Again, the use of adjuvant chemotherapy is under investigation.

High-dose radiotherapy and chemotherapy are used for tumors that cannot be removed surgically (in the head and neck or abdomen, for example). In some centers, radiotherapy is given during surgery for abdominal sarcomas (intraoperative radiotherapy).

Five-Year Survival 70 percent

Investigational
♦ Preoperative regional chemotherapy, combined with limb-sparing surgery.
♦ Adjuvant chemotherapy following surgery.
♦ The use of various special types of radiotherapy beams.
♦ Radiotherapy after limb-sparing surgery.

STAGE III
These are poorly differentiated or undif-

ferentiated (high-grade) tumors that have not spread to nearby lymph nodes or to distant sites. This stage is further divided into IIIA and IIIB according to the size of the primary tumor.

Standard Treatment Stage IIIA sarcomas are highly treatable and often curable but have an increased chance of metastatic spread. The standard treatment is surgery with radiotherapy or chemotherapy, or sometimes all three.

Sarcomas of the arms or legs are treated in a similar way to Stage II tumors. Sarcomas of the abdomen, trunk, and head and neck are treated with surgery followed by high-dose radiation. Radiotherapy is also sometimes given before surgery, and high-dose radiation combined with chemotherapy is given if the tumor cannot be completely removed surgically.

Stage IIIB sarcomas are treated much like Stage II and IIIA tumors. Because these tumors are larger, however, in many cases of tumors of the arms or legs amputation will be necessary. In some cases, preoperative radiotherapy or combination chemotherapy may allow tumors to be surgically removed when it would not have been otherwise possible.

Stage IIIB sarcomas of the abdomen, trunk, and head and neck are treated with surgery, often followed by high-dose radiotherapy. If the tumor cannot be completely removed, high-dose radiotherapy combined with chemotherapy may relieve symptoms.

Five-Year Survival 20 to 50 percent

Investigational
♦ Investigational treatments similar to those for Stage II.
♦ Intraoperative radiotherapy for Stage IIIA abdominal sarcomas.

STAGE IV
This stage is divided into two groups. Tumors of any grade or size that have

spread to regional lymph nodes but not to distant sites are Stage IVA. Tumors that have spread to distant sites beyond the lymph nodes draining the area of the cancer (most commonly to the lung) are Stage IVB.

Standard Treatment In Stage IVA, local control of the primary tumor is best obtained with surgery (including removal of lymph nodes) followed by radiotherapy. This may require amputation in some patients with sarcomas of the arm or leg. In some centers, radiotherapy is given both pre- and postoperatively. If the tumor cannot be surgically removed, radiotherapy and chemotherapy are used.

In Stage IVB, if the lung is the only site of spread, cure may be possible in up to 30 percent of patients by aggressive treatment of the primary tumor similar to earlier stages and removal of the lung metastases, even if there are several.

If lung metastases are not removed or there are other sites of metastasis, palliation may be provided by radiotherapy to the primary tumor combined with chemotherapy. Various combinations are used, generally containing doxorubicin and dacarbazine, sometimes with other agents as well. Combinations including ifosfamide are also used.

Standard therapy is not curative, so patients should be considered candidates for clinical trials.

Five-Year Survival Up to 20 percent

SUPPORTIVE THERAPY

Physical therapy with active and passive range-of-motion and strengthening exercises for the arms and legs is extremely important for people with primary bone and soft tissue tumors of the extremities. Exercise programs and elastic stockings can help prevent stiffness and swelling of the extremities.

TREATMENT FOLLOW-UP

Patients with malignant bone and soft tissue sarcomas have to be followed on a regular basis.

♦ Routine physical examinations look for any mass or recurrence of pain.

♦ X-rays and CT scans look for evidence of local tumor recurrence.

♦ Routine chest X-rays are done every two months for the first two years, with CT of the lungs done every six months. If there is any evidence of metastatic disease, it is important that it be found early so that chemotherapy can be started and surgical removal of the metastases can lead to successful or curative treatment.

RECURRENT SOFT TISSUE SARCOMAS

Treatment depends on the initial situation and treatment. Local recurrences often require aggressive local therapy, which means more surgery and radiotherapy. A recurrence in the same area as the original tumor makes another recurrence even more likely.

♦ If previous treatment was aggressive, amputation may be needed for tumors of the arm or leg.

♦ If lung metastasis is the first area of recurrence, treatment is the same as for Stage IV disease.

♦ If tumors recur after chemotherapy treatment, clinical trials using new agents are appropriate.

THE MOST IMPORTANT QUESTIONS YOU CAN ASK

♦ What will my limitations be after treatment of the bone or soft tissue tumor?

♦ Can I save my limb?

♦ How sick will I become from chemotherapy? Will I lose my hair?

♦ What is my overall chance of survival?

♦ Will it be possible for me to have a family after this treatment?

SKIN

Jill R. Slater-Freedberg, MD, and Kenneth A. Arndt, MD

◇

Skin cancer is the most common form of cancer found in humans. Over 600,000 cases were diagnosed in the United States in 1990, and the number is growing by 3.4 percent a year. One in every three new cancers is a skin cancer. It is estimated that 40 to 50 percent of fair-skinned people who live to be 65 years old will have at least one skin cancer (*see also* "Melanoma"). Ten years ago, skin cancer was unusual in those under 40, but now it is seen regularly in younger people. It is not uncommon in people in their twenties.

The most prevalent types of skin cancer—basal cell and squamous cell—are two to three times more common in men

than in women. Both are almost always curable.

Types Basal cell cancer (BCC) (*see* Melanoma, page 428) is the most common form of all skin cancers, affecting more than 400,000 people each year. It develops in the outermost layer of the skin, the epidermis, on hair-bearing surfaces. The appearance of BCC can vary considerably. The most common type is the nodular basal cell carcinoma, a flesh-colored (cream to pink) round or oval translucent nodule with overlying small blood vessels and a pearly-appearing rolled border. This tumor slowly grows sideways. It may eventually ulcerate and form a crust over the center as it outgrows its blood supply.

A second type of BCC is the pigmented lesion. This is darker than the nodular type, appearing blue, brown or black. It may be similar in appearance to the very aggressive malignant melanoma tumor. Naturally, it is very important to distinguish between malignant melanomas and pigmented BCC.

A third type of BCC is the superficial type that appears as a red, often scaly, localized plaque. It is frequently confused with psoriasis or eczema. There is also a morphea or sclerosing type, a single, firm, ill-defined, slightly raised lesion that tends to be more subtle to recognize than the nodular, superficial and pigmented forms. If untreated, basal cell carcinomas may crust, ulcerate and sometimes bleed.

Squamous cell carcinoma (SCC) is the second most common form of skin cancer, affecting between 80,000 and 100,000 people each year in the United States. It arises from the cells that make the protective keratin of the epidermis (keratinocytes).

These tumors usually occur in areas of sun-damaged skin and at sites of previous burns, scars or chronic ulcers. SCC usually appears as a red, scaling, well-defined plaque and may gradually develop an ulcer, a scaly crust or a wart-like surface. Eventually it can spread into the deeper or surrounding tissues.

Squamous cell cancers are considered superficial when the upper part of the dermis is involved and infiltrative when the lower dermis and fat tissues under the skin (subcutaneous) are invaded. These cancers are also described based on how differentiated the cells are—well-differentiated, moderately differentiated and poorly differentiated. The less differentiated the lesion, the least amount of normal tissue is preserved and the more aggressive the cancer.

Verrucous carcinoma is a cauliflower-like (fungating) type of SCC found in the mouth, on the membranes lining the anus and genitals or on the bottom surface of the foot. There are also a number of lesions that are precancerous. Actinic keratoses, for example, are multiple red, crusty discolored areas on sun-exposed areas of fair-skinned individuals that tend to scratch off but come back. Cutaneous horns are hard, funnel-shaped lesions extending from a red base on the skin. Also potentially precancerous is leukoplakia, a white patch on the oral and genital membranes.

How It Spreads Basal cell cancer usually remains unchanged for years or grows very slowly. It rarely spreads to distant sites. One study reported less than 0.01 percent occurrence of metastatic disease. The lesions that tended to spread were large, involved the head and neck with extensive local invasion and had recurred after treatment. When metastatic disease occurs it spreads to local lymph nodes and less often to bone, the lungs and the liver. Survival is less than one year once such spread has been discovered.

Squamous cell cancer has a higher rate of metastatic disease, with studies reporting a 3 percent rate of spread to distant sites. The most likely lesions to spread are large, invasive, greater than 1/10 in. (4 mm) thick and poorly differentiated.

Squamous cell cancer spreads via the lymph system and can involve bone, liver and brain. Metastases increase to a rate of 11 percent when SCC involves the oral and genital membranes and to 10 to 30 percent when the lesions are on areas of the skin previously injured from burns.

What Causes It Most skin cancers are caused by excessive exposure to sunlight. Genetic background is also a factor, since light-skinned people suffer a more adverse reaction to the sun's ultraviolet radiation.

RISK FACTORS

The two major risk factors for developing skin cancers are the amount of exposure to ultraviolet light (usually as sunlight) and the individual's response to ultraviolet light, which depends on skin type and the amount of melanin skin pigment that protects against ultraviolet light absorption.

At Significantly Higher Risk
♦ People who live in areas with high sun exposure and at high altitudes.
♦ People with fair skin (with less melanin in their skin).
♦ Males have a slightly higher incidence than females.
♦ Squamous cell carcinoma is most prevalent in people over 55. Males predominate except on the lower leg sites, where women have a higher incidence.
♦ Outside workers, since most malignant skin tumors occur on sun-exposed areas of the body including the head, neck and the back of the hands.
♦ People with medical conditions involving suppression of the immune system—those infected with the HIV virus, people with cancer, those who have undergone an

organ transplant and are taking immune-modulating drugs, those with debilitating chronic diseases, the malnourished, the elderly and patients receiving chemotherapy drugs and steroid hormones.

♦ Individuals with genetic skin disorders that predispose to skin cancer, such as basal cell nevus syndrome, xeroderma pigmentosum and albinism.

At Slightly Higher Risk
♦ Exposure to chemical carcinogens such as coal tar, arsenic in insecticides and nitrogen mustard (chemotherapy) ointment, viral carcinogens (some warts), ionizing radiation (x-rays), and chronic irritation and inflammation.

PREVENTION

People can protect themselves against ultraviolet light damage by taking simple precautions.

♦ *Using Sunscreens* A sunscreen of at least SPF (sunlight protection factor) 15 is recommended. The sunscreen preparation should be applied frequently, and more often with sweating and when swimming. Sunscreen use should begin in infancy.

Regular use of sunscreens with an SPF of 15 during the first 18 years of life can reduce the lifetime incidence of skin cancer by as much as 78 percent. One serious childhood or adolescent sunburn doubles the chances of developing skin cancer, especially malignant melanoma.

Sunscreens absorb the ultraviolet light of the B wavelength and prevent it from penetrating the skin. The SPF number correlates with the amount of time one can spend in the sun before the skin becomes pink or red. For example, if an SPF 15 is worn, a person can remain exposed to the sun 15 times longer without the skin becoming pink.

Sunscreens do not protect against penetration of longer wavelength ultraviolet light of the A type. The screens actually allow more exposure to the A type radiation by allowing a person to remain outside longer. Therefore, *sun exposure should be kept at a minimum.*

♦ *Wearing Protective Clothing* People who work outside should wear clothing that protects their skin, including long-sleeved shirts, hats and pants. Outdoor recreational activities should be scheduled before 11:00 A.M. and after 2:30 P.M., when the concentration of ultraviolet light is decreased by 70 to 80 percent.

♦ *Avoiding Tanning Booths* Tanning booths have advertised that by using UVA (A type ultraviolet light) a "safe" tan is obtained. There is no such thing as a "safe" tan.

Tanning is a response of the skin to injury. UVA does cause less redness than UVB, but like UVB it may induce skin cancer and photoaging (drying, wrinkles and pigment changes). UVA is actually used experimentally to produce skin cancer in mice. Since 1986, about 2 million people a year have visited tanning booths. This will contribute to an increase in the number of skin cancers we will see over the next 10 to 20 years.

♦ *Being Aware of Skin Changes and Getting Early Treatment* Besides sunscreens, avoiding ultraviolet light and wearing protective clothing, preventive measures include early detection and swift removal of precancerous lesions.

SCREENING

The best screening test is an extensive examination of the skin. Part of a yearly physical should include a thorough examination of the skin including the mouth, behind the ears, around the nose, the scalp, the penis, the areas around the vagina and rectum, the palms of the hands and the soles of the feet. Lymph nodes should also be examined.

Everyone should be examined this way, but especially fair-skinned, blond-haired, blue-eyed individuals and people who have had previous skin cancers. Special attention should be given to areas where a previous skin cancer was removed. These people should also examine themselves often to assess any change or development of new lesions to bring to the attention of a physician. If a skin lesion changes in any way, a dermatologist should be consulted.

COMMON SIGNS AND SYMPTOMS

The most common sign is simply a sore or mark on the skin that changes in size, color and shape. It may become itchy or painful and may start to bleed or ulcerate.

DIAGNOSIS

During the initial doctor's appointment, a medical history will be obtained with particular attention given to previous skin lesions, genetic skin disorders and exposure to chemical carcinogens or radiation. The history of the lesion in question should also be clarified—how long it has been present and how it has changed.

Imaging

♦ X-rays, like blood tests, are not usually necessary during the initial doctor visit. They may be necessary to look for signs of bone destruction, however, if there is evidence that the skin lesion is fixed to or invading the bone.

♦ Chest x-rays should be considered with advanced cancers to look for lung metastasis.

Endoscopy and Biopsy

♦ A biopsy should be performed on all suspicious lesions and the specimen sent to a qualified pathologist. The biopsy result will help the physician choose the appropriate treatment.

Four biopsy techniques are employed for skin cancer, with the type used depending on the size and location of the lesion, the equipment available and the experience of the physician.

♦ Shave biopsy uses a scalpel to remove a thin slice of an area in question. This procedure is used when the lesion extends above the skin and the underlying skin is smooth, open and convex.

♦ Punch biopsy uses a cylindrical instrument that is rotated into the skin and removes a cylindrical specimen. This method is used when tissue at a greater depth is required for diagnosis.

♦ Incisional biopsy removes a portion of the tumor with a scalpel.

♦ Excisional biopsy removes the entire lesion.

Because of the ease and minimal complications of these procedures, they can all be performed in the office, with local anesthesia being used to eliminate discomfort. Rare adverse effects include bleeding and infection.

TREATMENT OVERVIEW

There are six widely used methods to treat skin cancer. Which method is chosen depends on the type of lesion, its size and location, the definition of its borders, how invasive it is, how long it has been present and whether more than one lesion is involved. The person's age and overall health are also considered, as is the potential effect of treatment on appearance.

All treatment methods have a cure rate of about 90 percent or more. Tumors that have less than a 90 percent cure rate include sclerosing or morphea basal cell cancers, poorly differentiated squamous cell cancers, lesions around the eye, ear, nose and the forehead-temple region, tumors larger than 3/4 in. (2 cm), older lesions and recurrent cancers.

Basal cell and squamous cell cancers are treated using similar procedures. A larger amount of apparently normal tissue may have to be removed when cutting out a SCC, since there is a higher rate of metastasis than with BCC.

STANDARD TREATMENTS

Curretage with or without Electrodesication (C&E) This is a two-step procedure in which a curet (sharp-tipped instrument) removes the softer cancer tissue from normal tissue and bleeding is controlled by a chemical agent or by electrical current. This cycle is repeated two to four times if necessary. Nodular and superficial BCC and non-invasive SCC can usually be treated effectively with C&E.

C&E is ideal for small tumors with distinct borders, for primary lesions and for lesions on surfaces with minimal excess tissue. It is not recommended for large tumors, tumors invading dermis or fat, lesions with poorly defined borders, poorly differentiated squamous cell carcinomas, recurrent lesions or lesions at certain anatomic sites that have lower cure rates.

C & E is a low-risk procedure that can be performed on an outpatient basis. It may cause damage to underlying structures and leaves an open wound, which can then bleed, become infected and form a scar. The site may take one to three months to heal and appear acceptable.

 Cryosurgery This technique uses liquid nitrogen at very low temperatures to freeze the skin. The nitrogen is applied with an aerosolized spray to achieve tissue temperatures below –58°F (–50°C). The tissue is then allowed to thaw for about two minutes. This cycle is repeated two to three times.

Like C&E, cryosurgery is a low-risk procedure. It can, therefore, be used for people who cannot tolerate surgery and is also useful for anyone who is having treatment to prevent blood clotting (anticoagulation therapy).

Cryotherapy is effective for removing lesions where there is minimal excess tissue and can be used for large primary tumors. It is not useful with poorly defined lesions, poorly differentiated SCC, morpheaform BCC, recurrent lesions,

lesions in areas of decreased cure rates or on the extremities (arms and legs) where there is decreased blood flow.

As in C&E, cryotherapy leaves an open wound that takes three to ten weeks to heal. The wound may "weep" for two or three weeks after the procedure. Antibiotic creams or ointments are often used to avoid infection. Nodular, superficial BCC and noninvasive SCC can usually be treated effectively with cryotherapy.

 Radiation When used to treat a skin carcinoma, radiation therapy has minimal complications and good immediate cosmetic results. Radiation treatments are given three to five times a week for up to five weeks.

It is useful for older people who cannot tolerate surgery, for multiple lesions or large superficial lesions and for lesions that are too inaccessible to be removed surgically. It is particularly useful in lesions of the eyelids, nose, lips and ears. It can also be used as a palliative measure rather than for cure on excessively large cancers.

It should not be used for patients under 50 years old because of the possibility of causing new cancers at the radiation site. Long-term cosmetic results may not be as good as with other treatments. For patients over 50, radiation therapy can be used to treat nodular, superficial BCC and all SCC.

 Chemotherapy 5-fluorouracil (5-FU) is a chemotherapeutic agent that blocks DNA synthesis, thereby preventing normal cell growth and ultimately causing cell death. Applied directly to the skin twice a day for four weeks or more, 5-FU can be used for superficial basal cell cancers. As it works it causes an inflammatory reaction, which heals after the treatment is stopped.

Advantages of 5-FU are that it is easy to use and has minimal adverse effects. Disadvantages are that it may cause redness and a change in the pigment of the skin. After treatment with 5-FU, the tumor may be controlled on the surface but may continue to invade at the base.

Intravenous 5-FU has been used for skin cancers that have spread to distant sites, but few data are available on how effective this is because of the limited number of cases involved.

Surgery Excision is a surgical procedure that removes the entire lesion. The area is then closed with sutures. This is a more invasive procedure than C&E. The sutures help the healing process, so this procedure is ideal for lesions on the feet or legs, where there is decreased blood flow, and on the hands, where frequent skin contact occurs. This procedure can be used effectively for all skin cancers with excellent cosmetic results.

Mohs Micrographic Surgery This technique was first described in 1936 by Dr. Frederick Mohs. It involves removing successive horizontal layers of the skin cancer and any surrounding tissue that may be involved. Each layer is microscopically examined and the section that involves tumor is marked. Subsequent horizontal layers remove the areas of tumor involvement, sparing the normal skin tissue.

Mohs surgery has the highest cure rate of all treatment methods. It is, therefore, recommended for poorly differentiated SCC, morpheaform BCC, invasive tumors, recurrent lesions, lesions with indistinct borders, large primary tumors of long duration, lesions at sites of decreased cure rate and in patients with nevoid basal cell syndrome.

The disadvantages of Mohs surgery are that a great deal of expertise is required by the physician, the procedure is time-consuming, it requires more equipment than the other methods and it leaves an open wound that may take a long time to heal if the lesion is large. Today Mohs surgery is often followed by a plastic reconstruction to close the wound.

INVESTIGATIONAL

Although the treatments now most widely used have greater than a 90 percent cure rate, other therapies are being investigated that may be more practical, effective and cosmetically elegant. Examples of the newer methods of treatment include:

Retinoids These are synthetic and natural derivatives of vitamin A. Patients with vitamin A deficiency may have an increased susceptibility to skin cancer. This deficiency causes a premalignant change of the skin that can be reversed by applying vitamin A.

How the retinoids work is not yet clear, but research findings suggest a role for vitamin A in cancer therapy. Recent investigations have used the retinoids to treat premalignant and malignant skin cancers. Use of the locally applied (topical) and internal (systemic) forms have demonstrated an adequate cure rate when treating basal cell cancers. Limited information exists for use in SCC, but one study reported a 70 percent response rate.

Since the retinoids are naturally occurring substances, they usually have minimal side effects.

Interferons Interferons are proteins produced by human cells in response to a viral infection. Interferons have an antiviral activity, they inhibit the growth of malignant cells and they promote cell maturation. There are three interferons—alpha, beta and gamma.
♦ Interferon-alpha is found in T and B lymphocytes and in macrophages.
♦ Interferon-beta is found in fibroblasts (connective tissue producing cells).
♦ Interferon-gamma is found in activated T cells.

Interferon-alpha has been the most frequently studied interferon for use with skin cancers as well as other types of cancer. Preliminary reports have shown significant results in short-term remission of basal cell carcinomas when interferon-alpha is injected into the tumor (intralesional injection). Interferon is also effective given as nine intralesional injections over three weeks or, in a sustained-release form, as one or three intralesional injections per week.

Interferon leaves no surgical wound, has good cosmetic results and avoids bleeding and infection. Short-term side effects include fever, chills, muscle aches, headaches and nausea.

Photodynamic Therapy (PDT) This treatment uses visible light in combination with a photosensitizer, a compound that attracts light. The photosensitizer now being used is a hematoporphyrin derivative, HPD.

Approximately 48 to 72 hours after HPD is intravenously injected, most of the compound is cleared by the normal skin and selectively retained in the cancerous cells. Upon exposure to different colors of light, HPD undergoes a photodynamic reaction that damages the tumor cells and spares the uninvolved tissue. In practice, HPD is given as an intravenous injection and followed 48 to 72 hours later by irradiation with red or blue-green light.

There are no well-controlled studies using HPD, but encouraging preliminary results have been reported in treating basal and squamous cell carcinomas.

A disadvantage of photodynamic therapy with HPD is that levels of HPD may stay in the normal skin for three to six weeks after the injection. During this time, patients need protection from all bright light, since exposure to light can result in severe redness and swelling of the skin. This adverse effect would be eliminated if an effective photosensitizer could be applied only to the affected area of skin.

The most appropriate method of curing a specific skin cancer is the most effective, least toxic, most efficient and most cosmetically elegant therapy, which may be a combination of any of these nine standard or investigational treatments.

TREATMENT FOLLOW-UP

Twenty percent of people with a single basal cell cancer will develop a second one at another site within a year. If there were two basal cell cancers, there is a 40 percent chance of developing a new one within one year. People who have had a skin lesion removed should, therefore, see their doctor twice a year for the first three years after treatment, followed by yearly visits.

THE MOST IMPORTANT QUESTIONS YOU CAN ASK

♦ What are the most important things I can do to lower my risk of getting skin cancers?
♦ Will my physician be carefully and regularly examining all my skin surface to look for any premalignant and malignant lesions?
♦ Has the biopsy been reviewed by a pathologist with special training in skin tumors?
♦ Which method of treatment will give me the best results?
♦ What is the chance of recurrence or spread with this lesion and your recommended treatment?

SMALL INTESTINE
Ernest H. Rosenbaum, MD

◇

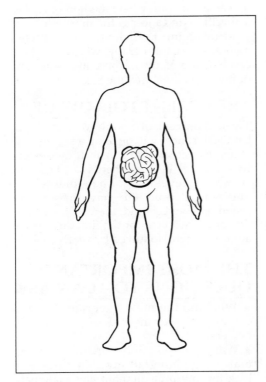

The small intestine is the longest segment of the gastrointestinal tract, making up three quarters of its total length. Yet malignant tumors are much less common in this organ than they are in the esophagus, stomach and large bowel. Of all the gastrointestinal tumors diagnosed, only 1.5 percent are found in the small intestine. In 1991 there are expected to be 2,900 new cases and 925 deaths due to cancer of the small intestine.

There are many reasons for the lower incidence. Cancer-causing agents have less contact with the surface membranes because of the rapid transit time of food through the small bowel compared with the colon. And, since the stool is still liquid, there is less mechanical injury to the membranes.

The inner surface of the small intestine secretes a large amount of gamma globulin that protects the lining against disease. Benzpyrene hydrolase, which can detoxify carcinogens, is found in large amounts in the lining (mucosa) of the small intestine. Finally, the contents of the small bowel are alkaline, which reduces the production of carcinogens from bile and prevents the formation of nitrosamines, environmental carcinogens that are formed only under acidic conditions.

Malignancies of the small bowel are almost always treatable and some may be curable. Their prognosis and treatment depend on the cellular origin.

Types Small intestinal malignancies are generally adenocarcinomas, sarcomas, carcinoid tumors and lymphomas.

The most common of all—half of small intestine tumors—are adenocarcinomas that develop in glandular tissue. Most people with adenocarcinomas have metastases to the lymph nodes, liver or peritoneum (abdominal lining) at the time of diagnosis.

Sarcomas are slow-growing tumors that account for 20 percent of small bowel cancers. Sarcomas can develop in any soft tissue such as fat cells (liposarcoma), blood vessels (angiosarcoma) or nerves (neural sarcomas, neurofibrosarcomas or malignant schwannomas, which develop from the nerve sheath, most commonly in the ileum). But 75 percent of the sarcomas, called leiomyosarcomas, originate in the smooth muscles encircling the bowel. These malignancies may reach a large size before diagnosis (many are larger than 2 in. (5 cm)). Only a third of smooth muscle tumors are malignant.

Carcinoid tumors account for 20 percent of small bowel malignancies. They are often small (usually 1/2 to 1 1/2 in./1 to 3 cm in diameter) and slow growing. There may be multiple lesions and may be present for years (*see* "Carcinoids of the Gastrointestinal Tract").

Lymphomas arising from lymphoid tissues in the wall of the small bowel make up 10 percent of small bowel tumors. They may occur in any part of the small intestine and 20 percent of them develop in multiple sites. Of all the lymphomas that start someplace other than in lymph nodes (extranodal lymphomas), 33 percent do so in the gastrointestinal tract, 10 percent in the small bowel. Most of these lesions are non-Hodgkin's lymphomas.

How It Spreads Small bowel cancers can spread directly through the bowel wall to adjacent tissues. Leiomyosarcomas grow in the muscle wall and extend to the surface (serosa). Sarcomas spread directly to the tissues supporting the bowel (mesentery), the retroperitoneum or the adjacent bowel. These cancers also spread through the lymphatic system and bloodstream to regional lymph nodes or to the liver, lungs or bone.

What Causes It There is an association with some inherited cancers and inflammatory bowel disease (Crohn's disease and celiac disease) and neurofibromatosis. Lymphomas are associated with immune deficiencies and celiac disease.

RISK FACTORS

At Higher Risk
♦ People older than 60, expecially those with a history of bowel disease.
♦ People with changes in the small intestine acidity, rapid transit and nitrosamine exposure.

♦ Those with inherited gastrointestinal disorders—Peutz-Jeghers syndrome, familial polyposis, inflammatory bowel disease, Crohn's disease and neurofibromatosis.
♦ Those with increased lymphoid deposits in the ileum and immune deficiency diseases are at a higher risk for lymphomas.

SCREENING

There are no general screening methods available, but if a tumor is suspected because of abdominal pain, anemia or some other symptom, a test for hidden blood in the stool is recommended.

COMMON SIGNS AND SYMPTOMS

Ten percent of people with small intestinal cancers have no symptoms. Most have abdominal pain or distention because of a partial or complete obstruction of the small bowel. There may also be weight loss, nausea and vomiting, fever, change in bowel habits and a general malaise, or weakness that may result from anemia caused by bleeding or malabsorption. The bowel may also become perforated, which can cause acute symptoms. With adenocarcinomas, jaundice may appear when the tumor is in the mid-duodenum, blocking drainage of the common bile duct. Blockage of the bowel may also be caused by what is called pseudolymphoma, a benign overgrowth of the lymph nodes.

DIAGNOSIS

Physical Examination
♦ Abdominal mass or painful distension.
♦ Rectal bleeding—possibly caused by ulcerations in the gastrointestinal tract—which may result in anemia.
♦ A partial or complete obstruction of the intestinal tract.
♦ Jaundice, which may be due to a tumor in the duodenum or to liver metastasis.

♦ Bowel kinking (intussusception).
♦ Often fatty fluid (chylous ascites) can collect in the abdomen.

Blood and Other Tests
♦ Blood counts usually show iron deficiency anemia when bleeding occurs.
♦ The level of carcinoembryonic antigen (CEA) in the blood is often elevated with adenocarcinomas.

Imaging
♦ The most useful x-rays are an upper gastrointestinal and a small bowel series. These can detect a small cancer (often a "napkin ring" deformity) or a polyp.
♦ X-rays showing small bowel thickening with ulceration may indicate a lymphoma.
♦ An abdominal CT scan can help identify lesions outside the bowel, including metastases.
♦ Angiography is helpful for evaluating the abdominal tumor blood vessels, displaced vessels and new blood vessels (neovascularization).
♦ A small bowel x-ray may locate a tumor. This procedure involves passing a small plastic tube through the nose to the duodenum and injecting barium and air to provide contrast.

Endoscopy and Biopsy
♦ Fiberoptic endoscopy is rarely possible unless it is done during surgery.
♦ A small part of the terminal ileum can be seen during a colonoscopic evaluation.
♦ Small bowel endoscopy is useful during surgery for additional evaluation.

STAGING

There is no staging system for primary small intestine cancer except for lymphomas. Cell type rather than stage is the major factor in prognosis and treatment decisions.

TREATMENT OVERVIEW

As in other gastrointestinal cancers, the standard treatment is to remove the tumor surgically whenever possible.

 Surgery The best chance for cure is offered by the surgical removal of a part of the small bowel with a wide margin around the tumor, along with the attached tissues supporting the bowel (mesentery) and its lymphatic drainage. If this cannot be done, surgical bypass and radiation can be considered as palliative measures for residual disease.

 Radiation The bowel is extremely sensitive to radiation, which limits the usefulness of this therapy. It may be poorly tolerated and may result in weakness, nausea, vomiting, and diarrhea with small bowel inflammation. It may lead to occasional remissions for sarcomas, but is usually used for relief of pain and obstructions. Small bowel lymphomas are highly responsive to radiation.

Radiation can complement surgery and is often recommended in lymphomas. Intraoperative radiotherapy (IORT) to the tumor or the tumor bed and area at risk may be done, because normal tissues can be moved aside and protected.

 Chemotherapy Like radiotherapy, chemotherapy is a less effective therapy than surgery and is recommended only for disease that can't be surgically removed or for metastases.

TREATMENT BY TUMOR TYPE

ADENOCARCINOMA
Standard Treatment If the tumor can be completely removed, radical surgery may lead to a cure. Simple excision of the tumor might be adequate for small malignancies, but for larger tumors the recommended procedure requires a segment of

the bowel with wide margins to be removed. If the cancer arises in the first part of the small bowel (duodenum), it should be noted that the duodenum is in a difficult location. It is behind the liver, pancreas and stomach, and the Whipple surgical procedure—involving the removal of the pancreas and duodenum—may be necessary.

 Palliation If surgical removal of the tumor is impossible, the symptoms of the disease may be relieved by a surgical bypass or palliative radiation therapy.

Five-Year Survival 20 percent (for resectable adenocarcinoma)

Investigational
♦ Radiation therapy with radiosensitizers and with or without chemotherapy.
♦ Various chemotherapy combinations have been tried such as 5-FU + leucovorin, 5-FU + streptozotocin or 5-FU + BCNU. Biologic response modifiers such as interferon are being evaluated.

SMALL INTESTINE LEIOMYOSARCOMA

Standard Treatment If the primary tumor can be removed, radical surgery similar to that for adenocarcinomas may lead to a cure. Isolated metastases in the liver and lung can also be removed.

If the primary tumor cannot be removed, any tumor that is obstructing the bowel can be surgically bypassed. Tumors that can't be removed may also respond to high-dose radiation therapy, occasionally with long-term survival.

 Palliation A combined approach using surgery and radiotherapy can help relieve symptoms of pain and obstruction in patients when metastases can't be removed.

Palliative chemotherapy with Adria-

mycin, cisplatin, ifosfamide, vincristine or dacarbazine (DTIC) can have response rates of up to 65 percent. Adjuvant chemotherapy may also be given after surgery if the tumor is high-grade, there is a high risk for local recurrence or there is a significant risk of metastasis (lymphatic or blood vessel involvement).

Five-Year Survival About 50 percent if the tumor can be removed surgically

Investigational
♦ Clinical trials are evaluating the value of new anticancer drugs and biologicals.
♦ Adjuvant radiotherapy in combination with chemotherapy is being studied.

SMALL INTESTINE CARCINOID
(*See* "Carcinoids of the Gastrointestinal Tract")

Five-Year Survival 54 percent

SMALL INTESTINE LYMPHOMA

Standard Treatment It is unusual to find a single lymphoma as a primary small bowel tumor, so it is mandatory that the standard lymphoma staging work-up be done to look for evidence of other areas of disease. The work-up will include abdominal and pelvic CT scans, a chest x-ray and bone marrow aspiration and biopsy. Depending on the stage and cell type, the standard treatment options include surgery, radiation and combination chemotherapy, all of which may lead to a cure.

For disease that is localized to the bowel wall or has gone beyond the wall (local extension), surgical removal of the tumor alone may be adequate if 12 or more nearby lymph nodes are removed and show no evidence of disease (a 40 percent five-year survival). But the addition of combination chemotherapy or radiation should also be considered. Radiation may lead to a cure, control tumor growth or relieve symptoms.

For disease that extends into the regional lymph nodes, the tumor should be removed at the time of diagnosis. Combination chemotherapy is then the treatment of choice (*see* "Non-Hodgkin's Lymphomas").

Combination chemotherapy is also the treatment of choice for disease that is extensive or cannot be removed surgically. Radiation therapy is often also used to eliminate any potential residual tumor cells, often in conjunction with chemotherapy.

 Palliation Radiation therapy can relieve the symptoms associated with large lymphomas that cannot be removed, often in combination with chemotherapy. Single liver metastases may respond well to radiation (survival chances decrease as the number of metastases increase).

Five-Year Survival 25 percent for diffuse lymphoma, 50 percent or more for nodular lymphoma

Investigational
♦ Adjuvant radiotherapy and chemotherapy are being studied.

SUPPORTIVE THERAPY

Nutritional support may be necessary after treatment of small intestinal cancers. This is especially so after a major portion of the small bowel has been removed or if the duodenum or terminal ileum have been removed or bypassed. These procedures result in poor absorption of iron, calcium, folate, vitamin B_{12}, fat and fat-soluble vitamins and pancreatic/biliary digestive secretions, leading to deficiencies in essential nutrients. Nutritional replacement programs can correct these deficiencies (*see* Chapter 18).

RECURRENT OR METASTATIC CANCER

Tumors may come back in the small bowel after treatment or may metastasize from cancers arising elsewhere, especially cancers of the colon, kidney, pancreas or stomach, which may extend directly into the small bowel. Symptoms include intestinal obstruction or bleeding from the tumor.

♦ If possible, surgery may be attempted for locally recurrent small intestine cancer, with removal of the lymph nodes if that is appropriate. Clinical trials are now evaluating ways of improving local control, such as the use of radiation therapy with radiosensitizers with or without chemotherapy.

♦ There is no standard chemotherapy for recurrent metastatic adenocarcinoma or leiomyosarcoma of the small intestine. Patients may be considered candidates for standard combination chemotherapy programs, or clinical trials evaluating the use of new anticancer drugs or biologicals in Phase I or Phase II trials.

THE MOST IMPORTANT QUESTIONS YOU CAN ASK

♦ What is the role of surgery for small bowel tumors?
♦ How do you tell the difference between benign and malignant tumors of the small bowel?
♦ How are small bowel lymphomas evaluated?
♦ Is there a role for radiotherapy?
♦ How does one select a chemotherapy program for small bowel cancer?
♦ What is the role for supportive nutritional therapy?

STOMACH

Ernest H. Rosenbaum, MD, and Malin Dollinger, MD

◇

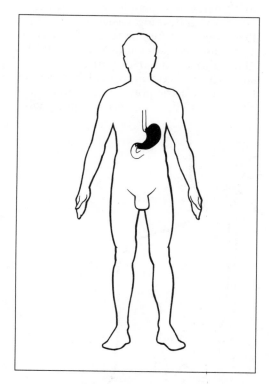

Stomach cancer was the leading cause of cancer deaths in the United States between 1900 and 1945, but is now the eighth most common cause of cancer deaths. The exact reason for the decline—which is greatest among the elderly and whites—is not understood, although dietary changes have been considered.

Types Stomach cancers are classified according to what sort of tissues they start in. The most common type arises in the glandular tissue lining the stomach. These tumors are called adenocarcinomas and account for over 95 percent of all stomach tumors. One particular form of this cell type, unusual in the United States but more common in Japan, is the superficial spreading adenocarcinoma that essentially replaces the lining (mucosa) of the stomach with sheets of malignant cells. Another rare subtype is scirrhous carcinoma (linitis plastica), a poorly differentiated mixture of mucin-producing carcinoma cells that infiltrates the muscle wall and turns it into rigid, leatherlike scar tissue that can't stretch or move during the normal digestive process (peristalsis).

Occasionally, a cancer may develop in lymph tissue (gastric lymphoma) or from the smooth muscles of the stomach wall (leiomyosarcoma). Carcinoids and plasmacytomas can also develop in the stomach.

How It Spreads The disease can spread directly through the stomach wall into adjacent organs and through the lymph system to nodes in the abdomen, the left side of the neck and the left armpit. Metastases through the bloodstream can spread to the liver, lungs, bone and brain. Metastases are also found in the lining of

Cancer of the stomach—also called gastric cancer or gastric carcinoma—is a treatable disease that can often be cured when it is found and treated at a local stage. Unfortunately, the general outlook for this type of cancer is poor because 80 percent of the cases diagnosed in the United States are already at an advanced stage, having spread to nearby or distant organs. In 1991, 23,800 Americans will be diagnosed with gastric cancer, and 12,400 of them will die because of the disease.

A more encouraging fact about this cancer, however, is that the death rate has dramatically decreased, falling approximately 60 percent between 1930 and 1970.

the abdominal cavity (peritoneum) and around the rectum.

What Causes It The exact cause is unknown, but most gastric cancers are believed to be caused by carcinogens, with diet as a major factor. Nitrites found in smoked meats, fish and other foods and the nitrates used as food preservatives have been strongly implicated, along with aflatoxin, a carcinogenic fungus contaminant that is present in some foodstuffs such as peanuts.

Various medical conditions are also associated with the development of stomach cancer. The lack of acid in stomach secretions (achlorhydria), for example, means that the bacteria responsible for converting nitrates to carcinogenic nitrosamines are not destroyed. About 5 to 10 percent of people with pernicious anemia will develop gastric cancer. And the chronic backup, or reflux, of stomach acids into the esophagus can irritate the glandular tissue at the junction of the stomach and esophagus, which may lead to cancer. Gastric polyps are another possibility, since they may become malignant.

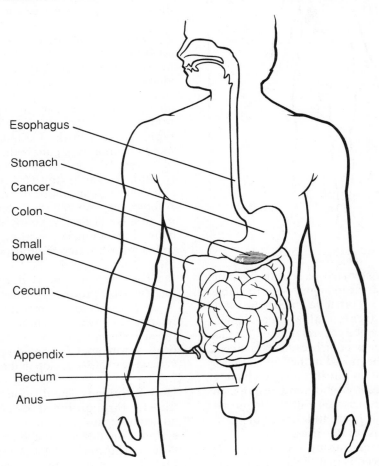

Esophagus
Stomach
Cancer
Colon
Small bowel
Cecum
Appendix
Rectum
Anus

Gastrointestinal tract, showing stomach cancer

RISK FACTORS

At Slightly Higher Risk
♦ People with type A blood and achlorhydria.
♦ Males living in colder climates.
♦ Those who have had part of the stomach removed because of peptic ulcers, leading to a decrease in stomach acids. There is a 6.5 percent incidence of tumors in the remaining stomach (gastric stump).
♦ Older people whose stomach lining produces less acid as it ages (atrophic gastritis).
♦ Slightly increased risk with alcohol or tobacco use.

At Significantly Higher Risk
♦ Those aged between 50 and 59.
♦ Twice as frequent in lower socio-economic groups in North America and Western Europe.
♦ Workers in various industries—coal mining, nickel refining (in Soviet Europe), rubber and timber processing.
♦ Workers exposed to asbestos fibers.
♦ People with pernicious anemia are 5 to 10 percent more likely to develop gastric cancer.
♦ People whose diet contains smoked, highly salted and barbecued foods. Japanese immigrants have a decreased incidence of this cancer when they adopt an American diet and lifestyle, a tenfold drop after two generations.

SCREENING

Screening would be helpful for finding early tumors that do not reach the outer wall of the stomach (serosa) or penetrate the serosa but have not spread to lymph nodes. By looking at the stomach through a lighted tube (fiberoptic endoscopy) or by using x-rays of the upper gastrointestinal tract, smaller tumors can be detected. These tests are especially pertinent for people with gastric complaints.

Although screening programs are available in countries such as Japan with high gastric cancer rates, they are not common in the United States. Screening is not cost-effective, given the dramatic decline in the incidence of stomach cancer. Upper gastrointestinal x-rays, for example, discover cancer in only 0.15 percent (1 in 600) of apparently healthy people.

COMMON SIGNS AND SYMPTOMS

The symptoms of stomach cancer are similar to the symptoms of a hiatal hernia or peptic ulcer, namely a vague pain aggravated by food, nausea, heartburn and indigestion. These symptoms are often thought to be due to the stress of psychosomatic illness and are treated with antacids or H-2 blockers. Unfortunately, the temporary relief this treatment brings often delays the tests that could diagnose cancer.

Loss of appetite, feelings of fullness after even a small meal and weight loss are common (upper abdominal pain, vomiting after meals and weight loss are seen in 80 to 90 percent of cases). There may also be mild anemia, weakness, gastrointestinal bleeding (40 percent of cases) and vomiting of blood. Both vomiting blood and rectal bleeding are seen in peptic ulcer disease, esophageal varices (varicose veins in the esophagus that grow and burst, a disease common in drinkers) and occasionally leiomyosarcomas.

DIAGNOSIS

Gastric cancers often seem to be benign ulcers, which are like pits in the stomach lining. Larger ulcers—more than 3/4 in. (2 cm) in diameter—that have borders raised above the level of the surrounding stomach are more likely to be malignant.

Physical Examination
There are few specific findings on a physical examination.
♦ Enlarged lymph nodes above the left collarbone (supraclavicular node).
♦ Nodal masses around the rectum, inside the navel or in the abdomen (involving the ovary).

♦ Enlarged liver (hepatomegaly).
♦ Increased fluid in the abdomen (ascites).

Blood and Other Tests
♦ Test for hidden blood in the stools.
♦ Complete blood count (CBC), which may indicate anemia from gastrointestinal bleeding.
♦ Serum chemistry profile to evaluate abnormal liver and bone chemistry enzymes, including tests for elevated levels of carcinoembryonic antigen (CEA) and levels of serum ferritin to indicate iron deficiency.
♦ Analysis of gastric acid to detect achlorhydria.

Imaging
♦ X-rays of the upper gastrointestinal tract (UGI series) by standard and double-contrast methods may find larger ulcer lesions.
♦ Chest x-rays.
♦ CT scan of the abdomen.
♦ Bone scan if the bone enzyme alkaline phosphatase is elevated in the serum.

Endoscopy and Biopsy
♦ Examination of the stomach through a gastroscope inserted through the esophagus (fiberoptic endoscopy) may find ulcers and masses. Seventy percent of early malignant ulcers may look benign and even heal, but are usually positive on biopsy.
♦ A small piece of tissue may be removed from any suspicious area for biopsy analysis by a pathologist, or a brush can be passed through the gastroscope to obtain cells in a way similar to a Pap smear. Tissue and brush biopsies can diagnose 98 percent of cases.

STAGING

Stages are defined according to the TNM classification. The major factor in defining the primary tumor is how deeply it invades through the stomach wall and whether it invades adjacent structures such as the spleen, small intestine or colon, liver, diaphragm, pancreas, kidney, adrenal gland or the abdominal wall. The stage is important in determining the initial treatment options as well as the prognosis.

TREATMENT OVERVIEW

Stomach cancer is a somewhat treatable disease, with over half the patients with early stage disease being curable. Early-stage disease accounts for only 10 to 20 percent of all cases diagnosed in the United States, however. Five-year survival for more advanced cancers range from around 20 percent for those with regional disease to almost nil for those with distant metastases. Treatment for metastatic cancer can relieve symptoms and sometimes prolong survival, but long remissions are not common.

Radical surgery is the only treatment that can lead to a cure, though lesser surgical procedures can play a significant role in therapy designed to relieve symptoms. Radiation and chemotherapy are also treatment options. Neither has been shown to improve the outlook for those with advanced tumors generally, although some patients with responsive tumors may benefit.

 Surgery The ideal treatment is radical surgery, meaning that most or all of the stomach is removed (subtotal or total gastrectomy) along with the surrounding lymph nodes. In early-stage disease (10 to 20 percent of all cases) over 50 percent are curable. But one-third of stomach cancers are inoperable at the time of diagnosis and require follow-up therapy with radiation and/or chemotherapy. About one-third can potentially be cured with surgery, although very radical operations may just increase the number of complications without increasing survival.

The decision about whether to remove the stomach depends on whether the tumor has invaded the adjacent bowel above and below the stomach, the lower part of the stomach near the duodenum

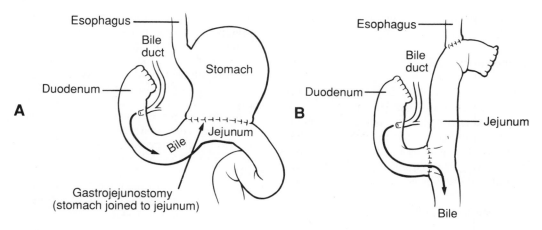

Surgical procedures for stomach cancer

or the junction of the esophagus and the upper part of the stomach. If it doesn't, up to 85 percent of the stomach is removed, along with the first portion of the small bowel (duodenum), nearby lymph nodes and the pad of fat (omentum) between the bowel and the lining of the abdominal cavity.

A CT scan may be helpful in detecting the margins of the cancer and lymph node involvement. Since it may seem to indicate more extensive disease than is really present, the CT result alone should not be a reason to avoid surgery.

This is major surgery. The incision may run from the chest down to the navel. All of the stomach must be removed if there is extensive stomach involvement. The esophagus may have to be connected to the mid-small bowel (esophagojejunostomy) and a gastric pouch constructed. With a total gastrectomy, 5 to 15 percent of patients may not survive the operation and there may be significant complications. One major complication is that the connection constructed during the esophagojejunostomy may break down. The surgical margin should be greater than 2 1/2 in. (6 cm) beyond the gross tumor. (A frozen section should be done to confirm that the margin has no cancer.)

When extensive surgery for cure is impractical or impossible, part of the stomach might still be removed as a palliative measure. Sometimes the tumor causes recurrent bleeding or becomes so large that it obstructs the gastrointestinal tract and causes nausea, vomiting or stomach distention. A partial gastrectomy can temporarily improve the quality of life, although total gastrectomies have a high rate of complications and have little benefit when all the tumor cannot be removed.

 Radiation The role of radiation therapy is mainly to relieve symptoms, not cure the cancer. Doses between 5,000 and 5,500 cGy can possibly help control tumors that can't be removed. Sometimes palliation is attempted over three to four weeks with 3,500 to 4,000 cGy, with infusions of 5-fluorouracil used as a radiation sensitizer during the first and often the fourth week. This combined therapy can increase survival. One study shows 23 percent of patients who had 5-FU and radiation still alive after five years while only 4 percent of those who had just radiation were still alive. Studies using 5-FU at the beginning of, during and after radiation therapy suggest possible advantages in response and an improved survival of from 6 to about 14 months.

Preoperative Radiation One Japanese trial showed that radiation given two weeks before surgery reduced the size and involvement of lymph nodes and improved survival by 12 percent. Another study showed that radiation before surgery increased the number of tumors that could be removed from 76 percent to 85 percent, although there was no increase in survival.

Intraoperative Radiation Giving radiation therapy directly to the tumor area during surgery for biopsy-proven residual cancer has been evaluated and shows survival increases. Some studies have shown five-year survival increases from nil to 50 percent.

 Chemotherapy While chemotherapy is occasionally useful in shrinking potentially operable tumors, its main role is in the treatment of advanced or metastatic disease. For almost 30 years, 5-fluorouracil (5-FU) has been the most common single drug used to treat advanced stomach cancer, with about 20 percent of patients responding to the treatment. Around the early 1980s, there were suggestions that using drug combinations was to become the "gold standard" of treatment, but results from recent trials question the value of routine combination chemotherapy.

One problem with combination chemotherapy is the poor complete response rate for *all* drug programs, with average survival varying between four and nine months. A second problem is that there has been little overall difference in survival for those receiving 5-FU alone or in combinations. The response rate may be higher for a combination, but the toxicity of the programs has to be assessed in light of the overall failure of chemotherapy to improve survival.

The standard combination recently had been FAM (5-FU + Adriamycin + mitomycin-C), with a response rate about 30 percent with little survival advantage and rare complete remission. Other combinations using 5-FU and a variety of drugs—including etoposide, Adriamycin and cisplatin—have higher reported response rates. Recent reports from Europe showed that three combinations were superior to FAM in both response and survival. These were the FAMTX combination (5-FU + Adria-mycin + high-dose methotrexate with leucovorin rescue), EAP (etoposide + Adriamycin + Platinol) and ELF (etoposide + leucovorin + 5-FU).

Investigational Combinations Some new combinations show promise. EAP, for example, has been reported to have a 57 percent response rate with 15 percent complete responses. For metastatic disease, the response rate was 49 percent with 8 percent complete response. The response was higher when the cancer had spread locally than when there were metastases in the peritoneum. The average overall survival, though, was only 17 months for those with a complete response.

If the surgical margin is found to be positive after gastrectomy on final pathology review, three courses of EAP followed by surgery for possible cure are being considered. Still, EAP is considered effective for locally advanced cancer, offering a surgical option to many who otherwise wouldn't have been able to have an operation.

Another effective and less toxic combination is ELF (etoposide + leucovorin + 5-FU). Response rates of 53 percent (12 percent complete) have been obtained for locally advanced disease, 49 percent (10 percent complete) for metastatic disease. Another combination EFP (etoposide + 5-FU + cisplatin) is being administered pre- and postoperatively with a reported increase in the surgical cure rate (including unresectable local/regional stomach cancers).

Another new combination using mitomycin-C + cytosine arabinoside + 5-FU given twice weekly for five weeks showed improved survival when tumors invaded the outer wall of the stomach—a 62 percent five-year survival versus 35 percent for those who did not have chemotherapy. The survival still remained high at 50 percent when there was possible lymph node invasion.

The combinations of EAP, ELF, EFP and FAMTX have proven to be of greater value than 5-fluorouracil alone, and chemotherapy modulators such as leucovorin may have the potential of improving drug effectiveness. A trial is ongoing comparing EAP and FAMTX for advanced gastric cancer.

Another avenue of research involves giving 5-FU by continuous catheter infusion through a central vein to patients with advanced gastric adenocarcinoma. One trial showed some positive results. The drug was continuously given each day until either the disease was seen to progress or there were signs of excess toxicity. The response rate was 31 percent, but there were no complete responses and half the patients had to have treatment interrupted because of side effects, mainly mouth sores and painful inflammation and swelling of the hands and feet (hand-foot syndrome, an uncommon side effect of 5-FU). The short remission time of five months was not terribly exciting.

Whatever drugs are used, chemotherapy should start as soon as possible. Waiting 40 to 60 days allows the tumor cell population to double. Primary stomach cancer appears to be more responsive to chemotherapy than metastatic cancer.

Adjuvant Chemotherapy Despite many ongoing American clinical trials evaluating the use of chemotherapy as an adjuvant therapy after surgery, there is not yet any conclusive proof of its effectiveness.

The Japanese have reported major benefits in adjuvant programs, but stomach cancer is different in Japan. The cancer is less differentiated and the surgery is more aggressive. Patients usually have fewer tumor cells left after the operation, which may explain the better results of adjuvant therapy.

 Biological Therapy Trials evaluating the use of radioactive tagged monoclonal antibodies or toxins such as ricin to kill cancer cells while sparing normal tissues are underway. Results so far have not been encouraging and more studies will have to be done to discover whether there is any benefit.

TREATMENT BY STAGE

STAGE 0
TNM Tis, N0, M0
An in situ tumor has not spread beyond the limiting membrane of the top level of the stomach lining (the mucosa).

Standard Treatment Experience in Japan, where this stage is diagnosed often, indicates that almost all patients who undergo a gastrectomy will survive beyond five years. An American series has recently confirmed these results.

Five-Year Survival Over 90 percent

STAGE I
TNM T1, N0, M0 (Stage IA)
T1, N1, M0 or T2, N0, M0 (Stage IB)
The cancer is confined to the stomach wall and no lymph nodes are involved.

Standard Treatment Surgery is the treatment of choice, although how extensive the operation has to be depends on the tumor's location and how much of the stomach is involved.

If the lesion is not in the area where the stomach joins the esophagus and does not diffusely involve the stomach, about three-quarters of the lower part of the stomach is removed (a radical subtotal gastrectomy). This treatment is associated with improved survival over other procedures.

When the lesion does involve the top of the stomach (cardia), cure may be attempted by removing most or all of the stomach, along with a sufficient length of the esophagus.

If the lesion diffusely involves the stomach, the entire stomach has to be removed along with, at a minimum, the greater and lesser omentum and nearby lymph nodes, the hepatic artery and the valve between the stomach and the duodenum (pylorus).

Five-Year Survival Up to 85 percent

Investigational
♦ Clinical trials of adjuvant combination chemotherapy are appropriate whenever the tumor invades to the serosa or local lymph nodes either grossly or microscopically (IB).

STAGE II
TNM T1, N2, M0 or T2, N1, M0 or T3, N0, M0
The cancer is confined to the stomach wall and does not involve adjacent tissues. The lymph nodes very close to the tumor or in the region around the stomach may be involved.

Standard Treatment This stage is sometimes curable with surgery. As in Stage I, the surgical procedure depends on the location and extent of the tumor. Procedures are the same as for Stage I cancers.

Five-Year Survival 52 percent (T2, N0, M0) 20 percent (T3, N0, M0)

Investigational Same as Stage I (adjuvant chemotherapy and/or radiotherapy).

STAGE III
TNM T2, N2, M0 or T3, N1, M0 or T4, N0, M0 (Stage IIIA)
T3, N2, MO or T4, N1, M0 (Stage IIIB)

The cancer involves tissues adjacent to the stomach and/or the lymph nodes very close to the tumor or in the region around the stomach.

Standard Treatment Cancer at this stage is treatable but not usually curable. All patients whose tumors can be removed should have surgery, but radical surgery for cure is limited to those who do not have extensive lymph node involvement at the time of exploratory surgery. Up to 17 percent of selected patients can be cured by surgery alone if the lymph nodes involved are confined to the immediate vicinity of the tumor (N1).

Overall survival is poor with either single or combined approaches to treatment, so all newly diagnosed patients with Stage III cancer should be considered candidates for clinical trials of new treatments.

Five-Year Survival 17 percent

Investigational
♦ Radiation therapy and/or adjuvant chemotherapy is being evaluated in patients with known residual disease or if the tumor invades the serosa.
♦ Adjuvant chemotherapy with 5-FU is being studied for those with no known residual disease who have a high risk of recurrence.

STAGE IV
TNM T4, N2, M0 (Stage IVA)
Any T, any N, M1 (Stage IVB)
The cancer has spread to adjacent tissue and to lymph nodes in the region around the stomach or has spread to distant sites, most commonly the liver or other organs.

Standard Treatment Because survival is so poor with all available single and combined treatment methods, no one approach can be considered state-of-the-art. Palliative surgery, combination chemotherapy and occasionally radiotherapy are all options.

When it is possible to remove the primary tumor, palliative surgery will at least reduce the risk of bleeding or obstruction and may lead to a longer survival.

When the tumor is so large that it blocks the entrance from the esophagus to the stomach, a gastroscope can be passed down the esophagus and a temporary hole created by using a laser beam or cauterization. A plastic tube can then be inserted through the hole to maintain a swallowing passage (*see* Chapter 9).

Chemotherapy—with 5-FU, FAMTX, EAP or ELF—can offer significant palliation to some patients and long-term remissions are sometimes possible.

Five-Year Survival Less than 5 percent

Investigational
♦ One trial suggested that by using EAP to shrink the tumor before surgery, some patients with Stage IV (T4, N3) cancer might be cured surgically.

TREATING OTHER TUMOR TYPES

GASTRIC LYMPHOMAS
These tumors, which may imitate primary adenocarcinomas of the stomach, are uncommon, making up only about 5 percent of gastric malignancies.

Patients with gastric lymphoma should have a general lymphoma evaluation including a chest x-ray, chest and abdominal CT scans, bone marrow biopsies and probably a pelvic CT scan to assess the major pelvic lymph node areas.

Standard Treatment Removing part of the stomach, if possible, may be the ideal treatment. In one series of 50 consecutive cases, a survival of 90 percent was obtained when the tumor involved only the mucosa, 80 percent when it involved the submucosa. A recent study for Stages IE and IIE (local tumor extension) lymphoma showed that patients who had four courses of CHOP

(Cytoxan + Adriamycin + Oncovin + prednisone) followed by radiation therapy and then additional chemotherapy did as well as patients who had surgery.

When the lymphoma fully penetrates the gastric wall and the lymph nodes in the region become involved, the survival is decreased to about 25 percent.

Radiation after surgery helps reduce the chance for local recurrences. The radiation therapy port usually covers the upper abdomen as well as the regional lymph nodes, and is given over several weeks.

LEIOMYOSARCOMAS
These tumors that start in the smooth muscles of the stomach wall account for only 1 to 3 percent of all gastric malignancies. Bleeding is common.

Standard Treatment The primary treatment is partial removal of the stomach, taking out just the area of the tumor and a rim of normal surrounding tissue. Radiation therapy and chemotherapy may be used after surgery or for metastatic disease. The most common chemotherapy combinations now used are Adriamycin + dacarbazine (DTIC) or Adriamycin + cisplatin. Ifosfamide may also be effective.

SUPPORTIVE CARE

Removing part or all of the stomach naturally produces many problems that require medical attention.
♦ Iron deficiency anemia often develops after a gastrectomy, since iron is absorbed mainly in the duodenum and stomach acids play a role in the process.
♦ Monthly doses of vitamin B_{12} should be given after a few years to prevent pernicious anemia.
♦ The dumping syndrome—with symptoms such as abdominal fullness, nausea, vomiting, a rapid heartbeat, weakness and dizziness—is quite common after surgery because food passes through the system so quickly that there is little time for absorption. The dumping syndrome often

resolves with time. Many treatments, including smaller meals and a lower-carbohydrate diet, and no chocolate or peppermint, can help. No food or fluid after 7:00 or 8:00 P.M. may help too.

◆ Symptoms of upset stomach (gastritis) may be related to the alkaline backup, or reflux, of bile and intestinal secretions into the esophagus. Symptoms can be controlled by antacids such as Maalox, Mylanta or Riopan, by sucralfate, which coats the stomach lining, or by a bile blocker such as Questran.

◆ Walking or simply staying upright after meals as well as sleeping with the head elevated can help control reflux by improving the drainage of the gastric pouch and help reduce symptoms.

◆ If the antrum—the gastrin-producing part of the stomach—is removed, there will be little need for gastric acid blockers. But if acid is still being produced, H-2 blockers such as Tagamet, Zantac, Pepsid or Losec will help.

◆ Bacteria can grow in the loop of the duodenum bypassed by a connection of the stomach to the small bowel, producing what is called the blind loop syndrome. This bacteria breaks down bile and the acids pouring in from the pancreas, resulting in diarrhea and poor absorption of fats. The blind loop syndrome can be treated with oral antibiotics.

RECURRENT CANCER

Survival is very poor with all available single and combined approaches to treatment, although an occasional patient might have a remission lasting several months or even a few years.

◆ All patients with recurrent stomach cancer should be considered candidates for Phase I and Phase II clinical trials testing anticancer drugs or biologicals. New agents such as triazinate and cisplatin analogues are being developed. There are also investigational programs using complex drug combinations and sequences (pharmacologic modulation).

◆ The only standard treatment option is palliative chemotherapy with 5-FU, FAM, EAP and ELF.

◆ For the patient with either local disease that couldn't be removed or local recurrent or residual disease after surgery, the use of radiation therapy in combination with chemotherapy has been considered the best palliative treatment, not only in helping to prevent and occasionally relieve an obstruction but also in reducing and controlling pain. This treatment has had no major benefits for survival, however.

One study of patients treated with 3,500 to 4,000 cGy with or without intravenous 5-FU during the first three days of radiation therapy showed an average survival of 12 months for the combination therapy versus 5.9 months for radiation therapy alone. The radiation therapy group had no five-year survivals, while 12 percent of the patients with the combination survived five years. Another study showed a combination of radiation therapy and methyl-CCNU + 5-FU had a disease-free interval of more than four years, which exceeds that of chemotherapy alone.

More recent programs under evaluation include a "sandwich" approach—giving chemotherapy such as 5-FU during the initial week of radiotherapy as well as during the fourth week—and, if surgery is done, intraoperative radiation therapy with or without chemotherapy.

THE MOST IMPORTANT QUESTIONS YOU CAN ASK

◆ How do you tell a benign ulcer from a malignant one?

◆ What is the best way to cure my gastric cancer? Does the stage make a difference?

◆ What disability might I have after surgery?

◆ Is there any role for radiation or chemotherapy?

◆ When will I know if I am cured?

TESTIS

Alan Yagoda, MD

◇

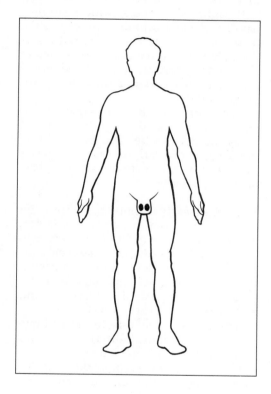

Testis cancer—also called germ cell tumors—accounts for about 1 percent of all male cancers, about 5,900 cases in the U.S. in 1991. Yet only 350 men will die of the disease because of earlier diagnosis and effective cisplatin-based chemotherapy.

In the past 35 years, the five-year survival rate has increased from 63 percent to more than 91 percent. This improvement reflects not only advances in treatment but also the fact that less than 15 percent of patients are now first seen with distant disease while more than 60 percent have only a testicular mass.

Types Testis cancers are broadly divided into two types—seminoma and non-seminoma. This arbitrary division was based on the better response and cure rates for seminoma resulting from radiation therapy, but with chemotherapy treatments this distinction is no longer of much importance.

Seminoma Pure seminoma, which makes up 25 to 40 percent of all testis tumors, is divided into three types—anaplastic, classic and spermatocytic. Anaplastic and classic seminomas seem to have a similar prognosis for each stage. Spermatocytic seminomas, a tumor frequently found in dogs, is a rare variety occurring in elderly men. It almost never spreads.

Seminoma is discovered generally in the fourth decade of life and has on occasion been confused with histiocytic lymphoma (the testis is the most frequent site of lymphomas that do not start in lymph nodes).

Non-seminoma Men with non-seminomatous testis tumors have an average age 10 years younger than that for seminoma, the mid-thirties. These tumors are composed of various cell types as seen under the microscope—embryonal carcinoma, teratoma, yolk-sac or endodermal sinus carcinoma and choriocarcinoma.

Most non-seminomatous germ cell tumors have more than one cell type in them—embryonal cell carcinoma with or without seminoma, embryonal cell carcinoma with or without yolk-sac tumor and with or without teratoma, and so on. Pure embryonal carcinoma accounts for only 3 percent of cases, pure teratoma for 2.7 percent, pure yolk-sac tumor for 2.4 percent and pure choriocarcinoma for 0.03 percent.

Embryonal cell carcinoma, a primitive cell type having the capacity to change into all the cell varieties listed above, is an aggressive tumor. But it is less aggressive than the choriocarcinoma variety, which is full of blood vessels and, therefore, spreads quickly by the bloodstream. Rapidly multiplying tumors like seminoma, embryonal cell and, to a lesser extent, teratocarcinoma are more solid masses that can outgrow their blood supply, producing cystic or "dead tissue" areas inside the tumor.

Teratocarcinoma is a mixture of embryonal cell carcinoma and teratoma, while so-called mature teratoma implies that embryonal cell carcinoma must have been present but has changed to a more mature (differentiated), more normal-appearing and less malignant cell form either spontaneously or because of therapy. There is also a very rare and aggressive teratocarcinoma variety called sarcomatous teratocarcinoma, which is not very responsive to the chemotherapy now available and is categorized as a poor-risk cancer.

Pure yolk-sac tumors are extremely rare and more frequently observed in the chest (mediastinum). The testes, which are derived from the yolk sac early in the embryo's development, move to an area called the urogenital ridge. Since the embryonic germ cells from this ridge travel almost the whole length of the developing body to their destination in the scrotum, bits of primitive tissue called embryonic rests can be left behind during the migration. This explains why some germ cell tumors are found in non-testicular (extragonadal) sites in the chest or abdomen.

How It Spreads There is a difference in the way cancers of the testis spread. Right-testis tumors spread by the spermatic cord and its associated blood and lymph vessels into lymph glands surrounding and between (interaortocaval) the large blood vessels, the aorta and the inferior vena cava.

Left-testis tumors drain via the spermatic cord vessels into the left kidney artery and venous lymphatic areas and to nodes just below the left kidney. They generally are not found in the interaortocaval nodal system as frequently observed with right-side tumors. Unless surgery has disturbed the scrotum—to remove the testis or repair an undescended testis through a scrotal incision—testis tumors always drain directly into the abdominal lymph nodes and not into the groin lymph nodes.

The most frequent site of organ metastases is the lungs, although in advanced cases the liver, bones and brain can be involved, particularly in cases of choriocarcinoma and, to a lesser extent, embryonal cell carcinoma.

What Causes It Unknown. There is no firm evidence that heredity is a factor, although a number of father and son cases have been described. There has been some association with a few uncommon genetic diseases such as hermaphroditism (mixture of male/female development) and Klinefelter's and Turner's syndromes.

The failure of the testis to descend into the scrotum (cryptorchidism) accounts for 10 percent of testicular cancers. But it is not known whether cryptorchidism is due to some underlying testicular abnormality that prevented the testicle's migration into the scrotum or to an anatomic abnormality that made an otherwise normal testis remain within the abdominal cavity, thereby leading to a cancerous change by, for example, raising the temperature of the testicle.

Other postulated causes are excessive maternal bleeding during pregnancy, testicular injury, mumps and the use of the synthetic female hormone diethylstilbestrol (DES) usually taken during pregnancy to prevent miscarriage. (DES has been implicated in the development of vaginal cancer.)

Each testis is surrounded by a thick fibrous capsule (tunica albuginea), lies in the scrotum and is composed of many small, thin, coiled tubes (called seminiferous tubules) packed into over 250 sections, or lobules.

Sperm is formed within these coiled tubules, then migrates to enter the straight tubules that make up the rete testis and the epididymis. These straight tubes then converge into one larger tube, the spermatic cord. From its attachment to the upper pole of the testis, the spermatic cord travels upward to enter into the body cavity through an opening called the inguinal ring (the area where inguinal hernias occur). From there the cord goes through the prostate, where it ends in the penile section of the urethra.

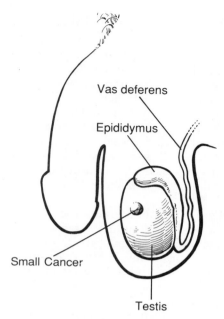

Cancer on the surface of testis

RISK FACTORS

At Significantly Higher Risk
♦ For men between 20 and 34 years old, testis tumors make up 22 percent of all cancers and rank first in cancer incidence. It is the second most common cancer for men aged 35 to 39 years and third for those 15 to 19.
♦ American white males have a rate four times that of black males.

At Slightly Higher Risk
♦ Uncommonly, tumors are found in men with fertility problems.

SCREENING

Testicular ultrasound is an accurate way to detect masses, but sonograms are too expensive to be used for screening. The most cost-effective screening method is simple physical examination of the testicles. Although a program has been developed in the Scandinavian countries to educate men about self-examination (simi-

lar to that for breast cancer in women), it has not gained acceptance in the United States. At the very least, men who have already had a testis cancer and those who had an undescended testicle should learn self-examination.

COMMON SIGNS AND SYMPTOMS

Swelling of the testicles, discomfort or masses are present in over 90 percent of cases. Such symptoms are sometimes ignored or misdiagnosed as being caused by an injury, as an inflamation of the testis (orchitis) or spermatic cord (epididymitis) requiring only antibiotic therapy or as enlarging veins of the spermatic cord.

Breast tenderness or enlargement because of high levels of HCG (human chorionic gonadotropin), and abdominal pain or cough with blood-tinged sputum, can be the main complaints, often due to metastases.

TESTIS TUMOR MARKERS

Testis cancers produce hormones that can be measured in the blood. These measurements are extremely reliable tumor markers. The three main markers are HCG, lactate dehydrogenase (LDH) and alpha-fetoprotein (AFP). They are so dependable that any increase above normal blood levels indicates a testis tumor recurrence. This is true even if there is no evidence of cancer by physical examination and x-ray examinations.

The Uses of Tumor Markers These markers are used to monitor the response to therapy. If the tumor markers decrease or return to normal levels after treatment, there is obviously a response. An increase is a sign of disease progression or failure to respond.

If the levels increase, signifying relapse, chemotherapy or sometimes surgery needs to be started (the cure rate for "marker relapse" is excellent, approaching 100 percent). But normal levels do not guarantee the complete absence of testis cancer, since microscopic deposits may still exist. This is why follow-up requires chest x-rays and CT scans. When masses are seen on CT scans and x-rays, particularly in the abdomen, they are assumed to be malignant when accompanied by an increase in the marker level, indicating that more treatment is necessary. If the markers are normal, such masses may well be only remaining scar tissue or benign teratoma.

The rate of disappearance of a marker from blood can also be predicted by its "half-life"—the time it takes for the amount of a marker in the bloodstream to be reduced by half. The half-life for HCG is about 30 hours, and five to seven days for AFP. Physicians using these formulas can determine to some degree whether the tumor is responding to treatment completely or partially. One study in the United States uses this information to plan for aggressive chemotherapy combined with autologous bone marrow transplantation.

Markers and Particular Tumor Types
Seminoma can have HCG and LDH, and about 80 percent of men with non-seminomatous germ cell cancer have an abnormality in one or more of the three markers.

HCG About 10 percent of patients with pure seminoma have a high HCG level, but never to the extent observed for those with choriocarcinoma or embryonal cell carcinoma.

HCG is produced by embryonal cells, by choriocarcinoma and by a tissue called syncytiotrophoblast found in seminomas, as well as in the normal placenta during pregnancy. In fact, HCG is used for pregnancy tests because it increases early within the first trimester.

It is a rather specific testis tumor marker associated with breast enlargement and nipple tenderness in males when markedly increased. Some unusual lung, liver and pancreatic cancers also can increase HCG levels although these are uncommon. One caution in using this marker is that marijuana smokers have increased HCG blood levels. So marijuana should not be used as an antinausea drug, since elevations that are not tumor-related may confuse physicians evaluating their patients after chemotherapy.

LDH This hormone—more specifically LDH-1, since there are five LDH enzymes—is increased in more than half of men with seminoma, but it is not as specific for testis cancer as HCG and AFP.

AFP This is called an oncofetal protein because it originates from the fetal liver and gastrointestinal tract and from the yolk sac of the embryo. AFP increases in a mother's blood during the second and third trimesters and disappears from a baby's bloodstream shortly after birth. AFP is found in 20 to 70 percent of testis tumor cases, and it is also seen in 70 percent of patients with a primary liver cancer (hepatoma).

New markers are being evaluated—seminoprotein for seminomas, blood group antigen H for non-seminomas and chromosome analysis for abnormalities in chromosome 12 (i12p), for example—but their accuracy has yet to be determined.

DIAGNOSIS

Physical Examination
♦ A testicular mass that can be felt, particularly a painless mass or one that does not completely clear within two weeks of antibiotic therapy, requires further tests. Some doctors now feel that all masses should be investigated by ultrasound.
♦ Enlarged lymph nodes in the abdomen and neck.

Blood and Other Tests
♦ Blood tests for markers such as LDH, AFP and HCG.
♦ Blood counts, biochemical screening profile, serum magnesium and urine collection for a creatinine clearance to evaluate kidney function.
♦ If bleomycin is to be used, lung function tests are performed as a baseline for future comparisons before additional treatment (bleomycin can cause lung scarring).
♦ Analysis of sperm and so-called sperm banking should be considered in most patients, since treatment can result in infertility. This might be the result of chemotherapy-induced toxicity or by loss of ejaculation if the surgical removal of lymph nodes requires cutting the nerves that control this function.

Imaging
♦ Ultrasound is extremely accurate, and any solid mass found on ultrasound should be considered cancerous until proven otherwise.
♦ Chest x-rays to evaluate lung metas-

tases. Many oncologists advise obtaining a baseline CT of the chest, even with a normal chest x-ray, to aid in follow-up.
♦ CT scans of the abdomen and pelvis are part of the staging procedure to evaluate the abdominal (retroperitoneal) and pelvic lymph nodes.
♦ Lymphangiography may help in about 10 percent of cases, but it is no longer routinely used because CT scans are more accurate.
♦ The role for MRI is undefined but probably adds little information concerning stage.
♦ X-ray tomograms of the chest have been largely replaced by the more accurate chest CT scan.
♦ Radionuclide bone and brain CT scans have to be done only when there are symptoms, although some doctors routinely order these scans for men with pure choriocarcinoma.

Endoscopy and Biopsy
♦ The removal of the testicle (orchiectomy) through an incision in the groin—never a scrotal incision or an aspiration biopsy—is required for diagnosis. Even when metastatic disease is found, the testis where the cancer started still has to be removed because the primary tumor does not always respond fully to chemotherapy.
♦ A recently recognized chromosomal abnormality found in many poor-risk non-seminomatous tumors is the presence of multiple copies of the short section (arm) of chromosome 12 (i12p). If a poor-risk case is suspected, fresh tumor may be sent for chromosome analysis. Such cases may require a more aggressive investigational approach to treatment.

STAGING

Several staging divisions are used for testis cancer, including the AJCC, based on the TNM classification. The stage depends on whether the primary tumor involves the testis, epididymis, spermatic cord and scrotum, whether a single node of various sizes or multiple nodes are involved and whether there are distant metastases to other organs, the most common being the lungs or lymph nodes above the diaphragm.

TREATMENT OVERVIEW

Surgery is necessary in all cases because the removal of the affected testicle is required for diagnosis. The use of further surgery, radiation and chemotherapy depends on the stage of the disease.

 Surgery For local tumors, the first step is to remove the testis, epididymis and spermatic cord (radical orchiectomy), performed by an inguinal approach, meaning that it is removed through the groin. This is never done through an incision in the scrotum because that would open up new lymph drainage areas to the groin.

When the cancer diagnosis is confirmed after orchiectomy, another operation is done to remove the lymph nodes in the back of the abdomen. This standard operation is known as a retroperitoneal lymph node dissection. Although recent studies suggest that in highly selected cases—those with small (T1) tumors and without spermatic cord or lymphatic and blood vessel invasion or embryonal components—simple surveillance can be used after the orchiectomy (in other words, watch until a relapse occurs), retroperitoneal lymph node dissection remains the "gold-standard" for treatment.

New surgical techniques have resolved many quality-of-life issues raised by this operation. The procedure is now much more acceptable, since the ability to have children is preserved in over 60 percent of cases. What is needed is more precise information to determine which tumors will ultimately relapse and then to evaluate by means of clinical trials the question of which patients need surgery or chemotherapy.

 Radiation For localized seminoma, radiation therapy to the pelvis and retroperitoneal lymph node areas is used as a preventive measure. Since most Stage I seminoma cases will probably never relapse, an investigational question is whether radiation (or even chemotherapy) is needed at all.

Chemotherapy There are many commonly used chemotherapy regimens for Stage III and, to some extent, for Stage II cases. Each agent has been found to be active against testis tumors when given alone, but prolonged, complete disappearance of tumors is best when other drugs are combined with cisplatin.

CHEMOTHERAPY COMBINATIONS USED FOR TESTIS CANCER

PVB	Cisplatin + vinblastine + bleomycin
VAB-6	Cisplatin + vinblastine + bleomycin + actinomycin + cyclophosphamide
PEB	Cisplatin + etoposide + bleomycin
EP	Cisplatin + etoposide
EC	Carboplatin + etoposide
IEC	Cisplatin + etoposide + ifosfamide
VIP	Cisplatin + vinblastine + ifosfamide

The earlier regimens of PVB and VAB-6 have mostly been replaced by PEB, EP and EC. There is some controversy concerning the need for bleomycin, since one study reported that the relapse rate is higher when this drug is not included in etoposide and cisplatin (or carboplatin) combinations.

While the older combinations are still sometimes given as so-called salvage therapy in relapsing cases, the ones containing ifosfamide (IEC and VIP), a derivative of cyclophosphamide, are the new salvage therapies. Because ifosfamide is a urinary bladder irritant that can produce blood in the urine, uroprotective drugs such as Mesna and NAC are required to prevent this complication. Such drugs do not affect the antitumor activity of ifosfamide.

Another role for this drug, as well as for etoposide and carboplatin, particularly in very high dosage, is in combination with autologous bone marrow transplantation as salvage therapy or as the primary treatment for very poor risk cases.

Bone Marrow Transplantation This procedure is replacing much more toxic salvage chemotherapy such as high-dose cisplatin and a combination named POMP/ACE. With complete responses seen in 20 to 40 percent of heavily pretreated men given bone marrow transplantation combinations, this therapy, rightly so, is now being used for early relapse after one or two programs containing cisplatin have failed, as well as immediately after one relapse in poor-risk cases.

TREATMENT BY STAGE

STAGE I

TNM Tis–T3, N0, M0

The tumor is limited to the testis (Tis, T1), the epididymis (T2) or the spermatic cord (T3). There are no lymph nodes involved nor distant metastases. In the AJCC staging system, spermatic cord (T3) involvement is placed together with scrotal (T4) invasion into Stage II.

Standard Treatment Radical (inguinal) orchiectomy—removal of the testis, epididymis and spermatic cord.

For pure seminoma, prophylactic radiation therapy is given to a total dose of 2,500 to 3,000 cGy to the pelvic and abdominal lymph node areas on the same side as the tumor.

For non-seminomatous germ cell tumors, retroperitoneal lymph node dissection is done to guarantee Stage I status. When Stage I is proved by surgery, the node dissection becomes both a diagnostic and prophylactic measure. Removal of microscopically involved nodes (really a Stage II case) is not only diagnostic but also therapeutic, for cure follows in almost all cases.

Five-Year Survival 95 to 100 percent

Investigational The concept of surveillance only—without lymph node surgery—has been investigated because 60 to 80 percent of Stage I cases will never relapse and effective cisplatin-based chemotherapy will cure almost all early relapses. At this time, surveillance must still be considered investigational.

In a recent study, the relapse rate varied from 20 to 40 percent. However, for good-risk patients or those with a true T1, N0, M0 tumor, the rate decreased to 15 to 25 percent.

In contrast, the relapse rate increased significantly to over 50 percent for poor-risk Stage I cases having tumor invasion of the epididymis, spermatic cord and lymphatic and/or blood vessels, particularly for the embryonal cell carcinoma variety.

If surveillance is the form of therapy chosen, it should be realized that this demands very careful follow-up, every four to six weeks for at least one to two years. Although almost all relapses will be found within the first 10 to 12 months, tumors have recurred as late as three years after diagnosis. With careful follow-up and starting chemotherapy immediately after detection of a relapse, less than 1 to 2 percent of men will die. For men not willing to make this type of follow-up commitment, the only (and correct) choice is surgery.

STAGE II

TNM Any T, N1–3, M0

The tumor involves the retroperitoneal lymph nodes either in a single node measuring 3/4 in. (2 cm) or less (N1), in a single node 3/4 to 2 in. (2 to 5 cm) or with multiple nodes all less than 2 in. (5 cm) (N2), or in any node larger than that (N3).

Stage II is also divided into non-bulky and bulky. Bulky disease indicates extensive retroperitoneal lymph node involvement with more than five nodes generally greater than 3/4 in. (2 cm), one node more than 2 in. (5 cm), or tumor that has spread to the fat surrounding the lymph node.

In the AJCC staging system, Stage III means only N1, M0 with Stage IV being N2, M0 or N3, M0 or any T, any N, M1 (organ invasion).

Standard Treatment Radical inguinal orchiectomy followed by therapeutic doses of radiation therapy (at least 4,000 cGy) will cure more than 90 percent of non-bulky seminoma cases. Because of the potential need for chemotherapy at relapse and the questionable benefit of preventive radiation to the chest and neck, further radiation therapy is not recommended.

For bulky Stage II seminoma (greater than 4 in./10 cm), chemotherapy may be preferred since older studies find the cure rate to be about 70 percent (admittedly, newer techniques and radiation equipment may produce better results).

Men with non-seminomatous germ cell Stage II cancer always used to have retroperitoneal lymph node dissection, but major controversies now exist as to the best form of therapy. For truly bulky masses (greater than 2 in./5 cm), chemotherapy may be a much better approach, with surgery as the salvage treatment for any remaining masses.

Surgery is appropriate for tumors less than 1 1/4 in. (3 cm) on abdominal and pelvic CT scans, but the value of prophylactic chemotherapy has to be discussed with each patient. One trial compared no additional immediate therapy versus two courses of PVB (BEP can be substituted) or VAB-6 (EP can be substituted) after surgery. Almost half of the patients with no additional therapy relapsed with tumor while less than 5 percent of those given two courses of prophylactic chemotherapy did so. Almost all relapsing cases completely responded when given the standard four courses of chemotherapy. What this means is that delayed chemotherapy given at relapse did not jeopardize curability, since overall survival was identical for both groups.

Relapse rates are very low for Stage II cases in whom there are less than six positive lymph nodes with none greater than 3/4 in. (2 cm). Consequently, chemotherapy can be withheld in such cases until relapse is found.

For non-seminomatous Stage II tumor masses between 1 1/4 and 2 in. (3 to 5 cm), urologists prefer surgery while some medical oncologists prefer chemotherapy, indicating that there are two possible and acceptable methods of treatment and we are not yet sure which is preferable. Both are correct choices. In any case, surgery is required for all patients who continue to show evidence of remaining masses after initial treatment with chemotherapy.

Five-Year Survival 90 to 95 percent

Investigational
♦ Prophylactic chemotherapy.

STAGE III

TNM Any T, any N, M1

The tumor invades other organs, most commonly the lungs or lymph nodes above the diaphragm.

Standard Treatment Radical orchiectomy followed by chemotherapy for both seminoma and non-seminomatous tumors.

The most frequently used drug combinations are cisplatin and etoposide (EP), each day for five consecutive days repeated every three weeks, or BEP, which uses the same doses and schedule of five days but adds bleomycin weekly.

Fluids are given by vein to prevent cisplatin-induced kidney toxicity. Nausea drugs are given by the same route to stop or minimize nausea and vomiting. A total of three to four cycles are given at no more than three- to four-week intervals, since it is harmful to delay therapy any longer. Only complete response is acceptable, and surgery is required when CT scans of the chest, abdomen and pelvis find any remaining disease, indicating a partial response.

If the remaining mass is less than 1 1/4 in. (3 cm), only scar tissue or benign teratoma may be found in the pathological specimen and no further treatment will be required because the relapse rate is less than 10 percent. But the relapse rate increases to 20 to 30 percent in men found to have viable (living) tumor (it is not unusual to find viable tumor in larger masses). In these cases, at least two more cycles of chemotherapy, preferably with a salvage regimen, must be given. Thereafter, careful follow-up is required to guarantee that treatment is begun at the very first sign of relapse, including only a marker relapse.

Five-Year Survival More than 90 percent

Investigational

♦ The etoposide + carboplatin (EC) combination is now being compared with EP. If results are identical, EC should become the new standard for good-risk cases, for it is significantly less toxic and so can be given completely in an outpatient setting. Depending on the definition used for poor risk, no more than 25 to 50 percent, at best, will attain complete response.

♦ For patients not attaining a complete response and whose AFP and HCG markers are not decreasing at the normal half-life rate, serious consideration should be given to either autologous bone marrow transplantation or experimental programs.

TREATMENT FOLLOW-UP

Follow-up is an integral part of testis cancer therapy, particularly since most relapses occur quickly within the first year.

♦ Marker levels (some doctors also include a complete blood and platelet count) and chest x-rays should be taken monthly—definitely no later than at six-week intervals—with CT scans at three- to four-month intervals during the first year.

♦ If abdominal or chest surgery has been performed, a repeat CT scan to serve as a new anatomic baseline can be done six weeks after the operation. Similar tests are then repeated every 8 to 10 weeks during the second year. Since relapse is very uncommon after two years, the same tests can be done every three to four months for the third year, every four months during the fourth year and every six months during the fifth year. Some doctors also do yearly examinations after that, but the value of such testing is uncertain.

♦ All men should be taught how to examine the remaining testicle and to seek advice when any change is found.

Long-Term Toxicity With almost all men being cured and having the expectation of a normal lifespan, therapy has been closely studied to evaluate any long-term toxicities.

♦ During therapy, nausea and vomiting can generally be prevented or minimized. Alopecia (hair loss) will occur but hair will return—sometimes thicker, darker and less wavy—within two to six months after chemotherapy is stopped.

♦ Low blood potassium, calcium and magnesium levels may be found but can generally be easily corrected and disappear after therapy.

♦ Lung scarring can occur when bleomycin is used, so pulmonary function tests are used to monitor any change. If lung function decreases, the drug must be stopped. This problem should soon disappear because new chemotherapy combinations may not use bleomycin.

♦ There have been rare reports of heart attacks and high blood pressure with some older combinations, but the newer EP, BEP and EC regimens that are given for a much shorter time—only three to four months—should alleviate this uncommon toxicity.

♦ The question of very delayed high blood pressure (hypertension) because of magnesium imbalance has not yet been resolved, so blood pressure has to be monitored at each follow-up.

♦ Following some chemotherapy combinations, particularly PVB, there have been reports of a chronic vascular disorder called Raynaud's phenomenon in 10 to 20 percent of cases. Again, this issue should be minimized with newer combinations.

♦ Sex drive (libido) is not changed by treatment and neither are erections. Chemotherapy may temporarily or permanently decrease the sperm count. Although most hormones correct themselves, fertility may or may not return.

♦ There is absolutely no evidence of any increased risk of abnormalities in children fathered by men who have had testis chemotherapy. Basically, either the sperm works or it doesn't. But it has been found that anywhere from 50 to 80 percent of men who have a testis cancer have low or zero sperm count before therapy, so a count should be done to document fertility *before* treatment is started.

RECURRENT OR NEW CANCER

Since 1 percent of patients may get another testis tumor, observation combined with self-examination and/or a baseline testicular sonography should always be done.

A new testicular cancer is treated according to the stages listed earlier. A relapse indicated only by an increasing HCG or AFP marker requires a completely new work-up.

♦ When the tumor is documented by CT scan, particularly in late relapsing cases, surgical debulking may be warranted to identify the type of tumor that recurred, followed by salvage chemotherapy.

♦ When markers are positive yet cancer cannot be found by any diagnostic test (including MRI), salvage chemotherapy should be started, since it is generally very successful in such cases. Some doctors, however, may recommend exploratory surgery first.

♦ For metastases to the spinal cord and bone, radiation therapy is the treatment of choice to control local symptoms. Brain metastases may be removed surgically, if possible, and should be followed by therapeutic full-dose radiation therapy.

THE MOST IMPORTANT QUESTIONS YOU CAN ASK

♦ What type of testis cancer do I have? What is the stage?

♦ Am I in the good-risk or poor-risk group?

♦ Will nerve-sparing surgery be possible?

♦ When should I sperm bank?

♦ What are the toxic effects and risks of chemotherapy?

♦ What are my tumor markers? What other tests are needed for follow-up?

♦ What is my chance of cure?

THYMUS

Malin Dollinger, MD, and Ernest H. Rosenbaum, MD

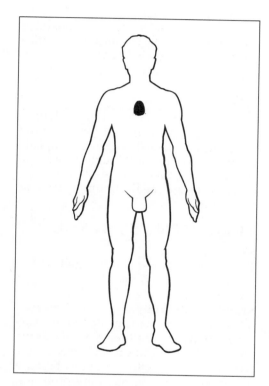

The thymus is a gland in the center of the chest (mediastinum) that has the important function during embryonic life of producing lymphocytes for the immune system. These thymus-derived, or T lymphocytes, are a major part of our immune system (cellular immunity) for our entire lives. Although these T lymphocytes look fairly similar under the microscope to the other major class of lymphocytes, B lymphocytes, they perform specialized immunologic functions to protect us from foreign organisms.

A variety of cancers can develop in the thymus—lymphomas, germ cell tumors, carcinoids, carcinoma and thymolipomas.

All are uncommon. The most common tumor is malignant thymoma, which originates in the covering, or epithelium, of the thymus gland.

Types Under the microscope, there are a number of cell sub-types of thymoma, but it is difficult to relate this microscopic appearance to how a tumor behaves. Some thymomas are non-invasive and appear to behave like benign tumors; others have all of the invasive characteristics of malignancy. So whether the tumors are called malignant depends not on their appearance but on their behavior (whether they have invasive characteristics). In the absence of invasion, the presence of a clearly defined covering, or "capsule," tends to classify the tumor as benign. But since all thymomas can become invasive and extend beyond the capsule, they should all be considered potentially malignant.

How It Spreads Most malignant thymomas grow slowly and have a tendency to recur in the chest at the site of origin. They seldom spread elsewhere, but if they do metastasize they often spread to the heart or lungs, especially to the covering over the heart (pericardium).

What Causes It The cause is unknown, but a number of systemic conditions, or syndromes, are associated with thymoma. Associated immune disorders include low red blood counts (pure red cell aplasia), low gamma globulins, signs and symptoms of connective tissue disorders, thyroiditis, ulcerative colitis, pernicious anemia, enteritis, sarcoid and, especially, a generalized muscle weakness called myasthenia gravis.

Various endocrine disorders are associated with thymoma, including hyperthyroidism, adrenal insufficiency (Addison's disease) and hypopituitarism.

RISK FACTORS

None known.

SCREENING

There are no general screening procedures for apparently healthy people. About a third of all thymoma cases are discovered during a routine or diagnostic chest x-ray. Myasthenia gravis, characterized by ever-worsening muscle weakness, is associated with a thymoma in up to 50 percent of cases. Removing the tumor will produce a complete remission of the myasthenia gravis in about one-third of patients, and at least half will improve.

COMMON SIGNS AND SYMPTOMS

People with thymoma usually have chest-related complaints such as a cough, shortness of breath, difficulty swallowing and chest pain or tightness. If the lesion is very large, the neck and face may be swollen because of an obstruction of the superior vena cava (superior vena caval syndrome).

The associated diseases or syndromes also produce a variety of symptoms. The predominant symptom of muscle weakness found with myasthenia gravis is especially noted in the eyelids. Severe depression of the red cells (pure red cell aplasia) in 5 percent of patients with thymoma leads to severe anemia, and 5 to 10 percent have a low gamma globulin level. Signs and symptoms of other autoimmune or endocrine disorders noted can lead to the diagnosis.

DIAGNOSIS

A thymoma can be suspected in a patient with myasthenia gravis or one of the other autoimmune or endocrine disorders noted above.

Imaging
♦ A thymoma can be strongly suspected if a mass is seen on a chest x-ray in the location of the thymus in the center of the chest.

Endoscopy and Biopsy
♦ The biopsy needed for a definite diagnosis may sometimes be obtainable with a fine needle aspiration (FNA) but may also require definite surgery.

STAGING

The most useful staging system defines three stages according to whether the tumor has remained within the capsule (limited), has broken through the capsule and spread either into adjacent tissues confined to the mediastinum or beyond these areas.

TREATMENT BY STAGE

STAGE I
The tumor cells remain confined within the capsule, which is intact.

Standard Treatment A non-invasive malignant thymoma is treated by the surgical removal of the tumor. Very specific and special precautions are needed for patients with myasthenia gravis because of the possibility of respiratory problems. Anesthesiologists experienced in this problem can dramatically reduce the rate of operative mortality.

If there is absolutely no evidence of spread through or beyond the capsule, no further therapy is needed. But if follow-up cannot be counted on, radiation therapy, possibly with adjuvant chemotherapy, may be given after surgery to try to improve the chances for long-term control.

There is a difference of opinion about the role of adjuvant radiotherapy for patients with encapsulated non-invasive thymomas. Since the recurrence rate is extremely low (about 2 percent), some physicians prefer to avoid the risks of radiation therapy. Others believe that radiotherapy is an essential part of treatment.

If, as sometimes happens, the mass is discovered at surgery to have invaded adjacent organs, radiation therapy is used in addition to or instead of surgery.

Five-Year Survival 83 percent (70 percent for people with myasthenia gravis, 90 percent for those without)

STAGES II AND III
The tumor has grown around the capsule into the adjacent fat (Stage III) or has spread farther into surrounding organs and/or elsewhere in the chest (Stage III).

Standard Treatment Invasive malignant thymoma is treated with surgical removal of the tumor if possible.

Radiation therapy is given postoperatively whether of not the tumor has been apparently completely removed. Fairly substantial doses, usually 3,500 to 4,500 cGy, are given and special techniques are necessary because of the large radiation ports required.

Drug therapy for locally invasive or advanced thymomas include the use of steroid hormones such as prednisone. These have caused regression of some thymomas that could not be removed and did not respond to radiotherapy.

Five-Year Survival 54 percent

Investigational
♦ Chemotherapy is under clinical evaluation, and a variety of drugs have been found to be useful in patients who have residual or recurrent disease following surgery or radiation therapy. The combi-

nation of cisplatin + doxorubicin + vincristine + Cytoxan produced a 91 percent response rate (47 percent complete) in one study.
♦ In one trial, almost half of the patients treated with a four-drug combination of vincristine + Cytoxan + lomustine + prednisone had complete responses. The combination of cisplatin + Adriamycin has produced a 70 percent remission rate.

TREATMENT FOLLOW-UP
♦ Periodic physical examinations, initially every two months during the first year.
♦ Routine x-rays and CT scans of the chest at intervals to detect recurrences.
♦ Routine blood chemistry tests are done every four to six months.
♦ Infections with unusual bacteria or fungi may occur, even if steroid hormones (prednisone) were not given.

RECURRENT CANCER
While the rate of recurrences is less than 2 percent for non-invasive tumors, it is 20 to 50 percent for invasive malignancies.

Local recurrences can be treated with repeat surgery, radiation therapy, drug therapy with corticosteroids (such as prednisone) or chemotherapy.

Chemotherapy programs include the multiple drug combinations mentioned above.

THE MOST IMPORTANT QUESTIONS YOU CAN ASK
♦ How safe is surgery? Are there special precautions?
♦ Do I need radiation therapy? What are the side effects?
♦ Should chemotherapy be used?
♦ If my tumor recurs, can I be cured?

THYROID

Malin Dollinger, MD

◇

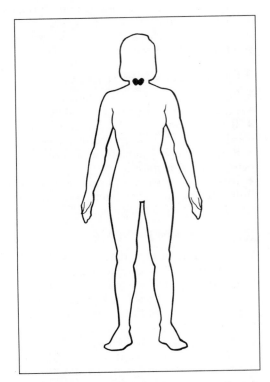

Cancer of the thyroid is the most common endocrine malignancy but is an uncommon cancer, comprising only about 1 percent of invasive cancers. It is estimated that there will be about 12,400 new cases in 1991, 9,100 in women and 3,300 in men. People with these malignancies are usually treated successfully.

Although invasive thyroid cancer is uncommon, doctors often have to diagnose and treat thyroid nodules, since about 4 percent of adults develop them. Thyroid cancer commonly appears as a "cold" nodule, meaning that it does not take up radioactive iodine. About 20 percent of cold nodules are cancer.

Most cases occur between 25 and 65 years of age, and the age at diagnosis is one of the most important factors in predicting prognosis. Men under 40 and women under 50 have significantly lower rates of recurrence and better survival rates than older patients.

Types There are three types of thyroid cancer: well-differentiated, undifferentiated and medullary carcinoma. Eighty percent are well-differentiated, and include papillary carcinomas and follicular carcinomas.

Papillary carcinomas are generally slow growing, with an 80 percent overall survival at 10 years. Even if tumor cells spread to regional lymph nodes or the lungs, survival may be more than 10 years. Tiny, clinically insignificant papillary carcinomas are found in 5 to 10 percent of thyroid glands examined at routine autopsies.

Follicular carcinomas occur in patients about 10 years older than those who get papillary carcinomas. Although these tumors are also usually slow growing, they behave somewhat more aggressively than papillary carcinomas.

Three percent of thyroid cancers are undifferentiated (anaplastic) carcinomas. They grow rapidly, behave aggressively and respond poorly to treatment.

Medullary carcinomas make up about 5 percent of thyroid cancers. These tumors secrete calcitonin, a tumor marker that is helpful in diagnosis and follow-up and also in screening relatives of those affected, since this tumor may occur on a familial, or inherited, basis. In the syndromes of multiple endocrine neoplasia (MEN), the cancer may be associated with tumors in other endocrine organs, such as pheochromocytoma of the adrenals, parathyroid cancer and islet cell cancer (*see* "Adrenal Gland," "Parathyroid" and "Islet Cell Carcinoma").

Other tumors that can arise in the thyroid gland include sarcomas, lymphomas, epidermoid carcinomas and teratomas. The thyroid gland can also be a site of metastasis from other cancers, especially cancers of the lung, kidney and breast, and melanoma.

How It Spreads Papillary carcinomas spread to nearby lymph nodes and the tissues in the neck, with metastatic lesions to the lungs and bones. With follicular carcinomas, local spread to lymph nodes is less common. These tumors spread through the bloodstream, with metastasis occurring more often to bone. Anaplastic carcinoma usually extensively invades surrounding tissue. Medullary carcinoma spreads to lymph nodes and may invade blood vessels.

What Causes It Thyroid cancer is associated with significant excess or deficiency of iodine in the diet, some inherited diseases and especially with exposure to radiation. There is an increased incidence of thyroid cancer among survivors of the atomic blasts in Japan.

The risk of radiation exposure to the neck is now well known, and radiation therapy to treat benign conditions of the head and neck—a common practice in the first half of this century—has been abandoned. This should eventually lead to a decrease in the incidence of thyroid cancer, but there is a long period between radiation exposure and the development of a tumor.

One new method of preventing thyroid cancer was used on a wide scale with children in the Chernobyl region of Russia after the nuclear reactor accident. Potassium iodide was given in an attempt to block the uptake of radioactive iodine in the fallout into the thyroid gland. It will probably take at least 30 years to know if this approach was effective.

RISK FACTORS

At Significantly Higher Risk
♦ Exposure to radiation therapy, especially between 1920 and 1950, for enlarged lymph nodes in the neck, mastoiditis, tonsils, whooping cough, acne, enlarged thymus gland, keloids and fungus infections. The incidence directly relates to the amount of radiation given. It generally takes 10 to 30 years after radiation exposure for a tumor to develop.

Thyroid cancer will develop in about 5 percent of children treated with low-dose radiation to the head and neck. Four percent of thyroid cancer patients have a history of such radiation therapy. Factors for increasing the risk after radiation exposure include female sex, younger age at exposure and a longer interval after radiation.

At Slightly Higher Risk
♦ Papillary carcinoma is increased in people with familial colon polyposis (multiple polyps of the colon), deficiency in the blood clotting Factor XI, and several other rare diseases.
♦ Risk for medullary carcinoma is inherited from one parent (autosomal-dominant) in 50 percent of patients.
♦ More anaplastic and follicular carcinomas develop in people from areas with endemic goiter. Eighty percent of patients with anaplastic carcinoma have a history of nodular goiter.
♦ Iodine deficiency is associated with follicular carcinoma, which is more common in iodine-deficient areas such as Switzerland.
♦ Iodine abundance is associated with papillary carcinoma, more common in areas using iodized salt (United States) or a high-iodine diet (Iceland).
♦ Patients with Hashimoto's thyroiditis have an increased incidence of lymphoma of the thyroid gland.

♦ There may be an increased risk of thyroid cancer in patients with chronic TSH (thyroid-stimulating hormone) elevation, usually as a congenital defect.

SCREENING

Physical examination is the best way to identify early-stage thyroid cancer. Two groups of people need special screening procedures:

♦ Those with a family history of thyroid cancer or multiple endocrine neoplasia (MEN). Serum thyroglobulin is useful in the former and serum calcitonin and carcinoembryonic antigen (CEA) are important tumor markers in the latter.

♦ Those who have had radiation therapy to the neck and who have no visible thyroid lumps should be examined at least every two years. A lump in the thyroid of these people generally suggests that the thyroid gland should be removed, since 40 percent will have cancer. To avoid surgery, nodules less than about 1/2 in. (1 cm) are sometimes treated with thyroid hormone for six months to see if they will disappear.

Patients with enlargement of the entire thyroid, without specific lumps or nodules, should have thyroid function tests and an ultrasound scan. If the thyroid is not overactive, thyroid hormone is given for six months. If a nodule grows, the thyroid lobe with the nodule is removed surgically. Otherwise, thyroid hormone treatment is continued. The risk of cancer in an enlarged thyroid with many nodules is significantly lower than in a thyroid with a single nodule.

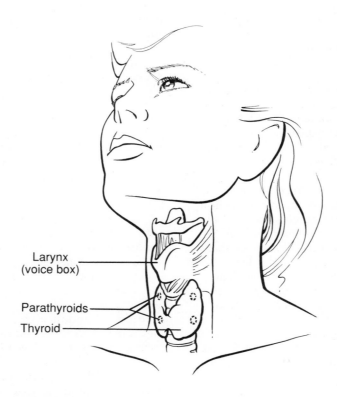

Larynx
(voice box)

Parathyroids

Thyroid

Thyroid and parathyroid glands

COMMON SIGNS AND SYMPTOMS

An enlargement of the entire thyroid, part of the thyroid or a lump or nodule is sometimes noticed while looking in the mirror while applying makeup or shaving. There may be enlarged lymph nodes in the neck that can be felt and there may be pain in the thyroid (especially with anaplastic carcinoma). These cancers also occasionally occur at the base of the tongue.

Pressure symptoms, including airway obstruction, hoarseness or difficulty swallowing, develop in fewer than 5 percent of patients.

DIAGNOSIS

When a thyroid nodule is found, administering thyroid hormone to suppress thyroid-stimulating hormone (TSH) may make it decrease in size. Benign nodules will commonly shrink while cancers won't, but exceptions occur in both situations. Suppression appears useful, however, in small nodules that have had fine needle aspiration (FNA) biopsy with benign findings. Surgery should be considered if there is any increase in size of the nodule during the suppression treatment. Biopsy is repeated after six months if the nodule has not shrunk.

Physical Examination
♦ Careful examination of the thyroid gland.

Blood and Other Tests
Blood tests are not generally useful to determine if a thyroid nodule is benign or malignant.
♦ Serum thyroglobulin levels are elevated in some well-differentiated thyroid cancers, but the level cannot indicate whether a lump is benign or malignant. The presence of thyroglobulin after a total thyroidectomy (surgical removal of the thyroid gland) or the recurrence of a high level after surgery suggests recurrent or metastatic disease.

♦ An elevated serum calcitonin after total thyroidectomy for medullary carcinoma suggests persistent disease. Families of all patients with medullary carcinoma should also be screened.
♦ CEA (carcinoembryonic antigen) levels are useful in predicting prognosis and discovering persistent disease in patients with medullary thyroid carcinoma.
♦ Blood tests, including serum alkaline phosphatase, are done to look for metastatic disease in the liver or bone. An elevated alkaline phosphatase level could suggest either liver or bone metastasis, leading to liver and bone scans.

Imaging
♦ Images of the thyroid can be taken after injection of a radioactive iodine tracer or of technetium 99M. Because thyroid cancers do not generally take up as much iodine as normal thyroid tissue, a cancer appears as a cold area on a scan. Only about 15 percent of cold nodules are cancer, however, and "warm" nodules can also be malignant, although infrequently. Though used extensively in the past to classify nodules as hot or cold, thyroid scans are used less and less because more information is provided by FNA.
♦ Ultrasound is a safe and simple way of determining if a mass is solid or filled with fluid (cystic). It can also detect multiple nodules where only one may be felt. High-resolution ultrasound can find nodules as small as 3 mm in diameter. It cannot distinguish benign from malignant tumors. Since it is non-invasive and sensitive, it is the most accurate way to measure and follow a suspicious nodule in a patient given thyroid hormone in an attempt to suppress the nodule. It may also be used to guide biopsy procedures.
♦ Standard x-rays, such as chest x-ray to look for metastases.

Endoscopy and Biopsy
♦ Indirect laryngoscopy if there is hoarseness, difficulty swallowing, shortness of

breath or if the patient has had a previous neck operation.

♦ Fine needle aspiration (FNA) biopsy is the initial step in evaluating thyroid nodules in patients who do not have a history of exposure to low-dose radiation therapy, as it provides more information than any other diagnostic technique. It is over 90 percent accurate for benign lesions and about 65 percent accurate for malignancies. FNA is not recommended for those with a history of radiation therapy because they usually have many nodules, only 40 percent have cancer, and the wrong one may be aspirated.

FNA is also very useful in selecting patients for surgery. Only about 3 percent of patients with benign findings on FNA will have thyroid cancer, so surgery can be postponed in these patients while the thyroid suppression trial is done. The TSH level must be suppressed by the dosage of thyroid hormone. If the nodule decreases, thyroid hormone is continued. If the nodule does not change after six months, aspiration is repeated. Malignant FNA results should lead to immediate surgery.

♦ Lesions larger than 1 1/4 in. (3 cm), especially rapidly growing ones, are more likely to be lymphoma or anaplastic thyroid carcinoma. FNA may be satisfactory for diagnosis of anaplastic cancer, but the diagnosis of lymphoma of the thyroid usually requires a larger cutting needle or open biopsy.

STAGING

The TNM staging system is not generally useful or uniformly accepted for thyroid cancers. Instead, staging systems have been designated for papillary and follicular carcinoma. There are no generally accepted staging systems for medullary carcinoma or anaplastic carcinoma.

TREATMENT OVERVIEW

A number of factors affect the prognosis for papillary and follicular thyroid cancers. A better prognosis can be expected with a pure papillary carcinoma, a tumor smaller than 3/4 in. (2 cm), small diffuse metastases, female sex and low-grade lesions.

A worse prognosis is related to age over 40, the degree of invasion of the thyroid capsule in follicular carcinoma, a primary tumor arising in thyroid tissue outside the thyroid gland, distant metastasis, a large tumor (especially over 1 1/2 in./4 cm), large nodular metastases, male sex and high-grade lesions (aneuploid).

 Surgery The primary treatment of thyroid cancer is surgery, but there are some differences in opinion about the best approach. A near-total thyroidectomy—removing almost all the thyroid—offers the best chance for cure, especially if the cancer is in several places within the gland. The removal of all functioning thyroid tissue also makes it easier to scan for metastatic disease with radioactive iodine.

One of the risks of a total thyroidectomy is the inadvertent removal of the parathyroid glands, which are situated, two on each side, at the edge of the thyroid. When a total thyroidectomy is done, an attempt is usually made to leave all four parathyroid glands in place. The surgeon must maintain an adequate supply of blood to the parathyroid glands to prevent the symptoms and signs of hypoparathyroidism or parathyroid hormone deficiency. Thyroid operations also have some risk of damage to the nerves in the neck that supply the larynx (voice box).

Removing one side of the thyroid (called a lobectomy) has fewer complications because only one nerve and two parathyroids are at risk. It is useful in selected cases. Tumor might remain, however, in a few patients.

The surgeon may select a procedure depending on the type of thyroid cancer as well as the size of the nodule and his or her own experience.

Radioactive Iodine Therapy It has been standard practice in many reputable cancer treatment centers to give radioactive iodine after surgery. Assuming that a scan demonstrates that the tumor takes up iodine, there is general agreement that this therapy is useful in patients over 45 years with papillary and follicular cancers if their tumors are multiple, locally invasive, larger than 1 in. (2.5 cm) or are associated with local or distant metastases.

This therapy has side effects, including temporary bone marrow suppression, inflammation of salivary glands, nausea and vomiting, scarring of the lung, pain in areas of metastasis and, rarely, leukemia.

The radioactive iodine is given when the patient is hypothyroid. After scanning or treatment, patients are again placed on thyroid hormone in order to avoid hypothyroidism and to suppress the TSH levels, which might stimulate residual tumor cells to grow. Some patients will require retreatment with radioactive iodine if the serum thyroglobulin level again becomes elevated or recurrent disease becomes evident.

TREATMENT BY TYPE AND STAGE

PAPILLARY THYROID CANCER
STAGE I
Tumor is confined to the thyroid gland. If it is on one side, it is considered Stage IA. If on both sides or there is more than one lump, it is Stage IB.

Standard Treatment The standard surgical procedure is removal of one side of the thyroid (lobectomy), but 5 to 10 percent of patients will have a recurrence. Enlarged lymph nodes are also removed. Thyroid hormone is then given to suppress the thyroid-stimulating hormone (TSH) from the pituitary gland, which decreases the chance of recurrence.

Other options are a near-total or total thyroidectomy. The rationale for this is that there is an increased chance of multiple tumors in both lobes and any tumor

left behind could change into the highly malignant (anaplastic) form. More important, scanning for metastases is possible once the thyroid is removed.

Five-Year Survival Over 95 percent

STAGE II
Cancer has spread to lymph nodes (IIA if to nodes on one side, IIB if to both sides or the mediastinal nodes—those in the center of the chest).

Standard Treatment The treatment is virtually identical to that for Stage I. The only difference between the two stages is the spread to lymph nodes. Removal of these metastases may reduce the chance of local recurrence and minimally improves survival.

Five-Year Survival Over 95 percent

STAGE III
The tumor has invaded the tissues of the neck.

Standard Treatment Total thyroidectomy, plus removal of all apparent areas of cancer that have spread to the neck (debulking). After surgery, radioactive iodine may be given if the tumor takes up this isotope. If the uptake is minimal, external radiation may be given.

Five-Year Survival 60 percent

STAGE IV
There are distant metastases, usually to lungs, bone and distant lymph nodes.

Standard Treatment Patients who have only distant lymph node metastasis may often be cured by radioactive iodine after a total thyroidectomy.

Solitary lung or bone metastases should be surgically removed, if possible. A therapeutic dose of radioactive iodine is then given; if there is no uptake, radiotherapy is given, if tolerated in the area involved. Taking thyroid hormone to suppress TSH may be effective in many metastatic tumors that are not sensitive to radioactive iodine.

Chemotherapy has produced occasional complete responses.

Ten-Year Survival Less than 20 percent

FOLLICULAR THYROID CANCER
STAGE I
The tumor is localized to the thyroid gland (IA if on one side, IB if on both sides or there are multiple lesions).

Standard Treatment Either a near-total thyroidectomy or a lobectomy may be done. This type of cancer has a higher risk of metastasis to lung and bone, and one disadvantage of leaving a remnant of thyroid is the difficulty in subsequent scanning with radioactive iodine (I-131). The residual thyroid rather than the metastasis will take up the isotope.

Sometimes, I-131 is used to eliminate any remaining thyroid tissue. Similarly, when therapeutic doses of I-131 are used, all or almost all of the thyroid gland should be removed first.

Less extensive operations such as lobectomy have fewer complications, but 5 to 10 percent of patients will have a recurrence in the thyroid.

As with papillary carcinoma, enlarged lymph nodes discovered at surgery should be removed without extensive surgery. In patients who have a limited surgical procedure (lobectomy), thyroid hormone is given postoperatively to suppress TSH and decrease the chance of recurrence.

Five-Year Survival 70 to 90 percent

STAGE II
The tumor has spread to lymph nodes (IIA if on one side, IIB if on both sides or to the mediastinal nodes—those in the center of the chest).

Standard Treatment Treatment is similar to that for Stage I. The only difference is the involvement of nearby lymph nodes, which affect only local recurrence and not survival.

Options include near-total thyroidectomy or lobectomy. The same considerations about hypoparathyroidism and multiple tumors apply.

Five-Year Survival 50 to 70 percent

STAGE III
The tumor invades the tissues of the neck.

Standard Treatment Total thyroidectomy and removal of local areas of tumor spread (debulking). If the tumor takes up radioactive iodine (I-131), the isotope is given in an attempt to treat all potential residual disease. When the I-131 uptake is low, external radiotherapy is given to the neck.

Five-Year Survival 20 to 60 percent (worse if blood vessels are involved)

STAGE IV
There are distant metastases, usually to lungs and bone.

Standard Treatment Treatment is usually not curative but may produce significant palliation.

The treatment options are similar to Stage IV papillary thyroid cancer, and include therapeutic doses of radioactive iodine if the metastases take up this isotope or external radiotherapy for localized lesions that do not respond to radioactive iodine. Tumors in many patients can be suppressed with thyroid hormone. A number of investigative chemotherapy protocols are being used for patients with metastatic disease that does not respond to these treatment programs.

Five-Year Survival Unusual

MEDULLARY THYROID CARCINOMA

In the sporadic form, the tumor is usually on only one side of the thyroid. In the inherited (familial) form, the tumor is almost always on both sides. It is usually a hard mass and blood vessels are often invaded microscopically.

Prognosis depends upon the size of the primary tumor, the involvement of nearby lymph nodes and how completely the tumor can be removed at surgery.

Standard Treatment A total thyroidectomy is done, with a central neck cleanout, meaning that all fibrofatty and lymphoid tissue is removed. If regional nodes are involved and the primary tumor is larger than 3/4 in. (2 cm), a modified radical neck dissection is done on the same side.

If the tumor is confined to the thyroid gland, almost all patients will be cured. In general, there is no benefit to radioactive iodine therapy, radiotherapy or chemotherapy, although occasional responses to these treatments are seen in metastatic disease.

Treatment for metastatic disease has generally been unsatisfactory, pointing up the need for detection and diagnosis while the tumor is confined to the thyroid and can be cured surgically. Patients with metastatic disease may have significant symptoms, especially severe diarrhea, related to the hormone produced by the tumor.

Five-Year Survival 40 to 95 percent. Survival may be better in patients with the sporadic rather than the inherited form.

ANAPLASTIC THYROID CARCINOMA

There are large cell and small cell types. Both grow rapidly and extend beyond the thyroid.

Standard Treatment This tumor has an extremely poor prognosis, most patients not surviving even one year after diagnosis. Most tumors cannot be surgically removed because of their size or the involvement of local structures.

After the diagnosis is established by FNA or a cutting needle biopsy, aggressive radiation therapy is often given. More useful is radiation therapy in combination with doxorubicin, a radiation sensitizer. In some cases, the combination of hyperfractionated radiation therapy (two treatments each day) and weekly doxorubicin has produced significant tumor shrinkage.

These patients frequently require a tracheostomy because of pressure symptoms and breathing difficulties.

Five-Year Survival About 5 percent, the average survival being less than six months

PRIMARY LYMPHOMA OF THE THYROID

Standard Treatment These patients have a rapidly enlarging thyroid mass, often with pressure symptoms. At least a third have thyroiditis (Hashimoto's disease) and most have limited-stage disease. The prognosis depends on the lymphoma subtype as well as on the stage.

Treatment is similar to that for any B-cell lymphoma arising outside lymph nodes. Since most patients have diffuse lymphomas, they tend to be treated with aggressive third-generation combination chemotherapy programs (*see* "Lymphomas: Non-Hodgkin's").

TREATMENT FOLLOW-UP

For well-differentiated thyroid cancers (papillary and follicular carcinoma), follow-up should include:

♦ Periodic physical examination, especially of the thyroid.
♦ Serologic marker (thyroglobulin).
♦ Periodic ultrasound examinations of the neck to identify recurrence in the thyroid area or lymph node metastases.
♦ Chest x-ray to detect metastases.

For medullary thyroid cancer, follow-up should include:

♦ Serum calcitonin level and CEA level every six months.

♦ Physical examination, emphasizing the thyroid, although calcitonin level is more accurate than physical examination for following persistent disease.

♦ Chest x-ray every six months until stable.

♦ Chemistry panel every six months.

RECURRENT AND METASTATIC DISEASE

When thyroid carcinoma is recurrent or metastatic and is also widespread or can't be removed, it is treated with radioactive iodine. If it does not take up radioactive iodine, it should be treated with radiation therapy.

♦ For the papillary and follicular types, an effort is made to scan for metastatic disease with radioactive iodine. After the thyroid gland is removed and thyroid hormone is stopped for an appropriate time, a tracer dose of radioactive iodine is given. If hot spots appear at sites outside the thyroid area, suggesting metastases, a therapeutic dose of radioactive iodine is given. Radioactive iodine effectively irradiates microscopic metastases. Larger metastases should be removed surgically before radioactive iodine is given. The thyroglobulin level should be determined, since if it is detectable or elevated after a total thyroidectomy, residual tumor is present.

♦ External radiation is used in patients whose tumors do not take up radioactive iodine or are undifferentiated.

♦ Some patients respond to chemotherapy, with regimens containing doxorubicin having the highest response rate. The combination of cisplatin and doxorubicin may produce some complete and partial remissions in metastatic thyroid cancer. In a few cases, the complete responders survived more than two years. Another combination (doxorubicin + bleomycin + vincristine + melphalan) was reported to show responses in about one-third of patients.

♦ In patients with anaplastic thyroid cancer, chemotherapy is occasionally effective and is usually combined with external radiation.

♦ Patients with metastatic thyroid carcinoma, especially if unsuitable or unresponsive to radioactive iodine, should be considered for entry into clinical trials in the hopes of finding a more effective chemotherapy program.

THE MOST IMPORTANT QUESTIONS YOU CAN ASK

♦ How extensive should my surgery be?

♦ What is the chance of complications of surgery, especially damage to the parathyroid glands and the risk of nerve malfunction?

♦ Why do I need to take thyroid hormone after surgery?

♦ Will I need radioactive iodine?

♦ What follow-up do I need?

♦ What is my chance of cure, and when can you be sure?

TROPHOBLASTIC DISEASE

Jeffrey L. Stern, MD

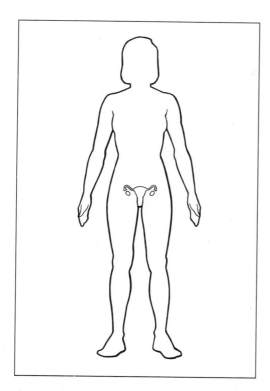

Gestational trophoblastic disease (GTD) is a rare cancer that develops from an abnormal fertilized egg. Of all the cancers that afflict women, it is one of the most commonly cured. Even when it is metastatic, the survival rate is extremely high.

The cure rate depends on the cell type, the extent of disease, the duration of time from the onset of the initial pregnancy to the start of therapy, the sites of metastases, the type of pregnancy before the development of GTD and earlier therapy. In some cases, it can also depend on the degree of elevation of the serum beta human chorionic gonadotropin (βHCG), a protein produced by a normal pregnancy as well as by all the different GTD cell types. It can be detected in the blood and urine and is an extremely sensitive tumor marker for GTD. It is measured often during both therapy and follow-up to measure the response to treatment and to detect recurrent disease.

Types There are three types of gestational trophoblastic disease—hydatidiform mole (also called a molar pregnancy), invasive mole (chorioadenoma destruens) and gestational choriocarcinoma, which is further divided according to whether it is metastatic or non-metastatic.

♦ A hydatidiform mole is essentially an abnormal embryo that contains many fluid-filled cysts. There are two types of hydatidiform moles, complete and incomplete (partial). The diagnosis of a complete hydatidiform mole is usually made during the first half of a pregnancy and is recognized by the health care provider about 50 percent of the time before the tumor cysts are expelled. A variety of clinical conditions may be confused with a molar pregnancy, but these can usually be distinguished on the basis of medical history, a physical exam and an ultrasound examination.

In contrast, a partial mole is associated with an embryo, umbilical cord and membranes. It occurs much less frequently than a complete mole. The embryo usually dies within nine weeks after the last menstrual period although occasionally it can survive to term. Partial moles are rarely associated with multiple ovarian cysts (thecolutein cysts), high βHCG titers and other accompaniments of a complete mole. There is also a lower incidence of malignant behavior (5 to 10 percent).

♦ An invasive mole (chorioadenoma destruens) is defined as a hydatidiform mole that invades the wall of the uterine muscle. It develops in 15 to 30 percent of all molar pregnancies.

♦ Choriocarcinoma is a very rapidly growing malignancy that tends to spread quickly. About 50 percent of all cases of gestational choriocarcinoma follow a hydatidiform mole, 25 percent follow a spontaneous abortion or tubal pregnancy and 25 percent follow a normal pregnancy. Choriocarcinoma follows a normal-term pregnancy in 1 in 40,000 pregnancies. GTD after a normal pregnancy is always a choriocarcinoma, never a mole or an invasive mole.

What Causes It A hydatidiform or invasive mole occurs when a single sperm fertilizes an egg without a nucleus. The chromosomes in the sperm duplicate, resulting in an abnormal embryo that has only male genetic material. A mole can also occur when two sperm fertilize a single egg. A mole develops from the abnormally fertilized egg and is characterized by a lack of a normal fetus and by many small fluid-filled cysts.

The cause of choriocarcinoma is uncertain. It can arise from a normal pregnancy, a miscarriage, a tubal pregnancy or from either type of mole.

How It Spreads Hydatidiform moles generally stay confined to the endometrial cavity. When it begins to invade the wall of the uterus, it is called an invasive mole. Occasionally a hydatidiform mole and an invasive mole can spread to distant sites, most typically to the lung.

An invasive mole can penetrate the full thickness of the uterine wall and rupture, resulting in severe intra-abdominal or vaginal bleeding. Invasive moles can also metastasize, most commonly to the vagina and lung. This may be confusing since women with proven invasive moles who have metastases may also have choriocarcinoma. Although an invasive mole is more aggressive locally than a non-invasive mole, it is no more likely to be complicated by choriocarcinoma.

Choriocarcinoma can spread virtually anywhere in the body but most commonly spreads to the lung, the lower genital tract (cervix, vagina and vulva), the brain, liver, kidney and the gastrointestinal tract.

RISK FACTORS

Gestational trophoblastic disease occurs only in women of reproductive age. An invasive mole develops in 15 to 30 percent of all complete moles and 5 to 10 percent of all partial moles. Choriocarcinoma develops in 3 percent of complete moles but rarely in partial moles.

At Significantly Higher Risk
Risks for the development of a hydatidiform or invasive mole or choriocarcinoma include:

♦ A prior mole (30 times the risk).

♦ Maternal age greater than 40 years (5 times) or less than 20 years (1.5 times).

♦ A previous spontaneous abortion (twice the risk).

At Slightly Lower Risk
♦ Eating a diet high in vitamin A and having one or more children without having a previous abortion is statistically correlated with a lower than average risk of developing a complete mole.

At Risk for Developing an Invasive Mole or Choriocarcinoma
For women with a molar pregnancy, there are several risk factors associated with the subsequent development of an invasive mole and choriocarcinoma. These include delayed hemorrhage after a dilation and curettage procedure (D&C), large ovarian cysts, acute pulmonary failure at the time of the D&C, a large uterus before the D&C, a serum βHCG level greater than 40,000 mIU/mL, a history of a previous mole and maternal age over 40.

SCREENING

Being so rare, GTD is not routinely screened for.

COMMON SIGNS AND SYMPTOMS

A molar pregnancy is usually associated with bleeding in the first half of a pregnancy, pain in the lower abdomen, high blood pressure before 24 weeks of pregnancy, excessive nausea or vomiting, a uterus larger than normal for the gestational age (50 percent of all cases), an absent fetal heartbeat and the expulsion of cysts.

Eighty to 90 percent of women with partial moles have abnormal uterine bleeding, a smaller than expected uterus for the gestational age of the pregnancy or the signs and symptoms of a spontaneous abortion.

The most common symptoms of choriocarcinoma are lack of a menstrual period, symptoms of pregnancy, abnormal vaginal bleeding or pelvic pain. Women with liver metastases may have bleeding within the abdomen because of a ruptured liver. Those with metastases to the lung may have a dry cough, cough up blood and have chest pain or shortness of breath. Spread to the intestinal tract may be associated with chronic blood loss and anemia or with massive hemorrhage. Brain metastases are often indicated by symptoms that suggest a brain tumor or stroke.

DIAGNOSIS

The diagnosis is usually suspected after an ultrasound examination of the uterus, but absolute diagnosis of a mole is made by examining the cysts under a microscope. A serum βHCG level far in excess of that of a normal pregnancy would support the diagnosis of a hydatidiform mole.

An invasive mole is seldom diagnosed definitively without a hysterectomy. The diagnosis is usually made after a hydatidiform mole is removed and the βHCG titers are persistently elevated and there is no evidence of metastases.

Confirmation of choriocarcinoma by removing cells for pathological analysis is not required and may be hazardous since this tumor bleeds easily. The diagnosis is made by the presence of metastases and an elevated βHCG level or, occasionally, on a D&C specimen.

Physical Examination
♦ When GDT is suspected or diagnosed, the physical examination pays particular attention to the pelvis, abdomen (specifically the liver), the lungs and the brain.

Blood and Other Tests
♦ Complete blood count.
♦ Tests for liver enzymes and kidney function.
♦ Serum chemistries.
♦ Serum βHCG.

Imaging
Studies before evaluation if a hydatiform mole include:
♦ Pelvic ultrasound.
♦ Chest x-ray.

STAGING

Gestational trophoblastic disease is not staged but is divided into non-metastatic or metastatic. Non-metastatic choriocarcinoma is defined as having no disease outside the uterus and has a survival rate of 100 percent. Metastatic choriocarcinoma is further divided into low-risk (good prognosis) and high-risk (poor prognosis) based on several factors.

TREATMENT OVERVIEW

Before starting chemotherapy for invasive mole or for non-metastatic and metastatic choriocarcinoma, certain diagnostic tests should be performed including a chest x-ray and a CT scan of the abdomen, pelvis and head. Even when the chest x-ray is normal, a CT scan of the lungs may reveal small metastases in up to 40 percent of women. These women have a 50 percent failure rate with single drug chemotherapy. A complete blood count, platelet count and kidney and liver function tests are also required before initiating chemotherapy.

An important aspect of treating women with GTD is to start therapy as quickly as possible after the diagnosis is made. It is also important to give chemotherapy as often as possible until the serum βHCG titers return to normal. A course of chemotherapy is generally given every 14 to 21 days, depending on the drug regimen used.

Depending on the extent of the disease, most physicians give one to three cycles of chemotherapy after the first normal βHCG level, then follow the titers monthly for 6 to 24 months after treatment. All women are advised to use oral contraceptives for one to two years after therapy.

TREATMENT BY TYPE AND STAGE

HYDATIDIFORM MOLE (MOLAR PREGNANCY)

Complications associated with a molar pregnancy include anemia because of blood loss, severe high blood pressure, an overactive thyroid gland, heart failure, hemorrhage, infection and acute pulmonary failure.

Standard Treatment As soon the diagnosis is made, a therapeutic suction dilatation and curettage (D&C) is performed in the operating room under anesthesia. For women who have completed childbearing, the removal of the uterus and cervix (a hysterectomy) is also an option.

Rhogam is given to women with Rh negative blood to prevent Rh sensitization. In about a third of women with a molar pregnancy, there may be enlargement of one or both ovaries because of multiple (thecolutein) cysts caused by the high levels of βHCG. Occasionally the cysts can rupture, bleed or become infected. In the vast majority of cases, these cysts do not have to be surgically removed because

they resolve with time, although sometimes it can take several weeks or months for them to disappear completely.

Chemotherapy may be given after the removal of the mole if there is a tissue diagnosis of choriocarcinoma, if the serum βHCG rises for two successive weeks or plateaus for three weeks or more (in the vast majority of women, the βHCG level plateaus or rises by seven weeks after the D&C), if metastases are found, if the serum βHCG rises again after reaching a normal level or if there is a hemorrhage not related to an incomplete D&C.

Five-Year Survival 100 percent

NON-METASTATIC GTD

Non-metastatic disease may be either an invasive mole or choriocarcinoma and is defined as having no disease outside the uterus.

Standard Treatment Chemotherapy for an invasive mole and non-metastatic choriocarcinoma is the same. All cases of non-metastatic GTD are considered curable, even if there is extensive local disease. If chemotherapy fails, a hysterectomy is usually performed.

The standard treatment is with a single chemotherapeutic drug. Most physicians use methotrexate if the liver functions are normal or actinomycin-D if they aren't. Methotrexate is given daily, either by injection into a muscle or intravenously, for five days. This schedule is repeated every 14 days until the βHCG level returns to normal. Three to four courses are usually required.

Methotrexate may also be given on days 1, 3, 5 and 7 with leucovorin given on Days 2, 4, 6 and 8. When used in this fashion, only one course of treatment is given (with a cure rate of around 80 percent). A second or third course is given only if the βHCG titer does not return to normal.

Actinomycin-D is usually given intravenously for five consecutive days and repeated every two weeks. If treatment with methotrexate fails to bring about titer remission, then actinomycin-D is given (or vice versa).

Five-Year Survival 100 percent for both invasive mole and non-metastatic choriocarcinoma

LOW-RISK METASTATIC GTD

Metastatic choriocarcinoma is considered low-risk when it is diagnosed less than four months after the onset of the pregnancy, when the βHCG titer is less than 40,000 mIU/ml, when there are no liver or brain metastases and when there has been no previous treatment with chemotherapy.

Standard Treatment Therapy for women with low-risk metastatic GTD is usually with a single chemotherapeutic drug as for non-metastatic disease. But many physicians use only single-agent chemotherapy for women who have an abnormal postmolar βHCG titer. All other cases with good prognostic features are treated with a combination of methotrexate + actinomycin-D + Cytoxan (MAC).

Those who fail chemotherapy with methotrexate alone (approximately 20 percent) are then treated with actinomycin-D or with MAC. MAC is given intravenously for five consecutive days every two to three weeks until the βHCG titer returns to normal.

Five-Year Survival 97 to 100 percent

HIGH-RISK METASTATIC GTD

Metastatic choriocarcinoma is considered high-risk when it is diagnosed more than four months after the onset of pregnancy, associated with a serum βHCG titer greater than 40,000 mIU/mL, liver or brain metastases, a history of chemotherapy or if it occurs after a full-term pregnancy.

Standard Treatment Poor-risk metastatic disease has to be treated as soon as possi-

ble with aggressive chemotherapy. Women with brain or liver metastases are often treated with radiation therapy to the brain or liver. Women with liver metastases have the worst prognosis.

Standard chemotherapy has been with MAC, but recently there has been a trend toward using a regimen known as EMA-CO, which includes the drugs etoposide, methotrexate, actinomycin-D, vincristine and Cytoxan.

Other drugs used in women who fail to respond to MAC and/or EMA-CO include vinblastine, cisplatin, bleomycin and ifosfamide. Once a negative βHCG level is obtained, most women are treated with three more courses of chemotherapy and are then followed with monthly βHCG titers for two years.

Five-Year Survival 75 percent

TREATMENT FOLLOW-UP

Regular measurements of the serum βHCG levels are the most important part of the follow-up surveillance for molar pregnancies. The levels are monitored weekly until normal—usually, the level progressively declines to normal within 14 weeks after the D&C—then monthly for 6 to 12 months.

♦ A gynecologic examination and careful physical examination is done one week after the D&C and then every four weeks until the βHCG titer returns to normal or unless symptoms develop.

♦ Contraception (preferably oral contraceptives) should be used for 6 to 12 months after the D&C.

The serum βHCG levels are also monitored for other types of GTD. Once the βHCG titer returns to normal after treatment, the levels should be measured monthly for one year in the case of non-metastatic disease or two years for metastatic disease.

Pregnancy After GTD Treatment No significant side effects of chemotherapy for

GTD affect future pregnancies. There do not seem to be a higher infertility rate, a lower chance for a successful term pregnancy or a higher rate of spontaneous abortion. But there is a higher incidence of subsequent GTD.

Most physicians recommend avoiding pregnancy for the first year after a hydatidiform mole is treated. This will prevent any confusion about the interpretation of elevated βHCG levels.

RECURRENT CANCER

Recurrent disease is usually treated with chemotherapy or occasionally surgery if the metastases are isolated. Chemotherapy for gestational trophoblastic disease automatically puts a woman in the high-risk group for recurrences.

Cure rates vary, depending on the site of metastases.

THE MOST IMPORTANT QUESTIONS YOU CAN ASK

♦ What type of gestational trophoblastic disease do I have, and what is its extent?
♦ What is the likelihood of cure?
♦ How was the chemotherapy decided upon?
♦ What are my prospects of having a normal pregnancy later on?
♦ Will a specialist in gynecologic oncology be involved in my care?

UTERUS: ENDOMETRIAL CARCINOMA

Jeffrey L. Stern, MD

◇

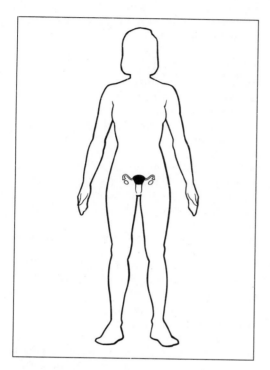

Endometrial cancer—carcinoma of the lining of the uterus—is the most common gynecologic malignancy and accounts for about 13 percent of all malignancies occurring in women. There are about 34,000 cases of endometrial cancer diagnosed in the United States each year but, encouragingly, there has been a significant decrease in the number of women who develop endometrial cancer each year since 1975.

Similarly, the death rate from endometrial cancer has steadily declined from 1950 to 1985, falling more than 60 percent. Since this cancer is usually diagnosed at an early stage, the cure rate is high, with a five-year survival of 83 percent in 1985.

Types All endometrial carcinomas arise from the glands of the lining of the uterus. Adenocarcinoma accounts for 75 percent of all endometrial carcinomas. Endometrial adenocarcinomas that contain benign squamous cells are known as adenoacanthomas and account for 17 percent of endometrial cancers.

The remaining three types of endometrial carcinoma have a poor prognosis. Approximately 15 percent of women have adenosquamous carcinoma, in which both the gland cells and squamous cells are malignant. Three percent have a clear cell carcinoma, and about 1 percent have a papillary carcinoma.

Uterine sarcoma is another kind of uterine malignancy. (*See* "Uterus: Uterine Sarcomas".)

How It Spreads From where it arises in the lining of the uterus, endometrial carcinoma eventually invades the wall of the uterus and may involve the cervix. With time, it can grow through the wall of the uterus into the surrounding tissues (the parametrium), the bladder and the rectum (*see* page 278).

It can also spread by the lymphatic system to the vagina, fallopian tubes, ovaries, the pelvic and aortic lymph nodes and to the lymph nodes in the groin and above the collarbone (supraclavicular). Like ovarian carcinoma, endometrial cancer can also spread throughout the abdominal cavity and occasionally through the bloodstream to the lung, liver and brain. How rapidly it spreads depends on the grade (histologic virulence) of the cancer.

Endometrial cancer is often associated

with a primary carcinoma of the ovary. (*See* "Ovarian Germ Cell Cancer.")

What Causes It Unknown.

RISK FACTORS

The use of birth control pills decreases the risk of developing endometrial cancer by half.

At Significantly Higher Risk
♦ Postmenopausal women.
♦ Menopause after age 52 (2.4 times as likely).
♦ Lack of children (twice as likely).
♦ Women with hypertension (twice as likely).
♦ Diabetics (2.8 times).
♦ Women who do not ovulate, in other words those with polycystic ovaries (Stein-Leventhal syndrome).
♦ Estrogen replacement therapy without supplemental progesterone (seven times as likely).
♦ History of pelvic radiation therapy (eight times).
♦ Obesity greater than 50 pounds (23 kg) over ideal body weight (10 times as likely).

SCREENING

Screening for endometrial carcinoma is not as satisfactory as screening for cancer of the cervix because of the inaccessibility of the uterine cavity. Pap smears detect only a small percentage of endometrial cancers.

There have been studies of other screening methods that can be performed in the doctor's office, with several showing the benefit of using endometrial biopsies to screen high-risk women who have no symptoms. This procedure is associated with some discomfort, however, and may not be cost-effective in the absence of risk factors. Routine annual screening for women without symptoms is not recommended by the American College of Obstetricians and Gynecologists.

COMMON SIGNS AND SYMPTOMS

In 90 percent of cases, there is abnormal uterine bleeding, from insignificant staining to a hemorrhage. There may also be pain in the pelvis, back or legs, bladder or rectal symptoms, weight loss and general weakness. Five percent of women will have no symptoms.

DIAGNOSIS
Physical Examination
♦ On a gynecologic examination, the external genitalia is usually normal. The cervix may be involved with cancer (Stage II), and the vagina may also be involved (Stage III).
♦ Occasionally the uterus will be enlarged or softened and masses may be detected in the pelvis (a rectal examination is an important aspect of the pelvic examination).
♦ Enlarged lymph nodes in the neck and groin.
♦ Enlarged liver, abdominal mass or excessive abdominal fluid (ascites).

Blood and Other Tests
♦ Complete blood count.
♦ Serum liver and kidney tests.
♦ Serum CA-125 is produced by a small percentage of women with endometrial carcinoma, which can be useful in follow-up to detect recurrences.

Imaging
♦ CT scan of the abdomen and MRI scan of the pelvis are both useful for determining the extent of cancer in the pelvis, the presence of ovarian disease and the presence of involved pelvic and aortic lymph nodes and liver metastases.
♦ Chest x-ray.

Endoscopy and Biopsy
♦ The definitive diagnosis is made on an endometrial biopsy, which involves a small scraping of the uterus and is usually

performed in the doctor's office. A dilation and curettage (D&C) is required for some women—those who have biopsy-proven endometrial hyperplasia (see below), who have an insufficient specimen on an office biopsy or who can't have an endometrial biopsy done in the office because of a small cervical opening or discomfort.

STAGING

Cancer of the uterus is surgically staged. Between 70 and 80 percent of all endometrial cancers are Stage I. In 1988, the International Federation of Gynecologists and Obstetricians (FIGO) staging was revised to include the grade of the cancer (degree of virulence) as determined on microscopic examination. The cancers are divided into three grades, with Grade 1 (well-differentiated) having the best prognosis and Grade 3 (least-differentiated) having the poorest.

ENDOMETRIAL CANCER PRECURSORS

Endometrial hyperplasia, an overgrowth of the lining of the uterus, is a precursor to the development of cancer. This disorder tends to progress from a simple, benign hyperplasia confined to the lining of the uterus, to more severe forms of hyperplasia and eventually to an invasive malignancy. The risk factors for endometrial hyperplasia are similar to those of endometrial carcinoma.

Abnormal uterine bleeding is usually the first symptom. The diagnosis is made by evaluating the lining of the uterus by biopsy or dilation and curettage (D&C).

Treatment depends on the degree of hyperplasia, the age of the woman and her reproductive desires. Total abdominal hysterectomy and removal of both tubes and both ovaries is recommended for post-menopausal women and women who have completed childbearing. Women who want to keep their reproductive organs can be treated with oral progestational hormones for several months. The cure rate depends on the degree of hyperplasia and the sensitivity of the endometrium to the progestational therapy.

TREATMENT OVERVIEW

Treatment of endometrial carcinoma is based primarily on the stage and grade of the cancer.

The standard therapy is an abdominal hysterectomy with removal of both fallopian tubes and ovaries, selective removal of pelvic and aortic lymph nodes and washings from the abdominal cavity to look for malignant cells.

Most gynecologic oncologists also recommend obtaining a specimen from the cancer for analysis of its estrogen and progesterone receptor content. The receptor content has prognostic value and may be useful in the selection of hormone therapy for recurrent or metastatic cancer.

 Surgery Most gynecologic oncologists recommend a midline abdominal incision to gain access to the upper abdomen. Complications of surgery can include infection, bleeding and injury to the bladder, rectum or ureter causing a leak, although this is rare. There may also be blood clots in the legs, occasionally dislodging and traveling to the lungs (pulmonary embolism).

 Radiation Women who have Stages Ib, Ic or IIa uterine cancers are frequently treated two to six weeks after surgery with radiation to the entire pelvis and upper vagina. Total dose is 4,000 to 5,000 cGy in divided doses given daily, five days a week for four to five weeks. Although pelvic external beam radiation therapy will decrease the frequency of recurrences in the pelvis and vagina, it does not statistically improve the five-year survival rate.

Side effects of radiation can include diarrhea, nausea and vomiting, bleeding from the bladder or rectum, vaginal scarring, intestinal obstruction, or leaks (fistulas) in the urinary or intestinal tracts.

 Chemotherapy Treatment with chemotherapy after surgery is being evaluated for later stages of the disease.

TREATMENT BY STAGE

ENDOMETRIAL HYPERPLASIA

Total abdominal hysterectomy and removal of both tubes and both ovaries is the treatment of choice when fertility is no longer an issue or when progestational hormone therapy is contraindicated. For those women who desire more children or preservation of the uterus, a D&C, therapy with oral progestational agents, induction of ovulation and avoidance of postmenopausal estrogen therapy without progesterone is frequently effective. Careful follow-up with an endometrial biopsy or a D&C is necessary.

STAGE Ia
The tumor is limited to the endometrium.

Standard Treatment Regardless of the grade, standard therapy is removal of the uterus and both tubes and ovaries. Postoperative radiation therapy is not usually required.

Five-Year Survival 90 to 95 percent

Investigational
♦ The most significant study in progress is whether postoperative pelvic radiation therapy improves survival.

STAGE Ib
The tumor invades the uterine wall but through less than half of its thickness.

Standard Treatment The abdominal removal of the uterus, both tubes and ovaries and sampling the pelvic and para-aortic lymph nodes is all that is required under certain conditions—namely, that

the tumor is Grade 1 or 2, involves the upper two-thirds of the uterus, does not invade the blood vessels of the uterus, invades the wall of the uterus by less than one-third and the abdominal washings contain no malignant cells.

If the tumor (any grade) invades more than one-third of the uterine wall or significantly invades the blood vessels, external beam radiation therapy is usually given to the pelvis and upper vagina after surgery. The total dose is 4,000 to 5,000 cGy, given daily in divided doses, five days a week for four to five weeks.

Five-Year Survival Up to 80 percent

Investigational
♦ The most significant study in progress is whether postoperative pelvic radiation therapy improves survival.
♦ Studies are looking at the role of adjuvant chemotherapy with Adriamycin, mitoxantrone, cisplatin, Cytoxan, carboplatin or progestational hormones in various doses and regimens.

STAGE Ic
The tumor invades the uterine wall by more than half of its thickness.

Standard Treatment Almost all gynecologic oncologists recommend whole pelvis radiation after surgery to decrease the frequency of recurrent disease in the vagina and pelvis. Although it does not statistically improve the five-year survival rate, it is effective in decreasing the incidence of local recurrences in the field of radiation.

Five-Year Survival Up to 70 percent

Investigational *See* Stage Ib.

STAGE IIa
The glands that line the cervix are involved.

Standard Treatment This stage is generally treated like Stage Ic—surgery followed by radiation. Sometimes, however, radiotherapy is given before surgery, with radioactive cesium temporarily placed in the upper vagina two weeks after external radiation treatment is finished.

Five-Year Survival Up to 60 percent

Investigational See Stage Ib.

STAGE IIb
The tumor cells invade the cervix.

Standard Treatment Before surgery, whole-pelvis external beam radiation therapy (total dose of 4,000 cGy) is given in divided doses, five days a week, over five weeks. After a two-week break, this is followed by a three-day application of radioactive cesium to the upper vagina, cervix and uterus. Six weeks later, an abdominal hysterectomy is performed, along with removal of both tubes and ovaries, selective pelvic and aortic lymph node sampling and cytological assessment of the abdominal cavity.

Alternative therapy for younger, non-obese women in good medical condition is a radical abdominal hysterectomy, removal of the tubes and ovaries, removal of all the pelvic lymph nodes and surgical staging.

Five-Year Survival Up to 60 percent

Investigational
♦ Studies are looking at the role of adjuvant chemotherapy with Adriamycin, mitoxantrone, cisplatin, Cytoxan, carboplatin or progestational hormones in various doses and regimens.

STAGE IIIa
This stage is defined by involvement of the uterine surface and/or the tubes and ovaries and/or the presence of malignant cells in the abdominal fluid (positive peritoneal washings).

Standard Treatment After surgery, any additional treatment is controversial and should be considered investigational. The chance of malignant cells being present within the abdominal cavity (Stage IIIa) increases with higher grades of cancer and with deeper invasion of the tumor into the uterine wall.

There is some controversy over the significance of malignant cells floating in the abdominal cavity, but most gynecologic oncologists recommend treatment with radiation therapy to the entire abdomen, intra-abdominal radioactive substances such as chromic phosphate, progestational hormone therapy or combination chemotherapy.

Which treatment is the most appropriate remains controversial because there is not enough information about the risk for recurrence and the prognosis.

Five-Year Survival Up to 30 percent

Investigational
♦ Postoperative pelvic radiation.
♦ Pelvic and whole-abdomen radiation.
♦ Intra-abdominal radiation (radioactive phosphorus.
♦ Pelvic radiation and intravenous combination chemotherapy with cisplatin or carboplatin + Adriamycin or mitoxantrone + Cytoxan.
♦ Intravenous combination chemotherapy alone.
♦ Intra-abdominal chemotherapy (cisplatin or carboplatin).
♦ Occasionally high-dose progestational hormones.

STAGE IIIb
Vaginal metastases.

Standard Treatment This stage is generally treated by abdominal hysterectomy, removal of the tubes and ovaries on both sides, thorough staging and, occasionally, surgical excision of the metastases.

These cases are then usually treated with external beam radiation therapy to the pelvis and vagina (total dose 4,000 to

5,000 cGy given in divided doses five days a week for four to five weeks). This is followed by either a temporary cesium insertion or the placing of radioactive iridium directly into the cancer (interstitial implant). Sometimes radiation therapy precedes surgery.

Endometrial cancer that extends locally outside the uterus is usually treated with radiation therapy—five weeks of external radiation therapy to the pelvis followed by two temporary cesium insertions two weeks apart or by a radioactive iridium interstitial implant—followed by surgery, if possible.

Five-Year Survival Up to 30 percent

Investigational See Stage IIb.

STAGE IIIc
Metastases to the pelvic and/or para-aortic lymph nodes.

Standard Treatment After surgery, women with positive pelvic and negative aortic lymph nodes receive external beam pelvic radiation therapy. If the para-aortic lymph nodes are involved, most gynecologic oncologists recommend radiation therapy to the aortic region as well.

Many gynecologic oncologists also recommend adjuvant chemotherapy such as cisplatin or carboplatin, Adriamycin or Cytoxan for women with positive aortic node metastases.

Five-Year Survival Up to 30 percent

Investigational See Stage Ib

STAGE IVa
The tumor invades the bladder or rectum.

Standard Treatment Treatment of cancer involving the bladder or rectum is usually by external radiation therapy to the pelvis followed by two insertions of radioactive cesium or interstitial radiation with iridi-

um inserted directly into the tumor.

Whole-pelvis radiation therapy followed by the surgical removal of the uterus, vagina, bladder and/or rectum (pelvic exenteration) is another acceptable therapy.

Five-Year Survival Up to 5 percent

Investigational
♦ Studies are looking at the role of adjuvant chemotherapy with Adriamycin, mitoxantrone, cisplatin, Cytoxan, carboplatin, ifosfamide or progestational hormones in various doses and regimens.

STAGE IVb
Distant metastases, intra-abdominal spread or disease in the lymph nodes of the groin.

Standard Treatment Treatment is based on the location of the distant metastasis, with the most common sites being the lungs or liver. Therapy is rarely curative and is usually palliative.

There is a 20 to 30 percent response rate to progestational hormones. If the metastatic cancer or the initial uterine tumor is sensitive to progestational hormones, as shown by the number of progesterone receptors it contains, then the response rate to hormone therapy will be significantly higher. The most commonly used progestational agent is Megace. Similarly, if the tumor contains many estrogen receptors, then antiestrogen therapy with tamoxifen may be effective with a response rate of 20 to 30 percent. Sometimes the two hormones are used together.

Chemotherapy with cisplatin + Adriamycin + Cytoxan every three to four weeks has been shown to be effective in some patients, with response rates in the range of 30 percent.

Chemotherapy is frequently given with hormones to many women and is given alone to those women whose tumors are estrogen or progesterone receptor negative. Women with intra-abdominal metastases can be treated with intra-abdominal chemotherapy (cisplatin or carboplatin).

Occasionally, palliative radiation therapy may be given to a localized distant metastasis.

Five-Year Survival Up to 5 percent

Investigational
♦ Chemotherapeutic drugs given in various doses and combinations are being studied. These include cisplatin, carboplatin, Adriamycin, mitoxantrone, Cytoxan, ifosfamide, 5-fluorouracil and methotrexate with or without progestational hormones or antiestrogenic drugs.

TREATMENT FOLLOW-UP

Most gynecologic oncologists recommend a general physical and pelvic examination including a Pap smear every three months for the first two years, then every six months for another three years.
♦ The serum CA-125 level can be monitored if it was elevated before therapy.
♦ X-ray studies are done whenever specific signs and symptoms warrant.

RECURRENT CANCER

Approximately 70 percent of recurrences take place within three years of the initial therapy. Symptoms of recurrent cancer may include vaginal bleeding or dis-

charge, pain in the pelvis, abdomen, back or legs, leg swelling (edema), weight loss and chronic cough.

Local recurrences—those in the pelvic wall, vagina and the tissue surrounding the cervix and uterus (parametrium)—are the most common sites in women who have not received pelvic radiation; distant metastases to the lung, liver or abdominal cavity are more common in women who have.

Radiation therapy, if not given previously, may cure those women with a vaginal or parametrial recurrence. In women who have a localized vaginal recurrence involving the bladder or rectum, the removal of the bladder and/or rectum and vagina (total pelvic exenteration) can be curative in 40 to 50 percent of cases.

Unfortunately, most women with recurrent endometrial cancer outside the pelvis cannot be cured. But symptoms may be relieved with progestational therapy, antiestrogen therapy or chemotherapy as noted above.

THE MOST IMPORTANT QUESTIONS YOU CAN ASK
♦ What qualifications do you have for treating cancer? Will a specialist in gynecologic oncology be involved in my case?
♦ Why do I need radiation therapy?
♦ Is chemotherapy of any benefit?
♦ Can I take estrogen replacement therapy?
♦ What symptoms of recurrent cancer should I be looking for after treatment?

UTERUS: UTERINE SARCOMAS

Jeffrey L. Stern, MD

◇

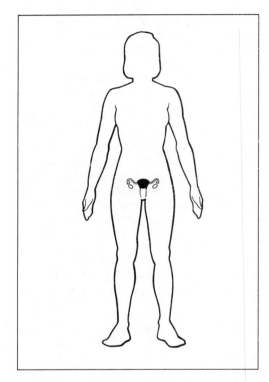

Uterine sarcomas are very rare. They are responsible for only 1 to 5 percent of all malignancies of the uterus (*see* "Uterus: Endometrial Carcinoma" for the much more common cancer of the uterus) and account for less than 1 percent of all gynecologic malignancies (*see*" Cervix", page 277).

Uterine sarcomas are treated like other uterine cancers, but the rate of cure is not high—50 to 75 percent for early-stage disease and less than 10 percent for advanced sarcomas.

Symptoms are similar to those of endometrial carcinoma, but some women are first diagnosed as having a benign uterine tumor called a fibroid. After this rapidly growing, presumably benign fibroid is surgically removed, the pathologist finds that it is a cancerous tumor.

Types There are two general categories of tumors, pure and mixed. Those pure tumors arising from the smooth muscle of the uterine wall or from a benign fibroid are known as leiomyosarcomas and account for about 30 percent of all uterine sarcomas. Leiomyosarcomas are considered benign if there are less than 5 dividing cells on microscopic examination and malignant if there are more than 10 dividing cells. If there are between 5 to 10 dividing cells, they are considered low-grade malignancies.

Another 15 percent of uterine sarcomas arise from the supporting stromal cells that surround the glands within the lining of the uterus (the endometrium) and are known as pure endometrial stromal sarcomas. They are classified according to grade, from the less virulent low-grade tumors to the extremely virulent high-grade tumors.

The most common type of uterine sarcomas—half of all cases—arise from both the endometrial glands *and* the supporting stromal cells of the endometrium. These are known as mixed mesodermal sarcomas, and are further subdivided into homologous and heterologous tumors. The homologous variety—also known as carcinosarcomas—contain malignant cells transformed from cells normally found in the uterus. The heterologous type—called malignant mixed mesodermal tumors—contain cellular elements not normally found in the uterus, including malignant bone, fat, cartilage and striated muscle.

Heterologous mixed mesodermal tumors are the most common type of uterine sarcoma and account for 1 to 3 percent of all uterine cancers. Homologous tumors are much less common.

How It Spreads Uterine sarcomas can grow locally to involve the tissue surrounding the uterus and cervix, to the rectum and bladder, to the groin, pelvic and aortic lymph nodes, to the surfaces of the abdominal cavity and distantly to the liver, lung and brain (*see* page 278).

Leiomyosarcomas spread by direct local extension, abdominal implantation or via the bloodstream. The lung is the most common site of metastases, followed by the liver, brain and bone.

Low-grade stromal sarcomas are usually slow growing and tend to remain confined to the uterus in about 70 percent of cases. Spread beyond the uterus occurs via the lymph system or via the bloodstream. High-grade stromal sarcomas spread in similar ways, but they behave much more aggressively and are usually advanced at the time of diagnosis.

What Causes It The exact cause is unknown. Like the more common endometrial carcinoma, heterologous mixed mesodermal tumors appear to be associated with diabetes, hypertension and obesity. There is also a significant association with previous pelvic radiation (10 to 30 percent of cases). The average time interval between pelvic radiation and the development of the sarcoma is 15 to 20 years.

Unlike other uterine sarcomas, leiomyosarcomas have no association with previous pelvic radiation.

RISK FACTORS

Heterologous mixed mesodermal tumors can occur in any age group, including infants, but they most commonly occur in postmenopausal women with a median age of 65. Homologous mixed mesodermal tumors can also occur in all age groups, but the median age is 57 years.

For leiomyosarcomas, the average age at diagnosis is 53.

Low-grade stromal sarcomas occur much more frequently in premenopausal women, with 70 percent occurring in women under 50. High-grade stromal sarcomas most commonly occur in postmenopausal women.

At Significantly Higher Risk
♦ Previous pelvic radiation.
♦ Women who are diabetic, hypertensive or obese.

SCREENING

Uterine sarcoma can occasionally be detected by a routine Pap smear, but screening for all uterine tumors is not as satisfactory as that for cervical cancer because of the inaccessibility of the uterine cavity. There is no screening program routinely used for women without symptoms.

COMMON SIGNS AND SYMPTOMS

With heterologous mixed mesodermal tumors, postmenopausal bleeding is the most common symptom. Abnormal uterine bleeding is also the first symptom of pure endometrial stromal sarcomas.

Most women with a leiomyosarcoma will have abnormal uterine bleeding, pressure or pain in the abdomen or pelvis, abnormal vaginal discharge or uterine fibroids, but many will have no symptoms.

DIAGNOSIS

Physical Examination
♦ A careful pelvic examination.
♦ Examination of the lymph nodes in the groin and above the collarbone.
♦ Examination of the abdomen to detect an enlarged liver, abdominal masses and excess fluid (ascites).

Blood and Other Tests
♦ Serum liver and kidney function tests.

Imaging
♦ Chest x-ray.
♦ Pelvic and abdominal CT scans to detect pelvic extension of tumor, pelvic and aortic lymph nodes and liver metastases.
♦ Pelvic MRI.

Endoscopy and Biopsy
♦ Cystoscopy and sigmoidoscopy (occasionally).
♦ The definitive diagnosis is made by a pathologist evaluating either an office endometrial biopsy, tissue removed during a D&C (dilation and curettage) or the tissue specimen after the uterus and cervix are removed (hysterectomy). Although stromal and mixed mesodermal tumors are diagnosed from an endometrial biopsy or D&C, most leiomyosarcomas are diagnosed after a hysterectomy for what is thought to be benign uterine fibroids. A preoperative diagnosis of leiomyosarcomas is uncommon.

STAGING

The International Federation of Gynecology and Obstetrics (FIGO) staging classification for uterine sarcoma is the same as that for endometrial carcinoma. Uterine sarcomas are surgically staged.

TREATMENT OVERVIEW

Surgery is the primary treatment and can lead to a cure if the tumor is confined to the uterus. Radiation and chemotherapy may also be used after surgery for some stages.

 Surgery Whenever possible, the uterus and cervix are removed (hysterectomy) along with the fallopian tubes and ovaries on both sides. The pelvic and aortic lymph nodes are selectively sampled, and fluid from the pelvis and abdomen is taken for analysis (peritoneal cytologic washings).

Complications of surgery can include infection, bleeding and, rarely, injury to the bladder, rectum or ureter causing a leak. There may be blood clots in the legs, which can occasionally dislodge and travel to the lungs (pulmonary embolism).

 Radiation External beam radiation therapy is often given to the pelvis after surgery to decrease local recurrences in early-stage disease. This does not appear to improve survival, however. Side effects of radiation can include diarrhea, nausea and vomiting, bleeding from the bladder or rectum, vaginal scarring, intestinal obstruction, or leaks (fistulas) in the urinary or intestinal tracts.

 Chemotherapy Although there is no definite proof of increased survival with adjuvant chemotherapy (treatment even if there is no obvious evidence of residual disease), many gynecologic oncologists and medical oncologists recommend its use even for early stages of disease. Metastatic sarcomas that have spread to distant organs are generally treated with chemotherapy.

TREATMENT BY CELL TYPE

MIXED MESODERMAL SARCOMAS
The prognosis depends mainly on the stage of the cancer. There does not seem to be any difference in survival between homologous and heterologous mixed mesodermal tumors.

Standard Treatment Hysterectomy, removal of tubes and ovaries on both sides, washings to check for malignant cells in the abdominal cavity and sampling of the pelvic and aortic lymph nodes on both sides.

After surgery, most women are treated with radiation therapy (total dose 4,000 to

5,000 cGy given in divided doses five days a week for five weeks) to the entire pelvis, including the upper vagina.

Chemotherapy is often used as an adjuvant therapy, although there is no documented proof of its benefit.

Investigational
♦ A clinical trial now being done by the Gynecologic Oncology Group is comparing ifosfamide with cisplatin versus ifosfamide without cisplatin for the treatment of mixed mesodermal tumors. Thirty-five percent of women respond to intravenous ifosfamide alone.
♦ Adriamycin in combination with DTIC or Cytoxan has been shown to be more effective than Adriamycin alone for advanced disease.
♦ Vincristine and Cytoxan have also been used in combination with actinomycin-D or Adriamycin, with or without DTIC, with some effectiveness.
♦ Mitoxantrone, a drug similar to Adriamycin, with ifosfamide is being studied.

LEIOMYOSARCOMA
Good prognostic factors for this tumor type include the presence of a small tumor, a tumor arising from a benign uterine fibroid (5 to 10 percent of all cases), a low number of dividing cells and being premenopausal.

Standard Treatment Abdominal hysterectomy, removal of the tubes and ovaries, washings to check for malignant cells in the abdominal cavity and selective sampling of the pelvic and aortic lymph nodes.

Any additional treatment for women with early-stage disease and less than 5 dividing cells per microscopic field has not been shown to be beneficial.

Women with 5 to 10 dividing cells are *sometimes* treated with postoperative pelvic radiation or adjuvant chemotherapy, while women with more than 10 dividing cells are *usually* given these treatments.

Postoperative whole-pelvis external beam radiation therapy (total dose 4,000 to 5,000 cGy given in divided doses five days a week for five weeks) is sometimes given to decrease the local recurrence rate in early-stage disease.

Although postoperative pelvic radiation and/or chemotherapy are often given, they have not been shown conclusively to increase survival. The most commonly used chemotherapeutic drugs include vincristine + Adriamycin or actinomycin-D + Cytoxan + DTIC.

Advanced leiomyosarcoma is treated with radiation therapy and/or chemotherapy.

Investigational
♦ Current studies include comparing postoperative pelvic radiation therapy versus no treatment, and chemotherapy.
♦ Cisplatin has been shown not to be of benefit.
♦ For women with advanced disease, Adriamycin in combination with DTIC or Cytoxan has been shown to be no more effective than Adriamycin alone.
♦ Vincristine has been used with actinomycin-D or Adriamycin and Cytoxan with or without DTIC with some effectiveness in advanced disease.
♦ Mitoxantrone, a drug similar to Adriamycin, and ifosfamide are being studied.

LOW-GRADE ENDOMETRIAL STROMAL SARCOMA
Standard Treatment As with the other types, the standard treatment for these sarcomas usually includes a hysterectomy, removal of the tubes and ovaries on both sides, selective pelvic and aortic node sampling and abdominal cytologic washings.

Early-stage disease can also be treated by a radical hysterectomy, removal of the pelvic lymph nodes and sampling of the aortic nodes, removal of the tubes and ovaries and abdominal cytologic washings.

Postoperative radiation therapy to the pelvis (4,500 to 5,000 cGy given in divided doses, five days a week for five weeks) is often given to decrease the chance of a pelvic recurrence. The frequency of recurrence depends primarily on the depth of uterine invasion.

Since these tumors frequently contain progesterone and/or estrogen receptors, hormone therapy with progestins or the antiestrogen tamoxifen is often given.

Investigational
♦ Various types and doses of progestins and antiestrogens are being studied.

HIGH-GRADE ENDOMETRIAL STROMAL SARCOMA
Standard Treatment For high grade stromal sarcomas, standard therapy is a hysterectomy, removal of the tubes and ovaries, selective pelvic and aortic node sampling and washings from the abdominal cavity to look for malignant cells.

For early-stage cancer, postoperative pelvic radiation therapy (total dose of 4,000 to 5,000 cGy given in divided doses, five days a week for five weeks) is recommended because it decreases the chance of a pelvic recurrence.

Adjuvant chemotherapy is sometimes given, but it should be considered experimental.

Investigational
♦ Since pelvic and distant recurrences are common and the prognosis of this malignancy is poor, many gynecologic oncologists and medical oncologists recommend adjuvant chemotherapy even though it has not yet been shown to be effective.
♦ Adriamycin in combination with DTIC or Cytoxan has been shown to be no more effective than Adriamycin alone.
♦ Vincristine and Cytoxan in combination with actinomycin-D or Adriamycin with or without DTIC may be somewhat effective.
♦ Mitoxantrone, a drug similar to Adriamycin, and ifosfamide are being studied.

TREATMENT BY STAGE

STAGE I
This early tumor is further divided into Stages Ia, Ib and Ic. In Stage Ia, the tumor is limited to the endometrium. In Ib, it invades the wall of the uterus by less than half of its thickness. In Ic, it invades the wall by more than half of the thickness.

Standard Treatment Surgery should include a hysterectomy, removal of both fallopian tubes and ovaries, washings from the abdominal cavity to look for malignant cells and selective sampling of the pelvic and aortic lymph nodes.

Postoperative radiation therapy is usually given to the entire pelvis (total dose 4,000 to 5,000 cGy given in divided doses, five days a week for five weeks).

Five-Year Survival 75 percent for Stage Ia, 50 percent for Stages Ib and Ic

Investigational *See* adjuvant chemotherapies under "Treatment by Cell Type."

STAGE IIa
The tumor involves the endocervical glands.

Standard Treatment Surgery as for Stage I and postoperative whole-pelvis radiation therapy.

Five-Year Survival 50 percent

Investigational Same as Stage I

STAGE IIb
Cervical stromal invasion.

Standard Treatment Surgery as for Stage I is standard. An alternative is whole-pelvis external beam radiation therapy (total dose 4,000 to 5,000 cGy given in divided doses five days a week for five weeks), followed two weeks later by the insertion of radioactive cesium into the uterus (intracavitary radiation) for one or two days. This will be followed six weeks later by the hysterectomy, removal of both tubes and ovaries, cytologic washings of the abdominal cavity and pelvic and aortic lymph node sampling.

Equally effective for young women or those in good medical condition is a radical hysterectomy, removal of both tubes and ovaries, complete removal of the pelvic lymph nodes and meticulous staging.

Five-Year Survival 50 percent

Investigational *See* adjuvant chemotherapies under "Treatment by Cell Type."

STAGE IIIa
The surface of the uterus and/or the tubes and ovaries are involved and/or there are malignant cells in the abdominal fluid (positive peritoneal washings).

Standard Treatment Surgery as for Stage I. Postoperative pelvic radiation therapy with or without whole-abdomen radiation therapy is given. Chemotherapy is also given sometimes.

Five-Year Survival 0 to 20 percent

Investigational *See* adjuvant chemotherapies under "Treatment by Cell Type."

STAGE IIIb
There are vaginal metastases.

Standard Treatment For women with vaginal metastases, the standard treatment is surgery as for Stage I cancer and postoperative external beam radiation therapy given to the whole pelvis and vagina. This is followed by one vaginal cesium insertion (a radioactive substance placed against the tumor) for one or two days or interstitial iridium (a radioactive substance placed directly into the tumor) for one or two days.

Women with disease that extends locally outside the uterus are treated with whole-pelvis radiation, one or two intracavitary cesium or interstitial iridium insertions, followed by surgery whenever possible.

Five-Year Survival 0 to 10 percent

Investigational *See* adjuvant chemotherapies under "Treatment by Cell Type."
♦ Interstitial radiation therapy with heat (hyperthermia) is being studied.

STAGE IIIc
Metastases to the pelvic and para-aortic lymph nodes.

Standard Treatment Surgery as for Stage I. Postoperative pelvic radiation therapy and radiation to the aortic lymph nodes (if they are involved) is usually given. Chemotherapy is sometimes given as well.

Five-Year Survival 0 to 10 percent

Investigational See adjuvant chemotherapies under "Treatment by Cell Type."

STAGE IVa
The tumor invades the bladder or rectum.

Standard Treatment Options include external beam radiation therapy to the entire pelvis and intracavitary or interstitial radiation therapy (in one or two insertions). Occasionally, the uterus, vagina, bladder and/or rectum are removed (pelvic exenteration).

Five-Year Survival 0 to 5 percent

Investigational
♦ Adjuvant chemotherapy.
♦ Interstitial radiation therapy with heat (hyperthermia) is under investigation.

STAGE IVb
There are distant metastases, with spread to organs within the abdomen and/or disease in the groin lymph nodes.

Standard Treatment Metastatic sarcomas are usually treated with chemotherapy. Commonly used drugs include Adriamycin or ifosfamide alone and the combinations of vincristine + actinomycin-D or Adriamycin + Cytoxan + DTIC.

Five-Year Survival 0 to 5 percent

Investigational
♦ Various doses and combinations of chemotherapy drugs are being evaluated.
♦ Mitoxantrone, a drug similar to Adriamycin, is being studied.

TREATMENT FOLLOW-UP

A general physical and pelvic examination is performed every three months for the first two years after treatment, then every six months for the next three years.
♦ A Pap smear is performed at each visit.
♦ Diagnostic x-ray studies are performed as specific symptoms and signs warrant.

RECURRENT CANCER

Uterine sarcomas usually recur within three years of treatment and may develop in the vagina, pelvis, lymph nodes, liver and lungs. Recurrences of leiomyosarcomas are usually distant, with only 5 percent confined to the pelvis. Recurrences of low-grade stromal sarcomas can occur late, sometimes 10 years after initial treatment. Although pelvic recurrences are the most common, it can recur in the abdominal cavity or in the lungs.

Common symptoms of recurrent cancer include vaginal bleeding or discharge, pain in the pelvis, abdomen, back or legs, swelling in the legs or abdomen, chronic cough or weight loss.

Treatment There is no standard therapy for recurrent disease.
♦ Chemotherapy has been used with variable effectiveness but rarely leads to a cure.
♦ Women with localized disease in the pelvis sometimes benefit from radiation therapy and occasionally by the removal of the pelvic organs (pelvic exenteration).
♦ Women with low-grade endometrial stromal sarcomas might benefit from progestational hormone or antiestrogen therapy.

THE MOST IMPORTANT QUESTIONS YOU CAN ASK

♦ What qualifications do you have for treating cancer? Are you a specialist in gynecologic oncology?
♦ What kind of sarcoma do I have?
♦ What is the stage?
♦ What benefit is there to having radiation therapy after surgery?
♦ Is there any benefit from chemotherapy?

VAGINA

Jeffrey L. Stern, MD

◇

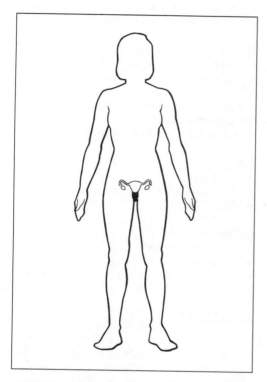

Carcinoma of the vagina is a relatively uncommon disease, affecting only about 2,000 women in the United States each year. It accounts for only 1 to 2 percent of all gynecologic malignancies. Cancer arising in another organ that spreads to the vagina is much more common.

Types The most common type of vaginal cancer develops in the surface (squamous) cells lining the vagina. About 85 percent of all vaginal cancers are squamous cell tumors. About 5 percent develop in glandular tissues (adenocarcinoma). Other cell types include melanoma (3 percent), sar-

comas (3 percent) and endodermal sinus tumor (1 percent).

Squamous cell carcinomas, leiomyosarcomas and melanomas generally arise in older women. Adenocarcinomas and rhabdomyosarcomas usually occur during adolescence. The very rare sarcoma botryoides and endodermal sinus tumors most frequently occur in infants.

How It Spreads Squamous cell carcinomas that originate in the skin lining of the vagina can remain confined to the lining for some time. At this stage it is known as vaginal intraepithelial neoplasia (VAIN) or dysplasia. Eventually it will invade the vaginal wall. With time, the tumor can extend directly to the tissue surrounding the vagina, the pelvic walls, the bladder or the rectum.

Lymphatic invasion and metastases is another avenue of spread. Carcinomas arising in the upper vagina can spread to the pelvic lymph nodes, and those in the lower vagina can spread to the lymph nodes in the groin.

Adenocarcinomas spread in a similar fashion, but they may have a higher incidence of metastases to the pelvic lymph nodes (*see* "Cervix", page 277).

What Causes It The human papilloma virus (HPV), a sexually transmitted virus responsible for genital warts, is believed to cause vaginal intraepithelial neoplasia and invasive squamous cell carcinoma of the vagina. The time from infection to the development of an invasive cancer is thought to be from 5 to 10 years.

Most cases of adenocarcinoma of the

vagina used to be associated with exposure to diethylstilbestrol (DES) in embryonic life. DES was given in the 1950s to women who were thought to be at risk for a miscarriage. The incidence of DES-related adenocarcinoma is highest for those women who were exposed during the first three months of their mother's pregnancy. The peak incidence is between age 17 and 21. The incidence of this disease peaked in the early 1970s and is now uncommon, since DES use during pregnancy fell out of favor during the 1960s and was banned in the early 1970s.

What causes other vaginal tumors is not clear.

RISK FACTORS

Squamous cell carcinoma of the vagina is associated with a previous history of genital warts or of intraepithelial or invasive carcinoma of the cervix or vulva. In 10 to 20 percent of women with squamous cell carcinoma of the vagina, there is a history of vaginal radiation therapy, usually for a cervical cancer.

SCREENING

Screening for malignancies of the vagina is similar to screening for cervical cancer. A careful annual pelvic examination and Pap smear is recommended. Women who have been exposed to DES are followed more carefully with twice-yearly pelvic examinations, Pap smears of the cervix and vaginal wall and colposcopic (magnification) examination of the vagina.

COMMON SIGNS AND SYMPTOMS

The most common symptoms are abnormal vaginal bleeding and a foul-smelling vaginal discharge. There may be pain in the pelvis, back or legs, as well as leg swelling (edema).

DIAGNOSIS

Physical Examination
♦ A careful gynecologic, pelvic and rectal examination is performed to assess the local spread of the cancer.
♦ Examination of the lymph nodes in the groin and neck and an abdominal examination are important to detect masses.

Blood and Other Tests
♦ Complete blood count (CBC).
♦ Serum carcinoembryonic antigen (CEA).
♦ Serum alpha-fetoprotein (for an endodermal sinus tumor).
♦ Serum kidney and liver function tests.

Imaging
♦ Chest x-ray.
♦ CT scan of the pelvis and abdomen.
♦ MRI of the pelvis.

Endoscopy and Biopsy
♦ Cystourethroscopy.
♦ Proctosigmoidoscopy.
♦ The cancer is confirmed by a vaginal biopsy.

STAGING

Vaginal carcinoma is staged by either the FIGO system (International Federation of Gynecologists and Obstetricians) or the TNM classification. In the TNM system, N1 indicates pelvic lymph node metastases when the upper two-thirds of the vagina is involved or groin node metastases on one side when the lower two-thirds of the vagina is involved. N2 indicates groin node metastases on both sides.

TREATMENT OVERVIEW

Several factors are considered in choosing the most appropriate way to manage vaginal cancer, including the cell type, stage, size, location of the lesion, presence or absence of the uterus and whether the woman has had previous radiation to the pelvis.

Early carcinomas are generally treated with either surgery or radiation therapy— external radiation and one or two insertions of radioactive cesium placed against the cancer (intracavitary) or radioactive iridium placed directly into the cancer (interstitial radiation). The total dose of 4,000 to 5,000 cGy is given in divided doses to the pelvis five days a week for five weeks.

Advanced cancers are treated with radiation therapy alone or with the simultaneous administration of combination chemotherapy.

If the serum CEA or AFP (for endodermal sinus tumors) was elevated before therapy, it can be checked periodically to assess response to treatment or detect recurrent disease.

TREATMENT BY STAGE

STAGE 0 (*squamous cell carcinoma*)
TNM Tis, N0, M0
Carcinoma in situ or intraepithelial carcinoma.

Standard Treatment There are a number of effective treatments, including the partial or complete removal of the vagina (vaginectomy), which occasionally requires a skin graft. The tumor may also be treated with laser therapy, intravaginal chemotherapy with 5-fluorouracil cream or intracavitary radiation with a cesium implant.

Five-Year Survival 100 percent

Investigational None.

STAGE I (*squamous cell carcinoma or adenocarcinoma*)
TNM T1, N0, M0
The carcinoma is limited to the vaginal wall.

Standard Treatment Young women with lesions involving the upper third of the

vagina can be treated by a radical vaginectomy, radical hysterectomy and removal of the pelvic lymph nodes on both sides.

Equally effective for all Stage I tumors, regardless of age and site, are external beam radiation therapy and intracavitary or interstitial radiation therapy. Smaller lesions are sometimes treated with only intracavitary or interstitial radiation therapy.

Five-Year Survival 70 to 80 percent

Investigational
♦ Meticulous surgical staging before radiation therapy.
♦ Chemotherapy given simultaneously with radiation therapy. Chemotherapeutic regimens under investigation include mitomycin-C + 5-fluorouracil (5-FU) with or without cisplatin.
♦ Radiation therapy with heat (hyperthermia).

STAGE II (*squamous cell carcinoma and adenocarcinoma*)
TNM T2, N0, M0
The carcinoma involves the adjacent vaginal tissue but has not extended to the pelvic wall.

Standard Treatment External beam radiation and interstitial or intracavitary radiation.

Five-Year Survival About 50 percent

Investigational Same as Stage I.

STAGE III and STAGE IVa (*squamous cell carcinoma and adenocarcinoma*)
TNM T3 (or less), N1, M0 or T3, N0, M0 (Stage III)
The carcinoma has extended to the pelvic wall.
TNM Any T, N2, M0 or T4, N0, M0 (Stage IVa)

The carcinoma has extended beyond the true pelvis or involves the lining of the bladder or rectum.

Standard Treatment These carcinomas are generally treated with external beam, intracavitary or interstitial radiation therapy. Surgery is an option in selected cases.

Five-Year Survival About 30 percent for Stage III, about 10 percent for Stage IVa

Investigational Same as Stage I.

STAGE IVb
TNM Any T, any N, M1
There is spread to distant organs.

Standard Treatment Neither radiation nor surgery can cure women with distant metastases, but both are used for local relief of symptoms.

A number of chemotherapy regimens that are effective in the treatment of metastatic cervical cancer are also used to treat metastatic vaginal cancers—cisplatin, carboplatin and the combinations of mitomycin-C + vincristine + bleomycin + cisplatin and cisplatin + ifosfamide + etoposide.

Five-Year Survival Less than 10 percent

Investigational
♦ Various doses and combinations of chemotherapeutic drugs are being evaluated, including cisplatin, carboplatin, ifosfamide, etoposide, mitomycin-C, 5-FU, vincristine, vinblastine, mitoxantrone, bleomycin and methotrexate.

TREATING OTHER CELL TYPES

Endodermal Sinus Tumors These are extremely rare and are treated with surgery and combination chemotherapy programs such as cisplatin + bleomycin + etoposide.

Vaginal Sarcomas Sarcomas of the botryoid type are treated with chemotherapy, including vincristine, actinomycin-D, Cytoxan and dacarbazine (DTIC) followed by surgery or radiation therapy as indicated.

Malignant Melanoma These tumors are generally treated by aggressive surgery, but the overall survival rate is extremely poor—less than 15 percent. Advanced melanomas are treated with chemotherapy regimens including dacarbazine (DTIC) + cisplatin + Cytoxan + tamoxifen (*see* "Melanoma").

TREATMENT FOLLOW-UP

After therapy, women are followed every three months with a careful general physical examination, pelvic examination and Pap smear.
♦ A chest x-ray or an abdominal or pelvic CT scan may be obtained if symptoms warrant.
♦ If the serum CEA and/or AFP were elevated before therapy, they can be followed to detect recurrent disease.

RECURRENT CANCER

Vaginal cancer can recur in the vagina, pelvis, liver, lungs and lymph nodes. Symptoms of recurrent disease include weight loss, vaginal or rectal bleeding, bleeding from the urinary tract, pain in the pelvis, back or leg, leg swelling and the development of a chronic cough.
♦ If the tumor is confined to the vagina, bladder and/or rectum, a recurrent vaginal carcinoma may be treated by the removal of the vagina, bladder and/or rectum (pelvic exenteration).
♦ Locally recurrent unresectable and/or metastatic disease is treated with single chemotherapeutic drugs such as cisplatin or carboplatin, or combination chemotherapeutic drug regimens such as mitomycin-C + vincristine + bleomycin + cisplatin, or carboplatin/or cisplatin + ifosfamide + etoposide.

Investigational
♦ Various doses and combinations of the different chemotherapeutic drugs are being studied, including cisplatin, carboplatin, ifosfamide, etoposide, mitomycin-C, 5-FU, vincristine, vinblastine, mitoxantrone, bleomycin and methotrexate.

THE MOST IMPORTANT QUESTIONS YOU CAN ASK
♦ What qualifications do you have for treating cancer?
♦ Will a gynecologic oncologist be involved in my care?
♦ What stage of cancer do I have?
♦ What is the cell type?
♦ Was the cancer related to DES (diethylstilbestrol)?
♦ Will concurrent chemotherapy be of value in the treatment of my cancer?
♦ What signs and symptoms should I look for after I've been treated?

VULVA

Jeffrey L. Stern, MD

◇

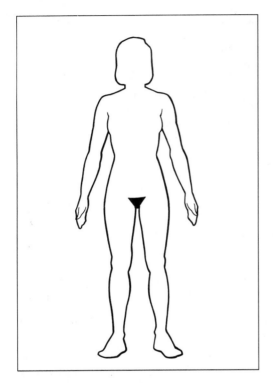

Malignant tumors of the vulva account for 3 to 5 percent of all cancers of the female genital tract and are easily cured when diagnosed at an early stage. And, because of better access to routine gynecologic care, these cancers are being diagnosed at an earlier stage.

Surgery has long been the mainstay of treatment, but views about the extent of surgery have changed over the years. In the 1940s, it was noted that the failure rate was much higher with conservative surgical measures. Since then, more radical operations have been performed with a marked improvement in the survival rate. But recently, as younger women with earlier disease are diagnosed with vulvar cancer, there has been a trend toward more conservative surgery with a greater emphasis on limiting the psychosexual consequences of therapy and preserving the normal female genital anatomy. Similarly, there has been a recent trend toward using local radiation therapy with chemotherapy in advanced cases either to reduce the amount of surgery needed or to improve the chance that the tumor can be removed.

Types Squamous cell carcinomas account for about 86 percent of all vulvar malignancies. Melanoma accounts for another 6 percent, adenocarcinoma of the Bartholin's gland for 4 percent, sarcomas for 2 percent, basal cell carcinoma for 2 percent and Paget's disease for 0.5 percent of all vulvar cancers.

Some physicians believe that the grade of the tumor cells as seen under the microscope is also significant. Immature, or undifferentiated, cells are more virulent and aggressive. Grade 1 (mature, or well-differentiated) cancers have a better prognosis than Grade 3 (poorly differentiated) tumors.

How It Spreads Squamous cell carcinoma arises in the skin of the genitalia and stays confined to the skin for an estimated 1 to 10 years. (At this stage, it is referred to as a carcinoma in situ or vulvar intraepithelial neoplasia—VIN.) Eventually it becomes invasive. With time it becomes locally destructive, growing to involve the urethra, vagina and the anus. It can also spread through the lymphatic system to the lymph nodes in the groin, then to the lymph nodes in the pelvis. Distant metastases, most frequently to the lungs and liver, are relatively rare (*see* "Cervix", page 277).

What Causes It Like carcinoma of the cervix, the risk factors for the development of vulvar cancer are primarily related to the likelihood of exposure to the sexually transmitted human papilloma virus (HPV).

RISK FACTORS

♦ The vast majority of women with invasive vulvar carcinoma are postmenopausal. But there has been a definite trend over the past two decades of an increasing incidence of carcinoma in situ and invasive squamous cell carcinoma in younger women. Forty percent of women with carcinoma in situ are under 40 years old.
♦ Five to ten percent of women with invasive vulvar carcinoma have a history of genital warts, and 15 percent have a history of or subsequent diagnosis of a cancer confined to the skin (carcinoma in situ) or invasive carcinoma of the cervix.
♦ Approximately 80 percent of the invasive squamous lesions of the vulva are associated with human papilloma virus types 16 or 18.
♦ Other sexually transmitted diseases such as syphilis, lymphogranuloma venereum and herpes simplex virus II also increase the risk for vulvar carcinoma.
♦ There is a higher incidence in women from lower socioeconomic groups, women with multiple partners and women with a history of infectious vulvitis or a history of vulvar dystrophy (abnormal benign or premalignant skin changes).

SCREENING

Careful visual and manual inspection of the external genitalia during an annual gynecologic examination is important. Women with a diagnosis of an HPV-related infection of any portion of the lower genital tract should undergo a careful col-poscopic (magnification) examination of the entire lower genital tract.

COMMON SIGNS AND SYMPTOMS

The most common signs and symptoms are a lump or an ulcer, itching, pain, burning, bleeding and discharge. Unfortunately, many women do not get medical attention when these signs appear. At the time of diagnosis, two out of three women with vulvar carcinoma have had symptoms for more than six months and one out of three has had symptoms for more than a year.

DIAGNOSIS

Physical Examination
♦ Careful visual and manual inspection of the external genitalia, anus and groin lymph nodes is crucial.
♦ Because of the association with precancerous and cancerous lesions of the cervix and vagina, a careful pelvic examination is also necessary.
♦ The majority of squamous cell carcinomas arise on the labia majora and minora and are frequently associated with vulvar dystrophy. The clitoris, outer vagina and the skin between the vagina and anus (perineum) may also be involved

Endoscopy and Biopsy
♦ The definitive diagnosis is made on a biopsy, sometimes under colposcopic direction (magnification) for smaller lesions.
♦ Upon diagnosis, a metastatic work-up is done, including a chest x-ray, CT scan of the pelvis and abdomen (occasionally), cystoscopy and proctoscopy (occasionally), a complete blood count and serum liver and kidney function tests.

STAGING

Staging is based on physical findings and x-ray results. Both the FIGO (Federation of International Gynecologists and Obstetricians) and the TNM classifications are used to stage vulvar cancer.

TREATMENT OVERVIEW

The prognosis for vulvar cancer depends on several factors—cell type, stage (which emphasizes local tumor extent), the presence or absence of groin node metastases, the size of the lesion, the depth of invasion, whether blood or lymphatic vessels are involved, the grade of the tumor and the pattern of invasion.

At diagnosis, about 35 percent of all vulvar carcinomas are Stage I, 30 percent of women have Stage II, 25 percent have Stage III and 10 percent have Stage IV disease. The overall five-year survival rate for all women with invasive squamous cell carcinoma of the vulva is 69 percent.

Surgery The standard therapy for the past four decades has been radical surgical excision of the vulva and the removal of the lymph nodes in the groin and, occasionally, the pelvis. External beam radiation therapy is frequently given to the groin and pelvis after surgery to women with positive groin and/or pelvic lymph nodes on one or both sides.

Over the past 15 years, less radical surgery and the removal of the groin nodes on one side has been shown to be equally effective in small, early-stage disease. Despite this trend toward conservative therapy, experience has taught that limiting surgery because of advanced age or frailty can result in overwhelming problems with locally advanced recurrent cancer in women who have lived longer than expected.

A radical vulvectomy and groin dissection is extraordinarily well tolerated and can be done in phases if the patient's medical condition warrants. Whether sexual function returns depends on the extent of

surgery and radiation therapy. Sexual function is also surprisingly more satisfactory than one would think.

Complications of radical surgery for vulvar cancer include wound breakdown or infection, chronic leg swelling, collection of lymphatic fluid in the groin (lymphocyst), scarring of the vaginal opening, vaginal or uterine prolapse, loss of urine when coughing (stress incontinence), blood clots in the leg that can dislodge and go to the lung (pulmonary embolism, which occurs in 1 to 3 percent of women), and death (approximately 1 to 2 percent).

 Chemotherapy and Radiotherapy In recent years, chemotherapy has been used in combination with local external beam radiation therapy and occasionally with interstitial radiation, in which radioactive iridium is temporarily placed directly into the cancer. This treatment has been used for women with advanced cancers, allowing subsequent surgical removal of the tumor or the preservation of the bladder or anus.

Currently, there is no standard chemotherapy for advanced or recurrent cancer, but drugs that are sometimes effective for other squamous cell carcinomas of the genital tract—such as cisplatin, mitomycin-C, 5-fluorouracil (5-FU), Cytoxan and bleomycin—have been used with some success.

TREATMENT BY STAGE

STAGE 0
TNM Tis, N0, M0
Vulvar carcinoma in situ, also known as intraepithelial carcinoma.

Standard Treatment Standard therapy has been either wide local excision or laser therapy. Occasionally a partial or total vulvectomy is performed with or without skin grafting.

Five-Year Survival 100 percent

Investigational None.

STAGE I
TNM T1, N0, M0
The tumor is confined to vulva and/or perineum, is less than 3/4 in. (2 cm) in diameter and there are no nodal metastases.

Standard Treatment For Grade 1 lesions with less than 2 mm of invasion or Grade 2 lesions with less than 1 mm of invasion and no vascular involvement, a wide local excision is adequate therapy.

For lesions that are clearly on one side of the vulva, a radical local excision with a complete groin node dissection on the same side is performed.

For other Stage I cancers involving the skin between the vaginal opening or the anus or clitoris, a radical vulvectomy and groin lymph node dissection on both sides is performed.

Five-Year Survival Over 90 percent

Investigational
♦ Conservative surgery.
♦ Treatment with radiation therapy with or without chemotherapy (5-FU + mitomycin-C + cisplatin).

STAGE II
TNM T2, N0, M0
The tumor is confined to the vulva and/or perineum and is more than 3/4 in. (2 cm) in diameter but has not spread to lymph nodes.

Standard Treatment Radical vulvectomy with removal of the groin lymph nodes on both sides.

Five-Year Survival 80 percent, up to 90 percent for those patients with surgically negative groin nodes

Investigational Same as Stage I.

STAGE III
TNM T3 or less, N1 or less, M0
The tumor may be of any size with either adjacent spread to the vagina, urethra or anus or metastases to the groin lymph nodes on one side.

Standard Treatment Radical vulvectomy with groin lymph node dissection on both sides is the standard therapy. Sometimes, a pelvic lymph node dissection is done at the time of surgery if the groin lymph nodes are positive.

External beam radiation therapy is frequently given postoperatively to the groin and pelvis if there are groin lymph node metastases. With two or more pathologically positive groin nodes, there has been a significantly better survival rate with pelvic radiation than with pelvic lymph node dissection in a study conducted by the Gynecologic Oncology Group.

Women with large vulvar lesions who have only a small margin of normal tissue around the tumor on microscopic examination of the surgical specimen may be treated with postoperative external beam radiation therapy to the remaining genital skin.

Five-year Survival About 50 percent

Investigational
♦ Preoperative external beam and interstitial radiation therapy (radioactive substances inserted directly into the tumor for one to two days) with or without chemotherapy (5-FU + mitomycin-C + cisplatin).
♦ Radiation therapy and heat (hyperthermia) have been used to improve resectability and to decrease the amount of surgery necessary in women with large cancers or cancers involving the urethra or anus.

STAGE IVa
TNM Any T, N2, M0 or T4, N0, M0
The tumor may involve the upper urethra, the bladder mucosa, the rectal mucosa, the

pelvic bone, and/or there are bilateral groin node metastases.

Standard Treatment Options include:
♦ Radical vulvectomy, removal of the lymph nodes on both sides and removal of the vagina, bladder and/or rectum (pelvic exenteration).
♦ Surgery followed by radiation therapy in those with close surgical margins.
♦ Radiation therapy with combination chemotherapy (5-FU + mitomycin-C + cisplatin), occasionally followed by radical surgery.

Five-Year Survival About 15 percent

Investigational
♦ External beam radiation therapy and interstitial radiation therapy with or without heat (hyperthermia) and with or without various doses and kinds of chemotherapeutic drugs are being evaluated.

STAGE IVb
TNM Any T, any N, M1a or M1b.
There are distant metastases including pelvic lymph nodes.

Standard Treatment Vulvar cancer that has spread to distant sites is treated with chemotherapy, but there is no standard chemotherapeutic regimen. Cisplatin, carboplatin, methotrexate, vincristine and bleomycin are all commonly used drugs.

Usually palliative local surgical removal or radiation therapy to the vulva is done for local symptom relief.

Women with metastases to the pelvic nodes are treated with pelvic external beam radiation therapy.

Five-Year Survival From 5 percent (metastases to the lungs or liver) to 25 percent (metastases to the pelvic lymph nodes)

Investigational
♦ Ifosfamide, carboplatin, 5-FU, mitomycin-C, methotrexate, vincristine,

bleomycin and cisplatin in various combinations and doses are being investigated.

RECURRENT CANCER

Recurrences are more common in women with large lesions or if treatment involved limited surgery. They usually occur within the first three years after treatment. The recurrence may be anywhere on the remaining external genitalia, in the groin or pelvic nodes or at distant sites. Symptoms of recurrent cancer may include bleeding, pain in the genitals, groin, pelvis or legs, leg swelling (edema), weight loss, chronic cough and chest pain.

Treatment options include wide local excision (for a local recurrence), radical local excision, pelvic exenteration, external beam radiation therapy, interstitial radiation therapy and chemotherapy.

TREATING OTHER VULVAR MALIGNANCIES

MALIGNANT MELANOMA OF THE VULVA
Although relatively rare, this is the second most common type of vulvar cancer. It occurs most commonly in women around the age of menopause and in postmenopausal women.

More than 80 percent of melanomas arise from the labia minora and clitoris. Most women seek medical attention because of itching, bleeding or a lump. Superficially spreading melanomas and mucocutaneous melanomas account for approximately 60 percent and 10 percent respectively of all vulvar melanomas and are somewhat slow growing until invasion occurs. Thirty percent are nodular melanomas, which behave much more aggressively.

Standard Treatment Radical vulvectomy and bilateral groin node dissection is the standard therapy, although over the past few years there has been a trend toward more conservative surgery.

Melanomas that are less than 0.7 mm in thickness without vascular space involvement can be treated by a wide local excision with a 3/4 in. (2 cm) skin margin, without a groin dissection.

The role of a pelvic lymph node dissection has not been determined, but if the groin nodes are involved, a pelvic lymph node dissection may be performed. The prognosis and survival is determined in large part by the depth of invasion and whether there are metastases.

Five-Year Survival 40 to 80 percent depending on the stage and the depth of invasion

BASAL CELL CARCINOMA
This type of vulvar cancer invades adjacent tissues but rarely metastasizes. It has an excellent cure rate and is managed with only a wide local excision.

ADENOCARCINOMA OF THE VULVA
This is a rare tumor and generally arises from the Bartholin's gland, located at the opening of the vagina. Survival is related to stage. Treatment is usually radical vulvectomy and bilateral groin node dissection.

PAGET'S DISEASE
This occurs most commonly in postmenopausal white women. Intense itching is the most common symptom.

About 30 percent of Paget's disease is associated with an underlying invasive adenocarcinoma, and for these the prognosis is quite poor. But Paget's disease confined to the vulvar skin has an excellent prognosis with only rare instances of subsequent invasion or death.

If there is no underlying adenocarcinoma, a wide local excision or total vulvectomy is all that is required.

If there is an underlying adenocarcinoma, radical vulvectomy and bilateral groin dissection is usually performed.

VULVAR SARCOMAS
These account for only 1 to 2 percent of all vulvar malignancies. The majority of vulvar sarcomas arise from the smooth muscle and are known as leiomyosarcomas.

Treatment is usually radical surgery followed by radiation therapy.

THE MOST IMPORTANT QUESTIONS YOU CAN ASK
♦ What type of cancer do I have?
♦ Is a radical vulvectomy and removal of the groin lymph nodes on both sides necessary if I have Stage I disease?
♦ Is there a role for radiation therapy with or without chemotherapy for my cancer?
♦ What is my prognosis?
♦ What qualifications do you have for treating cancer? Will a gynecologic oncologist be involved in my care?

GLOSSARY OF MEDICAL TERMS
Malin Dollinger, MD

◇

A

Absolute neutrophil count (ANC)
The actual count of the white blood cells (also called polys) that engulf and destroy bacteria. There is some concern about infection if the count is less than 1,000.

Acupressure
The use of finger pressure over various points on the body (the same points used in acupuncture) to treat symptoms or disease.

Adenocarcinoma
Cancer that arises from glandular tissues. Examples include cancers of the breast, lung, thyroid, colon and pancreas.

Adenoma
A benign (non-malignant) tumor that arises from glandular tissues, such as the breast, lung, thyroid, colon and pancreas.

Adjuvant chemotherapy
Chemotherapy used along with surgery or radiation therapy. It is usually given after all visible and known cancer has been removed by surgery or radiotherapy, but is sometimes given before surgery (neoadjuvant). Adjuvant chemotherapy is usually used in cases where there is a high risk of hidden cancer cells remaining and may increase the likelihood of cure by destroying small amounts of undetectable cancer.

Alkaline phosphatase
A blood enzyme commonly used in medical diagnosis. It is elevated in cases of bile obstruction (liver disease or cancer involving the liver) and in various bone diseases, including cancer involving bone. A variation of this test can distinguish between elevations due to bone and liver disease.

Alkylating agents
A family of anticancer drugs that combine with a cancer cell's DNA to prevent normal cell division.

Allogeneic transplant
A form of transplantation or transfer of a tissue—bone marrow, for example—from one individual to another. It is preferable that the tissue types match, but this is not always possible.

Alopecia
Partial or complete loss of hair. This may result from radiotherapy to the head (hair may not completely return after therapy) or from certain chemotherapeutic agents (hair always returns).

Alpha-fetoprotein
A protein that is elevated in the blood of patients with certain forms of cancer, such as liver or testis.

Ambulatory care
The use of outpatient facilities—doctors' offices, home care, outpatient hospital clinics and day-care facilities—to provide modern medical care without the need for hospitalization.

Ambulatory infusion
The administration of chemotherapy by a small pump device usually worn under the clothes. The pump delivers anticancer drugs slowly and gradually, with minimal or no side effects. Since there is no need to remain in the hospital or even at home, this method allows patients to work and carry on with their normal activities.

Amenorrhea
The temporary or permanent lack of menstrual periods. This may be a normal part of the menopause or is sometimes brought on by severe physical or emotional stresses. Some anticancer drugs can produce amenorrhea, especially if the woman is near the age when menopause would normally occur.

Amino acids
The building blocks of proteins, analogous to the freight cars making up a train.

Analgesic
A drug that relieves pain. Analgesics may be mild (aspirin or acetaminophen), stronger (codeine) or very strong (morphine). There are also a large number of mild, moderate or strong synthetic analgesics.

Anaplastic
A tumor that appears "wild" under the microscope, having no resemblance to the normal tissue of the organ involved. It is usually possi-

ble to tell where anaplastic tumors originate only by where the biopsy was taken or, knowing the area of involvement, by inference.

Anastomosis
The point where two hollow organs are joined together. In cancer therapy it usually refers to joining two portions of the bowel after a segment containing cancer has been removed.

Androgens
Male sex hormones. Testosterone is produced naturally and there are several synthetic ones used in treatment.

Anemia
Having less than the normal amount of hemoglobin or red cells in the blood. This may be due to bleeding, lack of blood production by the bone marrow or to the brief survival of blood already manufactured. Symptoms include tiredness, shortness of breath and weakness.

Aneuploid
Tumor cells that do not have the normal number of chromosomes—46—in a human cell. Tumor cells that do have 46 chromosomes are called euploid. Aneuploid tumors often have a worse prognosis.

Angiography
The taking of x-ray pictures of blood vessels by injecting a radio-opaque contrast agent into the blood vessel. Angiograms may be taken to determine a tumor's blood supply before surgery, to place a catheter or infusion pump or to determine the site for other intra-arterial procedures.

Antibody
A protein (gamma globulin) made by the body in response to a specific foreign protein, or antigen. The antigen may result from an infection, a cancer or some other source. If the same alien substance attacks again, the white blood cells are able to recognize it and reproduce the specific antibody to fight it.

Antiemetics
Drugs given to prevent or minimize nausea and vomiting.

Antigens
Substances that cause activation of the immune system.

Antimetabolites
A family of antitumor drugs that resemble normal vitamins or building blocks of metabolism. They bind to the tumor's enzymes and chemical pathways. The tumor cells "think" they are

getting the real vitamin and starve to the point where they can't grow or multiply.

Asbestosis
Scarring of the lungs and the lining of the chest cavity from the inhalation of asbestos dust. This increases the risk of lung cancer and cancer of the chest cavity lining (mesothelioma).

Ascites
An abnormal fluid collection in the abdomen from cancer or other causes.

Aspiration
Removal of fluid or tissue, usually with a needle or tube, from a specific area of the body. This procedure may be done to obtain a diagnosis or to relieve symptoms.

Atrophy
A withering or reduction in size of a tissue or a part of the body. This may result from lack of use during immobilization or prolonged bedrest or from pressure from an adjacent tumor.

Atypical
Not usual or ordinary. For example, cancer is the result of atypical cell division.

Autoimmunity
A condition in which the body's immune system fights and rejects its own tissues.

Autologous transplant
Removal of a patient's own tissue, especially bone marrow, and its return to the same patient after chemotherapy. This might more correctly be called bone marrow reinfusion rather than transplantation.

Autosomal
A non-sex-linked method of inheritance. The inherited characteristic does not depend on whether the person is male or female since the gene in question is not found on the sex (X or Y) chromosomes.

Axilla
The armpit. Lymph glands in the armpit are called the axillary nodes.

B

Barium enema
An x-ray study of the colon (large bowel) in which the patient is given an enema of a liquid barium mixture before the x-rays are taken. Laxatives and/or regular enemas are usually required beforehand.

Barium swallow
An x-ray study of the portion of the digestive

canal between the throat and stomach (esophagus) in which the patient swallows a barium mixture while the radiologist watches for signs of narrowing, irregularity or blockage. No preparation is required except fasting. Sometimes, in a procedure called an upper gastrointestinal (UGI) series, the barium is also observed after it enters the stomach to check for stomach problems or ulcers.

Basal cell carcinoma
A form of skin cancer that grows very slowly and is curable in almost all cases by surgery or other local treatment. The growth may be so slow that malignancy is not at first suspected.

B cell
Lymphocytes are the cells in the body that are intimately involved in the immune response. They occur in the blood, in lymph nodes and in various organs. The two types of lymphocytes are B cells and T cells. Special techniques are needed to tell them apart because they look the same when viewed by ordinary methods under the microscope. It may be essential to make this distinction in cases of lymphomas, since the treatment and prognosis of B cell lymphomas may be very different than that of T cell lymphomas.

BCG
A material prepared from killed bird tuberculosis bacteria. This has been widely used, especially in Europe, to vaccinate health care workers who work closely with tuberculosis patients and has been used in cancer treatment to stimulate the immune system.

Benign
A tumor that has no tendency to grow into surrounding tissues or spread to other parts of the body. In other words, it is not malignant. Under the microscope, a benign tumor does not resemble cancer.

Bilateral
Occurring on both sides of the body.

Biologic response modifiers
Substances or agents that may have a direct antitumor effect, and also affects tumors indirectly by stimulating or triggering the immune system to fight cancer. Examples include interferon, IL-2 and LAK cells.

Biopsy
The surgical removal of a small portion of tissue for diagnosis. In almost all cases a biopsy diagnosis of cancer is required before appro-

priate and correct treatment planning can take place. In some cases a needle biopsy may be enough for diagnosis, but in others the removal of a pea-sized wedge of tissue is needed. In many cases, the biopsy may be the first step of the definitive surgical procedure that not only proves the diagnosis but attempts to cure the cancer by removing the tumor.

Blastic
A bone lesion that appears on an x-ray to have more calcium (density) than normal.

Bleeding disorders
Blood clotting is a complex process involving the interaction of many substances in the blood that promote coagulation. A deficiency of any of these substances results in a bleeding disorder. Some disorders are inherited (hemophilia, for example) and some (such as liver disease) are acquired. A common disorder associated with cancer is a low platelet count (thrombocytopenia), which sometimes results from chemotherapy or radiotherapy and may make platelet transfusions necessary until the process subsides. Sophisticated tests are often needed to diagnose bleeding disorders.

Blood-brain barrier
A microscopic structure in the brain that separates blood capillaries from nerve cells. This prevents some substances from entering the brain. Many cancer chemotherapeutic agents, for example, cannot be used to treat brain tumors because they cannot pass through the barrier. Some others (CCNU, BCNU) are designed to penetrate it. There are techniques that can eliminate the barrier temporarily to allow the use of other antitumor drugs.

Blood cells
The red cells, white cells and platelets that make up the blood. They are made in the bone marrow.

Blood chemistry panel
Multiple chemical analyses prepared by an automatic apparatus from a single blood sample. These panels often include measurements of electrolytes (minerals) and proteins as well as tests of liver, kidney and thyroid function. The advantages of panels include less cost and greater accuracy and speed, with results often available the same or the following day.

Bolus chemotherapy
Administration of intravenous chemotherapy over a short time, usually five minutes or less. The other method is called infusion

chemotherapy, which may last from 15 minutes to several hours or days.

Bone marrow

A soft substance found within bone cavities. Marrow is composed of developing red cells, white cells, platelets and fat. Some forms of cancer can be diagnosed by examining bone marrow.

Bone marrow examination

The process of removing bone marrow by withdrawing it through a needle for pathological examination. It is usually withdrawn from the breast bone (sternum) or the hip bone. Both these bones are just under the skin, making the removal of marrow easy, safe and only momentarily uncomfortable with a local anesthetic. The procedure takes about ten minutes—nine and a half minutes for the anesthetic to take effect and 30 seconds for the actual procedure.

Bone marrow suppression

A decrease in one or more of the blood counts. This condition can be caused by chemotherapy, radiation, disease or various medications.

Bone scan

A picture of all of the bones in the body taken about two hours after injection of a radioactive tracer. "Hot spots" indicate areas of bone abnormality that may indicate tumors, although they can also be due to other causes such as arthritis. No preparation is required and the test is easy. The main problem is lying on a hard table for 15 minutes. This test can help determine if cancer has spread to the bones, if therapy is working and if damaged bony areas are healing.

Brachytherapy

The use of a radioactive "seed" implanted directly into a tumor. This allows a very high but sharply localized dose of radiation to be given to a tumor while sparing surrounding tissues from significant radiation exposure.

Brain scan

A picture of the brain taken after the intravenous injection of a radioactive tracer. CT and MRI scans have in most cases replaced such brain scans, since CT and MRI tend to discover smaller lesions and are more useful for following up the effects of therapy.

Bronchogenic carcinoma

Carcinoma of the lung.

Bronchoscopy

Inspection—and often biopsy—of the breathing tubes (bronchi) going to the lungs by means of a long tube inserted through the mouth or nose. The instrument usually used is a fiber-optic bronchoscope that is flexible and allows excellent visualization around corners. The procedure is often done on an outpatient basis after local anesthesia and sedation.

Bypass

A surgical procedure to "go around" an organ or area affected by cancer and allow normal flow or drainage to continue. In cancer of the pancreas, for example, the bile ducts may be blocked. A bypass procedure will allow the bile to drain into the small bowel, as it should.

C

Cachexia

The wasting away of the body, often due to malnutrition, disease or cancer.

Calcium

An important body mineral that is a vital component of bone. The calcium level may be elevated if tumors involve bone.

Candidiasis (Moniliasis)

A common fungal infection often seen as white patches on the tongue or the inside of the mouth.

Carcinogenesis

The development or production of cancer.

Carcinoma

A form of cancer that develops in the tissues covering or lining organs of the body such as the skin, uterus, lung or breast (epithelial tissues). Eighty to 90 percent of all cancers are carcinomas.

Carcinoma in situ

The earliest stage of cancer, in which the tumor is still confined to the local area, before it has grown to a significant size or has spread. In situ carcinomas are highly curable.

Cardiomyopathy

A condition in which the heart muscle is diseased. It may develop because of the toxic effect of a few anticancer drugs.

CAT scan

See CT scan

Catheter

A tube made of rubber, plastic or metal that can be introduced into a body cavity such as the bladder to drain fluid or to deliver fluids or medication.

Catheterization
The process of introducing a catheter. The term is also used when a tube is placed into an artery or a vein to take x-rays.

CEA (carcinoembryonic antigen)
A "tumor marker" in the blood that may indicate the presence of cancer. It may be elevated in some cancers, especially of the breast, bowel and lung. By monitoring the amount of CEA, doctors can detect the presence of these cancers and assess the progress of treatment.

Cell cycle
Each cell in the body, including a cancer cell, goes through several stages every time it divides. Various anticancer drugs affect the cell at different stages of this cell cycle.

Cell-cycle specific
Chemotherapeutic drugs that kill only cells that are dividing rather than resting.

Cell surface markers
Special proteins on the surface or edge of cells that can be used to identify them or their characteristics.

Cells
The fundamental unit, or building blocks, of human tissues.

Cellular immunity
Immunity brought about by the action of immune cells such as lymphocytes.

Cellulitis
Inflammation of the skin and underlying tissues.

Centigray (cGy)
A unit of measurement of radiation therapy that is replacing the older term *rads*.

Cervical dysplasia
The presence of abnormal—and possibly precancerous—cells in the mouth of the uterus (cervix).

Cervical (lymph) nodes
The lymph nodes in the neck.

Cervix
The lower portion of the uterus, which protrudes into the vagina and forms a portion of the birth canal during delivery. The Pap test is designed to check this area for cancer.

Chemoprevention
Attempting to prevent cancer through drugs, chemicals, vitamins or minerals.

Chemotherapy
The treatment of cancer by chemicals (drugs) designed to kill cancer cells or stop them from growing.

Choriocarcinoma
A carcinoma composed of cells arising in the placenta or the testes.

Chromosomes
The fundamental strands of genetic material (DNA) that carry all our genes. There are 23 pairs in each cell. Tumor cells sometimes have more or fewer than 23 pairs (*see* Aneuploid).

Clinical
Refers to the treatment of humans, as opposed to animals or laboratory studies. Also refers to the general use of a treatment by a practicing physician, as opposed to research done in cancer research centers ("preclinical").

Clinical trials
The procedure in which new cancer treatments are tested in humans. Clinical trials are conducted after experiments in animals and preliminary studies in humans have shown that a new treatment method might be effective.

Clone
A strain of cells—whether normal or malignant—derived from a single original cell.

Clonigenic assay
A test done by growing tumor cells in the laboratory and identifying which chemotherapy agents will prevent their growth. This information is sometimes useful in deciding which drugs to use or not to use in treatment.

Cobalt; cobalt treatment
A radiotherapy machine using gamma rays generated from the radioisotope cobalt 60.

Coin lesion
A single "spot" on a chest x-ray that may be a tumor, infection or other lesion. Given this name because it resembles the shadow of a coin.

Colonoscopy
A procedure to inspect the rectum and colon by means of a long fiber-optic telescope that is lighted and flexible. Biopsy specimens of suspicious tissue can also be obtained.

Colony stimulating factor (CSF)
A substance that stimulates the growth of bone marrow cells. Current clinical trials are using CSF to try to increase the dosage of chemotherapy that can be given safely.

Colostomy
An artificial opening in the abdominal wall created so that feces drains from the colon into a bag. A colostomy is sometimes necessary

after the removal of a diseased section of the large intestine, and can be either temporary or permanent (*see* Ostomy).

Colposcopy
A way to detect small lesions by inspecting the cervix with special binocular magnifying instruments after applying a solution to stain cancer tissue.

Combination chemotherapy
The use of several anticancer drugs at the same time. Most chemotherapy is now given this way, since it is a much more effective method.

Combined modality therapy
Treatment with two or more types of therapy—surgery, radiotherapy, chemotherapy and biological therapy. These may be used at the same time or one after the other. Surgery, for example, is often followed by chemotherapy to destroy random cancer cells that may have spread from the original site.

Computerized tomography
See CT scan

Cone biopsy
Removal of a ring of tissue from the opening of the cervix.

Congestive heart failure
Weakness of the heart muscle usually due to heart disease, but sometimes due to other causes, causing a buildup of fluid in body tissues.

Consolidation
A second round of chemotherapy to further reduce the number of cancer cells.

Contralateral
On the opposite side of the body. In cancer therapy it refers to a tumor or a site of disease. (*see also* Ipsilateral)

Cooperative groups
Clinical trials of new cancer treatments require many patients, generally more than any single physician or hospital can see. A number of physicians and/or hospitals form a cooperative group to treat a large number of patients in the same way so that the effectiveness of a new treatment can be evaluated quickly.

Cortisone
A natural hormone produced by the adrenal glands. The term is also loosely used to designate synthetic forms of the hormone (such as prednisone) that are used to treat inflammatory conditions and diseases, including certain cancers.

Cranial irradiation
The delivery of radiation to the brain to treat brain tumors.

Creatinine clearance
A sensitive test of kidney function that requires a 24-hour urine sample and a blood sample. The test is often required to make sure it is safe to give anticancer drugs that may be toxic to the kidneys.

Cruciferous vegetables
Vegetables such as cauliflower and Brussels sprouts that are high in beta carotene and are thought to help protect against colon cancer.

Cryosurgery
The use of a special cold probe as a surgical instrument. It is used to destroy cancer tissues.

CT scan
A CT (computerized tomography) scan creates cross-section images of the body, which may show cancer or metastases earlier and more accurately than other imaging methods. This type of x-ray machine has revolutionized the diagnosis of cancer and other diseases.

Cushing's syndrome
A condition characterized by swelling of the face and back of the neck and purple lines over the abdomen. It results from an excess of cortisone or hydrocortisone caused either by disease or by the administration of these substances or their synthetic derivatives.

Cyst
A fluid-filled sac of tissue that is usually benign but can be malignant. Cysts are sometimes removed just to be sure they are benign. Lumps in the breast are often found to be harmless cysts rather than cancer.

Cystitis
An inflammation and irritation of the bladder caused by bacterial infection, chemotherapy or radiation treatments. Symptoms include a burning sensation when urinating or a frequent urgent need to urinate.

Cytogenetics
Laboratory study or analysis of the chromosome pattern of a cell.

Cytokine
A substance secreted by immune system cells, usually to send "messages" to other immune cells.

Cytology
The study under a microscope of cells that have been cast off or scraped off organs such

as the uterus, lungs, bladder or stomach. Also called exfoliative cytology (*see* Pap smear).

Cystoscopy
Inspection of the inside of the bladder by means of a telescope. During the procedure a catheter may also be placed, biopsies taken or tissue removed.

D

Debulking
A procedure that removes a significant part or most of a tumor in cases where it is not possible to remove all of it. This may make subsequent radiotherapy or chemotherapy easier and more effective.

Differentiation
The process of maturation of a cell line of cancer cells. When they are fully differentiated or well-differentiated, they more closely resemble the normal cells in the tissue of origin.

Diuretics
Drugs that increase the elimination of water and salts in the urine.

DNA (deoxyribonucleic acid)
The building block of our genetic material. DNA is responsible for the passing of hereditary characteristics and information on cell growth, division and function.

Dose limiting
A side effect, complication or risk that makes it impossible or unwise to exceed a specific dose of a chemotherapeutic agent. A total dosage of bleomycin of more than 400 units, for example, may produce severe lung scarring. Lung toxicity is, therefore, dose limiting.

Drug resistance
The development of resistance in cancer cells to a specific drug or drugs. If resistance develops, a patient in remission from chemotherapy may relapse despite continued administration of anticancer drugs.

Dysphagia
Difficulty in swallowing; a sensation of food sticking in the throat.

Dysplasia
Abnormal developments or changes in cells, which are sometimes an indication that cancer may develop.

Dyspnea
Shortness of breath.

Dysuria
Difficult or painful urination; burning on urination.

E

Edema
The accumulation of fluid within tissues.

Effusion
A collection of fluid inside a body cavity, such as around the lungs (pleural), intestines (peritoneal) or heart (pericardial). This can be caused by cancer invading the cavity.

Electrolytes
Certain chemicals—including sodium, potassium, chloride and bicarbonate—found in the tissues and blood. They are often measured as an aid to patient care.

Electron beam
A form of radiotherapy in which the beam does not penetrate completely through the body as ordinary x-rays do. It is used for treating the skin or lesions beneath the skin.

Electrophoresis
See Serum protein electrophoresis

Emboli
Pieces of tissue, usually blood clots but sometimes tumor cells, that travel in the circulatory system until they lodge in a small artery or capillary, often in the lungs.

Embolization
A method of treating tumors in a localized area by blocking the blood vessels to the area. This is done by inserting a thin tube (catheter) into an artery and injecting tiny pellets or other materials, which then travel "downstream" and block the smaller arteries. The pellets may also carry chemotherapeutic agents for release in the area ("chemoembolization").

Emesis
A fancy word for vomiting.

Endemic
Refers to a disease process that is common in a particular community or population.

Endocrine glands
Glands—such as the pituitary, thyroid, ovaries and testes—that secrete hormones to control digestion, reproduction, growth, metabolism or other body functions.

Endometrial carcinoma
A cancer of the inner lining (endometrium) of the uterus.

Endoscope
An instrument (telescope) designed to allow examination of hollow organs or body cavities.

There are many specialized types such as the cystoscope for the bladder, colonoscope for the colon, gastroscope for the stomach and bronchoscope for the lungs.

Endoscopy
Examination of interior body structures with an endoscope. The physician is able to take photographs, obtain small samples of tissue or remove small growths during the procedure.

Enteral feeding
Administration of liquid food (nutrients) through a tube inserted into the stomach or intestine.

Enterostomal therapist
A medical professional specializing in the care of artificial openings in the abdominal wall and elsewhere—ileostomies, gastrostomies or colostomies, for example.

Enterostomy
The opening used for enteral feeding or for drainage if the bowel is obstructed.

Enzymes
Proteins that play a part in specific chemical reactions. The level of enzymes in the blood is often measured because abnormal levels may be a sign of various diseases.

Epidermoid carcinoma
A cancer arising from surface cells in an organ and resembling skin ("epidermis") when viewed under the microscope.

Epidural
The space just outside the spinal cord. Plastic catheters may be inserted in the space to deliver anesthetics or morphine for pain control.

Epstein-Barr (EB) virus
A virus known to cause infectious mononucleosis and associated with Burkitt's lymphoma and certain cancers of the head and neck.

ERCP (endoscopic retrograde cholagiopancreatography)
A specialized procedure in which a catheter is introduced through a gastroscope into the internal bile ducts.

Esophageal speech
A way of speaking used by people who have had their larynx (voice box) removed. As air is expelled from the esophagus, the walls of the pharynx and esophagus vibrate to produce sound.

Esophagitis
Soreness and inflammation of the esophagus due to infection, toxicity from radiotherapy or chemotherapy or some physical injury.

Estrogen
The female sex hormone produced by the ovaries. Estrogen controls the development of physical sexual characteristics, menstruation and pregnancy. Synthetic forms are used in oral contraceptives and in various therapies.

Estrogen-receptor (ER) assay
A test that determines whether the breast cancer in a particular patient is stimulated by estrogen.

Excision
Surgical removal of tissue.

Extravasation
Leakage into the surrounding tissues of intravenous fluids or drugs—especially cancer chemotherapeutic agents—from the vein being used for injection. Extravasation may damage tissues.

F

Familial polyposis
A hereditary condition in which members of the same family develop intestinal polyps. Also called Gardner's syndrome, it is considered a risk factor for colorectal cancer.

Fiber-optics
Flexible tubes that transmit light by means of glass fibers. They are used to inspect and treat internal parts of the body. Various types of endoscopes use fiber-optic technology.

Fibrocystic breasts
A condition, which may come and go in relation to the menstrual cycle, in which fluids normally absorbed by breast tissue become trapped and form cysts. There may be difficulty distinguishing between cysts and breast cancer.

Fine needle aspiration (FNA)
A simple and painless way to obtain small bits of tissue for diagnosis. After local anesthesia, a small needle is inserted through the skin directly into a tumor and a sample of tissue is drawn up inside the needle. In some cases—thyroid cancer, for example—FNA has become an integral part of the early diagnostic process. But the amount of tissue obtained this way may not be enough to diagnose lymphomas and some other cancers.

Fissures
Cracks or a splitting in the skin or an internal membrane.

Fistula
An abnormal opening between the inside of the body and the skin or between two areas inside the body.

Frozen section
A procedure done by the pathologist during surgery to give the surgeon an immediate answer as to whether a tissue is benign or malignant. Tissue is removed by biopsy, frozen, cut into thin slices, stained and examined under a microscope. This information is vital in helping the surgeon decide the most appropriate course of action.

G

Gamma rays
The form of electromagnetic radiation produced by certain radioactive sources. They are similar to x-rays but have a shorter wavelength.

Gene
A biological unit of DNA capable of transmitting a single characteristic from parent to offspring.

Grade of tumor
A way of describing tumors by their appearance under the microscope. Low-grade tumors are slow to grow and spread, while high-grade tumors grow and spread rapidly.

Graft-versus-host disease
After bone marrow transplantation or blood transfusion, immune cells in the donated (grafted) material may identify the patient's tissues (the host) as foreign and try to destroy them.

Granulocyte
The most common type of white blood cell. Its function is to kill bacteria (also called neutrophil, poly, PMN).

Guaiac test
A test to see if there is hidden blood in the stool. A positive result may be a sign of cancer, but many benign conditions also cause bleeding.

Gynecomastia
Swelling of the breast tissues in men. Although this can be caused by medications and other diseases, in the cancer field it is caused by certain cancers of the testis or by female hormones used to treat prostate cancer.

H

Hematocrit
A way of measuring the red cell content of the blood. The normal level is about 40 to 45 in men and from 37 to 42 in women. A low hematocrit is a sign of anemia.

Hematologist
A physician (internist) who specializes in blood diseases.

Hematoma
A blood lump under the skin that appears like a "black and blue" mark.

Hematopoietic
Pertaining to the blood-forming organs such as the bone marrow.

Hematuria
Blood in the urine. This may be obvious (gross hematuria) or hidden (microscopic hematuria).

Hemoglobin
A way of measuring the red cell content of the blood. The normal value in men is about 13 to 15 grams, in women from 12.5 to 14 grams.

Hemolytic anemia
Anemia resulting from the breakdown of red blood cells in the bloodstream before the end of their usual life span of 120 days.

Hemorrhagic cystitis
A bladder irritation, which may be caused by the anticancer drugs cyclophosphamide (Cytoxan) or ifosfamide.

Hepatic
Pertaining to the liver.

Hepatotoxicity
Adverse effects of drugs on the liver indicated by abnormal blood tests of liver function. It is also sometimes associated with jaundice.

Herpes simplex
A common acute viral inflammation of the skin or mucous membranes characterized by the development of blisters. This infection around the mouth is commonly called a cold sore.

Herpes zoster (shingles)
A painful eruption in the skin caused by a virus infection that affects nerves. The same virus that causes shingles causes chicken pox.

Histology
The appearance of tissues, including cancers, under the microscope.

Hormonal anticancer therapy
A form of therapy that takes advantage of the tendency of some cancers—especially breast and prostate cancers—to stabilize or shrink if certain hormones are administered.

Hormones
Naturally occurring substances that are released by the endocrine organs and circulate in the blood. Hormones control growth, metabolism, reproduction and other functions, and can stimulate or turn off the growth or activity of specific target cells. Some hormones are used after surgery to treat breast, ovarian and prostate cancers.

Hospice
A facility and a philosophy of care that stress comfort, peace of mind and the control of symptoms. Hospice care, provided on either an outpatient or inpatient basis, is generally invoked when no further anticancer therapy is available and life expectancy is very short. Hospice also helps family and friends to care for and cope with the loss of a dying loved one.

Humoral immunity
Immunity mediated by substances such as proteins (gamma globulins) produced by the immune system.

Hyperalimentation
Artificial feeding—temporary or permanent—by means of concentrated protein and fat solutions delivered intravenously. A special catheter is usually needed.

Hypercalcemia
High levels of calcium in the blood. It is a sign of some forms of cancer or of cancer spreading to bone and also occurs in some other benign conditions.

Hyperthermia
Increased body temperature. Generally used to mean the use of special devices to raise body temperature as a way of treating cancer. It is usually used along with radiation therapy.

Hypothermia
Excessively low body temperature.

Hysterectomy
Surgical removal of the uterus.

I

Ileostomy
An artificial opening in the skin of the abdomen, leading to the small bowel (ileum) (*see* Ostomy).

Iliac
The part of the lower abdomen just above the hip bone on each side of the body. Also refers to the iliac bone just above the hip joint.

Immune/immunity
A state of adequate defense against infections or foreign substances. Some cancers are also believed to produce immune responses.

Immune system
The body mechanisms that resist and fight disease. The main defenders are white blood cells and antibodies, which, along with other specialized defenders, react to the presence of foreign substances in the body and try to destroy them.

Immunoelectrophoresis
A way to separate serum gamma globulins—called IgA, IgG and IgM—into groups according to their immunologic qualities.

Immunosuppression
The state of having decreased immunity and thus being less able to fight infections and disease.

Immunosuppressive drug
A drug that modifies the natural immune response so that it will not react to foreign substances. This type of drug is most commonly given after organ transplants so that the new organ will not be rejected.

Immunotherapy
A method of cancer therapy that stimulates the body's defense mechanism to attack cancer cells or combat a specific disease.

Incontinence
Inadvertent loss of urine or feces, usually due to loss of nerve or muscle control.

Indirect laryngoscopy
Inspection of the lower throat, pharynx and larynx (voice box) by means of a small mirror placed in the back of the throat (*see* Laryngoscopy).

Induction
The initial treatment—usually of chemotherapy—to eliminate or control cancer. Usually applied to leukemia or lymphoma.

Induration
Firmness or hardness of tissues.

Inferior vena cava
The large vein draining the blood from the legs and abdomen back into the heart.

Infiltration
The leaking of fluid or medicines into tissues from a tube or needle. This can cause irritation or swelling (*see* Extravasation).

Inflammation
The triggering of local body defenses causing defensive white blood cells (leukocytes) to pour into the tissues from the circulatory system. It is characterized by redness, heat, pain and swelling.

Informed consent
A legal standard defining how much a patient must know about the potential benefits and risks of therapy before agreeing to receive it.

Infusion
Administration of fluids and/or medications

into a vein or artery over a period of time.

Infusion pumps
Small, preloaded mechanical devices used to continuously administer intravenous chemotherapy over a designated time.

Inguinal
Pertaining to the groin, the common site for hernias and the location of the inguinal lymph nodes, an area where cancer may spread.

In situ
A very early stage of cancer in which the tumor is localized to one area.

Interferons
Natural substances produced in response to infections. They have been created artificially by recombinant DNA technology in an attempt to control cancer.

Intra-arterial
Drugs directed into an artery through a catheter.

Intracavitary therapy
Treatment directed into a body cavity via a catheter.

Intramuscular (IM)
The injection of a drug into the muscle, whence it is absorbed into the circulation.

Intraperitoneal
Delivery of drugs and fluids into the abdominal cavity.

Intrapleural
Delivery of drugs and fluids into the space around the lung. Often employed when fluid collects there as a result of cancer.

Intrathecal
Administration of drugs into the spinal fluid.

Intravenous (IV)
The administration of drugs or fluids directly into the vein.

Intravenous pyelogram (IVP)
An x-ray of the kidneys taken after the intravenous administration of a radiopaque dye that is concentrated and excreted by the kidneys. This makes the kidneys and drainage system visible on an x-ray.

Invasive cancer
Cancer that spreads to the healthy tissue surrounding the original tumor site.

Ipsilateral
On the same side of the body (*see also* Contralateral).

J

Jaundice
The accumulation of bilirubin, a breakdown product of hemoglobin, which results in a yellow discoloration of the skin and the whites of the eyes. Jaundice is a sign of liver disease or blockage of the major bile ducts.

K

Kidney failure (renal failure)
Malfunction of the kidneys due to disease or the toxic effects of drugs or chemicals. Urine volume may or may not be diminished.

L

Laparotomy
An operation in which the abdominal cavity is opened.

Large cell carcinoma
A type of cancer of the lung, although large cell cancers may occur in other organs.

Laryngectomy
The surgical removal of the larynx (voice box) resulting in the loss of normal speech. A laryngectomee is someone who has undergone this operation.

Laryngoscopy
Inspection of the lower throat, pharynx and larynx by means of a small mirror placed in the back of the throat (indirect laryngoscopy) or by direct examination under anesthesia (direct laryngoscopy).

Leukocyte
White blood cell.

Leukocytosis
An increase in the number of leukocytes in the blood.

Leukopenia
A decreased white blood cell count (below 5,000).

Leukopheresis
A washing procedure that removes white blood cells from the blood.

Leukoplakia
White plaque on the mucous membranes of the mouth and gums. This may be precancerous.

Linear accelerator
A radiation therapy machine that produces a high energy beam.

Liver function tests
A group—panel—of blood tests to check if the liver is healthy.

Localized
A cancer confined to the site of origin without evidence of spread.

Lumbar puncture
Removal of spinal fluid for examination. This simple procedure—also called a spinal tap—involves numbing the skin of the back with a local anesthetic and placing a needle into the numbed area to remove the spinal fluid.

Lumpectomy
The removal of a breast cancer (lump) and the surrounding tissue without removing the entire breast. It is a less radical procedure than mastectomy and is usually followed by radiation treatment.

LVN
Licensed vocational nurse. A nurse trained to do more limited tasks than a registered nurse (RN).

Lymph nodes
Oval-shaped organs, often the size of peas or beans, that are located throughout the body and contain clusters of cells called lymphocytes. They produce infection-fighting lymphocytes and also filter out and destroy bacteria, foreign substances and cancer cells. They are connected by small vessels called lymphatics. Lymph nodes act as our first line of defense against infections and cancer.

Lymphangiogram
An x-ray picture of the abdominal lymph nodes obtained by injecting a contrast substance under the skin on the feet. This test helps to determine if cancer has spread to the abdominal lymph nodes.

Lymphatic system
The system of lymph nodes and the lymphatic vessels that connect them.

Lymphedema
Swelling, usually of an arm or leg, caused by obstructed lymphatic vessels. It can develop because of a tumor or as an unusual late effect of surgery or radiotherapy.

Lymphocytes
A family of white blood cells responsible for the production of antibodies and for the direct destruction of invading organisms or cancer cells.

Lymphokine
A specific protein (cytokine) secreted by lymphocytes.

Lytic
A bone lesion that has less calcium than normal. It may appear to be a "hole" in the bone.

M

Macrophages
White blood cells that destroy invading organisms by ingesting them.

Malaise
Tiredness or lack of "drive."

Malignant
An adjective meaning cancerous. Two important qualities of malignancies are the tendency to sink roots into surrounding tissues and to break off and spread elsewhere ("metastasize").

Markers (tumor markers)
Chemicals in the blood that are produced by certain cancers. Measuring the markers is useful for diagnosis, but especially useful for following the course of treatment (*see* CEA).

Mediastinum
The central portion of the chest, comprising the heart, large blood vessels, esophagus, trachea and surrounding tissues.

Metaplasia
Cells that appear abnormal under the microscope and do not yet show signs of malignancy.

Metastasis
The spread of cancer from one part of the body to another by way of the lymph system or bloodstream. Cells in the new cancer are like those in the original tumor.

Methadone (Dolophine)
A synthetic narcotic pain reliever related to morphine.

Milligrams/meter squared (mg/m²)
A formula for calculating dosages of chemotherapy drugs according to the surface area of the body. Since the amount of skin is hard to determine exactly, it is closely estimated from height and weight. An average person might have 1.7 square meters of body surface area. If the standard drug dosage were 650 mg/m2, then 650 x 1.7 = 1105 mg of drug to be given.

Mitosis
The process of cell reproduction or division. Cancer cells usually have higher rates of mitosis than normal cells. The number of divisions seen under the microscope reflects how aggressive the cancer is.

Modality
A general class or method of treatment. The basic modalities of cancer therapy include

surgery, radiation therapy, chemotherapy and immunotherapy.

Monoclonal antibodies

Highly specific antibodies, usually manufactured in a laboratory, that react to a specific cancer antigen or are directed against a specific type of cancer. Current research is studying their role in therapy. One potential use is to deliver chemotherapy and radiotherapy directly to a tumor, thus killing the cancer cells and sparing healthy tissue. Studies are also trying to find out if monoclonal antibodies can be produced to detect and diagnose cancer cells at a very early and curable stage.

Monoclonal gammopathy

An elevation in gamma globulin in the blood caused by a single clone of plasma cells or lymphocytes. Such a protein pattern may be associated with multiple myeloma.

Morbidity

Sickness; illness; symptoms and signs of disease. Not to be confused with mortality.

Mortality

Death as a result of disease.

MRI (Magnetic Resonance Imaging)

A method of creating images of the body using a magnetic field and radio waves rather than x-rays. Although the images are similar to those of CT scans, they can be taken in all three directions (planes) rather than just in cross-sections.

Mucosa (mucous membrane)

The inner lining of the gastrointestinal tract or other structures such as the vagina and nose.

Mucositis

Inflammation of the mucous membranes. Soreness—like "cold sores"—can develop in the mouth as a side effect of chemotherapy.

Multicentricity

A tumor that appears to start growing in several places at once.

Multimodality

Using a combination of two or more types of therapy—for example, radiotherapy plus chemotherapy, radiation plus surgery or chemotherapy plus surgery.

Mutation

A permanent change in a cell's DNA that alters its genetic potential. It may be a response to a chemical substance (mutagen) or result from a physical effect such as radiation. Sometimes the daughter cells may be cancerous.

Myelogram

An x-ray of the spinal cord after the introduction of radiopaque dye into the sac surrounding it. Used to see if a tumor involves the spinal cord or nerve roots.

Myeloma

A cancer of the protein-producing plasma cells of the bone marrow. Multiple bone lesions are common.

Myelosuppression

A fall in the blood counts caused by therapy, especially chemotherapy and radiotherapy.

N

Nadir

The lowest point to which white blood cell or platelet counts fall after chemotherapy.

Narcotics

A legal term defining euphoric and pain-relieving (analgesic) substances whose use is closely regulated by government. There are natural and synthetic types.

Nasopharynx

The part of the nasal cavity behind the nose and above the part of the throat that we can see.

National Cancer Institute

A highly regarded research center in Bethesda, Maryland, that conducts basic and clinical research on new cancer treatments and supervises clinical trials of new treatments throughout the United States.

National Surgical Adjuvant Breast/Bowel Project (NSABP)

A group of dedicated research and clinical physicians who have formed a large cooperative group to study new treatments. Many major advances in treatment are attributed to this group.

Necrosis

The disintegration of tissues caused by some physical or chemical agent or by lack of blood supply. Cancers treated effectively by chemotherapy, radiotherapy, heat or biological agents undergo necrosis.

Needle biopsy

Removing a tiny bit of tissue for diagnosis by placing a needle into a tumor. The procedure is usually done under local anesthesia.

Neoplasm

A new abnormal growth. Neoplasms may be benign or malignant.

Nephrotoxic

Toxic to the kidneys. The term is generally used to refer to a drug's effect.

Nerve block
Removing pain by numbing a nerve temporarily (with a local anesthetic) or permanently (with an alcohol injection).

Neuropathy
Malfunction of a nerve, often causing numbness (sensory nerve) or weakness (motor nerve). It is sometimes a side effect of anticancer drugs.

Neurotoxicity
Toxic effects (usually of drugs) on the nervous system.

Neutrophils
One of the white blood cells that fights infection. Also called granulocytes, polys or PMNs.

Nitrosoureas
A class of chemical compounds that can enter the brain through the blood-brain barrier. The anticancer drugs BCNU, CCNU and methyl-CCNU are nitrosoureas. (*See* Blood-brain barrier)

"No code"
An order, written in a hospital chart after careful and considered discussions, to *not* attempt to resuscitate a patient if breathing and/or the heartbeat should stop. This is usually considered if the patient, after all reasonable therapeutic efforts have been made and have failed, is suffering greatly and rapidly failing from a far-advanced malignancy. Also "Do Not Rescuscitate" (DNR).

Nodes
See Lymph nodes

Nodule
A small lump or tumor that can be benign or malignant.

Non-cell-cycle specific
Chemotheraputic drugs capable of destroying cells that are not actively dividing.

Nuclear Magnetic Resonance (NMR)
An old term for MRI.

O

Oncogenes
Specific stretches of cellular DNA that, when inappropriately activated, contribute to the transformation of normal cells into malignant ones.

Oncologist
A physician who specializes in cancer therapy. There are surgical, radiation, pediatric, gynecologic and medical oncologists. The term *oncologist* alone generally refers to medical oncologists, who are internists with expertise in chemotherapy and the handling of the general medical problems that arise during the disease.

Oncology
The medical specialty that deals with the diagnosis, treatment and study of cancer.

Oophorectomy
The surgical removal of one or both ovaries.

Opportunistic infections
Many common fungi and bacteria and a few microscopic parasites do not ordinarily cause infections in healthy people. But such ordinarily harmless organisms can produce severe, life-threatening and hard-to-contol infections in cancer patients by taking advantage of the reduced immune response resulting from the disease or therapy.

Ostomy
A surgically created opening in the skin, leading to an internal organ, for purposes of drainage (*see* Colostomy; Ileostomy).

Ototoxicity
Toxic effects on the ears, generally resulting in a ringing in the ears or hearing loss.

P

Palate
The roof of the mouth. The hard palate is in front, the soft palate just behind.

Palliative
Treatment that aims to improve well-being, relieve symptoms or control the growth of cancer, but not primarily intended or expected to produce a cure.

Palpation
Examination by feeling an area of the body—such as the breast and prostate—with the fingers to detect abnormalities. A palpable mass is one that can be felt.

Paracentesis
Removing fluid from the abdomen by inserting a small needle through the skin. This is usually done under local anesthesia.

Paraneoplastic (syndrome)
Various symptoms and signs—changes in body minerals, nerve function or water balance, for example—that indicate the presence of a tumor in the body but are not related to direct pressure by the tumor.

Parenteral nutrition
Artificial feeding by the intravenous administration of concentrated amino acid, sugar and

fat solutions (*see* Hyperalimentation; TPN).

Pathologist
A physician skilled in the performance and interpretation of laboratory tests and in the examination of tissues to provide a diagnosis.

Pathologic fracture
A fracture (break) in a bone through an area weakened by cancer. Usually little or no injury or trauma precedes the fracture, as is the case with the usual fracture of healthy bones.

Pathology
Study of disease through the examination of body tissues, organs and materials. Any tumor suspected of being cancerous must be diagnosed by pathologic examination. The physician who does this is called a pathologist.

PDQ (Physicians Data Query)
A comprehensive, up-to-date information service on state-of-the-art cancer treatment provided by the National Cancer Institute via computer.

Performance status
A measurement of how well a cancer patient is functioning. Index numbers from 0 to 100—increasing in steps of 10—are used to document and record functional status, as opposed to other measurements that indicate the size of a tumor. A person with a performance status of 80 functions better than one with a score of 50. Also called Karnofsky score.

Perineum
The part of the body between the anus and the genitals.

Perioperative
Occurring at or around the time of surgery. Often used with reference to chemotherapy or radiotherapy treatments.

Peritonoscopy
Inspection of the inside of the abdominal cavity by means of a telescope inserted under anesthesia through a tiny opening in the skin.

Petechiae
Tiny areas of bleeding under the skin usually caused by a low platelet count.

Phlebitis
Inflammation of the veins, often causing pain and tenderness (*see* Pulmonary embolism; Thrombophlebitis).

Photodynamic therapy
The injection of a light-sensitizing chemical or dye and the subsequent application of light, usu-ally laser, to a tumor. The chemical improves the effect of the laser treatment and thus minimizes or prevents damage to normal tissues.

Photosensitivity
Extreme sensitivity to the sun. Some medications—including a few anticancer drugs as well as tetracycline antibiotics—produce photosensitivity as a side effect, leaving the patient prone to sunburn.

Placebo
An inert substance, used in a research study or clinical trial, that resembles an actual medication. It is used to eliminate the improvement that may result from the *belief* that a medication is being given, rather than the actual effect of a medication.

Plasmapheresis
The replacement or "washing" of a patient's plasma by donor plasma or saline.

Platelet
One of the three kinds of circulating blood cells. The normal platelet count is about 150,000 to 300,000. Platelets are responsible for creating the first part of a blood clot. Platelet transfusions are used in cancer patients to prevent or control bleeding when the number of platelets has significantly decreased.

Plateletpheresis
Collection of platelets in a machine for transfusion into another person.

Pneumonectomy
Surgical removal of a lung.

Polycythemia
An excessively high red blood cell count. This may be caused by a primary blood disease or as a response to another type of disease.

Polyp
A growth that protrudes from mucous membranes, often looking like a tiny mushroom. Polyps may be found in the nose, ears, mouth, lungs, vocal cords, uterus, cervix, rectum, bladder and intestine. Some polyps occurring in the cervix, intestine, stomach or colon can eventually become malignant and should be removed.

Poorly differentiated
A tumor that under the microscope has little or only a slight resemblance to the normal tissue from the same organ (*see* Undifferentiated; Well-differentiated).

Port (infusion)
A small disc with a soft center (about the size of

a quarter) that is surgically placed just below the skin in the chest or abdomen. A tube coming out of the side is connected via a large vein directly into the bloodstream. By passing a small needle through the skin into the disc, fluids, drugs or blood products can be given without worrying about finding an adequate vein, making multiple venipunctures or causing leakage of the fluids into surrounding tissues.

Port-a-Cath
A venous access device that has nothing protruding from the skin. Injections are made into a chamber implanted just under the skin (*see* Port).

Potassium
An important mineral in the body that is often lost during illness, especially with diarrhea. Low potassium levels can cause weakness.

Precancerous
Abnormal cellular changes or conditions—intestinal polyps, for example—that tend to become malignant. Also called premalignant.

Primary tumor
The place where a cancer first starts to grow. Even if it spreads elsewhere, it is still known by the place of origin. For example, breast cancer that has spread to the bone is still breast cancer, not bone cancer.

Proctoscopy
See Sigmoidoscopy

Progesterone
One of the female hormones (the other is estrogen). It causes the buildup of the uterine lining in preparation for conception and performs other functions before and during pregnancy. Certain synthetic forms of the hormone are used in cancer treatment.

Progesterone-receptor (PR) assay
A test that determines if the breast cancer in a particular patient is stimulated by progesterone.

Prognosis
A statement about the likely outcome of disease in a particular patient. In cancer, it is based on all available information about the type of tumor, staging, therapeutic possibilities, expected results and other personal or medical factors. For example, breast cancer patients who are diagnosed early usually have a good prognosis.

Progression
The growth or advancement of cancer, indicating a worsening of the disease.

Prophylactic
Treatment designed to prevent a disease or complication that is likely to develop but has not yet appeared. Also may be called adjuvant treatment.

Prostate Specific Antigen (PSA)
A substance in the blood derived from the prostate gland. Its level may rise in prostatic cancer and is useful as a marker to monitor the effects of treatment.

Prosthesis
An artificial replacement or approximation of a body part—such as a leg, breast or eye—that is missing because of disease or treatment.

Protocol
A carefully designed and written description of a cancer treatment program. It includes dosages and formulas for any drugs to be administered.

Pulmonary embolism
A life-threatening condition in which a blood clot travels to the lungs from veins in the legs or pelvis, often from thrombophlebitis. The clots are diagnosed with a lung scan and treated with anticoagulants.

R

Radiation oncologist; radiotherapist
A physician who specializes in the use of radiation to treat cancer.

Radiation therapy
See Radiotherapy

Radical mastectomy
Removal of the entire breast along with underlying muscle and the lymph nodes of the armpit (axilla).

Radical neck dissection
An extensive surgical operation to remove all of the lymph glands on one side of the neck, usually in association with surgery to remove a primary tumor that may have spread to the lymph glands in the neck.

Radical surgery
An extensive operation to remove the site of cancer and the adjacent structures and lymph nodes.

Radioactive implant
A source of high-dose radiation that is placed directly into and around a cancer to kill the cancer cells.

Radioactive isotope
A radioactive substance used for diagnosis (tracer dose used for scans) or treatment (therapeutic dose).

Radiologist

A doctor who specializes in the use of x-rays as well as other imaging techniques such as ultrasound, MRI and radioactive tracers to diagnose and investigate disease. New radiology techniques are also used for treatment in some cases ("interventional radiology").

Radiosensitive

A cancer that usually responds to radiation therapy. The opposite is radioresistant.

Radiosensitizer

A drug or biological agent that is given together with radiation therapy to increase its effect.

Radiotherapy

The use of high-energy radiation from x-ray machines, cobalt, radium or other sources for control or cure of cancer. It may reduce the size of a cancer before surgery or be used to destroy any remaining cancer cells after surgery. Radiotherapy can be helpful in treating recurrent cancers or relieving symptoms.

Rads

A unit measuring radiation dosage. A newer unit is the centigray (cGy).

Recurrence

The reappearance of a disease after treatment had caused it to apparently disappear.

Red blood cells

Cells in the blood that bring oxygen to tissues and take carbon dioxide from them.

Regional involvement

The spread of cancer from its original site to nearby surrounding areas. Regional cancers are confined to one general location in the body.

Regression

The shrinkage of a cancer usually as the result of therapy. In a complete regression, all tumors disappear. In a partial regression, some tumor remains.

Rehabilitation

Programs that help patients adjust and return to a full productive life. Rehabilitation may involve physical measures such as physical therapy and prostheses, as well as counseling and emotional support.

Remission

The partial or complete shrinkage of cancer usually occurring as the result of therapy. Also the period when the disease is under control. A remission is not necessarily a cure.

Renal

Pertaining to the kidney.

Resection

The surgical removal of tissue.

Residual disease; residual tumor

Cancer left behind after surgery or other treatment.

Resistance

Failure of a tumor to respond to radiotherapy or chemotherapy. The resistance may be evident during the first treatment (primary) or, after an initial response, during the subsequent treatment (secondary).

Retroperitoneum

The area of the abdomen behind all the organs, including the bowel, near the back.

Reverse isolation

Isolation to prevent visitors or hospital staff from carrying an infection into a patient's room. This usually means that everyone must wear a gown, mask and gloves.

Ribonucleic acid (RNA)

A nucleic acid present in all cells and similar to DNA. It is the biochemical blueprint for the formation of protein by the cells.

Risk factors

The habits or conditions that promote the development of many cancers. Cigarette smoking, for example, is the major risk factor for lung cancer. The major risk factor for skin cancer is overexposure to the sun.

Risk reduction

Techniques used to reduce the chances of developing cancer. High-fiber diets, for example, may help reduce the risk of colon cancer.

RNA

See Ribonucleic acid

S

Salvage

The attempt to cure a patient by a second, third or later alternative treatment program after the first-line treatment has failed to produce a cure.

Sampling

Removal of a portion of a tissue for diagnostic tests.

Sarcoma

A cancer of supporting or connective tissue such as cartilage, bone, muscle or fat. Sarcomas are often highly malignant but account for only 2 percent of all human cancers.

Scans
Diagnostic procedures for assessing organs such as the liver, bone or brain. Radioactive tracers are introduced intravenously and if a malignant tumor or other foreign material is present pictures of the organ will show a filling "defect", corresponding to the tumor.

Screening
The search for cancer in apparently healthy people who have no cancer symptoms. Screening may also refer to coordinated programs in large populations.

Second-look surgery
Sometimes the only way to determine if aggressive therapy has worked is to explore the patient surgically some time after initial therapy. Second-look surgery can discover if there is any residual or recurrent cancer, which may help decide whether treatment is complete or if more radiotherapy or chemotherapy is needed. Residual tumor may also be removed during the operation.

Seizure (convulsion)
Shaking of a part or all of the body, often with loss of consciousness. This can be caused by an injury, a benign condition (such as idiopathic epilepsy) or a brain tumor.

Selective angiography
X-ray pictures of an organ taken after a catheter is passed through the artery to the organ and a dye, which shows on x-rays, is injected.

Sepsis (septicemia, bacteremia)
Bacterial growth within the bloodstream. This is a very serious situation and usually requires hospitalization for intravenous antibiotics.

Serum protein electrophoresis (SPEP)
A laboratory testing method that separates serum proteins into different groups—albumin, alpha globulin, beta globulin and gamma globulin. The different patterns produced are characteristic of various diseases.

Shingles (*see* Herpes zoster)

Sigmoidoscopy
An examination of the rectum and lower colon with a hollow lighted tube called a sigmoidoscope. It is used to detect colon polyps and cancer, to find the cause of bleeding and to evaluate other bowel diseases. A newer instrument using fiber-optics—the flexible sigmoidoscope—permits easier, safer and more extensive examination. Also called a proctoscopy.

Sodium
An important mineral in the body that helps maintain fluid balance. It is measured as part of an electrolyte panel.

Sonography
The use of ultrasound pictures in diagnosis.

Sphincter
A circular muscle that tightens around an organ or cavity to close it and to regulate the flow of material. If the sphincter around the rectum and the mouth of the bladder aren't functioning properly, for example, urine and stool might be lost involuntarily.

Spleen
An organ adjacent to the stomach, composed mainly of lymphocytes, which removes worn-out blood cells and foreign materials from the bloodstream.

Sputum
Material coughed up from the lungs. Also called phlegm.

Squamous cell (epidermoid) carcinoma
Cancer arising from the skin or the surfaces of other structures, such as the mouth, cervix or lungs.

Staging
An organized process of determining how far a cancer has spread. Staging involves a physical exam, blood tests, x-rays, scans and sometimes surgery. Knowing the stage helps determine the most appropriate treatment and the prognosis.

Stereotactic needle biopsy
A procedure often used in the diagnosis of brain tumors. A specialized "frame" is used to hold a patient's head or other body part stationary while the biopsy needle is directed to exactly the right spot. Usually a CT scanner or other computer-associated equipment is used to find the correct position. This method has also been applied recently to very small breast cancers.

Steroids
A class of fat-soluble chemicals—including cortisone and male and female sex hormones—that are vital to many different functions within the body. Some steroid derivatives are used in cancer treatment.

Stoma
A surgically created opening in the skin for elimination of body wastes. A stoma is made in the abdominal wall for elimination of wastes, for example, when the colon and/or rectum can no longer perform this function (*see* Colostomy).

Stomatitis
Inflammation and soreness of the mouth. This is sometimes a side effect of chemotherapy or radiotherapy.

Stool
Feces or bowel movement.

Stool for occult blood
A test to determine if bleeding has occurred. This may show signs of bleeding that are too mild to see with the naked eye (*see* Guaiac test).

Superior vena cava
The large vein draining the blood from the head, neck and arms back into the heart.

Suppository
A way to administer medications by absorbing the drug into a wax preparation, then inserting it into the rectum or vagina. Suppositories are used to treat local conditions such as vaginitis or hemorrhoids and are also used when pills cannot be swallowed or kept down because of nausea, sore mouth or narrowing of the esophagus. Antinausea suppositories such as Compazine and Tigan are often used to combat this side effect of chemotherapy.

Systemic disease
Disease that involves the entire body rather than just one area.

T

T cell
See B cell.

Teratogenic
A drug or toxin that, if taken during pregnancy, can cause the fetus to be malformed.

Terminal
This term has a number of definitions. Some people use it when cure is not possible, even if treatment can add years to the patient's life. Others say a patient is terminal when he or she has a specific short life expectancy, perhaps six months or one month. Still others mean that no other treatment can be given and "nature will take its course." If this term comes up, discuss with your doctor exactly what is meant by it.

Thoracentesis
Insertion of a needle or tube between the ribs and into the chest cavity to remove fluid. The procedure is done for diagnostic or treatment reasons and is performed under local anesthesia.

Thoracic
Pertaining to the thorax or chest.

Thoracotomy
A surgically created opening into the chest.

Thrombocytopenia
An abnormally low number of platelets (thrombocytes)—less then 150,000—due to disease, reaction to a drug or toxic reaction to treatments. Bleeding can occur if there are too few platelets, especially if the count falls to less than 20,000.

Thrombophlebitis
Inflammation of veins with blood clots inside the veins. Usually associated with pain, swelling and tenderness (*see also* Phlebitis; Pulmonary embolism).

Thrombosis
Formation of a blood clot within a blood vessel.

Tissue
A collection of cells of the same type. There are four basic types of tissues in the body: epithelial, connective, muscle and nerve.

TNM classification
A complex and exact system for describing the stage of development of most kinds of cancer. This system is not used for lymphomas, leukemias or Hodgkin's disease.

TPN (Total Parenteral Nutrition)
The use of complex protein and fat solutions to supply enough calories and nutrients to sustain life. The solutions can be delivered intravenously or in some cases orally through a tube to the stomach.

Tracheostomy
An artificial opening in the neck leading to the windpipe (trachea). The opening is created surgically to allow breathing when the trachea is blocked.

Tumor
A lump, mass or swelling. A tumor can be either benign or malignant.

Tumor necrosis factor
A natural protein substance produced by the body, which may make tumors shrink.

U

Ulcer
A sore resulting from corrosion of normal tissue by some irritating substance such as stomach acid, chemicals, infections, impaired circulation or cancerous involvement.

Ultrasound
The use of high-frequency sound waves to create an image of the inside of the body. Also called ultrasonography.

Undifferentiated

A tumor that appears "wild" under the microscope, not resembling the tissue of origin. These tumors tend to grow and spread faster than well-differentiated tumors, which do resemble the normal tissue they come from (*see* Anaplastic; Poorly differentiated; Well-differentiated).

Unilateral

On one side of the body.

Urostomy

A surgical procedure in which the ureters that carry urine from the kidneys to the bladder are cut and connected to an opening on the skin outside the abdomen. This allows urine to flow into a collection bag (*see* Stoma).

Uterus

The female reproductive organ, located in the pelvis; the womb in which an unborn child develops until birth.

V

Venipuncture

Inserting a needle into a vein in order to obtain blood samples, start an intravenous infusion or give a medication.

Ventricles

Four fluid-filled cavities in the brain all connected with each other. There are two lateral ventricles in the top part of the brain—one on each side—with the third and fourth ventricles in the center of the brain. Obstruction of the connections or the outflow tract leads to swelling (hydrocephalus). Also refers to the chambers in the heart.

Vesicant drugs

Chemotherapeutic agents that can cause significant tissue irritation and soreness if they leak outside the vein after injection.

Virus

A tiny infectious agent that is smaller than bacteria. Many common infections such as colds and hepatitis are caused by viruses. Viruses invade cells, alter the cells' chemistry and cause them to produce more viruses. Several viruses produce cancers in animals. Their role in the development of human cancers is now being studied.

W

Well-differentiated

A tumor that under the microscope resembles normal tissue from the same organ (*see* Poorly differentiated; Undifferentiated).

White blood cells

Cells in the blood that fight infection. These are composed of monocytes, lymphocytes, neutrophils, eosinophils and basophils. The normal count is 5,000 to 10,000. It may be elevated or depressed in a wide variety of diseases. Chemotherapy and radiotherapy usually cause low white counts.

ANTICANCER DRUGS AND THEIR SIDE EFFECTS

Adrenocorticosteroids (Prednisone) (Decadron)

Type of Cancer Acute and chronic lymphocytic leukemias, Hodgkin's and non-Hodgkin's lymphoma, myeloma, breast, brain metastases

Route Adminstered Oral, Intravenous, Intramuscular

Precautions Use of antacids, H-2 blockers, check for increased blood sugar (for diabetes), interferes with immune function, infection precautions, low salt diet

Side Effects Could lead to peptic ulcer or pancreatitis, edema (fluid and salt retention), headaches, sleeplessness, vertigo, psychiatric problems, muscle weakness (low potassium), osteoporosis, bone damage to hips, increased hair growth, increased blood sugar (diabetes), cataracts, malaise, increased infections

Aminoglutethimide (Cytadren)

Type of Cancer Breast, prostate, and adrenal

Route Administered Oral

Precautions Add salt to diet

Side Effects Unstable balance (ataxia), uncoordinated eye motion, sleepiness, dizziness, skin rash, low blood counts, eyelid swelling, low adrenal gland function (need cortisone replacement), loss of appetite, nausea, vomiting, constipation, gastric discomfort

Androgens (Testosterone) Fluoxymesterone (Halotestin)

Type of Cancer Breast

Route Administered Oral, Intramuscular

Side Effects Loss of menstrual periods, masculinization, hoarseness, acne, clitoral enlargement, increased hair growth, jaundice, leg swelling (edema), nausea, intestinal upset, fluid and mineral imbalance

Asparaginase (Elspar)

Type of Cancer Acute lymphoblastic leukemia and lymphomas

Route Administered Intravenous, Intramuscular

Precautions Use antihistamines, costeroids (have epinephrine available in case of allergic reaction). Retreatment at later time requires special precautions

Side Effects Fever, allergic reaction (anaphylaxis), neurologic problems (seizures, reduced level of consciousness, drowsiness), stroke, liver malfunction, weakness, increased blood sugar, pancreatitis, kidney failure, loss of appetite, nausea, vomiting, abdominal discomfort, sore mouth, malabsorption

Bleomycin (Blenoxane)

Type of Cancer Squamous carcinoma of head and neck, Hodgkin's and non-Hodgkin's lymphoma, testis, anus, vulva, uterus, cervix, malignant pleural effusions

Route Administered Intramuscular, Subcutaneous, Intravenous, Intracavitary

Precautions Allergic reactions (antihistamines), lung function tests to detect malfunction early, kidney failure requires reduced dose

Side Effects Darkening of skin, rash and thickening of skin of palms and fingers, lung scarring and decreased breathing function (limited life-time dosage), cough, shortness of breath, joint swelling, fever after first dose (test dose often used), sore mouth, anorexia, nausea/vomiting, difficulty swallowing, weight loss

Carboplatin (Paraplatin)

Type of Cancer Ovary, cervix, small cell lung, head and neck, bladder, testis, mesothelioma, brain

Route Administered Intravenous

Precautions Hydration

Side Effects Anemia, low blood counts, nerve toxicity, decreased hearing, kidney toxicity, nausea, vomiting, loss of appetite, diarrhea, constipation, sore mouth, altered taste

Carmustine (BCNU) (BiCNU)

Type of Cancer Brain, Hodgkin's disease, lymphomas, myeloma, melanoma, lung

Route Administered Intravenous

Precautions May add local anestethic to minimize pain on injection. Pulmonary evaluation if cough or difficulty breathing

Side Effects Anemia, low blood counts, pulmonary fibrosis, occasional liver toxicity, dizziness, loss of balance, skin darkening, vision changes, nausea, vomiting, pain on injection

Chlorambucil (Leukeran)

Type of Cancer Chronic lymphatic leukemia, Hodgkin's and non-Hodgkin's lymphoma, breast, ovary
Route Administered Oral
Side Effects Anemia, low blood counts, rash, hair loss, lung fibrosis (cough), joint pains, loss of menstrual periods, low sperm count, nausea, vomiting, increased uric acid (gout), secondary malignancies

Cisplatin (Platinol)

Type of Cancer Testis, ovary, head and neck, Hodgkin's and non-Hodgkin's lymphoma, sarcomas, bladder, lung, stomach, cervix, myeloma, prostate, mesothelioma
Route Administered Intravenous
Precautions Nausea program, watch for hearing loss, hydration to prevent kidney failure
Side Effects Anemia, low blood counts, nerve toxicity (numbness, tingling, hearing loss) wheezing, reduced blood pressure, fast heart rate, nausea, vomiting, anorexia, mineral imbalance, increased uric acid (gout), loss of taste

Cyclophosphamide (Cytoxan)

Type of Cancer Hodgkin's and non-Hodgkin's lymphoma, multiple myeloma, sarcomas, leukemias, neuroblastoma, breast, lung, testis, endometrium, mycosis fungoides
Route Administered Oral, Intravenous
Precautions Increased fluid intake, bladder emptying
Side Effects Hair loss, bladder irritation or hemorrhage, anemia, low blood counts, immunosuppression, water overload (antidiuretic effect), sterility, lung scarring, increased skin pigmentation, loss of appetite, nausea, vomiting, sore mouth (stomatitis), diarrhea, gastrointestinal ulcers, increased uric acid (gout), secondary malignancies

Cytarabine (Ara-C) (Cytosar)

Type of Cancer Acute leukemia, lymphomas, head and neck
Route Administered Intravenous, Subcutaneous, Spinal (intrathecal)
Side Effects Anemia, low blood counts, immunosuppression, liver malfunction with jaundice, dizziness, lethargy, rash, weakness, neuritis, imbalance (cerebellar toxicity), eye irritation (high dosage), nausea, vomiting, loss of appetite, sore mouth, diarrhea, difficulty swallowing, increased uric acid (gout)

Dacarbazine (DTIC)

Type of Cancer Hodgkin's disease, malignant melanoma, sarcomas, carcinoid, islet cell, medullary thyroid
Route Administered Intravenous
Precautions Nausea program
Side Effects Anemia, low blood counts, liver toxicity, light-headedness, nerve tingling, rash from sun (photosensitivity), hair loss, itching, rash, anorexia, nausea, vomiting, sore mouth (stomatitis), diarrhea, metallic taste

Dactinomycin (Actinomycin D)

Type of Cancer Testis, melanoma, choriocarcinoma, Wilms' tumor, neuroblastoma, retinoblastoma, Kaposi's sarcoma, sarcomas
Route Administered Intravenous
Precautions Severe skin reaction with IV leak
Side Effects Anemia, low blood counts, hair loss, skin lumps, increased skin sensitivity if given with or after x-ray therapy, weakness, sleepiness, nausea, vomiting, loss of appetite, sore mouth, diarrhea, inflamed tongue, sores in corner of mouth

Daunorubicin (Cerubidine)

Type of Cancer Acute lymphoblastic and myelogenous leukemias
Route Administered Intravenous
Precautions Severe skin reaction with IV leak
Side Effects Anemia, low blood counts, cardiac toxicity (limited lifetime dosage), increased sensitivity to radiation, joint pain, nausea, vomiting, sore mouth, diarrhea

Doxorubicin (Adriamycin)

Type of Cancer Lung, breast, bladder, prostate, pancreas, stomach, ovary, thyroid, endometrium, sarcoma, leukemias, Hodgkin's and non-Hodgkin's lymphoma, mesothelioma, myeloma, cancer of unknown primary site, Wilms' tumor
Route Administered Intravenous
Precautions Severe skin reaction with IV leak, monitor effects on heart with special studies
Side Effects Hair loss, anemia, low blood counts, cardiac toxicity (limited lifetime

dosage), skin cracking and increased nailbed pigmentation, increased skin toxicity when given with or after radiation, nausea, vomiting, sore mouth, diarrhea, iron loss, loss of appetite

Estramustine (Emcyt)

Type of Cancer Metastatic prostate.
Route Administered Oral
Precautions May irradiate male breast to minimize swelling
Side Effects Headaches, loss of coordination, liver enzyme elevation, enlarged tender breasts, anemia, low blood counts, heart failure, strokes, thrombosis and embolism, fluid retention, nausea, vomiting, diarrhea

Estrogens (Diethylstilbestrol) (DES)

Type of Cancer Prostate, breast metastases (women 5 or more years post-menopausal and receptor positive)
Route Administered Oral
Precautions Take multivitamins and iron, avoid constipation, use low salt diet. Fluid retention may aggravate heart disease. May irradiate male breast to minimize swelling
Side Effects Increased clotting, enlarged breasts, testicle atrophy, loss of libido, edema (fluid retention), water-soluble vitamin deficiency, iron deficiency, gall stones, sugar intolerance, increased serum calcium, constipation, loss of appetite, nausea, vomiting

Etoposide (VP-16) (Vepesed)

Type of Cancer Acute non-lymphocytic leukemia, lymphome, head and neck, testis
Route Administered Intravenous, Oral
Precautions Monitor blood pressure during infusion

Side Effects Low blood counts, nerve numbness and tingling, wheezing, shortness of breath (bronchospasm), rapid heart rate, hair loss, low blood pressure if IV rate too rapid,.loss of appetite, altered taste and smell, nausea, vomiting, sore mouth, diarrhea, loss of fluids and electrolytes

Fluorouracil (5-FU)

Type of Cancer Breast, stomach, colon, liver, pancreas, ovary, bladder, prostate. Topical use in skin cancer

Route Administered Intravenous, Topical
Precautions Reduce dosage if liver failure
Side Effects Rash, photosensitivity (sun rash), rare heart toxicity, hair loss, anemia, low blood counts, skin dryness, nail cracking and loss, increased tears (tear duct narrowing), hand foot syndrome, (redness of skin), eye irritation, loss of appetite, nausea, vomiting, sore mouth and throat, diarrhea, bile salt loss, thiamine and niacin deficiency

Flutamide (Eulexin)

Type of Cancer Prostate
Route Administered Oral
Side Effects Hot flashes, loss of libido and potency, enlarged tender breasts, liver toxicity, anorexia, nausea, vomiting, diarrhea, lactose deficiency

5-FUDR (Floxuridine)

Type of Cancer Liver (primary or metastatic), head and neck
Route Administered Arterial infusion
Precautions Four times more active than 5-FU, if liver failure occurs, reduce dose
Side Effects Hair loss, rash, anemia, low blood counts, loss of appetite, nausea, vomiting, sore mouth and throat, diarrhea, bile salt loss, thiamine and niacin deficiency

Goserelin (Zoladex)

Type of Cancer Prostate
Route Administered Subcutaneous
Precautions Temporary increased bone pain, use flutamide (Eulexin) to improve results and help prevent flare reaction
Side Effects Hot flashes, enlarged swollen and tender breasts, skin rash, testicular atrophy, peripheral edema, dizziness, headaches, tingling in extremities, loss of appetite, nausea, vomiting, constipation, diarrhea, difficulty swallowing, elevated blood pressure

Hydroxyurea (Hydrea)

Type of Cancer Chronic myelogenous leukemia, head and neck, kidney, brain, melanoma, ovary
Route Administered Oral
Precautions Drink extra fluids
Side Effects Low blood counts, nausea, vomiting, diarrhea, iron loss, loss of appetite, sore mouth, constipation, increased uric acid (gout)

Ifosfamide (Ifex)

Type of Cancer Non-Hodgkin's lymphomas, lung, ovary, testis, sarcomas, melanoma, chronic lymphocytic leukemia
Route Administered Intravenous
Precautions Requires uroprotector (Mesna); bladder catheter often needed during treatment
Side Effects Bladder bleeding and inflammation, cystitis, kidney malfunction, low blood counts, sleepiness and confusion, hair loss, liver malfunction, phlebitis, antidiuretic effect (water overload), lung scarring, nausea, vomiting

Interferon-alpha
Intron-A
Roferon-A

Type of Cancer Melanoma, kidney, myeloma, chronic myelogenous leukemia, hairy cell leukemia, Kaposi's sarcoma, lymphoma
Route Administered Intramuscular
Side Effects Sweating, fever, nerve numbness and tingling, arthralgias, dizziness, rash, skin itching, high blood pressure, flu syndrome, muscle aching, weight loss, loss of appetite, nausea, vomiting, diarrhea, altered taste and smell, sore mouth

Leucovorin (Folinic acid)

Type of Cancer To reverse clinical toxicity of methotrexate and to potentiate and modulate 5-FU
Route Administered Oral, Intramuscular, Intravenous
Precautions May counteract antiepileptic effect of phenobarbital
Side Effects Will increase symptoms of pernicious anemia, allergic reactions, nausea, vomiting

Leuprolide (Lupron)

Type of Cancer Prostate
Route Administered Subcutaneous
Precautions Temporary increased bone pain, use flutamide (Eulexin) to improve results and help prevent flare reaction
Side Effects Hot flashes, enlarged swollen and tender breasts, skin rash, testicular atrophy, peripheral edema, dizziness, headaches, tingling in extremities, loss of appetite, nausea, vomiting, constipation, diarrhea, difficulty swallowing, elevated blood pressure

Levamisole (Ergamisole)

Type of Cancer Colon
Route Administered Oral
Precautions Has been reported to produce "antabuse-like" effects when given concomitantly with alcohol. No alcohol on days one takes levamisole
Side Effects Mild diarrhea, nausea, vomiting, stomatitis (sore mouth), altered taste and smell, abdominal discomfort and diarrhea (especially when combined with 5-FU), low blood counts, fatigue, weakness, and flu-like symptoms. Occasional headaches, confusion, insomnia, excitement and convulsions

Lomustine
CCNU

Type of Cancer Hodgkin's and non-Hodgkin's lymphoma, brain, melanoma, kidney, lung
Route Adminstered Oral
Precautions Nausea program
Side Effects Low blood counts, hair loss, confusion, liver toxicity (jaundice), lung toxicity (cough, shortness of breath), skin rash, itching, pre-leukemia and bone marrow scarring, loss of appetite, nausea, vomiting, diarrhea, sore mouth

Mechlorethamine (Mustargen) (Nitrogen mustard)

Type of Cancer Hodgkin's and non-Hodgkin's lymphoma, malignant pleural effusions, lung, mycosis fungoides
Route Administered Intravenous, Intracavitary
Precautions Antinausea program, severe reaction with IV leak
Side Effects Low blood counts, thrombophlebitis, tissue reaction, second malignancies, hair loss, skin rash (rare), sterility, anorexia, nausea, vomiting, gastrointestinal bleeding and ulcers, increased uric acid (gout), secondary malignancies

Melphalan (Alkeran)

Type of Cancer Multiple myeloma, ovary, breast
Route Administered Oral.
Side Effects Low blood counts, second malignancies, pulmonary scarring, loss of menstrual periods, low sperm count, dermatitis, nausea, vomiting, sore mouth, increased uric acid (gout)

Mercaptopurine (Purinethol) (6-MP)

Type of Cancer Acute leukemia, chronic myelogenous leukemia, immunosuppression

Route Administered Oral

Precautions Reduce dosage if allopurinol also given

Side Effects Low blood counts, liver scarring and abnormal function, lung scarring, shortness of breath, cough, pneumonia, kidney failure, headaches, stroke, mental changes, hair loss, loss of appetite, nausea, vomiting, diarrhea, sore mouth, abdominal discomfort, increased uric acid production (gout)

Mesna (Mesnex)

Type of Cancer To prevent bladder irritation (hemorrhagic cystitis) from ifosfamide and high-dose Cytoxan

Route Adminstered Intravenous

Side Effects Nausea, vomiting, diarrhea

Methotrexate (Mexate)

Type of Cancer Acute leukemia, sarcoma, choriocarcinoma, head and neck, breast, lung, stomach, esophagus, testis, lymphoma, mycosis fungoides

Route Administered Oral, Intravenous, Intramuscular, Subcutaneous, Spinal (intrathecal)

Precautions Maintain good fluid intake, alkaline urine

Side Effects Low blood counts, skin rash, liver enzyme abnormalities and jaundice, kidney toxicity, lung scarring, shortness of breath, seizures, coma, dizziness, confusion, tiredness, joint pains, anorexia, nausea, vomiting, diarrhea, gastrointestinal bleeding and ulcers, lactose intolerance, iron and protein loss, fat-soluble vitamin loss

Mitomycin-C (Mutamycin)

Type of Cancer colon, stomach, pancreas, esophagus, anus, breast, lung, cervix, bladder

Route Administered Intravenous

Precautions Take care not to leak outside of vein, vitamin B6 (pyridoxine) will reduce tissue damage from extravasation, infections, bleeding

Side Effects Weakness, lung scarring (interstitial pneumonitis), renal failure with severe blood platelet reaction (hemolytic-uremic syndrome), hair loss, liver toxicity, synergistic heart toxicity with Adriamycin, loss of appetite, nausea, vomiting, diarrhea, sore mouth, loss of protein and salts, severe skin reaction with IV leak

Mitotane (Lysodren)

Type of Cancer Adrenal cortical carcinoma

Route Administered Oral

Side Effects Lethargy, sleepiness, dizziness, vertigo, skin rash, headaches, high blood pressure, blurred vision, bladder bleeding, anorexia, nausea, diarrhea

Mitoxantrone (Novantrone)

Type of Cancer Acute leukemia, breast, ovary, lymphomas

Route Adminstered Intravenous

Side Effects Low blood counts, heart toxicity, muscle damage, heart failure, liver toxicity, nausea, vomiting, diarrhea, sore mouth, gastrointestinal bleeding and ulcers, urine may turn green

Myleran (Busulfan)

Type of Cancer Chronic myelogenous leukemia, bone marrow transplantation

Route Administered Oral

Precautions Lung function tests

Side Effects Anemia, low blood counts, lung scarring (fibrosis), shortness of breath, loss of menstrual periods, impotence, fever, bruising, skin pigmentation, weakness, enlarged breasts, cataracts, anorexia, nausea, vomiting, diarrhea, dry mouth, sore mouth, increased uric acid (gout)

Progestins (Megace, Provera)

Types of Cancer Breast, prostate, uterus, kidney

Route Adminstered Oral, Intramuscular

Precautions History of thrombophlebitis, contraindicated in the first four months of pregnancy, low salt diet (fluid retention), which may worsen pre-existing epilepsy, migraine, asthma, cardiac or renal problems

Side Effects Vaginal bleeding, spotting and change in menstrual cycle, lack of menstrual periods, edema, (diuretics may be necessary), jaundice, allergic rash, itching, nausea, vomiting, weight gain and mental depression. When used in combination with estrogens, increased cerebral thrombosis and embolism. Occasional glucose intolerance. Increased excretion of salt: a sodium restricted diet may be essential

Tamoxifen (Nolvadex)

Type of Cancer Breast, endometrial, ovary, prostate (under investigation)
Route Administered Oral
Side Effects Hot flashes, low blood counts, vaginal bleeding, itching, anorexia, nausea, vomiting, taste changes, weight gain, dehydration. Bone pain initially may signify response

Thioguanine

Type of Cancer Acute non-lymphocytic leukemia
Route Administered Oral.
Side Effects Low blood counts, liver failure (jaundice), bleeding, rash, anorexia, nausea, vomiting, diarrhea, increased uric acid (gout), niacin and amino acid deficiency

Thiotepa (Triethylenethiophosphoramide)

Type of Cancer Breast, bladder, ovary, Hodgkin's disease, bone marrow transplantation
Route Administered Intravenous
Side Effects Low blood counts, headaches, fever, bronchoconstriction, dizziness, local pain., loss of appetite, nausea, vomiting, potential secondary malignancies

Vincristine (Oncovin)

Type of Cancer Acute lymphocytic leukemia, Hodgkin's and non-Hodgkin's lymphoma, neuroblastoma, testis, sarcomas, lung, breast, cervix, Wilms' tumor
Route Administered Intravenous
Precautions Take care not to leak from IV site (irritating), constipation program
Side Effects Severe reaction with IV leak, numbness, tingling fingers and feet, hair loss, loss of nerve function (foot drop and partial paralysis), low blood counts, nausea, vomiting, constipation, sore mouth and throat, difficulty chewing or swallowing, dry mouth, altered taste and smell, increased uric acid (gout)

Vinblastine (Velban)

Type of Cancer Hodgkin's disease, choriocarcinoma, testis, breast, lung, Kaposi's sarcoma
Route Administered Intravenous
Precautions Take care not to leak from IV site, constipation program
Side Effects Severe skin reaction with IV leak, low blood counts, peripheral neuropathies, headache, rash, hair loss, anorexia, nausea, vomiting, sore mouth or throat, constipation, abdominal discomfort

DIRECTORY OF CANCER CENTERS, ASSOCIATIONS AND SUPPORT GROUPS

American Cancer Society
National Headquarters
1599 Clifton Road NE
Atlanta, GA 30329
800-ACS-2345

Bosom Buddies
CanCare
2929 Selwyn Avenue
Charlotte, NC 28209
704-372-1232

Breast Cancer Advisory Center
11426 Rockville Pike
Suite 406
Rockville, MD 20859
301-984-1020

Cancer Guidance Institute
5604 Solway Street
Pittsburgh, PA 15217
412-521-2291 or 412-782-4023 (hotline)

Cancer Information Service
National Cancer Institute
Bethseda, MD
1-800-4-CANCER

Cancer Support Network
802 East Jefferson
Bloomington, IL 61701
309-829-2273

Candlelighters Foundation
National Headquarters
2025 Eye Street NW
Suite 1011
Washington, DC 20006
202-659-5136

The Concern for Dying
250 West 57th Street
New York, NY 10019
(non-profit organization distributes

will, a document that records patient wishes concerning treatment)

Corporate Angel Network
Building One
Westchester County Airport
White Plains, NY 10604
914-328-1313
(long distance transportation service)

Encore
National Board YWCA
726 Broadway
New York, NY 10003
212-614-2700
(exercise and discussion program for women who have had breast cancer)

International Association for Enterostomal Therapy
505-A Tustin Avenue
Suite 282
Santa Ana, CA 92705
714-972-1725

International Association of Laryngectomies
777 Third Avenue
New York, NY 10017
212-371-2900

Let's Face It
Box 711
Concord, MA 01742
508-371-3186
(for people who have facial disfigurements)

Leukemia Society of America
800 2nd Avenue
New York, NY 10017
212-573-8584

The Lost Chord
(contact a local chapter of the American
Cancer Society)

Make Today Count
PO Box 303
Burlington, IO 52601

Make-a-Wish Foundation of America
1624 East Meadowbrook
Phoenix, AZ
602-248-9474

**National Coalition for Cancer
Survivorship**
323 8th Street SW
Albuquerque, NM 87102
505-764-9956

The National Hospice Organization
1901 N Fort Meyer Drive
Suite 307
Arlington, VA 22209
703-243-5900

National Leukemia Association, Inc.
585 Stewart Avenue
Suite 536
Garden City, NY 11530
516-222-1944

Ronald McDonald Houses
Golin/Harris Communications, Inc.
500 N Michigan Avenue
Chicago, IL 60611
312-836-7114

Share
817 Broadway
6th Floor
New York, NY 10003
212-260-0580
(self-help for women with breast cancer)

Sunshine Foundation
4010 Levick Street
Philadelphia, PA 19135
215-335-2622 or 1-800-767-1976

Sunshine Kids
2902 Ferndale Place
Houston, TX 77098
713-524-1264

The Skin Cancer Fund
Box 561
New York, NY 10156

United Ostomy Association
36 Executive Park
Suite 120
Irvine, CA 92714
714-660-8624

Vital Options
4419 Coldwater Canyon Avenue
Studio City, CA 91604
818-508-5657
(support group for young adults
with cancer)

**Wellness Community National
Headquarters**
1235 5th Street
Santa Monica, CA 90401
213-393-1415
1-800-PRO-HOPE
(comprehensive program to encourage
and support active participation by
patients in improving their quality of life
and their chances of recovery)

Y-ME Breast Cancer Support Program
18220 Harwood Avenue
Homewood, IL 60430
312-799-8338 or 1-800-221-2141 (hotline)
312-799-8228 (24-hour hotline)
(provides support and counselling)

SUGGESTED READINGS

◇

Anderson, Greg. *The Cancer Conqueror: An Incredible Journey to Wellness.* Andrews and McMeel, Kansas City, 1990.

Benjamin, H. *From Victim to Victor.* Jeremy Tarcher, 1987.

Brinker, N. and Harris, C.E. *The Race is Run One Step at a Time.* Simon and Schuster, 1990.

Bruning, N. *Coping with Chemotherapy.* The Dial Press, 1985.

Cox, B.G. *Living with Lung Cancer: a Guide for Patients and their Families.* Triad Publications Co., 1987.

Love, Susan. *Dr. Susan Love's Breast Book.* Addison-Wesley, 1990.

Fiore, Neil A., PhD. *The Road Back to Health: Coping with the Emotional Side of Cancer.* Bantam, 1984.

Graham, Jory. *In the Company of Others: Understanding the Human Needs of Cancer Patients.* Harcourt Brace Jovanovich, 1982.

Larschan, E.J., and Larschan, R.J. *The Diagnosis is Cancer.* Bull Publishing, 1986.

Laszlo, J. *Understanding Cancer.* Harper and Row, 1987.

Morra, Marion, and Eve Potts. *Choices: Realistic Alternatives in Cancer Treatment.* Avon, 1987.

Ramstack, J., Rosenbaum, E.R., and Carter, B. *Nutrition for Cancer Patients.* Bull Publishing, 1990.

Rosenbaum, E.H. *Can You Prevent Cancer?* Mosby Medical Library, 1983.

Rosenbaum, E.H. *Decision for Life: Portrait of Living.* Bull Publishing, 1980.

Rosenbaum, E.H., and Rosenbaum, I.R. *A Comprehensive Guide for Cancer Patients and their Families.* Bull Publishing, 1980.

Rosenbaum, E.H. *Living with Cancer.* Mosby Medical Library, 1982.

Rosenbaum, E.H. and Rosenbaum, I.R. *Going Home - a Home Care Training Program.* Bull Publishing 1980.

Rosenbaum, E.H., Stitt, C.N., Drasin, H., and Rosenbaum, I.R. *Nutrition for the Cancer Patient.* Bull Publishing, 1980.

Young People with Cancer: a Handbook for Parents. Office of Cancer Communi-cations, National Cancer Institute and National Candlelighters Foundation. Department of Health and Human Services, 1988.

MEDICAL BOOKS

The American Cancer Society Cancer Book: Prevention, Detection, Diagnosis, Treatment, Rehabilitation, and Cure. Arthur I. Holleb, ed. Doubleday, 1986.

Cancer Nursing: Principles and Practice. Susan L. Groenwald et al, ed. Jones and Bartlett, 1990.

Cancer: Principles and Practice of Oncology. Vincent T. DeVita, Jr. et al. ed. 3rd edition. Lippincott, 1990.

Cancer Chemotherapy: Principles and Practice. Bruce A. Chabner et al., ed. Lippincott, 1990.

Cancer Chemotherapy Handbook. David S. Fisher and M. Tish Knobf, ed. 3rd edition. Year Book Medical Publishers, 1990.

Cancer Treatment. Charles M. Haskell, ed. W.B. Saunders, 1990.

Diagnosis and Management of Breast Cancer. Marc E. Lippman, MD, et al, ed. W.B. Saunders, 1988.

Handbook of Oncology Nursing. Bonny Libbey Johnson and Jody Gross. Wiley, 1985.

Handbook of Pediatric Oncology. Roberta A. Gottlieb and Donald Pinkel, ed. Little, Brown & Co., 1989.

Handbook of Psychooncology: *Psychological Care of the Patient with Cancer.* James C. Holland and Julia Rowland, ed. Oxford University Press, 1989.

Manual of Clinical Concology. Dennis Albert Casciato and Barry Bennett Lowitz, ed., 2nd edition. Little, Brown & Co., 1988.

Manual of Clinical Problems in Oncology. Carol S. Portlock and Donald R. Goffinet. 2nd edition. Little, Brown & Co., 1986.

Manual of Oncologic Therapeutics 1989/1990. Robert E. Wittes, ed. Lippincott, 1990.

Principles of Cancer Biotherapy. Robret K. Oldham, ed. Raven Press, 1987.

AUDIOTAPES

c/o Cancer Care Associates
3440 Lomita Boulevard
Torrance, CA 90505

Dollinger, M. *Understanding Cancer.* 1990.

Dollinger, M. *Coping with Cancer.* 1991.

INDEX

Petterle, Elmo A., 183
Peutz-Jeghers syndrome, 511
P-glycoprotein, 54, 58
Pharmacists, 22
Phenacetin, 222
Phenobarbital, 237
Pheochromocytoma, 204-8
Pheoxybenzamine, 208
Philadelphia chromosome, 195
Phosphosoda (Fleet's), 125
Photocoagulation, 301
Photodynamic therapy, 70, 227-28, 509
Physical examination, 11-12; *See also* Diagnosis, under cancer type
Physical fitness, 41, 164-66
  isometric exercises, 165
  isotonic exercises, 165
  program planning, 165
Physical therapists, 22
Physician's Desk Reference, 36
Pinealoma, 230
Pineal tumors, 294-95, 299
Pituitary gland cancer, 483-84
  causes, 483
  diagnosis, 483
  questions to ask, 484
  spreading, 483
  symptoms, 483
  treatment, follow-up, 484
  treatment, overview, 484
  treatment, by type, 484
  types, 483
Planning, for future, 183-85
Plasma cell leukemia, 449
Plasma cell myeloma, 7, 449
Plasmapheresis, 454
Pleural effusion, 414, 457
Pneumonia, 84, 145
Polycythemia, 376
Polymorphonuclear leukocytes, 62
  basophils, 63
  eosinophils, 63
  neutrophils, 62, 65
Polyneuropathy, 449
Polyps, 308
"Porcelain" gall bladder, 335
Port-a-Cath catheter, 291
Ports, 39-40, 55
Posterior fossa, of brain, 294, 298
Potentials unlimited, Inc., 170
Pre-cancerous conditions, 37
Precision Low Residue, 126
Prednisone, 123, 142, 237, 259,

275, 292
Preleukemia, 384
Pressure sores, 179
Prevention, 186
  dietary, 191
  environmental, 191
  guidelines, 190
  lifestyle, 191
Primitive neuroectodermal tumors, 285, 295
Procarbazine, 234, 275
Proctitis, radiation, 490
Progesterone, 53, 247, 253
Progestins, 261, 263, 491
Progression, of tumor growths, 53
Prophylactic surgery, 37
Propoxyphene, 140
Prostate cancer, 10, 32, 49, 128, 158, 187, 190
  causes, 486
  diagnosis, 487
  impotence, treatment, 494
  incontinence, treatment, 494
  metastatic, 495
  questions to ask, 495
  recurrence, 495
  risk factors, 486
  screening, 487
  spreading, 485
  staging/grading, 488
  symptoms, 487
  treatment, follow-up, 494
  treatment, overview, 488
  treatment, by stage, 491
  tumors, other, 494
  types, 485
Prostatectomy
  radical, 489-90
  transurethal, 493
Prostate-specific antigen, 190, 487, 494
Prostatic intraepithelial neoplasia, 485
Prostheses, 72
Protein needs, 132
Protein tyrosine kinase, 195-96
Proto-oncogenes, 193, 195
Pruritis, 471
Psychologists, 22
Psychometric testing, 292
Psychoneuroimmunology, 171, 174
Psyllium, 125
Pulmonary complications, 43
Pulmonary embolism, 44, 459
Pumps, 40, 55

ambulatory, 55
balloon, 55
infusaid, 56

Q
Quadrantectomy, 248
Quadriplegia, 252

R
Radiation enteritis, 136
  management of, 137
  medications for, 138
  symptoms, 137
Radiation oncologists, 22, 46
Radiation therapy, 10, 30-31, 40, 45-51
  afterloading, 49
  clinical modifiers, 50
  dosage, 46
  external, 45, 47-48
  fractionation schedule, 46
  high linear energy transfer, 50
  hyperthermia, 49-50
  internal, 45, 47-48
  interstitial, 45, 48
  intracavity, 45, 49
  intraluminal, 49
  intraoperative radiation, 48, 235, 442
  megavoltage machines, 47
  mixed beam, 47
  nurse training in, 103
  nutritional problems, 135-38
  orthovoltage machines, 47
  planning of, 45
  radiation enteritis, 136
  radiation port, 46
  side effects of, 50-51
  simulation, 46
  stereotactic radiosurgery, 48
  therapeutic ratio, 46
  See also Treatment, under cancer type
Radiation Therapy and You, 202
Radioactive iodine (I-131), 48
Radioactive seeds, 37, 45, 48-49
Radioemitter, 40
Radiography. *See* X-rays
Radioprotectors, 50
Radiosensitizers, 215
Radiotherapy. *See* Radiation therapy
Radol, 93
Rads, definition, 46
Ramstack, Janet, 61

A Smithsonian Book of

COMIC-BOOK COMICS

Edited by
Michael Barrier
and
Martin Williams

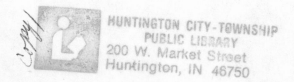
Copublished by
Smithsonian Institution Press and
Harry N. Abrams, Inc., New York

Printed in the United States

**Library of Congress Cataloging in
Publication Data**
Main entry under title:

A Smithsonian book of comic-book
comics.
Bibliography: p.
1. Comic books, strips, etc.—United
States. I. Barrier, J. Michael. II.
Williams, Martin T. III. Smithsonian
Institution. PN6726.S58 741.5'973
81-607842   AACR2
ISBN 0-87474-228-5 (SIP)
ISBN 0-8109-0696-1 (HNA)

All of the stories in this volume
have been reproduced from their first
comic-book printings.

Printed in the United States of America

Contents

About E.C. 295

A Selective, Annotated Bibliography 334

Acknowledgments

The names of the copyright holders who have generously contributed to this volume appear on the comics pages that follow. And we owe special thanks to the following individuals, for help of many kinds.

C. C. Beck, Glenn Bray, Steve Brewster, Steve Brumbaugh, Pete Costanza, Ann Durell, Will Eisner, Harlan Ellison, William M. Gaines, Steve Geppi, Don Glut, Wallace I. Green, Mary C. Janaky, Barbara Johnson, Jenette Kahn, Bob Kane, Selby Kelly, Jim Lawson, Paul Levitz, Chuck McCleary, Mercy Macabeo, Sheldon Mayer, Wendall Mohler, Eileen Opatut, Ethan Roberts, Joe Shuster, Jerry Siegel, Bill Spicer, Terry Stroud, J. R. Taylor, Bill Tighe, Larry R. Vasquez, Kim Weston, John C. Worrell, Craig Yoe.

And the following have an especially strong claim on our gratitude.

John Benson, Rick Durell, Don and Maggie Thompson.

Introduction

The comic book as we know it today—with its slick covers, newsprint-paper insides, and crude colors, all in a package measuring about seven by ten inches—was a long time in being born.

The comic book was the child of the newspaper comic strip, and the comic strip was born in the United States late in the nineteenth century. Several elements that had been separately present in European culture for centuries—drawings in sequence that told a story, "balloons" filled with dialogue, caricature—were combined by American cartoonists, as what quickly came to be called comic strips, in American newspapers beginning in the 1890s. Within a few years, daily comic strips and Sunday comics sections in color were widely featured in American newspapers.

Some newspaper comics offered extended narratives—stories that were told over many days, and in many drawings—almost from the start. And although the full-color Sunday comics were often presented in a grid pattern—rows of boxed drawings, or panels, of the same size—cartoonists sometimes dealt with the comics page as a whole, giving their panels different shapes and arranging them in unusual ways.

Many ingredients of the comic book—the comic-strip form, the extended narrative, the page as a basic unit along with the panel—were thus present in newspaper strips from around the turn of the century. (The Sunday comics section—very thick and colorful in those early days—was itself a comic book of a sort.) But just as the comic strip took a curiously long time to assume its definitive shape, so too did the comic book.

For about three decades, publishers experimented with formats of many kinds. They first reprinted newspaper strips in books (both hard and soft covers), making what one might call early comic books. In 1929, one publisher tried something different—a weekly publication made up of completely new comics. Called *The Funnies,* it died after a few issues, perhaps because it was tabloid size (twice as large as a modern comic book) and so looked too much like a Sunday comics section.

In 1933, comic books of approximately the modern size and shape were published by Eastern Color Printing Company—but as premiums, to be given away by retailers and manufacturers to their customers. No one thought about selling these comic books directly to readers until M. C. Gaines, a salesman at Eastern Color, tested the market by putting ten-cent price stickers on a few copies and leaving them at two newsstands. The comic books quickly sold out, and this led—after a few false starts—to the publication of

Famous Funnies No. 1 in May 1934. *Famous Funnies* was sold on newsstands for a dime, and it was soon being published on a monthly schedule. It was the first true comic book in the modern sense.

But, like the premium comic books that preceded it, *Famous Funnies* was composed of reprinted newspaper strips. The first comic book made up entirely of new material did not appear until early in 1935; this was *New Fun* No. 1. In later years, comic books with new material came to dominate the field, eclipsing the comic books made up of reprints.

So, depending on the definition one uses, the first comic book was published anywhere from early in the century to as late as 1935. But the real turning point in the comic book's history probably came in the summer of 1932.

Jerry Siegel, a student at Glenville High School in Cleveland, and his classmate, Joe Shuster, had become friends because of a shared interest in comic strips, particularly heroic fantasies like *Tarzan* and *Buck Rogers*. They began to make comic strips of their own; Siegel wrote and Shuster illustrated. As Siegel later told the story to a writer for the *Saturday Evening Post,* the idea for the new strip came to him one hot night in 1932, as he was trying to fall asleep:

"I am lying in bed counting sheep when all of a sudden it hits me. I conceive a character like Samson, Hercules, and all the strong men I ever heard tell of rolled into one. Only more so. I hop right out of bed and write this down, and then I go back and think some more for about two hours and get up again and write that down. This goes on all night at two-hour intervals, until in the morning I have a complete script."

That morning, Siegel rushed to Shuster's house, and they whipped up the script and the drawings for twelve installments of a daily newspaper strip—two weeks' worth—to submit to newspaper syndicates. The strip was called *Superman.* The established syndicates were uniformly unflattering in their assessments of Siegel and Shuster's samples and *Superman* gathered a large pile of rejection slips. When *Superman* finally found a home, in 1938, it was in the first issue of a monthly comic book, *Action Comics,* wherein the strips had been cut up and the panels rearranged to make a thirteen-page feature.

Within a short time, *Action Comics*—with *Superman* in each issue—was selling almost a million copies every month, the bimonthly *Superman* comic book was selling well over a million copies per issue, and the character had spread from comic books to radio and the movies. And to the

10

newspapers—by 1941, *Superman* as a daily strip signed by Siegel and Shuster, was running in 230 papers.

If, in the mid-1930s, just one syndicate editor had come to a different decision and given *Superman* a test run, the history of comic books would surely have been different. Had *Superman* squeezed onto the newspaper comics pages before 1938, the strip probably would have wound up in a reprint comic book, and a second-hand *Superman* of that kind could not have changed comic books the way that *Action Comics* and the *Superman* bimonthly did.

Superman alerted publishers to the riches to be gained from offering readers the larger-than-life costumed super-hero, and within a couple of years the newsstands were filled with comic books starring such characters, and comic books themselves had become big business. Some of the new heroes were super-human, like Superman, although they usually had fewer powers than Superman did, and some of them had powers that Superman did not (the ability to burst into flame, for example, or to stretch one's body into all sorts of improbable shapes). Other heroes were not super-human, but had well-developed muscles and specialized skills; they were not the heirs of Superman so much as of the masked, law-into-their-own-hands vigilantes (the Phantom, the Lone Ranger, the Green Hornet, and others) who had become popular through comic strips, radio, and pulp fiction. However, the new comic-book vigilantes were clad in costumes far more garish than simple masks. The exemplar was Batman, whose adventures became the lead feature in *Detective Comics* (published by National, the company that brought out the *Superman* titles) a year after Superman's debut. Batman quickly became the second most popular of the super-heroes; his bimonthly comic book was selling 800,000 copies per issue by 1941.

Not all comic-book heroes had the sustained success of Superman and Batman, but starting in the early 1940s other kinds of comic books, from many different publishers, found favor with millions of readers. The Walt Disney characters Mickey Mouse and Donald Duck began appearing monthly in *Walt Disney's Comics and Stories* in the fall of 1940, and other comic books with animated-cartoon characters soon followed. Another genre was the comic book with teenage characters; the *Archie* feature, which first appeared in 1941 as a filler in a super-hero comic book, spawned a multitude of imitators. The western—that staple of Americana—made the transition to comic books with ease, and cowboy movie stars like Roy Rogers and Gene Autry became comic-book stars as well. Romance comic books flourished in the postwar years, sharing the appeal of radio soap operas and confession magazines.

Of the many new genres, the one that ultimately had the greatest effect on the industry was the crime comic book. Crime was always present in the super-hero comic books—the heroes usually proved themsleves to be heroes by defeating criminals—but in the new crime comics, the emphasis was on the crimes themselves. A wave of such comic books started with *Crime Does Not Pay* in 1942 and crested in the postwar years. The success of the frequently lurid and violent crime comic books encouraged one publisher, E. C., to go a step further, and in 1950 it introduced three horror titles—*The Crypt of Terror, The Vault of Horror,* and *The Haunt of Fear.* Other publishers quickly scented a bonanza, and the comic racks filled up with bloody axes, severed heads, and rotting corpses.

Comic books had been criticized in print since 1940 or so; because most of the readers were children, some people worried that comic books—crude and violent as many of them were—might be damaging young minds. The crime and horror comic books were found especially alarming, and a storm of indignation finally struck the industry with full force in 1954. Comic books were dumped on bonfires; comic books were denounced in Congress; comic books were solemnly condemned by psychiatrists as the root of a host of social evils. (And, more important for business, distributors started refusing to accept some comic books from the publishers.) As the movie producers had done twenty years earlier, the comic-book publishers responded to charges of immorality by drawing up an extremely strict code and entrusting its enforcement to a panel recruited from outside the industry. Only one major publisher—Dell, whose comic books starred such licensed characters as Donald Duck and the Lone Ranger and had attracted little criticism—could afford to shun the new Comics Code.

The adoption of the Comics Code in October 1954 marked the end of sixteen years of flamboyant success for the comic-book industry. Many publishers left the business in the 1950s, and total circulation fell sharply. Despite occasional bursts of prosperity (like the one that accompanied the public's interest in the *Batman* television show of the 1960s), comic books have never come close to equaling their popularity in the 1940s and early 1950s. Once ubiquitous on newsstands and in drug stores, variety stores, and supermarkets, comic books in recent years have been slipping slowly out of sight.

Even when comic books were at the peak of their success,

very little of that success trickled down—in the form of money or artistic freedom—to the writers and cartoonists who were producing the magazines.

For the most part, comic books did not attract established, main-line magazine publishers. They attracted publishers that were already on the fringes—companies that specialized in pulp fiction or movie-fan magazines or, at best, mass-market children's books. Such publications were produced mostly according to formulas, with the formulas determined by whatever sold well. The publishers were accustomed to dealing with formula writers, and everything that passed through their hands was therefore treated like hackwork. In such an atmosphere, there was not much incentive to try to make comic-book stories into artistic statements.

And if a feature turned out to have great commercial value, it was the publisher, not the artist or writer, who profited. (Siegel and Shuster were paid only ten dollars a page for the *Superman* story that was published in *Action Comics* No. 1—and they were required by the publisher to sign away all rights to the character. Although they continued to work on the *Superman* comic books and strips, it was as employees only.) The artists and writers who worked on comic books were often not allowed to sign their work, and many saw comic books only as a rung on the ladder leading up to a contract for a syndicated newspaper strip, or to writing for radio or slick magazines, or to a career in commercial art.

In short, there was no reason to believe that the comic book, when it was flourishing in the 1940s and 1950s, would give birth to stories of enduring value. But it did.

The comic books' readers can take part of the credit. Readers often responded with delight to those few comics that broke free of the formulas or turned them to new purposes. *Captain Marvel, Uncle Scrooge, Little Lulu,* and the early *Mad* won the allegiance of hundreds of thousands of readers. But of course the readers could not bring such comic books into being by themselves.

On at least one occasion, a group of comics creators—supported by an enlightened publisher—set out to do work well above the industry norm. That happened in the early 1950s at E.C., the company that spawned the horror-comic boom. Cushioned by the profits from E.C.'s crime and horror titles, the company's editors and artists put their best efforts into science-fiction and war comic books that were aimed at more mature readers (and did not sell as well as crime and horror). E.C.'s patience with slow-selling titles paid off spectacularly when the satirical *Mad,* edited and written by Harvey Kurtzman, became a best seller after a rocky start.

Another cartoonist did not have to seek out a mature audience; it came built in. Will Eisner's *Spirit*—the adventures of a masked crime-fighter—was distributed as a small comic-book section with Sunday newspapers, and as such was read by adults as well as by children—perhaps more by adults than by children. Although Eisner worked under severe deadline pressures—turning out a seven-page story every week—he worked under few pressures of any other kind, and many episodes of *The Spirit* were so formula-free that the title character played only a limited role in them.

But outstanding stories usually emerged in another way. A single cartoonist was hired to perform a specific, limited task; often—but not always—he was hired to both write and draw his stories. The cartoonist set out to do the work in the spirit of a craftsman; and slowly, he became something more than a craftsman.

For example, a few cartoonists started with conventional super-heroes—C. C. Beck with Captain Marvel, Jack Cole with Plastic Man—and put them at the center of stories that were far more witty and charming than comic-book conventions had seemed to permit. Other cartoonists, like Walt Kelly and George Carlson, found havens in comic books intended for very young children. Many such comic books were published in the 1940s, especially by Dell, which brought out *Animal Comics, Fairy Tale Parade, Raggedy Ann and Andy,* and *Santa Claus Funnies.* It was in these low-key Dell comic books that Kelly perfected the skills that he put to use in his famous *Pogo.* Unlike Kelly, who worked in comic books in the early stages of his career, Carlson came to comic books—to *Jingle Jangle Comics*—after many years as a cartoonist and illustrator. He saw—and seized—an opportunity to cap his career with very free and inventive stories about such zanies as the Pie-Face Prince.

Other cartoonists wrote and drew humorous features to be used as "comic relief" in titles that were dominated by characters meant to be taken more seriously. Both Sheldon Mayer and Basil Wolverton filled this role in the 1940s—Mayer with this *Scribbly* feature, Wolverton with *Power house Pepper* and other features. Since they worked on the edges of the spotlight, Mayer and Wolverton could indulge comic fancies even to the point of mocking the super-heroes that were the mainstay of the industry.

In the 1940s, it was common for a cartoonist to be paired with an existing character and to draw the stories with that character in issue after issue, perhaps for years. Such pairings did not lead inevitably to distinguished work; but sometimes, a gifted cartoonist could find unsuspected possibilities in an established character. That happened when Carl Barks was assigned to the *Donald Duck* feature in *Walt Disney's Comics and Stories,* and when John Stanley was asked to write and draw the new *Little Lulu* comic book. Both cartoonists turned out brilliant stories in which the familiar characters were transformed and enriched.

Other cartoonists, too—far more than could be represented in this book—did comic-book work that reflects high levels of both craft and caring.

Comic books did not seek out truly original talents. But in its heyday, the field was so large and so fluid that talented people could find ways to do exceptional work—and, sometimes, extraordinary work.

Our volume is intended to be not so much a survey or a sampler as a statement about the comic book at its best. Therefore, most of our choices are here because of our own convictions about their quality. We considered several thousand stories in making our selections. One or the other or both of us read all, or almost all, of the comic-book work of some of the creators represented here (Barks, Stanley, Kelly, Carlson) and large selections from the others. We also sought and received valuable advice from several people whose names you will find in our acknowledgments. But the choices here are our own.

To reduce the criteria for our selections to a few words would be difficult, but perhaps we can say that we have looked for compelling stories whose creators have made use of the medium itself—who have made their words and pictures work together to achieve results not possible in any other medium.

It will not come as a surprise, to anyone who has glanced at this volume's table of contents, that we think most highly of the humor features, even those that treated the conventions of the comic book itself and the concept of the super-heroes themselves with humor. And it will soon be evident also that our own list of the major talents of the comic book would begin with Carl Barks, Walt Kelly, John Stanley, C. C. Beck, Will Eisner . . .

Our cut-off date for this collection has been the adoption of the Comics Code in October 1954 (the first comic books that had been subjected to the Code's requirements were published in the spring of 1955). Nothing published after the Code took effect will be found here. The adoption of the Code marked a distinct change in the industry, although some comic books with real vitality—like Stan Lee's collaborations

15

with Jack Kirby and Steve Ditko in the Marvel super-hero comics (*Fantastic Four, Amazing Spider-Man*) of the mid-1960s—have been published under the Code.

Inevitably there are dozens of popular features that are not included in this volume; *Blackhawk* and *The Heap* are two much-admired examples. We have been forced to exclude the work of many highly regarded artists; Alex Toth, for one. Many artists were not well served by the writers whose scripts they illustrated, and we have felt that the features included in this book should be distinguished in writing as well as drawing. There are also genres and types of comics that we have not represented. We have no romance comics and no westerns. There are no teenage comics here, and hence no examples from the very durable *Archie* magazines. We include no examples of the comics based on classic novels, plays, and poems, and none of the comics based on movies or—except for the Disney ducks—on the supposed adventures of movie stars, such as Bob Hope, Jerry Lewis, or others. We have also avoided those comics that were based on newspaper strips—those that offer not reprints but new material about their characters.*

All of the features in this book are, of course, comic-book originals. And it is our conviction that although some may show the work of assistants, none were in any sense ghosted, and all are ultimately the work of the men we have identified as the authors.

But enough. It is high time for the reader to begin to enjoy that work.

Michael Barrier
Martin Williams

---

* Those latter magazines, incidentally, were often turned out by the syndicate that distributed the strip and were probably never seen by the newspaper strip's author or authors. A few conscientious strip artists did directly supervise their comic-book ghosts. And a small few even worked, with assistants, on the comic-book adventures of their characters.

About "Superman"

As we have seen, comic-book originals began to appear in 1935; the first was a magazine called *New Fun.* In its first issue, *New Fun* (its name was soon changed to *More Fun*) was anything but impressive. Some of its features had a professional look; more of them looked like the work of promising amateurs; and some seemed to be the work of amateurs of little promise. Many of them were indeed the work of eager teenagers in their conception, their scripting, and their drawing. But from *More Fun* came the magazines *New Adventure, Detective Comics,* and *Action Comics,* and from these came the whole line of National Periodical Publications, now called DC Comics and now part of a huge conglomerate.

Two things intervened to make all that possible: the arrival of the feature called *Superman* in 1938 and the one called *Batman* in 1939, both in comic books published by National Comics. Indeed, at second hand, the sustained success of these features probably made a whole industry possible and, thus, at third hand made the contents of this book possible.

Superman, as we have said, came from Jerry Siegel, who wrote it, and Joe Shuster, who drew it. They had been contributing to *More Fun* and *Detective Comics* since 1936, but they originally intended *Superman* to be a newspaper strip and had submitted it unsuccessfully to almost every syndicate there was. Harry Donenfeld purchased it for *Action Comics* and had its daily-format panels pasted into a thirteen-page feature. Three years later *Superman* was appearing in three comic books simultaneously and still other *Superman* adventures had newspaper distribution as well.

The idea of a secret identity for Superman (he is otherwise, of course, Clark Kent, "mild-mannered reporter") could have come from such heroes of pulp fiction as the Shadow and the Spider or their radio counterparts like the Green Hornet or from the several films based on the Zorro character—but, in the Scarlet Pimpernel of the British novelist Baroness Orczy, the idea dates back earlier than they.

Philip Wylie's 1930 science-fiction novel, *Gladiator,* has often been suggested as Superman's inspiration. An equally handy suggestion could have come from John Carter, the hero of Edgar Rice Burroughs's Martian adventures. Carter was an American mysteriously teleported to Mars in the 1860s. There he discovered that the lesser pull of Martian gravity made his earthling's muscles exceedingly powerful: he could leap to great heights, run in great strides, and fight with superior strength. Substitute Krypton for Mars, reverse the idea, and one has Kryptonian Clark Kent-Superman on earth, "able to leap tall buildings at a single bound." Indeed, in his initial conception, superior strength and leaping power on earth, plus a skin impenetrable to bullets, were Superman's super powers. The ability to fly unlimited distances and X-ray vision—such powers came later.

On the other hand, one does not have to look for conscious sources for *Superman* or look too far to account for his appeal. The promotional material for the 1978 *Superman* movie made the matter virtually specific in the blurb, "with Marlon Brando as Jor-El, who gave his only son to save the world." Intended or not (and the allusion would not *have* to be conscious), only the word "begotten" seems to be missing from the sentence.

Superman: conceived in a magic land in the sky (the planet Krypton), from a superior group of beings and fathered by a wise and powerful member of that group (Jor-El), threatened in his infancy with death (the destruction of Krypton), sent to earth, raised in humble surroundings (the farming Kent family), the possessor of great powers that he uses to save mankind.

Superman is one version of the hero with a thousand faces—to employ the title of Joseph Campbell's excellent book on the subject—and his appeal should therefore not surprise us. But Superman is a crude version of the hero; if you will, an elementary one. Unlike his more developed analogues in all the world's great religions, Superman does not offer love or goodwill, self-knowledge or contemplation as keys to man's salvation. He offers his own physical powers. Ultimately Superman's message for man rests only in his own superior strength and lies in his power to be an enforcer of his own judgement of what is good and what is evil.

For our Superman choice here, rather than jump forward to his later appearances in his own *Superman* comics, we have chosen the less frequently reprinted first appearance in *Action Comics* No. 1, with Siegel's episodic scripting (designed for daily newspapers, remember) and Shuster's cartoon-oriented drawing style. Superman's origin is barely sketched; Krypton is unnamed; Kent's newspaper is called the *Daily Star;* and although there is a "Lois," there is no Perry White and no Jimmy Olsen.

M.W.

SUPERMAN

JEROME SIEGEL & JOE SHUSTER

As a distant planet was destroyed by old age, a scientist placed his infant son within a hastily devised space-ship, launching it toward Earth!

When the vehicle landed on Earth, a passing motorist, discovering the sleeping babe within, turned the child over to an orphanage

Attendants, unaware the child's physical structure was millions of years advanced of their own, were astounded at his feats of strength

When maturity was reached, he discovered he could easily:

Leap ⅛th of a mile; hurdle a twenty-story building....

Raise tremendous weights...

...Run faster than an express train....

—and that nothing less than a bursting shell could penetrate his skin!

Early, Clark decided he must turn his titanic strength into channels that would benefit mankind. And so was created....

SUPERMAN!

Champion of the oppressed, the physical marvel who had sworn to devote his existence to helping those in need!

A SCIENTIFIC EXPLANATION OF CLARK KENT'S AMAZING STRENGTH

Kent had come from a planet whose inhabitants' physical structure was millions of years advanced of our own. Upon reaching maturity, the people of his race became gifted with titanic strength!

—Incredible? No! For even today on our world exist creatures with super-strength!

The lowly ant can support weights hundreds of times its own.

The grasshopper leaps what to man would be the space of several city blocks.

From *Action Comics* No. 1, June 1938.
© 1938 Detective Comics, Inc.
Renewal © 1965 DC Comics, Inc.

21

THE *DAILY STAR* OFFICE IS REACHED...

YOU WANTED TO SEE ME?

YES, BE SEATED

34

DID YOU EVER HEAR OF *SUPERMAN*?

WHAT!

35

REPORTS HAVE BEEN STREAMING IN THAT A FELLOW WITH GIGANTIC STRENGTH NAMED *SUPERMAN* ACTUALLY EXISTS. I'M MAKING IT YOUR STEADY ASSIGNMENT TO COVER THESE REPORTS. THINK YOU CAN HANDLE IT, KENT?

LISTEN, CHIEF, IF *I* CAN'T FIND OUT ANYTHING ABOUT THIS *SUPERMAN NO ONE CAN*!

36

HURRY, KENT— A PHONED TIP... WIFE-BEATING AT 211 COURT AVE!

I'M ON MY WAY!

37

AT 211 COURT AVE. — — 38

HOLD IT!

WHAT D'YOU WANT?

DON'T GET TOUGH!

TOUGH IS PUTTING *MILDLY* THE TREATMENT YOUR GOING TO GET!

YOU'RE NOT FIGHTING A WOMAN, NOW!

40

BUTCH FORCES LOIS'S TAXI INTO A DITCH!

PULL OVER THERE!

LET ME GO!

GET IN THAT CAR AND SHUT UP!

WHAT BURNS ME UP IS THAT I LET HER YELLOW BOY FRIEND OFF SO EASY!

WELL, MAYBE YOU TWO MAY MEET AGAIN

THEN I HOPE IT'LL BE SOON!

HEY — WATCH OUT! SOME ONE'S STANDING IN THE ROAD AHEAD OF US!

HA! HA! WATCH ME SCARE HIM OUT OF HIS WITS!

LOOK OUT! YOU'LL HIT HIM!

SUPERMAN HURDLES THE ONCOMING AUTO!

IT'S THE DEVIL HIMSELF!

BUTCH! STEP ON THE GAS! HE'S CHASING AFTER US!!!

BUTCH'S CAR LEAPS FORWARD LIKE A RELEASED ROCKET, BUT IS EASILY OVERTAKEN BY SUPERMAN

THE OCCUPANTS OF THE CAR ARE SHAKEN OUT ——

NEXT, SUPERMAN OVERTAKES BUTCH IN ONE SPRING..

——AND THE CAR, ITSELF, SMASHED TO BITS!

JUST A MINUTE, BUTCH!

DO YOU MIND?

THIS WILL TAKE BUT A FEW SECONDS

About "Batman"

Just as we have included Superman's first appearance, we have also selected Bob Kane's first six-page account of *The Bat-Man* (as it was called) from *Detective Comics* No. 27. And even less than the first Superman appearance is it concerned with its hero's fictional origin.

The details of the Batman's creation are somewhat obscure and even controversial. National Comics editor Whitney Ellsworth frankly wanted a bizarre character who would be as popular as the company's Superman. He went to Kane, who had been working regularly with writer Bill Finger, and between them they worked out the Batman.

A bat-costumed night-stalker had appeared more than once in pulp magazines—on either side of the law. And Kane, incidentally, points to a striking analogy in his early Batman depiction and Leonardo's notebook designs for his flying devices.

Batman was, by day, Bruce Wayne, a man with inherited millions, a rather bored character who was friend to the city's Police Commissioner Gordon. Acting on information he casually gathered from Gordon, Wayne became the Batman by night, a self-trained strongman, gymnast, and acrobat, with high intelligence—a costumed vigilante who preyed on the fears, superstitions, and insecurities of criminals to stalk them and turn them over to the police (or occasionally, in the early days, to shoot them himself).

Wayne, it was later revealed, had been orphaned when his well-to-do parents were killed in a street holdup, and he decided to devote his life to fighting crime, or rather, of course, to one-man vigilante justice. The feature's other regular characters, Alfred, Kane's butler, and Robin, the Boy Wonder (a young orphaned circus acrobat whom Wayne adopted), came later.

So did the colorful recurring criminals: The Joker, the Penguin, the horrifying Two-Face, and the rest. And there the inspiration, like the inspiration for the feature's flat, angular, poster-like drawing style, was in part Chester Gould's *Dick Tracy* newspaper strip. As *Batman* evolved, a brooding, threatening quality was sustained in its predominantly black, night-time panels.

Kane had begun his comic-book career at age twenty; at first it was mostly devoted to humor strips, plus a couple of thrillers he worked on with Bill Finger. He remained with *Batman* well into the 1960s. Meanwhile, the feature's quick success had led to several comic books, to the employment of artist Jerry Robinson to share the work, to a newspaper strip version, to two movie serials—long before the campy TV version of the 1960s.

M.W.

From *Detective Comics* No. 27, May 1939.
© 1939 Detective Comics, Inc.
Renewal © 1966 DC Comics, Inc.

About "Scribbly" and Sheldon Mayer

The following early sequence from Sheldon Mayer's *Scribbly* is heartening evidence that the implicit pomposity of the costumed super-heroes received romping, low-comic comment almost from the moment of their arrival (and in a comic book from National, the home of the most popular super-heroes).

The *Scribbly* feature did not quite begin with this uninhibited super-hero buffoonery. In the first issue of *All-American Comics,* it introduced the adventures of a would-be boy cartoonist, and it developed and explored that premise for ten subsequent years, not only in *All-American* but in the young protagonist's own magazine. Mayer was also editor of *All-American,* and *Scribbly* was a comic interlude among the more earnest doings of *The Green Lantern, The Atom,* and a *Rescue on Mars.* Predictably, perhaps, Scribbly sometimes confused his own life with the events in his cartoonist's fantasies.

Mayer was born in 1917 in New York City, where he worked as an assistant (and occasional ghost) to several established cartoonists, beginning in 1932. By 1936, in addition to his other work, Mayer had begun to help with the editing of a new comic-book line for Dell, and thus he was a founding professional of the comic book. He held the editorship of *All-American* and its related titles for ten years, and he continued to write features of all kinds for National Comics after that. After *Scribbly,* however, Mayer's most respected feature was another humor strip, *Sugar and Spike,* begun in 1956 and continued through 1971. It was his own reaction to the many derivative comic-book imitations of Hank Ketcham's newspaper feature, *Dennis the Menace,* and his own determination not to do another one. In *Sugar and Spike,* Mayer came up with two spunky infants, merrily observing and involving themselves in the adult world, but communicating in a gibberish baby talk that only they (and the reader) understood.

As we join the *Scribbly* saga, the formidable Ma Hunkel has bought a grocery store, and some racketeers have made the mistake of trying to collect "protection money" from her. She has mussed them up and they have fled in their car—not knowing that Ma's daughter Sisty and Scribbly's brother Dinky have locked themselves in the rumble seat.

M.W.

44

WHO IS THIS MYSTERIOUS FIGURE WHO HAS COME TO THE RESCUE OF SISTY AND DINKY? WHOEVER HE IS, HE CERTAINLY PICKED THE RIGHT TIME TO SHOW UP! DON'T MISS THE NEXT ISSUE KIDS—

From *All-American Comics* No. 21, December 1940

47

48

49

150-85A

From *All-American Comics* No. 22, January 19...
© 1940 All American Comics, I...
Renewal © 1968 DC Comics, I...

53

From *All-American Comics* No. 23, February 19
© 1940 All American Comics,
Renewal © 1968 DC Comics,

56

From *All-American Comics* No. 24, March 19
© 1941 J.R. Publishing

59

EXTRA! EXTRA! RED TORNADO A HOAX! READ ALL ABAHT IT!

In practically no time at all, an extra edition of the Morning Despatch is spread all over town announcing the Red Tornado Hoax!

③

HEY, SMOKEY, DIDJA READ THIS? NO MORE RED TORNADO!

YEAH, I GUESS DERE AINT NOTHIN' TO BE AFRAID OF NOW.... WE KIN ROUND UP TH' GANG, AN' START COLLECTIN' PROTECTION MONEY FROM TH' SUCKERS AGAIN!

AND SO, BEFORE THE EXTRA EDITION IS MORE THAN AN HOUR OLD, THE RACKETEERS WHOM THE RED TORNADO HAD SCARED INTO HIDING, ARE OUT OF THEIR RAT-HOLES, AND BUSY AT WORK!!

C'MON—PAY UP OR ELSE!!

D-DON'T HIT ME—I'LL PAY!

BUT I DON'T WANT A SLOT MACHINE IN MY STORE!

YOU'LL TAKE IT, AN' LIKE IT, BUD!

By evening, everyone is talking about the sudden crime wave--- within twelve hours, it has been felt all over town!

DIDJA HEAR WHAT THEY'RE SAYIN' ABOUT TH' RED TORNADO, DINKY?

YEAH--IT'S AWFUL, AINT IT? I JUS' CAN'T BELIEVE TH' RED TORNADO WUS A FAKE!

WELL, WHETHER HE'S A FAKE OR NOT, THEM PUNK GANGSTERS ARE STILL MAKIN' PESTS OF THEMSELVES! SOMEBODY OUGHTTA STOP 'EM!

YEAH—WHAT THIS COUNTRY NEEDS IS MORE AN' BETTER MYSTERY MEN

YOU GOT IT! C'MON!

I GOT IT? I GOT WHAT? HEY!! WHO YA PULLIN'?

YOU, YA DOPE! YA GOT A IDEAR! STAND STILL!

HEY! WHADDAYA DOIN'?

WHAT AM I DOIN', HE ASKS ME! I'M CREATIN' TWO OF TH' COUNTRY'S BEST MYSTERY MEN! THE CYCLONE KIDS!!

?

160-95A

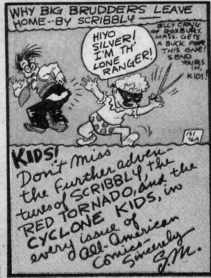

About "Plastic Man" and Jack Cole

Plastic Man was the creation of Jack Cole, a man whose life came close to true tragedy.

Cole was born in 1918 in New Castle, Pennsylvania. He once took a correspondence course in cartooning, but he was a man with the natural talents of a cartoonist. By 1937, he was already at work in comic books, turning out gag features built around more or less traditional "big foot" characters. Within two years, however, he was meeting the demand for super-heroes and adventure by editing, drawing, and writing several features, including the durable *Daredevil.* Cole also worked as an assistant to Will Eisner, particularly on the daily newspaper version of *The Spirit* that ran in the early 1940s.

Meanwhile, the magazine *Police Comics* had appeared in 1941, and in it Cole's inventive *Plastic Man,* a light-hearted feature with a crime-fighting hero who did have a super-power, but a super-power with decidedly comic implications. Clearly, *Plastic Man,* featuring what Joe Brancatelli has called "breathless story telling and a refined, semi-slapstick," combined elements of Cole's "realistic" present and his "big foot" past in a single feature. The balance was not perfectly achieved, however, until the appearance of *Police Comics* No. 13 and the arrival of a maladroit sidekick in Woozy Winks, an out-and-out traditional clown, right down to his costume.

By 1943, Plastic Man ("Plas" to his admirers) had his own comic book, and the feature thrived under Cole's guidance through 1950. Others took over the comic book, and it lasted until 1956. (And there have been revivals since, including an animated TV version in 1979.)

Cole meanwhile had begun a career as a panel cartoonist in such publications as *Collier's* and the *Saturday Evening Post.* By 1955, he had begun a regular collection of *Females by Cole* in *Playboy.* In 1958, a humorous Cole "family strip" called *Betsy and Me* began daily newspaper syndication by the Chicago *Sun-Times.* But on August 15th of that year, Jack Cole took his own life. He left no note and gave no explanation.

We have chosen Plastic Man's first appearance for inclusion here, and the adventure of the arrival of Woozy Winks.

M.W.

From *Police Comics* No. 1, August 194
© 1941 Comic Magazine

TH' YELLOW #$#$%!! GOTTA GET AWAY... SOMEHOW... SOME-PLACE!! CURSE THIS ACID! IT'S IN THE WOUND AND STINGIN' LIKE BLAZES!!!

LATER IN A DAZE THE EEL WANDERS THROUGH SWAMPS:

MUST... KEEP GOING!! COPS COMING!!

THEN UP A MOUNTAIN SIDE:

LEGS WON'T WORK..... HEAD REELING!! CAN'T GO ON!

THEN, UNCONSCIOUSNESS:

SOME TIME LATER HE AWAKENS:

OH, MY HEAD! WHERE AM I? WHO ARE—??

YOU ARE IN REST-HAVEN, SON!

IN HEAVEN?? ME? QUIT TH' KIDDIN'! WHERE I'M GOIN, THE COLDEST DAY IS °300 ABOVE!

REST-HAVEN, MY BOY... A MOUNTAIN RETREAT FAR FROM THE TROUBLED WORLD!

I FOUND YOU ON THE TRAIL THIS MORNING EEL O'BRIAN!

HOW DO YOU KNOW MY NAME?

THE POLICE TRAILED YOU HERE, BUT I TURNED THEM AWAY!!

YOU... YOU DID THIS... TOOK A CHANCE LIKE THAT FOR ME? WHY??

BECAUSE SOMETHING TOLD ME THAT HERE IS A MAN WHO COULD BECOME A VALUABLE CITIZEN IF HE ONLY HAD THE CHANCE!

COME, WON'T YOU TELL ME YOUR STORY?

WELL, Y'SEE, MY FOLKS DIED WHEN I WAS TEN, LEAVING ME ALONE IN THE WORLD. I TRIED TO WORK HARD BUT PEOPLE KEPT PUSHING ME AROUND—ALWAYS PUSHING!! UNTIL FINALLY I GOT TIRED OF IT AND STARTED PUSHING THEM AROUND!!

EEL TELLS HIS STORY

I'D COMPLETELY LOST FAITH IN MANKIND UNTIL.... WELL, YOU'VE GIVEN ME A NEW SLANT ON THINGS!

BUT THE IMPORTANT THING RIGHT NOW IS TO REST AND GET WELL!

68

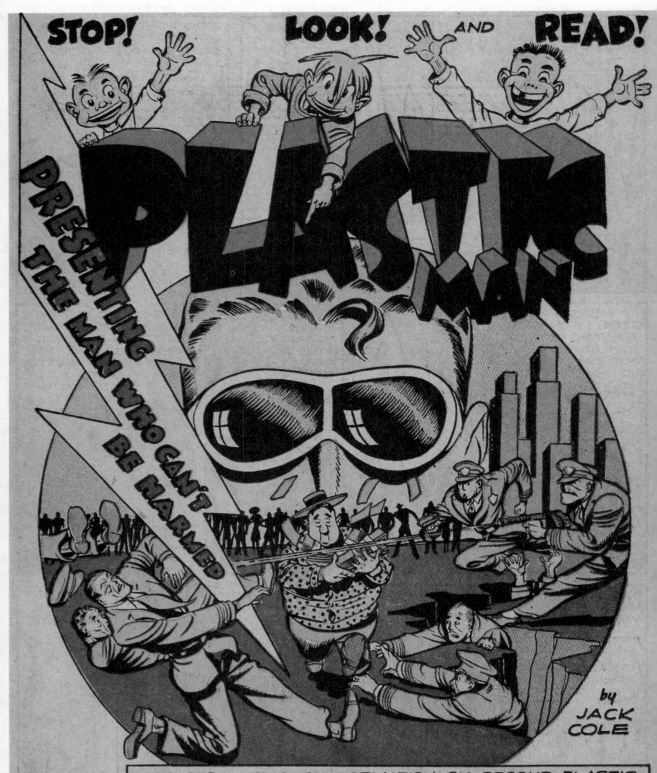

From *Police Comics* No. 13, November 1942.
© 1942 Comic Magazines.

THIS IS HOMER TWITCHEL, THE GREAT SCULPTER.. COME QUICKLY.. MY PRICELESS STATUES HAVE BEEN STOLEN!

OKAY, HOMER ..DON'T GET SO UPSET ABOUT IT!!..

DON'T GET UPSET, HE SAYS!

HEY PLASTIC! THINK YOU CAN STOP RUBBERING OUT THE WINDOW LONG ENOUGH TO ANSWER A CALL?

OH, OH.. GOTTA GO MIKE!

C*!!# JUS' WHEN I HAD Y'LICKED!

BUT WHEN PLASTIC MAN REACHES HOMER'S STUDIO, HE FINDS...

?? THE PLACE IS EMPTY!! IF THIS IS A JOKE..!

THAT'S QUEER.. THE WORD "HELP" SPELLED OUT IN CLAY ON THIS BOOK..

HANS Y GRETHEL
HELP

BUT WHY ON A BOOK ?? AND WHY, "HANS AND GRETHEL"?? ..UNLESS..

HANS AND GRETHEL DROPPED BREAD CRUMBS TO MARK A TRAIL.. PERHAPS HOMER TWITCHEL DROPPED CLAY!

AH, HERE'S A PIECE!

OUT INTO THE STREET HE FOLLOWS THE TRAIL.

HERE'S ANOTHER!

PLASTIC MAN, GUTTER SNIPING! TCH! TCH! TCH!!

WHY, DADDY?

MEANWHILE NOT FAR AWAY...

OHHHHH.... MY LIFE'S WORK.. RUINED! WHY DID YOU DO IT? WHY KIDNAP ME?

BOSS' ORDERS!.. NOW WHERE DID I PUT THAT SAW?

73

NOW FOR A FEW JOBS TO CONVINCE THE SKEPTIC..

THUS BEGINS A SERIES OF DARING ROBBERIES, THE LIKE OF WHICH IS SELDOM SEEN..

IN BANKS

IF THEY ONLY KNEW I'M SHOOTING BLANKS!

BAM! BAM!

IN JEWELRY STORES..

IT'S EEL O'BRIAN!

STOP THIEF!

THE THINGS I HAVE TO GO THROUGH JUST TO GET IN THE GOOD GRACES OF A CROOK!

NO ONE IS SAFE FROM HIS GRASP

WUXTRY!! ANOTHER BANK LOOTED BY THE EEL! WUXTRY!!

HMM.. THE LAD'S REALLY GOOD! HMMM..

EEL O'BRIAN ON THE LOOSE

HOT-TEMPERED POLICE CAPTAIN MURPHEY IS IN A DITHER..

FINE FORCE YOU ARE.. LETTING THE EEL MAKE GOOPS OF YOU!!

WE KNOW!

DON'T RUB IT IN CHIEF!

WHEN TWO WEEKS ARE UP EEL MEETS WOOZY..

..AND AFTER DUE CONSIDERATION, FRIEND, I'VE DECIDED TO TAKE YOU ON AS MY JUNIOR PARTNER

SWELL! WHEN DO WE START!

TONIGHT! HOW ARE YOU ON SWIPING MARBLE STATUETTES??

JUST TRY ME, PAL!

WE'RE GOING TO STEAL EVERY ONE OF HOMER TWITCHEL'S BUSTS FROM THE CITY MUSEUM!

BUT WHY?

IT'S A SECRET, CHUM! MEET ME HERE AT EIGHT!

AS PLASTIC MAN, HE GOES TO THE POLICE..

AND WHERE WERE YOU WHEN EEL O'BRIAN WAS TEARING THE CITY APART, MISTER PLASTIC MAN?

BANK YOUR FIRES, MURPHEY.. I'VE JUST FOUND OUT THAT EEL AND THE THUG WHO STOLE HOMER TWITCHEL'S SCULPTURE PIECES ARE PULLING A REPEAT TONIGHT!

YEAH?

BULLETIN BOARD

WHAT DO YOU CARE AS LONG AS YOU GET A THOUSAND FOR THE JOB? I'LL PAY YOU AS SOON AS THE BOSS PAYS ME!

SEE YOU TOMORROW!!

WHAT A CAGY CUSS! HAVEN'T SQUEEZED A BIT OF INFORMATION OUT OF HIM! BETTER TRAIL HIM AND SEE WHERE HE GOES!

HE'S HEADING FOR THE MIRE MANSION

WELL?

EVENING, MIRE! JUST DROPPED BY TO TELL YOU I DESTROYED THREE MORE TWITCHEL BUSTS TONIGHT!

BLUNDERING IDIOT! I HEARD ALL ABOUT IT OVER THE RADIO! THOSE BUSTS WERE ONLY PLASTER!! THE COPS HID THE REAL ONES! HOW DO YOU EXPECT ME TO INCREASE THE VALUE OF MY OWN TWITCHELS IF THE REST AREN'T DESTROYED ?!!?

I'VE BEEN TRICKED!

DEAR ME! THIS IS BAD! IT MUST HAVE BEEN EEL O'BRIAN!

GET OUT!!

BUT THE CHAIR SUDDENLY COMES TO LIFE

GOT YOU THIS TIME!

PLASTIC MAN!!

?

BLACKIE! COME OUT!

IMMEDIATELY A DOOR OPENS

OH, OH! WE'LL HAVE TO POSTPONE OUR SCRAP, WINKS!!

AFTER HIM!!

RRRRRRR

IT'S NO USE.. I'LL HAVE TO TRY REASONING WITH HIM!

LOOK, WOOZY, YOU'RE NOT A BAD GUY AT HEART.. WHY DON'T YOU PAY YOUR DEBT TO SOCIETY AND START OFF FRESH?

THINK OF YOUR MOTHER..WHAT WOULD SHE SAY IF SHE KNEW ABOUT YOUR CRIME CAREER?

WHY, IT'D BREAK HER HEART! YOUR CONSCIENCE WILL PLAGUE YOU THE REST OF YOUR LIFE!!

STOP IT! STOP IT! I CAN'T BEAR IT.. TAKE ME AWAY!

LATER.. HERE YOU ARE, MURPHEY.. THE SCULPTURE THIEF AND ALL OF EEL O'BRIAN'S LOOT!

WELL!

SN'FF I'M NO GOOD?!..

THAT'S GOOD AS FAR AS YOU WENT BUT WHERE'S EEL, HIM- SELF?

GOT AWAY!

LOOK HERE, PLASTIC..WE'VE LET THE EEL RUN LOOSE LONG ENOUGH! I WANT HIM CAPTURED IF IT'S THE LAST JOB YOU EVER DO FOR THE FORCE!!

PSST..CAN I HELP YOU NAB HIM? I'VE GOT A PRIVATE SCORE TO SETTLE WITH O'BRIAN!

SORRY, WOOZY.. BUT YOU'VE A SENTENCE TO SERVE!

VERY WELL, I QUIT!

WAIT! ALL RIGHT, YOU CAN HELP ME..BUT COME BACK HERE!

POLICE

SO I'VE GOT TO CAPTURE MYSELF, EH?.. AND WITH WOOZY WINKS AS A HELPER!! THIS SHOULD BE A VERY INTERESTING EXPERIENCE!

DON'T MISS NEXT MONTH'S EPISODE WHEN PLASTIC MAN BATTLES EEL O'BRIAN (CHIMSELF) AIDED BY THE NEW COMIC FIND, WOOZY WINKS, THE MAN WHOM NATURE PROTECTS !!!!!

About "Captain Marvel" and C. C. Beck

Captain Marvel was the result, first, of an executive decision, and, following on that, of the fortuitous coming together of exceptional talents.

The decision came when Fawcett Publications declared itself a relatively late entrant into the highly profitable comic-book field. C. C. Beck, a cartoonist who had contributed gag panels to Fawcett's humor magazines, was brought together with writer Bill Parker. They came up with an orphaned big-city newsboy who could transform himself into a super-being. Billy Batson was lured into an abandoned subway station by a mysterious figure, led past grotesque depictions of the Seven Deadly Enemies of Man (actually the Seven Deadly Sins of medieval Catholic theology), and taken to an ancient, enthroned magician who was somehow Egyptian. This sage gave Billy a magic word, "Shazam," based on the initials of a polyglot of Biblical characters, Greek and Roman deities, and mythic heroes. Uttering this word, Billy would invoke a lightning bolt and convert himself into Captain Marvel. (And, incidentally, as if to domesticate the whole picture, the Captain was physically modeled on the actor Fred MacMurray, and the Captain's archenemy, Dr. Sivana, on C. C. Beck's neighborhood pharmacist.)

Beck's graphic renderings were simple, uncluttered, cartoon-oriented, and appropriately humorous. And Captain Marvel was a huge success. He was soon appearing in a whole group of magazines and had spun off a Captain Marvel, Jr., a Mary Marvel—even a Marvel Bunny.

Beck needed a whole roomful of assistants to help out. The foremost of these was Pete Costanza, who worked directly with Beck and also supervised the other helpers. Meanwhile, in 1941, the feature had found its perfect author in the fanciful Otto Binder. Binder understood that the *Captain Marvel* stories were best treated as light-hearted children's fare, and knew that strong rationalizations and pseudo-scientific explanations of its magic events and magic powers were not only unnecessary, they might simply get in the way of the psychological truths the magic imparted. Binder's introduction of Tawky Tawny, a "civilized," talking jungle tiger, was indicative: Billy befriends him and he becomes a sports-jacketed American suburbanite, confirming for the feature's readers that the savage impulse can be domesticated—with a sense of humor.

Both Charles Clarence Beck and Otto Binder came from the American Midwest. Beck was born in Zumbrota, Minnesota, in 1910. He studied at the Chicago Academy of Fine Arts and the University of Minnesota, and was a humor illustrator for Fawcett by 1933. Binder was born a year after Beck in

Bessemer, Michigan, and had been writing for pulp and short-story magazines and, beginning in 1939, for comic books.

The various Marvel-family comic books continued with high success until 1953. National Comics had brought legal action against Fawcett, claiming that the Captain infringed upon its Superman copyrights, and Fawcett finally decided that fighting the suit wasn't worth the money and the effort. (Insiders insist, incidentally, that there were other, less successful super-heroes that were closer to Superman in conception than was Captain Marvel.)

Our selection, *Captain Marvel Battles the Plot Against the Universe,* comes from 1949 and the one-hundredth issue of *Captain Marvel Adventures.* Its title is perhaps the only awkward moment in this little masterpiece of breakneck whimsy, as Binder's plotting is rendered and embellished in Beck's and Costanza's drawings. The elements are, as usual, wonderfully preposterous: pseudo-science, traditional myth, space travel, time travel—all are invoked with no inhibition, and the feature's pseudo-heaven (the Rock of Eternity) is prominently featured. If a new magic metal is needed to get the story started, let's have one: shazamium. If another is needed to keep it going, let's have another: sivanium. If a third is required to resolve things, so be it: marvelium. Most indicative of the tone of it all, the artists give us Captain Marvel's torture at the hands of Sivana in the "splash panel" to Part 3—he gets some ink on his red suit from a squirt gun, some itching powder, and (torture of tortures!) a swift kick in the behind.

The story is sustained by an innocent, unapologetic fascination with its own willful fancy, and by our delight in following that fancy—those things, plus an absolute refusal to take itself seriously. And to bring it all off involves a balance of attitudes, of story elements, of pictures—and balances within balances—that are not nearly so easy to achieve and to sustain as they seem.

Otto Binder died in 1974, but C. C. Beck has remained active, and he illustrated the first few issues of a revived *Captain Marvel* comic book (titled *Shazam!*) in the 1970s. Ironically, the comic book was published by National, the company that had put the Captain out of business twenty years earlier.

M.W.

CAPTAIN MARVEL ADVENTURES

Executive Editor
WILL LIEBERSON

Editor
WENDELL CROWLEY

The following outstanding magazines are easily identified on their covers by the words A FAWCETT PUBLICATION.

CAPT. MARVEL ADVENTURES • WHIZ COMICS • CAPT. MARVEL JR. • MASTER COMICS • WESTERN HERO
OZZIE AND BABS • THE MARVEL FAMILY • TOM MIX WESTERN • MONTE HALE WESTERN • HOPALONG CASSIDY
FAWCETT'S FUNNY ANIMALS • ROCKY LANE WESTERN • NYOKA THE JUNGLE GIRL • GABBY HAYES WESTERN

Every effort is made to insure that these comic magazines contain the highest quality of wholesome entertainment.

W. H. Fawcett, Jr. President

Captain MARVEL

BATTLES THE PLOT AGAINST THE UNIVERSE

WHENEVER BILLY BATSON, FAMOUS BOY NEWSCASTER, SAYS THE WORD "SHAZAM" HE IS MIRACULOUSLY CHANGED INTO POWERFUL CAPTAIN MARVEL, THE WORLD'S MIGHTIEST MORTAL, WHO COMBINES IN HIS MAGNIFICENT PHYSIQUE THE POWERS OF SIX OF THE MIGHTIEST HEROES OF ALL TIME!

SOLOMON....WISDOM
HERCULES....STRENGTH
ATLAS....STAMINA
ZEUS....POWER
ACHILLES....COURAGE
MERCURY....SPEED

PART 1 DR. SIVANA STRIKES AT SHAZAM

NO GREATER EVIL GENIUS THAN DR. SIVANA, THE WORLD'S WICKEDEST SCIENTIST, HAS EVER EXISTED ON THIS EARTH OF OURS! HIS SINISTER AMBITION IS TO RULE NOT ONLY EARTH, BUT THE ENTIRE UNIVERSE! THE VERY EXISTENCE OF CAPTAIN MARVEL HIMSELF IS THREATENED AS THE WILY SCIENTIST SETS IN MOTION HIS LATEST AUDACIOUS PLOT TO GIVE HIM POWER OVER ALL THE UNIVERSE! READ ON, FOR 100 THRILLS, CHILLS, AND EXCITING EPISODES COMPLETE IN THIS 100th ANNIVERSARY ISSUE!

LET US PEER INTO THE SECRET LABORATORY OF DR. SIVANA, THE GREATEST ENEMY OF CIVILIZATION EVER KNOWN, AS HE REPEATS A DREAD VOW!

I VOW TO WEAR THAT CROWN YET! SOMEHOW---SOMEDAY--- I'LL BECOME *RIGHTFUL RULER OF THE UNIVERSE!* HEH, HEH, HEH!

THE WORLD'S MADDEST SCIENTIST HAS NEVER GIVEN UP THIS ALL-CONSUMING AMBITION, BUT THERE HAS ALWAYS BEEN ONE GREAT STUMBLING BLOCK!

CURSES! HOW CAN I WIN OUT WITH THAT BIG RED LOUT, *CAPTAIN MARVEL,* AGAINST ME? HE SMASHES MY BEST PLOTS EVERY TIME! BAH!

AND I CAN'T EVEN GET *BILLY BATSON,* THE BOY THAT CAPTAIN MARVEL CHANGES BACK INTO! EVERY TIME I GO FOR BILLY, HE SOMEHOW CHANGES TO CAPTAIN MARVEL IN TIME! *BAH!*

ZING

AND CAPTAIN MARVEL CAN'T BE DEFEATED--- NOT WITH THOSE POWERS FROM SIX ELDER HEROES, GRANTED TO HIM BY SHAZAM, THE ANCIENT EGYPTIAN WIZARD! BAH, BAH!

SOLOMON-WISDOM
HERCULES-STRENGTH
ATLAS-STAMINA
ZEUS-POWER
ACHILLES-COURAG[E]
MERCURY-SPEED

WAIT! THAT GIVES ME A GREAT IDEA! THE ONE WAY TO CRUSH CAPTAIN MARVEL IS THROUGH *SHAZAM!* I'VE GOT TO FIND SHAZAM HIMSELF AND WORK ON HIM! HEH, HEH, HEH!

BUT WHERE *IS* SHAZAM? THAT'S ONE SECRET I NEVER FOUND OUT! I CAN'T JUST GO AND ASK BILLY OR CAPTAIN MARVEL! BUT I'VE GOT TO FIND OUT! LET ME THINK... THINK... THINK!

MEANWHILE, LET US LOOK INTO THE MODEST HOME OF MR. TAWKY TAWNY, THE WELL-KNOWN TALKING TIGER!

I'M WRITING MY MEMOIRS! LET'S SEE... CAPTAIN MARVEL, MY GREAT FRIEND, IS THE WORLD'S MIGHTIEST MORTAL! HE GAINED HIS POWERS FROM SHAZAM, THE WIZARD! THIS ALL HAPPENED WHEN.....?

DEAR ME! I CAN'T FINISH! IT JUST OCCURS TO ME NOW THAT I REALLY KNOW NOTHING OF CAPTAIN MARVEL'S ORIGIN AT ALL!

[BI]LLY BATSON OFTEN DROPS IN ON HIS [TI]GER FRIEND, AND...

[H]ELLO, [M]R. TAWNY! [H]OW ARE [Y]OUR MEMOIRS GOING?

I'M STUCK, BILLY! TELL ME, WHEN, WHERE AND HOW DID CAPTAIN MARVEL COME INTO EXISTENCE?

THIS IS A SECRET THAT BILLY TELLS ONLY TO TRUSTED FRIENDS!

IT'S A LONG STORY, MR. TAWNY! BUT COME WITH ME! I THINK IT'S TIME YOU KNEW ALL ABOUT CAPTAIN MARVEL, SINCE YOU'VE HAD SO MANY ADVENTURES WITH HIM!

BILLY LEADS THE WAY TO AN OLD FORGOTTEN SUBWAY TUNNEL!

MANY YEARS AGO, AS A RAGGED NEWSBOY, I WAS LED TO THIS TUNNEL MYSELF! DOWN AT THE END OF IT I MET THE EGYPTIAN WIZARD!

[AL]THOUGH HE IS GONE FROM EARTH AND LIVES AT [TH]E ROCK OF ETERNITY, I CAN STILL SUMMON [H]IS SPIRIT BY LIGHTING THIS BRAZIER!

I AM HERE, MY SON!

FOR THE FIRST TIME, MR. TAWNY MEETS SHAZAM!

GREETINGS, MR. TAWNY!

I AM HONORED, SHAZAM! BUT I DON'T UNDERSTAND! HOW CAN YOU EXIST IN SPIRIT FORM?

BY MEANS OF THIS BRACELET, MADE OF AN ELEMENT UNKNOWN TO EARTHLY SCIENCE! IT'S CALLED **SHAZAMIUM**! WITHOUT IT, I WOULD VANISH UTTERLY! WHOEVER WEARS THIS CAN ADOPT ETHEREAL FORM! AND IT ALSO ENABLES ME TO WHISK BACK AND FORTH FROM THE ROCK OF ETERNITY, IN THE WINK OF AN EYE!

NOW I MUST GO! YOU HAVE DONE WELL, MR. TAWNY, AIDING CAPTAIN MARVEL IN THE GREAT FIGHT AGAINST EVIL!

THANK YOU, GREAT SIR!

LATER, BACK AT MR. TAWNY'S HOME ...

NOW I CAN FINISH MY MEMOIRS! THANKS, BILLY!

JUST ONE THING, MR. TAWNY--- DON'T WRITE DOWN **WHERE** THAT FORGOTTEN TUNNEL IS! NOBODY ELSE MUST EVER FIND THAT OUT! GOOD NIGHT!

BUT MEANWHILE, SIVANA HAS COME TO THE HOME OF MR. TAWNY!

I'VE FINALLY FIGURED IT OUT! MR. TAWNY IS A CLOSE FRIEND OF BILLY AND CAPTAIN MARVEL! HE OUGHT TO KNOW **WHERE SHAZAM IS!** AFTER BILLY IS OUT OF SIGHT, I'LL STRIKE!

FOR THE FIRST TIME, SIVANA AND MR. TAWNY MEET!

SIVANA! I RECOGNIZE YOU FROM YOUR PICTURES! YOU'RE THE MOST EVIL GENIUS ON EARTH!

GREETINGS, MR. TAWNY! I SEE MY REPUTATION PRECEDES ME! HEHHHH!

YOU MADE A MISTAKE COMING HERE!

DID I?

HEH, HEH, HEH!

HOLY MOLEY! SIVANA HAS KIDNAPPED MR. TAWNY!

SHAZAM!

SPOKEN ALOUD BY BILLY, THE HONORED NAME SENDS DOWN A CRASH OF MAGIC LIGHTNING WHICH CHANGES BILLY TO CAPTAIN MARVEL!

BOOM!

WHAT ARE YOU UP TO, YOU LITTLE WEASEL? WHAT DO YOU WANT WITH MR. TAWNY?

NONE OF YOUR BUSINESS YOU BIG RED CHEESE!

OH COME, SIVANA! PULLING A GUN ON ME WON'T HELP YOU! YOU SHOULD KNOW BY NOW THAT BULLETS CAN'T HARM ME!

OH, YEAH?

THIS GUN WILL COVER YOU ALL OVER WITH STICKY ROPE AND GIVE ME TIME TO ESCAPE! HEH!

HOLY MOLEY!

CAPTAIN MARVEL WILL BE FREE IN A MOMENT--- BUT THAT'S ALL I NEED TO GET INTO MY SHIP!

I'M FREE! AND YOU OUGHT TO KNOW I CAN OUTFLY ANY SHIP, SIVANA!

SNAP

WHOOSH

BUT THIS IS A **TIME SHIP**, DUMMY! I'M FADING OUT OF THE **PRESENT**, INTO THE **PAST**! HOW CAN YOU CHASE ME **THERE**? HEH, HEH, HEHHHH!

BEFORE CAPTAIN MARVEL'S EYES, THE TIME SHIP FADES AWAY INTO NOTHINGNESS!

HOLY MOLEY! HE GOT AWAY... WITH MR. TAWNY AS HIS PRISONER!

WHERE DID HE GO? HOW FAR INTO THE PAST? AND WHAT DOES HE WANT FROM MR. TAWNY? I DON'T LIKE THIS ONE LITTLE BIT! AND YET, WHAT CAN I DO? *HOW CAN I CHASE HIM THROUGH TIME?*

RUISING INTO THE PAST, SIVANA REVEALS HIS GHASTLY PLOT TO HELPLESS MR. TAWNY!

I'M GOING BACK TO THE TIME APTAIN MARVEL WAS FIRST ALLED FORTH BY SHAZAM! BUT I'M GOING TO ARRIVE A LITTLE **BEFORE** THAT AND AMBUSH BILLY IN THE TUNNEL!

BUT I'LL NEVER TELL YOU HOW TO FIND THE TUNNEL, YOU FIEND!

OH, YES, YOU WILL! UNDER THE INFLUENCE OF THIS **HYPNO RAY**, YOU HAVE NO WILL TO RESIST MY QUESTION! *WHERE IS THE TUNNEL?*

I WON'T TELL! I---UH--- UH---

NDER THE POWERFUL HYPNO RAY, MR. AWNY IS FORCED TO ANSWER!

I OBEY! THE TUNNEL IS AT THE CORNER OF SLUMM STREET AND NINTH, BEHIND THE OLD WAREHOUSE!

THE TIME SHIP LANDS IN THE PAST, AND...

HERE'S THE OLD WARE- HOUSE! NOW TO FIND THE SUBWAY ENTRANCE!

HERE IT IS! WE'RE BACK IN TIME **BEFORE** BILLY BATSON FIRST ENTERED! I'VE TIMED ALL THIS PERFECTLY!

SUBWAY

THE SEVEN DEADLY ENEMIES OF MAN, EH? WE'LL HIDE BEHIND ONE OF THOSE STATUES!

THE SEVEN DEADLY ENEMIES OF MAN

PRIDE · ENVY · GREED · HATRED · SELFISHNESS · LAZINESS

I WANT YOU TO SEE THIS, MR. TAWNY! SOON BILLY WILL COME! I'LL NAB HIM HERE, **BEFORE** HE REACHES THE THRONE OF SHAZAM --- AND **BEFORE** CAPTAIN MARVEL IS CREATED! AND YOU WON'T BE ABLE TO YELL TO WARN HIM! HEHHH!

MEANWHILE, OUTSIDE, THE BILLY BATSON OF THE PAST IS MET BY A MYSTERIOUS, DARK FIGURE!

HE'S BECKONING ME TO FOLLOW??

WHY ARE YOU TAKING ME INTO THIS OLD ABANDONED SUBWAY TUNNEL?

THIS IS THE BILLY BATSON OF YEARS BACK --- A YOUNG NEWSBOY WHO DOES NOT KNOW THAT HE HAS BEEN SELECTED BY SHAZAM TO BECOME THE FUTURE CAPTAIN MARVEL! HE DOES NOT YET KNOW OF THE GREAT AND BLAZING CAREER FOR WHICH HE IS DESTINED AS THE WORLD'S MIGHTIEST MORTAL!
    THIS IS BILLY BATSON **BEFORE** CAPTAIN MARVEL EVER EXISTED!

AS IT ALL ONCE HAPPENED IN THE PAST, BILLY IS LED THROUGH THE CAVERN OF THE SEVEN DEADLY ENEMIES OF MAN!

THE SEVEN DEADLY ENEMIES OF MAN

PRIDE · ENVY · GREED · HATRED · SELFISHNESS · LAZINESS

OW LURKING SIVANA IS READY TO TRIKE!

HAH! NOW TO CAPTURE AND KILL BILLY! CAPTAIN MARVEL WILL NEVER COME INTO EXISTENCE AT ALL! HEH, HEH!

I'M HELPLESS TO STOP HIM! WAIT...

I GOT MY TAIL FREE! NOW I HAVE A CHANCE TO SAVE BILLY!

AWRKKK!

BONG!

HE'S OUT COLD! NOW ALL WILL GO ON AS BEFORE --- BILLY WILL REACH THE THRONE, MEET SHAZAM, AND...

AND MR. TAWNY IS NOW THRILLED TO WITNESS, WITH HIS OWN EYES, THE ACTUAL EVENTS THAT LED TO THE FIRST APPEARANCE OF CAPTAIN MARVEL, THE WORLD'S MIGHTIEST MORTAL!

BILLY BATSON, I AM SHAZAM, AN ANCIENT EGYPTIAN WIZARD! I HAVE FOUGHT EVIL, BUT MY TIME IS NOW UP! YOU SHALL BE MY SUCCESSOR!

M-ME, SIR?

YES! YOU ARE PURE OF HEART! YOU HAVE BEEN CHOSEN! SPEAK MY NAME!

SHAZAM!

FOR THE FIRST TIME, THE AMAZING MAGIC LIGHTNING THUNDERS DOWN!

BOOM

AND FOR THE FIRST TIME IN HISTORY CAPTAIN MARVEL, THE WORLD'S MIGHTIEST MAN, APPEARS!

BUT NOW, THE BLOCK OF STONE, THAT HAD HUNG BY A THREAD ABOVE SHAZAM'S THRONE, CRASHES DOWN UPON THE WISE WIZARD!

SNAP

SO IT IS WRITTEN THAT I MUST GO!

CRASH!

BUT A MOMENT LATER, THE SPIRIT OF SHAZAM ARISES, AND...

I NAME YOU--- CAPTAIN MARVEL! THROUGH MY NAME YOU ARE GIVEN THE POWERS OF THESE SIX MIGHTY HEROES! HENCEFORTH, YOU WILL FIGHT EVIL ON EARTH!

SOLOMON — WISDOM
HERCULES — STRENGTH
ATLAS — STAMINA
ZEUS — POWER
ACHILLES — COURAGE
MERCURY — SPEED

YES, GREAT SIR!

THAT WAS SIMPLY WONDERFUL! I SAW THE ACTUAL ORIGIN OF CAPTAIN MARVEL! THERE HE GOES NOW, OUT INTO THE WORLD, TO BEGIN HIS BLAZING CAREER AGAINST EVIL AND INJUSTICE! BUT WHAT'S GOING TO HAPPEN TO ME NOW? SIVANA IS COMING TO!

PRIDE ENVY GRE...

YES, WHAT WILL HAPPEN TO MR. TAWNY? UNAWARE OF THEIR PRESENCE, THE NEW CAPTAIN MARVEL PASSES THEM BY! FOILED IN HIS FIRST MOVE, WHAT WILL WICKED SIVANA TRY NOW? THE NEXT STORY IN THIS ISSUE WILL GIVE YOU THE AMAZING ANSWER!

Captain MARVEL

BATTLES THE PLOT AGAINST THE UNIVERSE

FROM HERE I SHALL **RULE THE UNIVERSE!** HEHHHHHHH!

NOT IF I CAN STOP YOU, SIVANA!

PART 2
THE INVASION OF THE ROCK OF ETERNITY

ROCK OF ETERNITY

IN THE PREVIOUS STORY, SIVANA FAILED TO DESTROY BILLY BATSON AND CAPTAIN MARVEL! BUT THE EVIL GENIUS IS STILL ARMED WITH VITAL KNOWLEDGE OF THE SECRETS OF SHAZAM, THE SHAZAMIUM BRACELET, AND THE ROCK OF ETERNITY! SO NOW THE MAD SCIENTIST LAUNCHES ANOTHER CUNNING PLAN THAT THREATENS TO GIVE HIM CONTROL OF THE ROCK OF ETERNITY ITSELF, HUB OF THE UNIVERSE!

SIVANA HAS NOW REGAINED HIS SENSES AND IS FILLED WITH MAD RAGE AT MR. TAWNY'S INTERFERENCE WITH HIS EVIL PLAN!

CURSES! YOU KNOCKED ME OUT AND LET THE CREATION OF CAPTAIN MARVEL OCCUR! I'LL GET YOU FOR THAT, MR. TAWNY!

GULP! I'M SUNK! WAIT...

...BY SHIFTING MY WEIGHT I CAN ROLL AWAY! NOW, IF I COULD JUST GET OUT OF THESE ROPES...

92

GET IN THERE AND WORK THE CONTROLS!

WHEN WE GET TO 1949 I'LL HAVE TO ESCAPE---SOMEHOW! WAIT, I KNOW! THIS WILL BE CLEVER!

WHEN THEY STEP OUT IN 1949...

TO THE POLICE!

HEH, HEH! NOW'S THE TIME TO TURN THE TABLES! TAWNY HAS NO CLOTHES ON, SO...

[H]ELP! [W]ILD TIGER! [M]E ESCAPED [F]ROM THE ZOO!

WHAT?

OMIGOSH! LOOK!

NOT REALIZING IT IS TAME MR. TAWNY, A MOB TURNS ON HIM!

KEEP THAT WILD TIGER AT BAY! CORNER HIM!

POW

STOP! WAIT! OH, THEY WON'T LISTEN!

[IN] THE EXCITEMENT, [NO]BODY NOTICED ME [A]T ALL! I'M FREE! [N]OW BACK TO MY [S]HIP! HEH, HEH. HEHHHHH!

MEANWHILE, FROM A HIGH WINDOW IN STATION WHIZ, BILLY BATSON SEES THE SCENE...

HOLY MOLEY! LOOKS LIKE AN ESCAPED TIGER DOWN THERE! BEFORE SOMEBODY GETS HURT... SHAZAM!

HELP!

GET HIM!

MAGIC LIGHTNING FAITHFULLY THUNDERS DOWN AT THE NAME, AND CAPTAIN MARVEL REPLACES BILLY!

BOOM!

CAPTAIN MARVEL RECOGNIZES HIS TIGER FRIEND!

HOLY MOLEY! STOP, FOLKS! THIS IS MR. TAWNY, THE CIVILIZED TIGER!

THUMP

AM I GLAD TO SEE YOU, CAPTAIN MARVEL!

SIVANA GOT AWAY!

WHERE DID SIVANA TAKE YOU, MR. TAWNY YOU'VE BEEN GONE HOURS!

I'LL TAKE YOU TO YOUR HOME AND YOU CAN TELL ME THE WHOLE STORY! WE HAVE TO FIGURE OUT WHAT SIVANA'S NEXT MOVE WILL BE!

LATER, THE FIGURE OF BILLY BATSON AGAIN ENTERS THE FORGOTTEN TUNNEL, BUT THIS IS IN 1949, NOT THE PAST!

PAST THE STATUES, TO THE THRONE...

PRIDE   ENVY   GREED   HATRED SELFISHNESS LAZINESS

NOW TO LIGHT THE BRAZIER AND SUMMON THE SPIRIT OF THE OLD MAGICIAN!

YES, MY SON? WHAT IS IT?

GREAT SIR, TELL ME MORE ABOUT THAT SHAZAMIUM BRACELET YOU WEAR!

SHAZAMIUM IS A WONDER ELEMENT WHICH ALLOWS ITS WEARER TO ADOPT ETHEREAL FORM, LIKE MINE! IT ALSO GIVES ONE THE POWER TO TRAVEL BACK AND FORTH FROM THE ROCK OF ETERNITY INSTANTANEOUSLY!

DO YOU WISH TO SEE IT CLOSELY, BILLY? HERE, TAKE IT--- BUT RETURN IT QUICKLY! WITHOUT IT ON MY ARM, I WOULD FADE AWAY INTO NOTHINGNESS IN 24 HOURS! IT MEANS LIFE TO ME!

BUT NOW, THERE ARISES AN OMINOUS, MOCKING CHUCKLE!

HEH, HEH, HEH, HEH, HEH, HEH, HEHH!

BILLY! THAT EVIL CHUCKLE! YOU SOUND LIKE SIVANA!

STARTLING REVELATION!

I AM SIVANA, SHAZAM! HEH, HEH! OF ALL MY CLEVER DISGUISES, THIS HAS BEEN THE MOST CUNNING OF ALL! IT WAS THE ONE WAY I COULD GET THE GREAT SHAZAMIUM BRACELET IN MY HANDS! HEHHHHHH!

OH, WHAT HAVE I DONE? WITHOUT THAT BRACELET, I AM POWERLESS!

EXACTLY WHAT I FIGURED! HEH! I FAILED TO STOP THE CREATION OF CAPTAIN MARVEL, BUT NOW I HAVE YOU IN MY POWER, SHAZAM! I'LL PUT ON THE BRACELET!

THE AMAZING SHAZAMIUM BRACELET GIVES SIVANA THE SAME ETHEREAL FORM THAT SHAZAM HAS!

MY HAND PASSES RIGHT THROUGH SOLID MATTER! HEH, HEH! THIS IS BETTER THAN BEING A GHOST!

AND YOU'RE MY PRISONER, SHAZAM! NOW OFF TO THE ROCK OF ETERNITY!

I AM HELPLESS TO RESIST!

IN THE WINK OF AN EYE, THROUGH THE POWER OF THE SHAZAMIUM BRACELET, THEY ARE HURLED BEYOND SPACE AND TIME TO THE ROCK OF ETERNITY, WHERE SHAZAM HAS DWELLED!

FROM HERE, I WILL SOON RULE THE UNIVERSE! HEH, HEH, HEHHHHH!

SHORTLY AFTER, THE REAL BILLY BATSON VISITS THE SECRET TUNNEL!

MR. TAWNY TOLD ME THE WHOLE STORY OF SIVANA'S VISIT TO THE PAST, AND HIS ATTEMPT TO DESTROY ME! I THINK SHAZAM HIMSELF MAY BE IN DANGER NOW! I'D BETTER WARN HIM!

NOW, AS USUAL, I LIGHT THE BRAZIER TO SUMMON HIS SPIRIT!

HEH, HEH!

BILLY BATSON RECEIVES THE SHOCK OF HIS LIFE!

HOLY MOLEY! THAT'S NOT THE EGYPTIAN WIZARD! IT'S SIVANA!

YES, MY SON! WHAT CAN I DO FOR YOU? OH HEH, HEH, HEH, HEH, HEH, HEH!

CAPTAIN MARVEL WILL TAKE CARE OF YOU! SHAZAM!

GO AHEAD! CHANGE TO THAT RED OX! I'M NOT WORRIED! ♪ HUM DE DUM ♪

THE MAGIC LIGHTNING COMES AS USUAL, FOR AS LONG AS SHAZAM EXISTS, THE WORD WILL NOT FAIL BILLY!

BOOM!

I'LL GRAB YOU AND --- HOLY MOLEY! IT'S LIKE GRABBING SMOKE!

SURE! I'M IN ETHEREAL FORM NOW, JUST LIKE OLD SHAZAM! ALL YOUR MIGHTY STRENGTH CAN'T HARM ONE HAIR OF MY HEAD --- IF I HAD ANY! HEH, HEHHHHHH!

AND LOOK! WITHOUT THIS SHAZAMIUM BRACELET, OLD SHAZAM WILL FADE AWAY INTO LIMBO, IN 24 HOURS! AND WITH HIS PASSING, YOU, TOO, WILL VANISH! IN 24 HOURS THERE WON'T BE ANY MORE CAPTAIN MARVEL! HEHHH!

HOLY MOLEY!

SIVANA PRONOUNCES A DREAD DOOM FOR THE WORLD'S MIGHTIEST MORTAL!

Captain MARVEL

BATTLES THE PLOT AGAINST THE UNIVERSE

PART 3
THE EVIL ELEMENT

Sivana makes a strange bargain with Captain Marvel!

BAH, SIMPLE! DON'T FORGET THAT THIS ROCK OF ETERNITY IS THE **CENTER** OF THE UNIVERSE! FROM HERE, I CAN ATTACK IN ANY DIRECTION THROUGH **SPACE AND TIME!** BUT WAIT TILL YOU SEE MY NEXT STEP! *HEHHHHHH!*

FOR THAT, WE GO BACK TO MY SECRET LABORATORY ON EARTH! *COME ALONG, SLAVE!*

BACK ON EARTH, IN HIS SECRET LAB, SIVANA REVEALS AN AMAZING ELEMENT OF HIS OWN CREATION!

I'VE NAMED THIS **SIVANIUM** IN MY OWN HONOR! IT IS *LIVING METAL!*

SIVANIUM
SIVANIUM

LIVING METAL? WHAT DO YOU MEAN?

I MEAN THAT IT CAN EASILY BE FASHIONED INTO HUMAN SHAPE, DUPLICATING EVERY ORGAN, AND THEN IT WILL LIVE! *THUS I CAN MAKE* **DUPLICATES OF MYSELF!**

BRAIN
LUNGS
MUSCLE
HEART
GIZZARD
HEART
NERVE
TOE

HOLY MOLEY! DUPLICATE SIVANAS TO OVERRUN THE UNIVERSE!

BUT OF COURSE, IN MY ETHEREAL FORM, I CAN'T HANDLE SOLID OBJECTS MYSELF! THAT'S WHY I NEED YOUR HELP! NOW GET TO WORK AND BUILD ME AN ARMY OF SIVANAS!

NO, I WON'T! I...UH....

WITH CARE

BUT NOW CAPTAIN MARVEL REMEMBERS THE WORDS OF SHAZAM!

OBEY HIM, MY SON! OBEY HIM IN ALL THINGS!

SHAZAM TOLD ME TO **CARRY OUT** SIVANA'S ORDERS! *IF I ONLY UNDERSTOOD WHY!*

AND TO ADD TO CAPTAIN MARVEL'S MENTAL TORMENT, SECONDS ARE SLOWLY TICKING BY, BRINGING HIM CLOSER AND CLOSER TO THE AWFUL MOMENT OF EXTINCTION!

ONLY 18 MORE HOURS LEFT FOR SHAZAM AND ME! IF I'M GOING TO HELP SIVANA, I'D BETTER WORK AT TOP SPEED!

SCREWS
NAILS

TICK TICK

THE WORLD'S MIGHTIEST MORTAL IS ABLE TO DO THE WORK OF HUNDREDS OF MEN, IN FASHIONING THE WEIRD **SIVANIUM** INTO HUMAN FORM!

THIS **SIVANIUM** CAN BE WORKED AND WELDED LIKE METAL, IN FORMING HUMAN SHAPE!

NOW PUT IN THE **SIVANIUM** BRAINS! MY DUPLICATES WILL BE EQUAL TO ME IN THINKING POWER! THOSE BRAINS ARE EXACT DUPLICATES OF MINE!

BUT WILL THEY REALLY COME ALIVE?

OF COURSE, IDIOT! WATCH! **ARISE, SIVANA NUMBER ONE!**

HELLO, DR. SIVANA AND CAPTAIN MARVEL! HEH, HEH, HEH, HEH, HEH, HEH!

HOLY MOLEY! SIVANA'S EXACT TWIN, EVEN TO THE DIRTY LAUGH!

HEY!

YES, AND I ALSO HATE YOU, YOU BIG RED CHEESE! HEHHHH!

HEH, HEH!

SLAP!

WHY, YOU LITTLE RODENT! I'LL KNOCK YOU CLEAR INTO NEXT FRIDAY!

SLAP!

CLANG!

Captain MARVEL
BATTLES THE PLOT AGAINST THE UNIVERSE

IF SIVANA CAN HAVE DUPLICATES, WHY CAN'T I? I TOOK AN X-RAY OF MY BRAIN AND MADE AN EXACT DUPLICATE OUT OF SIVANIUM!

HELLO, CAPTAIN MARVEL!

HELLO YOURSELF! HOLY MOLEY! THIS IS JUST LIKE LOOKING INTO A MIRROR!

THE WORLD'S MIGHTIEST MORTAL EXPLAINS HIS CLEVER PLAN!

MY IDEA IS THIS! YOU, THE DUPLICATE, WILL KEEP WORKING HERE! SIVANA WON'T KNOW THAT I --- THE REAL CAPTAIN MARVEL --- AM GONE!

RIGHT! BUT WHAT ARE YOU PLANNING TO DO NOW?

I'VE GOT TO FIND SOME WAY TO GET THAT BRACELET AWAY FROM SIVANA! THERE'S ONLY 8 HOURS LEFT! I'VE GOT TO SAVE THE EGYPTIAN WIZARD --- AND MYSELF --- AND THE UNIVERSE!

GOOD LUCK!

A LITTLE LATER, SIVANA'S ETHEREAL FORM SUDDENLY RETURNS FROM THE ROCK OF ETERNITY!

JUST WANTED TO CHECK UP ON YOU, CAPTAIN MARVEL, IN CASE YOU'D TRIED TO SKIP!

I'M HERE, SIVANA!

I GUESS YOU'VE GIVEN UP ALL HOPE OF DEFEATING ME, EH? HEH, HEH!

JUST ABOUT, SIVANA! I HATE TO ADMIT IT, BUT I THINK THIS TIME YOU'LL WIN!

THE DUPLICATE CAPTAIN MARVEL PLAYS HIS PART TO THE FULL, LULLING ALL SUSPICION!

EVEN CAPTAIN MARVEL HAS GIVEN UP HOPE! HEH, HEHH! HOW CAN I LOSE? NOW BACK TO THE ROCK OF ETERNITY, TO FINISH OUR PLANS TO CONQUER THE UNIVERSE!

107

SCIENTISTS HAVE CREATED FOUR NEW ELEMENTS SO FAR ... SIVANA MADE SIVANIUM, THE BRACELET IS MADE OF SHA--THIS NEXT ELEMENT, AND NOW, LATEST OF ALL, IS MARVELIUM, THE HEAVIEST AND STRONGEST ELEMENT OF ALL!

NEW ELEMENTS
No. 93 NEPTUNIUM
No. 94 PLUTONIUM
No. 95 AMERICIUM
No. 96 CURIUM
No. 97 Sivanium
No. 98 Shazamium
No. 99 Marvelium

IN FACT, IT'S THE WORLD'S MIGHTIEST ELEMENT! THERE IS NO KNOWN FORCE IN THE UNIVERSE THAT CAN WORK IT--- EXCEPT ME! THAT'S WHY I'VE CALLED IT MARVELIUM!

IN A SHORT TIME CAPTAIN MARVEL BUILDS A MYSTERIOUS BOX OUT OF THE NEW ELEMENT, AND THEN PROCEEDS TO TEST IT WITH EVERY FORCE KNOWN TO HUMAN SCIENCE!

I'M CONVINCED THAT NOTHING CAN PENETRATE THAT MARVELIUM SHELL---ABSOLUTELY NOTHING!

ZAP!

WHAT DOES CAPTAIN MARVEL PLAN TO DO WITH THIS AMAZING WONDER ELEMENT?

NOW TO STATION WHIZ WITH IT! HOW MUCH TIME HAVE I LEFT?

ONLY ONE HOUR! HOLY MOLEY! ONE HOUR TO CARRY OUT MY PLAN TO SAVE THE UNIVERSE! I'LL LEAVE THIS HERE AT STATION WHIZ!

TICK TICK TICK TICK TICK TICK TICK TICK TICK

ONLY ONE HOUR REMAINS...ONE HOUR IN WHICH CAPTAIN MARVEL MUST DEFEAT SIVANA AND SAVE THE UNIVERSE! NOT ONLY THAT, BUT IT MEANS LIFE ITSELF TO CAPTAIN MARVEL! FOR IF THE SHAZAMIUM BRACELET IS NOT RETURNED TO SHAZAM, THE WIZE WIZARD WILL VANISH---AND WITH HIM WILL VANISH CAPTAIN MARVEL! IT IS A GRIM RACE AGAINST TIME NOW!

SIVANA IS UP ON THE ROCK OF ETERNITY! I'VE GOT TO PLAY MY HAND CAREFULLY AND LURE HIM BACK TO EARTH! BUT HOW? WAIT! I KNOW HOW! ALL I NEED ARE THE PROPER DISGUISE MATERIALS!

A FEW MINUTES LATER...

I'VE GOT THE STUFF! NOW OFF TO THE ROCK OF ETERNITY!

BY EXCEEDING THE SPEED OF LIGHT, ACCORDING TO THE EINSTEIN FORMULA, CAPTAIN MARVEL IS FLUNG OUT OF SPACE-TIME TO THE DISTANT ROCK OF ETERNITY IN THE WINK OF AN EYE!

HEH, HEH!!

HEH, HEH!

HEH, HEH!

SIVANA AND HIS DUPLICATES ARE STILL PLOTTING! GOOD! I'LL FLY INTO A CORNER OF THE CASTLE!

CAPTAIN MARVEL! WHAT ARE YOU DOING HERE?

O GREAT SIR, I'M SORRY, BUT I THINK IT WAS A MISTAKE FOR ME TO HELP SIVANA AS YOU DIRECTED! NOW I'M GOING TO WORK **AGAINST** HIM!

SHAZAM!

MAGIC LIGHTNING THUNDERS DOWN AND RETURNS CAPTAIN MARVEL TO THE FORM OF BILLY BATSON!

BOOM!

SIVANA DISGUISED HIMSELF AS **ME** ONCE! NOW I'M DISGUISING MYSELF AS **HIM**! WE'RE ABOUT THE SAME SIZE!

UNNOTICED, DISGUISED BILLY JOINS THE MULTIPLE SIVANAS IN THE CONFERENCE ROOM!

OUR PLANS ARE MADE! WE ARE READY TO START **CONQUERING THE UNIVERSE!** HEH, HEH, HEHHHH!

HEH, HEH, HEHHHH!

I HOPE MY CHUCKLE IS AS NASTY AS IT SHOULD BE! BUT NOW...

HEH, HEHHH!

HEH, HEH!

HEH, HEH!

WAIT, MASTER! DON'T YOU THINK YOU OUGHT TO VISIT YOUR LAB ON EARTH AGAIN, RIGHT NOW? MAYBE THAT BIG RED CHEESE, CAPTAIN MARVEL, IS UP TO SOMETHING DESPERATE!

YOU'RE RIGHT! WON'T HURT TO CHECK ON HIM!

13

THAT FOOLED HIM! HE'LL RETURN TO EARTH, WHERE I WANT HIM! NOW--- SHAZAM!

HURRY, MY SON! I GROW WEAK! ONLY HALF AN HOUR REMAINS TO ME!

MAGIC LIGHTNING AGAIN BRINGS THE WORLD'S MIGHTIEST MAN!

BOOM!

BACK TO EARTH! BY NOW, SIVANA MUST HAVE ALREADY REACHED THE LAB! THIS IS ALL CLOSE TIMING! I'VE GOT TO GET TO STATION WHIZ FAST!

IN SIVANA'S LAB, ON EARTH...

CAPTAIN MARVEL IS STILL BUSILY WORKING! THEN HE DIDN'T TRY ANY TRICKS AT ALL! HE GAVE UP! HEH, HEH, HEHHH! AND IN 20 MINUTES, HE AND SHAZAM WILL DISAPPEAR FOREVER!

I'M LICKED, SIVANA!

OR AM I?

HELLO, FOLKS! THIS IS BILLY BATSON, YOUR BOY NEWSCASTER...

WHAT???? CAPTAIN MARVEL IS IN FRONT OF MY EYES! HOW CAN BILLY BATSON BE BROADCASTING? THE TWO OF THEM NEVER EXIST TOGETHER AT THE SAME TIME!

SIVANA GETS THE SHOCK OF HIS LIFE!

WE TRICKED YOU, SIVANA! I'M ONLY A DUPLICATE CAPTAIN MARVEL!

WHAT'S THIS ALL ABOUT? I'LL FIX THAT BILLY BATSON! I'LL GET HIM AT STATION WHIZ!

BUT WHAT AM I WORRYING ABOUT? SHAZAM AND CAPTAIN MARVEL WILL BOTH VANISH IN 15 MORE MINUTES! AND CERTAINLY YOU CAN'T DO ANYTHING TO ME, BILLY BATSON!

YOU'RE RIGHT, SIVANA!

111

NOW TO GET THIS BRACELET TO THE WIZARD... HOLY MOLEY! ONLY A FEW SECONDS LEFT!

IN MEMORIUM TO CAPTAIN MARVEL

I'LL WEAR THE BRACELET MYSELF! IN ETHEREAL FORM I CAN WHISK TO THE ROCK OF ETERNITY INSTANTLY!

CAPTAIN MARVEL ARRIVES AT THE VERY ZERO MOMENT!

FAREWELL, MY SON......

NO! I'VE GOT THE BRACELET! PUT IT ON! HURRY!

MY STRENGTH IS BACK! ALL IS WELL! WE HAVE WON!

SHAZAM IS SAVED!

YES, BUT WHEW!--- THAT WAS CLOSE! I WISH YOU HADN'T ADVISED ME TO HELP SIVANA FIRST, SIR! I WOULD HAVE DEFEATED HIM SOONER!

THE WISE OLD WIZARD REVEALS HIS SUPREME WISDOM!

NO, MY SON! YOU WOULD HAVE LOST! THINK BACK--- ONLY BY HELPING SIVANA DID YOU USE THE SIVANIUM AND THUS DISCOVER THE WAY TO MAKE A DUPLICATE OF YOURSELF, LEAVING YOU FREE TO MAKE MARVELIUM! OTHERWISE, OPPOSING SIVANA, YOU WOULD HAVE WASTED YOUR TIME IN USELESS DIRECT BATTLE!

FORGIVE ME, GREAT SIR! I SHOULD NEVER HAVE DOUBTED YOU FOR A MOMENT!

IT WAS SO WRITTEN--- AND SO IT CAME TO PASS!

BUT WAIT--- THOSE DUPLICATE SIVANAS! I MUST DESTROY THEM!

YOUR DUPLICATE ALSO CAME, AND IS TAKING CARE OF THAT, MY SON!

113

About Basil Wolverton

Powerhouse Pepper was the work of Basil Wolverton, who also produced one of the best known and most widely distributed caricatures ever drawn by an American. Only a few of the millions who saw that drawing bothered to retain its artist's name, however, and fewer still learned much about his other work. Finally, although Wolverton has a high reputation among the aficionados of the comic book, he produced at least two kinds of features, and thus his admirers have trouble deciding which represented the best Wolverton, or the "real" Wolverton.

Basil Wolverton (1909-1978) was born in the Oregon town of Central Point. With no formal art training, he sold his first cartoon to *America's Humor* in 1926. He was long established as a newspaper artist in the Northwest by the time he started contributing to comic books in 1938. His first regular feature was *Spacehawk,* an interplanetary adventure with a far-larger-than-life hero, begun in *Target* comics in mid-1940. Spacehawk's adventures were often brutal and violent, and (not uniquely) they tended to equate retribution with justice.

Wolverton's depictions of realistic figures in *Spacehawk* and his other space fantasies were often stiff and posturing, and his panels occasionally cramped. But his grasp of depth and perspective was almost uncanny, and resulted in one of the most compelling visual fantasies ever seen in the comics idiom. Indeed, Wolverton's 1940s drawings of space-suited figures, adrift, attached umbilically to their motherships, craftily predict the realities of the space shots of the 1960s and 1970s.

Wolverton's most famous cartoon, mentioned earlier, appeared on a cover of *Life* in 1946. It came about as the result of a contest held by United Features Syndicate for the best depiction of a character alluded to but never seen in Al Capp's *Li'l Abner,* Lena the Hyena, "Lower Slobbovia's ugliest woman." Wolverton won with a drawing that managed to be ingeniously hideous and compellingly gleeful all at once. The drawing more or less established Wolverton as a master of comic grotesques and he contributed more of them to *Mad* in the 1950s and to the short-lived *Plop!* in the 1970s.

Beginning in 1942, meanwhile, Wolverton had contributed *Powerhouse Pepper,* an example of which we have chosen for inclusion here. Powerhouse Pepper was conceived, somewhat along the lines of Popeye or Alley Oop, as a relatively innocent comic hero who could outpunch anyone who pushed him too far. His adventures frequently involved him in the kind of broad burlesque of standard plots and situations depicted here.

115

In these explosive, low-comic stories, Wolverton's talent for grotesques was always there but always latent. His comparative ease with cartoon figures of keenly exaggerated anatomy, Wolverton's engaging silliness, his sight-gag ornamentation of his silliness in his drawings, his elementary energy in depicting comic attitudes—all of these resources thrived in *Powerhouse Pepper*. In addition, he sprinkled his *Powerhouse* dialogue with engaging doggerel rhymes and alliterations.

The feature lasted nearly a decade after Powerhouse's initial appearance in *Joker Comics*, and there were five intermittent issues of a *Powerhouse Pepper* comic book as well.

M.W.

DR. DIMWIT

by BASIL WOLVERTON

From *Sub-Mariner* No. 4, 1942.
1942 Timely Comics, Inc.

117

From *Tessie the Typist* No. 8, January 194
© 1947 Twentieth Century Comic Cor

119

120

124

I THINK YOU SHOULD TRY A LITTLE MILK! IT'LL BE GOOD FOR YOU!

MILK!? NO! NO! NOT THAT! I CAN'T STAND IT!

WELL - IF YOU CAN'T STAND IT, YOU CAN LEAVE! OTHERWISE, I'M GOING TO CRAM IT DOWN YOUR CRAW, McCLAW!

ZIP!

SWISH

HAIRY PRAIRIE

YIPPEE! McCLAW HAS SCRAMMED!

SO WHAT? HE'LL BE BACK SOME OTHER TIME!

DON'T WORRY! IF HE COMES BACK, YOU CAN ALWAYS SCARE HIM AWAY WITH MILK!

STRANGER, YOU'VE SAVED OUR TOWN!

YA-HOO!

HOO-RAY!

RIGHT! AS MAYOR OF THIS DUMP, I HEREWITH PRESENT YOU WITH THIS KEY TO OUR CITY!

BUT THIS IS A PIANO KEY!

SURE! IT'S THE KEY OF C FOR CHASING OUT McCLAW!

HEY! I'LL BET A BUCK THAT THIS BOY IS A SECRET UNITED STATES MARSHALL!

IS THAT RIGHT, STRANGER?

ER-THAT'S RIGHT! HERE'S MY BADGE!

I KNEW IT! WHO EVER HEARD OF A WESTERN STORY WITH A STRANGER THAT DIDN'T TURN OUT TO BE A U.S. MARSHALL?

FOLLOW ME FOR FURTHER FLOCKS OF FUNNY BUSINESS, FRIENDS!

About George Carlson

The first thing that strikes one about George Carlson is the uniqueness of his drawing style, all curves and circles and flow, all boldness in its comic figures. The second is his swirling ingenuity in designing and filling the individual comic-book page. And the third, which comes as one begins to read him, is the apparently absolute sureness Carlson has in what he is doing—whatever that may turn out to be.

In 1970, Harlan Ellison (science-fiction author, screenwriter) offered an appreciation of Carlson's work as a "comic of the absurd," and in the course of his essay he invoked most of those modern writers whose work is apt to involve and move us before we are quite sure what they are up to—Pirandello, Kafka, Genêt, Beckett, Pinter, Ionesco.

Ellison was writing in the anthology *All in Color for a Dime,* and both his subject and his approach must have come as a surprise to the book's readers and some of its other contributors, preoccupied as most of them evidently were with the *sock-baram-powie-shoosh* of the super-heroes. Ellison's awe, his enthusiasm, and his careful recounting of one of Carlson's best strip episodes could, of course, have been no substitute for the real thing, and most of the book's readers probably had not seen the real thing.

George Carlson (1887-1962) came to comics rather late in a long and varied career. In the 1930s and 1940s he was a prolific illustrator of popular children's books, chiefly for the Platt and Munk company (he illustrated eight collections of Uncle Wiggily stories). He also did the illustration for the original dust jacket for *Gone With the Wind,* and he was puzzle editor for the *National Girl Scouts Magazine* (that later aspect of his career was revived for the short-lived *Puzzle Fun Comics*).

Between the February 1942 and December 1949 issues, the full life of *Jingle Jangle Comics,* George Carlson worked on that magazine. He contributed the plotting and drawing to one *Jingle Jangle Tale* and one adventure of *The Pie-Face Prince of Pretzelburg,* Dimwitri by name, in almost every issue.

Jingle Jangle Comics, like its contemporary *Animal Comics* (and like our contemporary *Casper the Friendly Ghost*), was a comic book intended for small children, and I expect that the virtues of Carlson's work will not occur to us unless we remember that fact. Carlson's wonderful silliness and follow-your-nose whimsy functioned best when it was uninhibited by any demands of a well-rounded plot (which he did occasionally set for himself). Like another American tale-spinner/illustrator for small children, Johnny Gruelle, the creator of Raggedy Ann, Carlson functioned best when he improvised—that is, free-associated—incident upon incident to an ending, rather in the manner of small children playing an adventure game among themselves, and making it up as they go along.

All of which leads me here to invoke another name. Enough of litterateurs and playwrights of the absurd. George Carlson was a kind of George Herriman for little children, and the achievement of his work in *Jingle Jangle Comics* is like Herriman's *Krazy Kat,* but on the level of a small child.

I realize that this is praise indeed. And if it is valid praise, then surely what is called for next is a book collection of Carlson's best comics work—a book all to himself.

M.W.

136

CONTINUED NEXT PAGE

142

From *Jingle Jangle Comics* No. 24, December 1946.

144

145

146

147

148

About "Little Lulu" and John Stanley

Late in 1934, there was a small crisis at the *Saturday Evening Post*. The magazine was losing Carl Anderson's popular weekly panel cartoon, *Henry*, to King Features Syndicate. An editor at the *Post* asked a regular contributor to the magazine, Marjorie Henderson Buell—she signed her cartoons "Marge"—for help in coming up with a replacement for *Henry*. The *Post* wanted a child like Henry, but a girl this time. "The editors noodled out the name," Mrs. Buell told an interviewer more than thirty years later. "I was too busy thinking about how she'd look and what she'd do."

The name the editors "noodled out" was "Little Lulu." For a design, Mrs. Buell essentially added a skirt and corkscrew curls to Henry's shoe-button eyes and up-turned nose. The new character was a devilish child, heiress to a long line of such characters that in newspaper comics extended back to the Yellow Kid, Buster Brown, and the Katzenjammer Kids. Like theirs, her mischief, as displayed in a weekly panel, often bordered on the malicious.

Lulu first appeared in the *Post* for February 23, 1935, and ran there until the end of 1944. By that time, Lulu was also appearing in animated cartoons and in ads for Kleenex tissues. "The *Post* didn't want me to go into large-scale business with Lulu," Mrs. Buell has said, "but I wanted to see what she could do in all forms. We parted amicably."

A few months after Lulu left the *Post,* she made her debut in a comic book. That first issue of *Little Lulu* was written and drawn by a cartoonist named John Stanley. (*At the Beach,* the first of the four stories we have chosen for his book, is from that issue.) Stanley also wrote and illustrated the second issue of *Little Lulu.* After that, he drew only the covers, but he wrote everything in each issue for thirteen or fourteen years—about 150 issues, all told—and his writing made *Little Lulu* an extraordinary comic book.

John Stanley was born on March 22, 1914, in New York City, and he worked briefly at the Max Fleischer animation studios, made drawings for Disney merchandise, and held down other jobs before he began writing and drawing stories for Western Printing and Lithographing Company (which produced comic books for publication by another company, Dell) in the early 1940s. At that time, Western produced many comic books for small children, most of them edited by Oskar Lebeck. Lebeck ruled with a light hand, and cartoonists like Walt Kelly, Dan Noonan, Morris Gollub, and, of course, John Stanley did charming and funny work for him. It was Lebeck who assigned Stanley to *Little Lulu.* "I'm sure it was due to no special form of brilliance he thought I'd lend to it," Stanley told Don Phelps. "It could have been handed to Dan Noonan, Kelly, or anyone else. I just happened to be available at the time."

To say that Stanley "wrote" *Little Lulu* is actually a little deceptive, since he was responsible for more than the plots and the dialogue. He sketched each story in rough form, so that he controlled the staging within each panel and the appearance and the attitudes of the characters. The finished drawings were made by other cartoonists (the three later stories in this book were illustrated by Irving Tripp). Stanley himself disliked the published drawings—"too static for me"—but in fact, the "static" style seems appropriate for such highly stylized characters.

Like the panel cartoons, Stanley's stories had a strong flavor of the 1930s. Most obviously, the children—especially the boys—dressed in styles of that decade (knickers, shorts, and so on). Lulu's home town was not suburban, but looked like an eastern city of the Depression years: small, plain houses, with tiny yards or none at all (many front doors opened directly onto the sidewalk). Families were small—one or two children—and the parents usually middle-aged or close to it. Like the *Archie* stories, whose trappings were similarly dated, Stanley's *Lulu* stories remained frozen in time, with only a few concessions to postwar changes. The anachronisms seem never to have been bothered *Little Lulu*'s readers.

At first, Stanley's conception of Lulu herself owed quite a bit to Marge's. But Stanley's Lulu was not so much mischievous as single-minded. She had a very clear idea of what was important to *her,* and she wasn't distracted by irrelevancies like what adults thought was important. Children are, after all, very serious about their own concerns, and Stanley's stories abound in collisions between adults and children all of whom are behaving reasonably—on their own terms.

For the first few years, Stanley worked mainly with Lulu herself and her friend Tubby (who was, like Lulu, inherited from the magazine cartoons). Other children appeared in more or less interchangeable roles until, around 1950, Stanley gave Tubby a group of friends—Willie, Eddie, and Iggy—and a clubhouse, and gave Lulu some other girls to play with, including a buck-toothed gamine named Annie. The rivalry between boys and girls—an element in the series from the start—was magnified by the presence of so many children from both sexes. Lulu herself became a "good little girl" who outsmarted the boys, instead of triumphing through sheer brass as she had in the past. Many of the stories built around the rivalry theme are ingenious and funny, and the best of them spiral upward until the boys

150

become the victims of a comic catastrophe like the one at the climax of *Five Little Babies,* which follows here.

Stanley found other ideas that could be nursed into comic life and exploited in one story after another. For example, Tubby assumed Lulu's old role as the serenely egocentric child, resenting all adult efforts to deflect him from his course; he played that role brilliantly in a string of stories in which he became "the Spider," a detective wreaking all the havoc necessary to solve a case. (Lulu's father was invariably the culprit—although he was of course no culprit at all by adult standards.)

Stanley's most striking departure from the feature he inherited from Marge was in the stories that Lulu told to Alvin, a vicious little next-door neighbor whose personality was not far removed from that of the magazine-cartoon Lulu. Beneath the laughter, Stanley's mock fairy tales could be as strong as real fairy tales. Lulu was the featured player, as well as the narrator, and she often took the part of a cheerful Candide in a world otherwise filled with greedy and stupid people. In *The Little Rich Boy,* a story we have chosen for this book, the fairy-tale Lulu is an ingénue indeed—until she gets rich. Then she takes revenge, with a chilling thoroughness, on the boy who has scorned her love.

While he was writing *Little Lulu,* Stanley contributed scripts to many other Dell comic books, and in the 1960s, after leaving *Lulu,* he both wrote and illustrated a few, like *Melvin Monster.* But he left comic books years ago (his comments on comic books—even his own work—have become rather sour), and he has worked recently for a silk-screening company in upstate New York.

M.B.

154

155

159

From *Little Lulu* No. 38, August 1951.
© 1951 Western Publishing Company, Inc
Used by permissio

164

165

174

175

WHEN HE WANTED WALNUTS HE BOUGHT A WHOLE WAREHOUSE FULL OF THEM...

HERE'S YOUR MONEY! SCRAM!

...AND THEN HE BOUGHT A HERD OF ELEPHANTS TO CRACK THE WALNUTS FOR HIM...

HE EVEN TRIED TO BUY THE *ATLANTIC OCEAN* TO SAIL HIS SAILBOAT IN!

OBOY!

AFTER BUYING IT, HE WAS GOING TO MAKE ALL THE OTHER SHIPS GET OFF OF IT BECAUSE THEY MIGHT BUMP INTO HIS SAILBOAT!

HERE'S YOUR MONEY! GIMME THE ATLANTIC OCEAN!

BUT UNCLE SAM WOULDN'T SELL HIM THE ATLANTIC OCEAN BECAUSE HE SAID HE MIGHT NEED IT ONCE IN A WHILE...

HOW ABOUT A *SMALLER* BODY OF WATER—LIKE *LAKE SUPERIOR*?

NO!

THIS MADE HIM AWFUL MAD, AND FOR A LITTLE WHILE HE WAS *VERY* ANGRY WITH THE UNITED STATES...

GRRRR!

BUT HE GOT EVEN BY GIVING THE UNITED STATES A GOOD BEATING WITH THE BIGGEST STICK HE COULD FIND!

TAKE THAT! AN' THAT, AND THAT!

AFTER THAT HE FELT BETTER AND WENT AND BOUGHT HIMSELF A FREIGHT CAR FULL OF YO-YOS...

OBOY!

ONE DAY WHILE THIS VERY RICH LITTLE BOY WAS STROLLING DOWN THE STREET ON A PAIR OF GOLD-PLATED STILTS, HE SAW A POOR RAGGEDY LITTLE ORPHAN GIRL LOOKING INTO A BAKERY STORE WINDOW FULL OF GOODIES...

HE FELT AWFUL BAD FOR THE POOR LITTLE GIRL BECAUSE SHE DIDN'T HAVE ANY MONEY TO BUY ANYTHING, AND COULD ONLY *LOOK* AT THE THINGS IN THE WINDOW...

SNIFF!

SO HE GOT RIGHT DOWN OFF HIS STILTS, WALKED INTO THE BAKERY STORE AND BOUGHT IT, LOCK, STOCK AND BARREL...

I'M TAKING OVER NOW!

WOW!

THEN HE CLIMBED INTO THE WINDOW WHERE ALL THE TASTIEST BUNS AND CAKES WERE...

STANDING ON TOP OF A BIG WEDDING CAKE, HE COULD JUST BARELY REACH THE BIG WINDOW SHADE...

IN A TWINKLING HE PULLED THE SHADE DOWN TO THE VERY BOTTOM OF THE WINDOW...

THEN HE WALKED OUT OF THE STORE AND LOCKED THE DOOR...

CLICK!

AS HE STROLLED DOWN THE STREET ON HIS GOLD-PLATED STILTS, HE FELT VERY HAPPY, BECAUSE NOW THE POOR LITTLE GIRL WOULDN'T HAVE TO LOOK AT THINGS SHE COULDN'T BUY...

LATER, THE LITTLE BOY WAS RIDING DOWN THE STREET ON HIS SIX-WHEEL CYCLE (HE DIDN'T LIKE *THREE*-WHEEL CYCLES BECAUSE *ANY* KID COULD HAVE ONE OF THOSE)...

JUST AS HE WAS PASSING AN AMUSEMENT PARK HE SAW THE POOR LITTLE GIRL AGAIN — SHE WAS STARING UP AT THE HUGE FERRIS WHEEL...

THE POOR LITTLE GIRL WISHED VERY MUCH THAT SHE WAS RIDING ON IT WITH ALL THE OTHER HAPPY KIDS...

THE RICH LITTLE BOY FELT *VERY* SORRY FOR HER! HE GOT RIGHT DOWN OFF HIS SIX-WHEEL CYCLE AND BOUGHT THE FERRIS WHEEL...

THEN HE GOT SOME MEN TO UNSCREW THE BOLT THAT HELD THE FERRIS WHEEL...

WHEN THE FERRIS WHEEL WAS FREE HE ORDERED THE MEN TO PUSH IT DOWN THE HILL...

NOW THE POOR LITTLE GIRL WOULDN'T HAVE TO LOOK LONGINGLY AT THE FERRIS WHEEL...

THIS GOOD DEED MADE THE RICH LITTLE BOY VERY HAPPY... HE GOT BACK ON HIS SIX-WHEEL CYCLE AND RODE OFF WHISTLING A MERRY TUNE...

NOW DON'T THINK THE POOR LITTLE GIRL DIDN'T NOTICE ALL THE GOOD DEEDS THE RICH LITTLE BOY WAS DOING FOR HER...

GOSH! HOW C'N ANYBODY BE SO *GOOD*?

SHE WAS VERY GRATEFUL...SO GRATEFUL, THAT SHE JUST COULDN'T HELP FALLING IN LOVE WITH THE RICH LITTLE BOY...

?

SHE FELL SO MUCH IN LOVE WITH HIM THAT SHE FOLLOWED HIM AROUND WHEREVER HE WENT...

BUT THE RICH LITTLE BOY WAS VERY ANNOYED...HE TOLD HER IF SHE DIDN'T STOP FOLLOWING HIM AROUND HE'D GIVE HER SUCH A SOCK—

OH, YOU'RE SO KIND! BUT COULDN'T YOU GIVE ME *TWO* OF THEM? *BOTH* MY SOCKS ARE ALL HOLES!

THIS DIDN'T STOP THE LITTLE GIRL AT ALL—SHE WAS EVEN MORE IN LOVE WITH HIM THAN *BEFORE*!

FINALLY THE RICH LITTLE BOY WAS SO ANNOYED THAT HE DECIDED TO GO TO THE POLICE STATION...

HE WANTED THE POLICEMEN TO ARREST THE LITTLE GIRL AND PUT HER IN JAIL FOR THE REST OF HER LIFE...

SORRY, CAN'T DO IT!

...AT FIRST THE POLICEMEN WOULDN'T DO IT...BUT THEY CHANGED THEIR MINDS WHEN THE RICH LITTLE BOY PULLED OUT A BIG BUNDLE OF MONEY AND BOUGHT THE POLICE DEPARTMENT!

WOW!

RIGHT AWAY THE POLICEMEN SAW THEIR DUTY AND QUICKLY SNAPPED FOUR PAIRS OF HANDCUFFS, SIX PAIRS OF LEGCUFFS AND ONE PAIR OF EARCUFFS ON HER...

THEN THEY DRAGGED HER PAST A LONG ROW OF CELLS AND THREW HER INTO A LITTLE GIRL'S CELL...

IN YOU GO!

THE POOR LITTLE GIRL WAS VERY HAPPY! THIS WAS THE FIRST TIME IN HER LIFE SHE EVER HAD A ROOF OVER HER HEAD!

WOW! A REAL ROOF!

THIS WAS *ANOTHER* GOOD DEED THE RICH KIND LITTLE BOY HAD DONE FOR HER... *GOSH*, HOW SHE LOVED HIM NOW!

SHE LOVED HIM *SO* MUCH THAT SHE WAS WILLING TO SACRIFICE THE ROOF OVER HER HEAD JUST TO FOLLOW HIM AROUND...

I'VE JUST *GOT* TO BE NEAR HIM!

SO SHE GOT RIGHT TO WORK WITH THE LITTLE METAL END OF HER SHOELACE AND BEGAN PICKING AWAY AT A HUGE STONE IN THE WALL...

SHE WORKED ALL NIGHT PICKING AWAY AT THE STONE... NEXT MORNING THE STONE WAS LOOSE...

OBOY! I THINK IT'S MOVING!

WITH ONE GOOD SHOVE THE LITTLE GIRL WAS FREE...

WOW!

IN A LITTLE WHILE SHE WAS STANDING OUTSIDE THE DOOR OF THE GREAT BIG HOUSE THE LITTLE BOY LIVED IN...

THE LITTLE BOY HAD JUST COME DOWN FROM HIS ROOM...

THERE YOU ARE, MASTER!

WHAT'S THE MATTER WITH YOU, ANYWAY, DOPEY? I DECIDED WHEN I WOKE UP THIS MORNING THAT I WOULDN'T *HAVE* ANY BREAKFAST!

THREE BUTLERS OPENED THE BIG FRONT DOOR FOR HIM AND HE STEPPED OUT ON THE PORCH...

GOSH, HE WAS SURPRISED WHEN HE SAW THE POOR LITTLE GIRL AGAIN!

HE RUSHED RIGHT BACK INTO THE HOUSE AND SLAMMED THE DOOR...

AS QUICK AS HE COULD HE RAN TO THE BACK DOOR...

BUT WHEN HE PEEKED OUT THE BACK DOOR THERE WAS THE LITTLE GIRL AGAIN!

HE SLAMMED THE DOOR, FELL ON THE FLOOR AND HAD A GOOD TANTRUM FOR HIMSELF!

YOW! YOW! YOW! YOW! YOW! YOW!

WHEN HE QUIETED DOWN HE WENT TO THE TELEPHONE AND CALLED THE DOG-CATCHERS...

...I WANT TO **BUY** THE DOG-CATCHERS' DEPARTMENT!

IN A FEW SECONDS HE WAS THE SOLE OWNER OF THE DOGCATCHERS' DEPARTMENT!

I'LL SEND THE MONEY TO YOU!

...NOW, I'LL TELL YOU WHAT I WANT YOU TO DO—

FIVE MINUTES LATER A DOGCATCHERS' TRUCK DROVE UP TO THE DOOR...

A DOGCATCHER JUMPED OUT OF THE TRUCK AND RAN AROUND TO THE BACK OF THE BIG HOUSE...

...NEXT THING THE POOR LITTLE GIRL KNEW, A NET WAS THROWN OVER HER HEAD...

GOTCHA!

THEN SHE WAS CARRIED TO THE TRUCK AND DUMPED INTO THE BACK WITH A BUNCH OF STRAY DOGS...

THEN THE TRUCK RACED OFF TO THE DOG POUND WITH HER...

WHEN THEY GOT TO THE DOG POUND THE LITTLE GIRL WAS THROWN INTO A BIG CAGE THAT WAS FULL OF ALL KINDS OF DOGS...

GOSH, SHE WAS HAPPY! SHE LOVED DOGS, ALL KINDS OF DOGS...AND SHE WAS SURE THAT THIS WAS ANOTHER GOOD DEED THE KIND LITTLE BOY HAD DONE FOR HER....

BUT, THOUGH SHE LOVED DOGS VERY MUCH, SHE LOVED THE KIND LITTLE RICH BOY EVEN MORE!

I'VE GOT TO GET OUT OF HERE!

SO, THAT NIGHT WHEN THE GUARD WAS ASLEEP SHE PICKED THE LOCK ON THE CAGE WITH A HAIRPIN AND TIP TOED TO THE BACK DOOR...

NEXT MORNING SHE WAS WAITING AT THE FRONT DOOR OF THE RICH LITTLE BOY'S HOUSE....

WHEN THE LITTLE BOY OPENED THE DOOR AND SAW THE LITTLE GIRL A-GAIN HE ALMOST FAINTED FROM SUR-PRISE...

HE SCREAMED AND HOLLERED AT HER AND TOLD HER HOW MUCH HE HATED HER...

I HATE YOU! I HATE YOU! I HATE YOU!

I HATE YOU! I HATE YOU! I HATE YOU!

THEN HE TOLD HER TO GO DIG A DEEP, DEEP HOLE AND CRAWL INTO IT...

...AND I'LL BE GLAD TO LEND YOU THE SHOVEL!

GOSH, THE POOR LITTLE GIRL WAS SHOCKED! THERE WAS NOTHING ELSE FOR HER TO DO BUT GO DIG A DEEP, DEEP HOLE AND CRAWL INTO IT...

...AND DON'T FORGET TO RETURN THE SHOVEL!

SO SHE WENT TO A LONELY PLACE IN THE WOODS AND STARTED TO DIG...

SNIFF!

SNIFF!

DAY AND NIGHT SHE DUG...

SNIFF!

UNTIL FINALLY SHE DECIDED SHE WAS ALMOST DEEP ENOUGH...SHE DUG ONE LAST SHOVELFUL AND—

WHOOM!

SUDDENLY SHE WAS SHOT HIGH INTO THE AIR! SHE HAD *STRUCK OIL!*

WOW!

THE LITTLE GIRL WAS *RICH!* NOW SHE COULD BUY ANYTHING SHE WANTED!

I'M RICH!

I'M RICH!

THE FIRST THING SHE DID WAS BUY A GREAT BIG HOTEL SO THAT SHE COULD TAKE A BATH AND WASH ALL THE THICK, BLACK OIL OFF HERSELF...

OBOY!

THEN SHE BOUGHT A *TWELVE* WHEEL CYCLE...

AND A PAIR OF *SOLID* GOLD STILTS...

Marge's Little Lulu

the "Spider" spins again

OH, GEORGE! YOU LOOK SO *DIFFERENT* WITH YOUR MUSTACHE SHAVED OFF!

MAKES ME LOOK *YOUNGER*, DON'T YOU THINK?

WAIT TILL *LULU* SEES YOU!

I HOPE SHE *LIKES* ME THIS WAY!

I'M *HUNGRY*, LULU! DO YOU MIND IF I LOOK IN YOUR *REFRIGERATOR?* THERE MAY BE SOMETHING THERE THAT'S GETTING *BAD*...

I THINK THERE'S A WILTED CARROT THERE..

HI, LULU! NOTICE ANYTHING *DIFFERENT?*

WHY, POP! YOU *SHAVED* YOUR *MUSTACHE* OFF!

?

DO YOU *STILL* 'LOVE YOUR OL' POP?

GOSH, POP, AN OL' *MUSTACHE* DOESN'T MAKE ANY DIFFERENCE.

LULU! CAN I SPEAK TO YOU FOR A MINUTE? *ALONE!*

WHAT IS IT, TUB?

LULU, I HATE TO TELL YOU THIS, BUT I FEEL IT'S MY DUTY...

...YOUR *POP* IS *GUILTY* OF SOMETHING!

WH-WHAT DO YOU MEAN, TUB?

HE SHAVED HIS MUSTACHE OFF 'CAUSE HE DOESN'T WANT TO BE *RECOGNIZED* BY THE *POLICE!*

WHAT?

From *Little Lulu* No. 81, March 1955.
© 1955 Western Publishing Company, Inc.
Used by permission.

About "Donald Duck" and Carl Barks

In the late 1930s, the Walt Disney characters were appearing not in a comic book but in a children's magazine called the *Mickey Mouse Magazine.* In 1940, this magazine was converted into a monthly comic book called *Walt Disney's Comics and Stories;* it was the first of dozens of comic books based on animated-cartoon characters. The comic books with major characters like Donald Duck, Bugs Bunny, Woody Woodpecker, and Tom and Jerry were produced by Western Printing and Lithographing Company and published under the Dell label. Other publishers used less popular characters, like Mighty Mouse and the Fox and the Crow, or invented their own. The "funny animal" comic books, as they were often called, remained consistently popular throughout the 1940s and 1950s. They faded only in the 1960s, when the super-heroes made a comeback. The Disney comic books were always the most popular of the "funny animal" comic books; and of the Disney comic books, the most popular—and easily the best—were written and drawn by Carl Barks.

Barks was born in Oregon on March 27, 1901, and he passed through a variety of jobs—heating rivets in a railroad yard, editing a men's humor magazine in Minneapolis—before going to work for the Disney Studios in 1935. He was a "story man," thinking up gags for Donald Duck cartoons, until he left Disney in 1942 to work as a free-lance cartoonist. He started his new career by illustrating the ten-page *Donald Duck* feature for the April 1943 issue of *Walt Disney's Comics and Stories;* for the next issue, he wrote, as well as illustrated, *Donald Duck* and he continued to write and illustrate that feature in almost every issue of *Walt Disney's Comics* for the next twenty-three years.

Barks of course never signed his work, but his crisp, precise drawing style was so distinctive—in comic books otherwise filled with soft, broad drawings—that he was recognized by many children as "the good artist." Barks's *Donald Duck*—the lead story in each issue of *Walt Disney's Comics*—was so popular that when Barks was taken off the feature in 1950 to handle stories in other Disney comic books, reader protests quickly led to his reinstatement. At one point in the early 1950s, *Walt Disney's Comics* was selling three million copies per issue, making it one of the most successful comic books ever published; and a very large part of that success was due to Barks.

During his first ten years in comic books, Barks also wrote and illustrated longer stories—usually thirty-two pages—for the *Donald Duck* comic book. Most of these stories were comic adventures—mixtures of laughter and thrills. Barks sent Donald and his three nephews, Huey,

Dewey, and Louie, to many exotic places, like the jungles of Africa, the outback of Australia, and the desolate moors of Scotland. The best-remembered of these stories is probably *Lost in the Andes,* in which Donald and his nephews went to South America in search of mysterious square eggs. Deep in the Andes, they found not only the eggs but a block-shaped race of people who spoke in the accents of the American Deep South and called their homeland "Plain Awful."

When he started writing and drawing *Donald Duck,* Barks had only Donald and his nephews (and occasionally Donald's girlfriend, Daisy) to work with. For one 1947 story in *Donald Duck,* Barks gave Donald a wealthy, miserly uncle, Scrooge McDuck. Scrooge was a supporting character in the *Donald Duck* stories for the next few years; he was always trying to get more money or protect what he had, and this made him a fertile source of plot ideas. Scrooge finally became so popular that he was given his own comic book in 1952. Like the Barks issues of *Donald Duck,* the quarterly *Uncle Scrooge* combined comedy and adventure; Scrooge's money could—and did—take the ducks any place, from the sunken continent of Atlantis to outer space. *Uncle Scrooge* was tremendously successful, outselling those Disney comic books with characters—like Mickey Mouse—who were more famous but who did not have the good fortune to have their adventures recounted by Carl Barks.

Along the way, Barks created other characters who became more or less established residents of the Disney universe: Donald's incredibly lucky cousin, Gladstone Gander; the eccentric inventor, Gyro Gearloose (a chicken); the Junior Woodchucks of the World (a spoof of the Boy Scouts); the villainous Beagle Boys; the sorceress Magica de Spell.

Barks's stories were so popular, and so good, because he took pains where most writers and cartoonists for "funny animal" comic books did not. He used the ducks in everything from purest slapstick to hair-raising adventures that had only a light flavoring of comedy—but always, he worked to give his stories plausibility. Plausibility in the way the plots and gags were constructed, in the detailed and accurately drawn settings (he made sure that an ancient Persian city *looked* like an ancient Persian city), and above all, in the way his characters talked and behaved. Barks's characters were never puppets; the ducks were always propelled by passions so comically powerful that they could scarcely be contained even within exaggerated faces and bodies. In Barks's stories, the world is very different from the one we know—it is a world of talking ducks, and of huge "money bins" filled with Scrooge's coins and greenbacks—but "duck nature" is really human nature, and very much the same as in our own world. It was by making his characters so completely recognizable as people, despite their orange beaks and webbed feet, that Barks won the devotion of so many readers.

Barks's work was at its richest and funniest in the late 1940s and early 1950s. *Letter to Santa,* the story we have included here, was published in 1949, in the first issue of a "giant" comic book—it cost twenty-five cents, instead of the usual dime—called *Walt Disney's Christmas Parade. Letter* is a rarity among Barks's longer stories because it is not a mixture of comedy and adventure but is instead completely comic from start to finish, like most of the ten-page stories in *Walt Disney's Comics.*

Letter to Santa was the first story with the "classic" version of Uncle Scrooge—the cranky old capitalist who is bursting with energy, and who has so much cash that it spills around his desk. In the earlier stories, Scrooge was not as rich or as egomaniacal; in later stories, after he had gotten his own comic book, Scrooge became a bit more likable but a bit less funny.

Santa Claus himself appears in *Letter to Santa,* and this is unusual, because Barks usually avoided characters who were wholly fanciful even on the terms set by the ducks' fanciful universe. But when Barks did use such characters—Santa Claus, or a witch, or a dragon—he presented them with the same care, the same concern for plausibility, that he gave to the other elements in his stories; Barks's Santa is one we can almost believe in. For one thing, Barks has figured out a way to get his Santa down even narrow chimneys. Note too that this Santa is a very practical fellow; he gives the nephews exactly what they want, but only that—there's no flood of unrequested gifts. And, typically for Barks, this Santa, by his very existence, creates more problems than he solves.

Carl Barks retired from comic-book work in 1966, although he wrote a few stories for the *Junior Woodchucks* comic book until 1973. He lives now in southern California, where he has carved out a new (and successful) career as a painter in oils and water colors.

M.B.

201

204

206

209

MEANWHILE, THE KIDS HAVE BEEN COUNTING THE HOURS, THE MINUTES, AND THE SECONDS AS THEY WAIT FOR MIDNIGHT AND SANTA CLAUS!

HALF PAST ELEVEN!

THIRTY MORE MINUTES TO WAIT!

YEAH! EIGHTEEN HUNDRED SECONDS!

I'M WORRIED ABOUT UNCA' DONALD! HE SHOULDA BEEN HOME HOURS AGO!

I'M WORRIED, TOO, BUT SANTA CLAUS IS MORE IMPORTANT!

SOME DISTANCE DOWN THE STREET!

JINGLE!

JINGLE!

TELL ME, UNCLE SCROOGE! WHAT IS THE IDEA OF THIS SCREWBALL MASQUERADE?

YOU'RE GOING TO BE SANTA CLAUS, LOUT! AND SANTA ALWAYS DRIVES UP IN A REINDEER BUGGY, DOESN'T HE?

JINGLE JINGLE

FOR HIRE

PHONE CR. 1-6157

I HEAR SLEIGH BELLS!

IT CAN'T BE SANTA!

IT'S TOO EARLY!

MAYBE THE CLOCK IS SLOW!

GET INTO THAT SANTA COSTUME AND BE READY TO GO INTO YOUR ACT!

WHAT AM I SUPPOSED TO DO?

YOU'RE GOING TO TELL THE KIDS A **HARD LUCK** STORY!

TELL 'EM YOU'RE SANTA CLAUS AND THAT YOU'RE ALL OUT OF STEAM SHOVELS THIS YEAR, BUT THAT **NEXT** CHRISTMAS —

SAY! THAT'S A **SWELL** WAY OUT OF THIS JAM! UNCLE SCROOGE, YOU'RE A **GENIUS!**

YOU'VE CALLED ME WORSE NAMES, BUT, FOR NOW, PUT ON YOUR PUTTY NOSE! WE'RE HERE!

WHOA, DONNER! WHOA, BLITZEN! WHOA, DASHER AND PRANCER!

IT **MUST** BE SANTA!

HE STOPPED IN THE ALLEY

WHERE WE CAN'T SEE HIM!

QUICK! PUT OUT THE FIRE, SO HE CAN COME **DOWN** THE CHIMNEY!

UH, OH!

212

213

I DON'T KNOW WHAT I'D DO WITHOUT UNCLE SCROOGE'S HELP!

RED BEANS

PINTO BEANS

ALL RIGHT, BOYS! PUSH OUT THE SCALES, AND LET'S GO!

ONE HUNDRED AND SIX POUNDS! GEE! YOU'RE **HEAVY**, SANTA!

HERE'S OUR TREE, SANTA! WE WANT YOU TO SEE HOW NICE WE FIXED IT UP!

DOGGONE! THOSE SLICK BOOTS AGAIN!

FIRE !

JUMP IN THE SHOWER, SANTA! WE'LL PUT THE FIRE OUT!

EVERYTHING HAPPENS BUT THE **RIGHT** THING!

216

About "Pogo" and Walt Kelly

It will probably come as a surprise to some readers to find
Pogo and Walt Kelly in this collection. It will probably come
as a surprise to more readers to learn that Kelly actually
began Pogo as a comic-book character, first in *Animal
Comics* from 1942 to 1947, and then in the *Pogo Possum*
comic book, which ran for sixteen issues between 1949 and
1954. By the time that the fine, farcical adventures
presented here first appeared in *Pogo Possum*, Kelly's *Pogo*
had already become a widely syndicated, much-loved
newspaper feature, and softcover collections of those
newspaper strips were best sellers.

In discussing his own past, Walt Kelly sometimes
indulged in the same talent for whimsy that he brought to
the animal adventures in the Okefenokee. So it has become
difficult to be sure of the biographical details. But the main
facts seem clear enough. Kelly was born August 25, 1913, in
Philadelphia, but his family had moved to Bridgeport,
Connecticut, within two years. Kelly on occasion described
his father as a painter of theatrical scenery, but that seems
doubtful, particularly as the profession of a citizen of
Bridgeport in the 1930s. In any case, Walt contributed
drawings to his high school newspaper (which he also
edited) and yearbook. On graduation, he went to work for
the Bridgeport *Post*.

By 1935, Walt Kelly had been hired by the Walt Disney
Studios, where he animated parts of *Fantasia* and *Dumbo*. In
1941, Kelly moved to New York, where he worked for
Western Printing and Lithographing Company on Dell comic
books, chiefly *Animal Comics* and *Our Gang*.

For the former he created a feature that was probably
derived to some extent from the Uncle Remus stories. At
first it had no continuing title but it centered around a
comically ravenous alligator named Albert and a black
youngster named Bumbazine who visited with Albert and the
animals in a southern swamp. The swamp's anthropomorphic
inhabitants included a Pogo Possum whose role became gradually more prominent as Bumbazine's waned. (Incidentally,
the drawing of Pogo that appears in the collection *Ten Ever-
Lovin' Blue-Eyed Years with Pogo* captioned, "Pogo circa
1943," is another example of Kelly whimsy, circa 1959.
Pogo did look different in his early appearances but he
didn't look like that.)

During World War II, Kelly worked as a civilian
employee for the Army, contributing drawings to language
manuals. He continued to work for Western Printing, too,
contributing to comic books like *Raggedy Ann and Andy,
Santa Claus Funnies,* and *Easter with Mother Goose*—along
with *Animal Comics* and *Our Gang*—well into the postwar

years. The charming illustrated parodies of standard nursery rhymes and nursery tales that were later featured in Kelly's books were first tried out in *Raggedy Ann and Andy* and other comic books.

In 1949, Kelly became art editor for the idealistic enterprise known as the New York *Star,* a newspaper for which he did editorial cartoons and spot drawings, and for which he revived Pogo in a daily comic strip. When the *Star* died, *Pogo* was taken over by the New York *Post* and its Post-Hall Syndicate, then by Field Enterprises. The success of that strip was rapid and book collections of *Pogo* strips quickly followed. Kelly remained the steward of the strip until his death on October 18, 1973.

Walt Kelly's work in *Animal Comics,* with its audience of small children, is particularly interesting in retrospect. The early Albert Alligator was a comic villain who actually intended to make his lunches of the swamp's other inhabitants. That fact gives another dimension to one of the adventures that follows: the one about Albert's accidental cannibalism. Many fine variations on that idea appeared in Kelly's daily and Sunday *Pogo* strips.

Kelly found himself and found the nature of his talent when *Pogo* became a four-panel, daily comic strip. But the *Pogo* Sunday feature gave Kelly's improvisational fancy a larger yard to play in, and the contemporaneous comic book, so unduly neglected as it was, gave him virtually an open field.

The comic-book treatment of *Pogo* was curiously different. Despite more panels and larger panels, the characters dominate the strip and the backgrounds are sparser. (Incidentally, Kelly's comic-book stories, like those of John Stanley's *Little Lulu,* would thus make superb storyboards for cartoons—particularly TV cartoons—just as they are.)

The three vaudeville-like comic-book sketches that follow, with their comic delight in the humanized attitudes and reactions of their characters, their verbal games and fun, and their detached but passionate observations on us all—these *Pogo* sketches suggest that Walt Kelly's sensibility was perhaps closest to that of another gifted and whimsical twentieth-century Irishman, James Joyce.

In addition to the three stories from *Pogo Possum,* we have included the very first Pogo story, published in *Animal Comics* in 1942.

M.W.

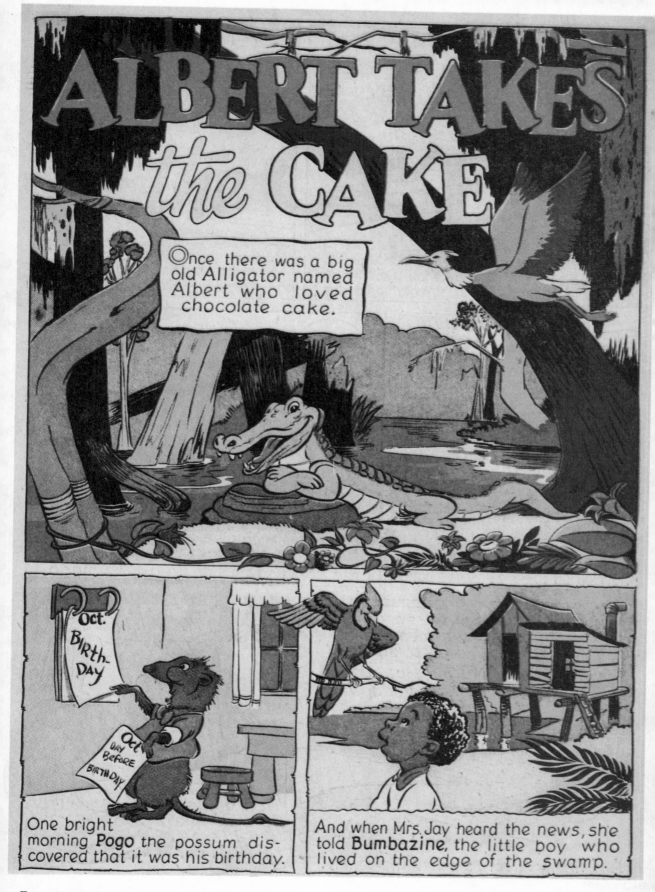

ALBERT TAKES the CAKE

Once there was a big old Alligator named Albert who loved chocolate cake.

One bright morning **Pogo** the possum discovered that it was his birthday.

And when Mrs. Jay heard the news, she told **Bumbazine**, the little boy who lived on the edge of the swamp.

From *Animal Comics* No. 1, 1942.
© 1942 Oskar Lebeck.

Bumbazine decided to bake a chocolate birthday cake for his friend Pogo. So he took flour and water and salt and pepper and sugar and molasses—

and three chocolate bars and a piece of bacon rind. He mixed them all together and baked the mixture into a cake.

Man alive! This is a powerful **heavy** *cake!*

When it was all done, Bumbazine hurried off to Pogo Possum's house.

Mmmm!

Mmmm!

And though it **was** a heavy cake, it had the most beautiful smell that the swamp creatures had smelled in a blue moon.

Well, bless my soul if that doesn't smell like chocolate cake!

It is! Bumbazine is taking it to Pogo Possum for his birthday!

And finally Albert smelled the smell!

There he goes!

But he won't have the cake long—I'll see to that! Heh-heh!

Congratulations on your birthday, Pogo!

Thank you, Beetle!

Pogo was receiving greetings from his neighbors—

Hi, there, Pogo! I'm coming across on this log!

Oh, hello, Bumbazine! I didn't recognize you in your new hat.

when he heard Bumbazine hailing him.

This isn't a hat! It's a cake and it's for you, because today is your birthday!

Gosh— look out, Bumbazine! That's not a log, either!

Ow! It's Albert!

Not so fast—Bumbazine!

Pogo, give me that cake or I'll eat Bumbazine!

But the cake was so heavy that it pulled Albert to the bottom and there he stayed for a week.

So Pogo and Bumbazine celebrated the birthday in peace.

234

THAT FOR YOU!

WHILE YOU IS STIRRIN' MY CAKE BATTER, I'LL GIT ON A DIS-GUISE, AN' GO FERRET OUT MY OWN INFORMATION.

HOT DOG!

I SHOULD OF BEEN A BEAUTIFUL SPY QUEEN. NOBODY WILL KNOW WHO I IS— MY DISGUISE IS INPENATROUBLE.

OOMPH— LOOKY THERE!

UGH!

HULLO THERE, UNCLE ALBERT.

HOWDY, UNCLE ALBERT.

HEY, UNCLE ALBERT, HOW IS YO'?

HI, UNCLE ALBERT!

HULLO, UNCLE ALBERT.

NATURAL, THEY MUS' OF MISTOOKEN ME FO' A LI'L GAL RABBIT NAME OF "UNCLE ALBERT."

MAN ALIVE! THAT IS THE SMELL OF CATFISHES FRYIN'!...SEEMS TO ME SOMEBODY IS HAVIN' A PARTY, AND I ISN'T INVITED.

I'LL JUST TICKY-TOE OVER TO THE LI'L SHACK AN' SEE WHAT'S COOKIN'!

WHY—LOOKY THERE, MAMMY MUSKRAT, OL' UNCLE ALBERT SNEAKIN' UP ON US IN A DISGUISE.

SO HE BE!

RUN AROUND TO THE SIDE OF THE HOUSE AN' SNIP OFF THE HORNETS' NEST HANGIN' ON THE TREE—ALBERT IS UP TO NO GOOD.

HE GONE TO SNEAK UP AN' SWIPE OUR FISH PIE FOR THE BIG FISH FRY—WE'LL FOOL HIM.

238

239

THIS LETTER IS FROM ME—I DICK-TAKIN' IT TO THE FOLKS AT THE FRY.

SAY: "GOOD-BYE, CRUEL WORLD. I GONE DO WAY WITH MYSELF 'CAUSE YO' DIN'T TELL ME 'BOUT THE ANNUAL FRY AN' YOU TRY TO POISON ME— *HAIL AN' FAREWELL.*"

GREAT!

GREAT! WHAT YOU MEAN GREAT—?

I MEAN GREAT HOW YOU FRAMES THE LITERATURE AN' GREAT 'CAUSE NOW OL' MAIL-MAN GOT A REASON TO GO TO THE FRY.

GIT ALONG AN' DEE-LIVER THAT TO POGO POSSUM.

I HOPES YO' PASSIN' IS QUIET, ALBERT.

'COURSE I ADMIT THAT I TOLE EVERYBODY LAST YEAR THEY DIN'T NEED TO INVITE ME SPECIAL. THE ANNUAL FRY IS OPEN TO ALL.

BUT I WISH FOLKS WOULD RE-MEMBER WHAT I MEAN AN' NOT WHAT I SAY—MM-CAKE DONE.

241

ONLY ONE THING! TAKE THE FIRE PUMP WHAT WE HAD IN CASE THE BONFIRE GIT OUT OF CONTROL.

QUICK, ALBERT! OPEN YO' MOUTH AN' LET THE PULMOTOR WHICH I IS PULLIN' PUMP OUT THE POISON. IT'S YO ONLY CHANCE.

A UNFORESEEN CALAMITY!

SWALLER DOWN THE INTAKE PUMP HOSE AND I PUMPS YO'.

ONE, TWO, ONE, TWO—

SPOOIE! POGO SURE PICKS OUT UNCOMFORTABLE WAYS TO PROVE HE'S MY BEST FRIEND.

I'LL JUST STICK THIS HOSE IN THE LAGOON AND THAT'LL SATISFY POGO—THEN I CAN BE SICK IN PEACE.

MY SAKES, ALBERT, YOU TRIED THE MOST HORRIBOBBLE DEATH OF ALL..."DRINKIN' SWAMP WATER.

244

From *Pogo Possum* No. 8, Jan.-Mar. 1952

WELL, IT SEEM LIKE THEY WAS THIS BEAUTIFUL YOUNG GAL GO BY NAME CINDEROLA.

SHE LIVE IN A HOUSE WITH HER STEP-MOTHERS AN' SISTERS AN' THEY MAKE HER SLEEP IN THE CINDERS SO THAT HOW SHE GIT THE NAME.

SHH!

....

HER MOTHER WAS A MEAN OL' FIERCE OL' MAN BEAR NAME OF STEPMOTHER.

HER SISTERS WAS A LADY MA BEAR AN' A BABY BOY BEAR CALLED BIG SISTER AN' LI'L SISTER.

WHILST CINDEROLA HERSELF WAS A LI'L HE POSSUM NAME OF POGO.

ONE DAY COMES A KNOCK AT THE DOOR.

BLESS MY HARD-WORKIN' LI'L SELF.

DING DING

PAGE FROM THE KING IS HERE WITH A BLOWIN' HORN!

FRAMP!

248

251

MOOM? WHY, YOU GOGGLE-GAITED OL' GULL, I COULDN'T PULL A GNAT'S TOOTH, LET ALONE A PICNIC-SIZE PUMPKIN FULL OF PASSENGERS.

ALA-GA-ROO-GA-ZAM! THERE! YOU'RE A HORSE!

IF I'M A HORSE, HE'S A BEAUTIFUL GAL!

THAT SETTLES THAT.

'N JUS' A WUFFY THIS COACH WILL BE READY FOR YOU, CINDEROLA.

IF I'M PULLIN', LADY, YOU IS PUSHIN'!

THINK ANYBODY WILL NOTICE MY SHOES IS STICKIN' OUT?

YOU WANT THE FRONT DOOR OR THE BACK, MISS?

LET'S TRY TO SNEAK IN A WINDOW.

POORADE! POO-RADE!

YOU SHOULD BE HOME IN BED!

ME, TOO.

254

HA!

THAT MUST BE THE PRINCE, AN' YOUR DISMAL STEPSISTERS IS GETTIN' READY TO POUNCE ON HIM.

RUSH IN, CHILE, YO' FURRY GODMOTHER KNOWS BEST.

HELLO, PRINCEY, I IS READY TO MARRY YOU!

ME, TOO!

BUT I IS UNDECIDED WHICH OF YOU IS THE MOST BEAUTIFUL!

COME BACK, HON!

HALP!

GANGWAY, YO' RAGABONES!

PHOO! WHAT A PRINCE!

YOU IS TRIPPED ME!

RIGHT OUT THE DOOR.

IT'S SNOWIN'! YOU IS THE ONLY ONE WITH SNOWSHOES! YOU CAN HELP ME ESCAPE.

HA! YOU BACK THERE, YOU IS ALL FOILED!

AND SO THE HANDSOME PRINCE MARRIED GOLDY-LONKS AND THEY LIVES HAPPY EVER AFTER.

GOLDY-LONKS? HOW SHE GITS INTO THE CINDEROLA STORY?

MAN, YOU DON'T THINK THE HANDSOME PRINCE WAS GONE MARRY-UP THAT NO-COUNT CINDEROLA AN' ALL THEM FAT OL' BEARS?

BUT WHERE'D THIS PRINCE FIND GOLDY-LONKS?

HE GOT INTO ANOTHER STORY, HOW ELSE?

A SECOND-STORY MAN, HUH? LET'S GIT ON HOME, CHILLUN, AFORE YOU HAS TO HEAR THE OTHER ONE, TOO.

EM'LY SAY SHE ENJOYED THE FIRST BY SLEEPIN' **ENTIRE** THROUGH IT.

THE BIG Rock Candy quarry

WHAT'S THIS OL' CHEST YOU KEEPS, UNCLE ALBERT?

THIS HERE IS KNOWED AS A HOPE CHEST.

Albert

HOPE CHEST? THAT'S A KIND OF THING WHAT GAL TYPES KEEPS DOILIES AN' TOWELS AN' STUFF IN— HOPIN' THEY'LL GIT MARRIED.

WELL, GALS ISN'T THE ONLY ONES WITH HOPES.

WELL, WHAT SORT OF HOPES AN' JUNK IS YOU STORED AWAY?

ALL KINDS OF KEEPSAKES, CURIOS—

AN' MEDALS GUV AT ME BY KINGS AND QUINGS AN' CROWNED HEADS—MEMENTOS OF MY GLORIOUS PAST, WHEN I WAS A HERO IN TWELVE AN' A HALF LANGUAGES.

HOW 'BOUT THIS UGLY GREEN SAUSAGE? WHAT WAS IT GUV YOU FOR?

GREEN SAUSAGE? MUST OF BEEN GUV ME FOR SOME HEROIC DEED LIKE RESCUIN' A ARMY OR FIGHTIN' OFF A FEW GIANTS.

Albert

From *Pogo Possum* No. 8, Jan.-Mar. 1952.

257

258

263

IT'S THE ALTITUDE HAS AFFECTED YOU, SON—YOU IS IN A STATE OF DELERIUMS.

HOWDY, SIR, THAT'S A MIGHTY FINE-LOOKIN' MESS OF ROCK CANDY.

ROCK CANDY?

I'M GOIN' HOME AN COUNT SUGAR.

DON'T GO! MAYBE A WITCH HAS CONJURED UP A SPELL TO MAKE THIS HERE OL' CANDY LOOK LIKE GARBAGE.

WELL, THAT SOUNDS MORE REASONABLE.

SURE!

US GOT A MAP WHAT POINTS OUT THIS SPOT AS A ROCK CANDY MOUNTAIN.

IT DOES? OH, YES! WHY, IT DOES INDEED!

YOU OWN IT?

YEP, BUT I IS WILLIN' TO SELL.

I SEE YOU GOT IT DISGUISED AS A PILE OF GARBAGE.

YEP—OTHERWISE FOLKS WOULD STEAL IT.

WELL, SAM, IT LOOKS LIKE BOTH OF US IS LOST OUR FORTUNES.

WAS THAT THE ROCK CANDY WHAT HIT ME?

YEP—EASY COME, EASY GO.

NOW WE IS BOTH RUINED.

I ISN'T SO RUINED THAT I CAN'T SMELL A PARTY A-BREWIN'.

MMMMMM!

MMMMMM, INDEED!

HEY, ALBERT, WE FOUND A BIG BOOK OF RECIPES IN YO' HOPE CHEST AN' US IS A-TRYIN' 'EM.

YOU GITS HEAD OF TABLE 'CAUSE WE IS USIN' FOOD OUTEN YO' PANTRY TO TEST THE REE-SIPPYS!

OOP!

OH WELL—I'LL JES' RESTOCK THE WAY I IS DID AFORE, BY HEAVY OL' BORRY-FYIN'!

I KNOWED YOU WOULDN'T MIND, YOU OL' ALBERT, YOU.

About "The Spirit" and Will Eisner

As comic books boomed in the prewar years, some newspaper syndicates began trying to take advantage of their popularity. The Register and Tribune Syndicate of Des Moines offered a sixteen-page (later eight-page) comic book that newspapers could distribute along with their Sunday comics sections. The comic book first appeared on June 2, 1940, and ran for a little more than twelve years, until October 5, 1952; it appeared in relatively few newspapers, mostly in large eastern cities.

The comic book's lead feature, *The Spirit*, was written and drawn by Will Eisner (with some help from other writers and cartoonists). Eisner was one of the principals in the small firm that assembled the comic book every week; unlike most comic-book creators, Eisner has always owned at least part of his feature.

Eisner, who was born in New York City on March 6, 1917, had already spent several years producing comic books—complete packages, ready to print—for several publishers by the time he started *The Spirit*. A number of well-known features, like *Sheena, Queen of the Jungle,* had been originated by Eisner and the men who worked for him. As Eisner told John Benson, "I was running a shop in which we made comic-book features pretty much the way Ford turned out cars. So perhaps the reason that the Register and Tribune consented to distribute *The Spirit* in the first place was because I had demonstrated my ability as a producer...." Throughout his career in comic books, Eisner remained that rare combination: an artist who was also a capable businessman.

The Spirit himself was a hero from the vigilante mold. His costume, however, amounted to nothing more than a mask and gloves. Eisner resisted pressure from his business partners to make the Spirit a costumed hero of the Batman variety, and so the Spirit remained a cross between a super-hero and a pulp-fiction detective. He was a criminologist named Denny Colt—supposedly dead, but actually living in a hideout in Wildwood Cemetery.

The Spirit, in its first year or so, was not far removed from conventional comic-book stuff of the period. But in 1941, Eisner started making very free and inventive use of the comics medium, as in the first of the three stories included here, and the emphasis began to shift away from the title character.

More than most comics creators, Eisner had the freedom to strike out in new directions; his partners and his syndicate made few demands on him, except that he meet his deadlines. Eisner explained the evolution of *The Spirit* to Benson: "I began to realize who I was writing for"—that is, an audience dominated by adults, rather than children—and "I suddenly found an opportunity to do what I had really always wanted to do, which was to write 'seriously' or write good material, and at the same time stay within the medium I knew and had developed skills for."

Eisner was drafted in 1942, and *The Spirit* was left in the hands of other cartoonists during the war. When Eisner returned to *The Spirit,* he became pre-eminently a short-story writer who wrote mostly with pictures instead of entirely with words. Probably no other cartoonist has ever made such fluent use of his medium. John Benson, writing in *Panels* magazine, speaks of Eisner's "effortless visual narrative style, which is so unlabored that most readers are unaware of how much more his pictures tell us than do the pages of most comic books. Like Alfred Hitchcock, Eisner *shows* his stories instead of telling them. And Eisner's pictorial sense, like Hitchcock's, is so integral to his sense of narrative that it's often overlooked: the type of story favored by the artist is more likely to be recognized—the 'Hitchcock story' or the 'Eisner story'."

Eisner is, for one thing, a master of the "silent panel" (a panel without dialogue or captions), placing each such panel at the point where its dramatic effect is greatest. And Benson cites as an example of Eisner's virtuosity his use of "indirect portrayal: we are shown a reaction, or the aftermath of an action, rather than the action itself—and are thereby forced, usually without being aware of it, to imagine bits of action and story elements that Eisner has not actually shown."

The "Eisner story" could be playful, or serious, or sentimental—or all three at once, like the 1948 story about Gerhard Shnobble that we have included here. But it was always a big-city story (in its atmosphere if not in its setting) and, like city life, it was always flavored with the grotesque.

The other postwar episode that follows originated in a script by Jules Feiffer, who was one of Eisner's assistants before beginning his own highly successful career as a newspaper and magazine cartoonist; Feiffer told John Benson that the script was "an autobiographical fantasy based on my Bronx upbringing." (It is also one of the many comic-book stories that shows the influence of radio drama; Feiffer cites *Suspense* as a source.) Eisner always remained the dominant partner in such collaborations, of course, often rewriting a script until it was mostly his own work.

The Spirit himself is not much to be seen in the two postwar stories we have included, and that is true of many of the best postwar *Spirit* stories. Sometimes Eisner had to shoehorn the Spirit into what could have been complete and satisfying short stories without him. Although Eisner depicted his hero in an appealingly tongue-in-cheek manner, the Spirit remained a conventional character in many ways (he was, for example, preternaturally resilient when shot or beaten), and the postwar stories tended to be more interesting the less of the Spirit himself there was in them. Richard Kyle has said of Eisner, "He remained bound to a hero smaller than the truth he had to tell."

Eisner gave less and less of his time to *The Spirit* in the early 1950s, finally abandoning the feature to produce comics for the educational market. But in recent years *The Spirit* has been revived in a bimonthly magazine, now published by Kitchen Sink Enterprises. *The Spirit* magazine includes new material by Eisner as well as reprints of old stories.

M.B.

SUNDAY, AUGUST 10, 1941

"...To condemn a thing false or impossible is to assume unto himself the advantage and the power of our common mother nature ~ ~ ~ ~

If we term those things monsters or miracles to which our reason cannot attain, how many such do daily present themselves into our sight ??? "

Montaigne

BY WILL EISNER

IF AT SOME TIME YOU HAPPEN TO BE IN CENTRAL CITY AND YOU PERCHANCE WALK BY THE OLD MANSION ON CARVEL STREET, PAUSE A SECOND AND SEE IF THE LIGHT BURNS IN THE THIRD STORY WINDOW.. FOR, IF IT DOES, THEN YOU MAY BE SURE THAT OLD PROFESSOR CORDA IS STILL WORKING.. WORKING TO CREATE A NEW ELEMENT ... TIME!!

IT WAS ON A HOT SUMMER NIGHT THAT PROFESSOR CORDA FLUNG OPEN HIS LABORATORY AND ABOVE THE ROAR AND FLASH OF THE THUNDER STORM, SCREAMED ...

MRS. LEARY!! MRS. LEARY!! I'VE GOT IT!!

GLORY BE... WHAT IS WRONG? WHAT'S HAPPENED?

MRS. LEARY, YOU SEE BEFORE YOU A MAN WHO HAS JUST CONDENSED TIME INTO AN ELEMENT !!!

YOU MEAN LIKE CONDENSED MILK..??

BAH.. YOU'VE A PEASANT'S MIND.. LOOK AT THIS VIAL.!! SEE THIS LIQUID.?! THAT IS TIME!!!! OH, HOW CAN I MAKE YOU UNDERSTAND?... LIKE.. WELL, LIKE MILK.. MILK GIVES YOU CALCIUM... THIS WILL GIVE ONE TIME!!

DO YOU REALIZE THE POTENTIAL POWER OF THIS ELEMENT?? TIME IS THE MOST PRECIOUS THING IN THE WORLD... WITH IT MAN CAN CONTROL THE UNIVERSE!!

?

HOW OFTEN HAS MAN SAID, "IF ONLY I HAD THE TIME..".?.WELL, I CAN GIVE IT TO HIM ... HA..HA..HA.. NOW.. DO YOU SEE WHAT I MEAN ?!!

?

I DON'T GET IT !!

HOW DOES IT WORK?.. HOW DO YOU KNOW THAT IT DOES WORK? HAVE YOU TRIED IT OUT ON SOMEONE..?! FAITH, WHIN I MAKE STEW, I LET SOMEONE TASTE IT AFORE I CALL IT STEW!!

AH ..YES!

I WILL TRY IT ON SOMEONE... THIS VERY NIGHT.. YES, I MUST KNOW !!!

AT THAT SAME MOMENT IN ANOTHER PART OF THE CITY...

TOMMY!! TOMMY, WHAT ARE YOU DOING?!

WHAT D'YA THINK?!

TOMMY!!..PLEASE.. NO MORE CRIME.. YOU'RE ON PAROLE NOW...IF THEY CATCH YOU AGAIN.. IT'LL BE JAIL FOR LIFE.. PLEASE, TOMMY!!!

NICK ENNIS SQUEALED ON ME AND HE'S GONNA PAY FOR IT!!!!

NO..NOT MURDER! TOMMY, THINK OF ME!! THE BABY!! YOU'LL BE CAUGHT!!!

THEY WON'T GET ME.. I'VE GOT IT ALL FIGURED OUT! GIT OUTA MY WAY!!

NO!! I WON'T!!

GIT OUTA MY WAY I SAID!!

NO ONE SQUEALS ON ME AND LIVES!! *÷!!☆*?₵

HELLO, JUSTIN??..YEH, TOMMY... NICK ENNIS IN?? GOOD.. GET ALL THE SERVANTS OUTA THE HOUSE...YEH, I'M GONNA SLIP 'IM THE BIZNISS TO-NIGHT.. I'LL WAIT IN THE PARK FIVE MINUTES.. THAT'LL GIVE YOU A CHANCE TO CLEAR THE GROUNDS.. RIGHT!!

THUS, ON SUCH THIN COINCIDENCES, THE WEB OF LIFE IS SPUN...

AH, THE PARK.. I'LL FIND SOMEONE THERE TO TEST MY ELEMENT.. AH.. THERE!! I SAY, MY GOOD MAN...

!?

I WILL PAY YOU THIS FIVE THOUSAND DOLLARS IF YOU WILL ALLOW ME TO INJECT 4 CENTIMETERS OF THIS FLUID INTO YOUR VEINS... IT'LL ONLY TAKE 5 MINUTES TO WEAR OFF!!

5000 BUCKS!!! WHEW! I COULD MAKE MY GETAWAY WITH THAT MUCH ... YEH.. WHAT A BREAK!!

YEAH, SURE MISTER, I'LL TAKE Y'R OFFER!!

275

THIRTY-FIVE YEARS OF SWEAT AND WORK FOR **NOTHING!**

HEY! WHAT ABOUT MY DOUGH!?

OH. YES. HERE!

BAH!

BUT I'M NOT BEATEN!! I'M A SCIENTIST... I WILL CONTINUE MY WORK ... SOMEDAY I WILL FIND IT...PASTEUR DID NOT GIVE UP AT HIS FIRST FAILURE...

A FEW FEET AWAY..

FIVE MINUTES ARE UP...I ..GOSH .. SOMEHOW I DON'T WANNA KILL NICK NOW!

THAT DREAM... IT WAS LIKE LIVIN' IN THE FUTURE... IT WAS REAL ... I COULD FEEL IT! THAT WASN'T AN ORDINARY DREAM, I'M SURE!! FUNNY, HOW CLEAR THE SPIRIT WAS ...YET I HAVE NEVER SEEN HIM BEFORE ... WONDER WHAT HE REALLY LOOKS LIKE ??!

WELL, ANY-WAY I GOT 5000 BUCKS! BY GOLLY, I'M GONNA GO STRAIGHT... I CAN OPEN AN HONEST BUSINESS ... TAKE MARY WITH ME... YES SIREE ... I'M STARTIN' LIFE OVER AGIN !!

AT THAT MOMENT IN WILD-WOOD CEMETERY ...

WAKE UP, MIST' SPIRIT BOSS..YO' IS TALKIN' IN YO' SLEEP!!

WHY ..?! OH.. OH. EBONY... YAWWWNN...WHAT A HORRIBLE DREAM I HAD!!!

SEEMS THAT A CERTAIN TOMMY MORAN KILLED A MAN NAMED NICK ENNIS. NEVER SAW OR HEARD OF EITHER IN MY LIFE ... WELL, SIR, I GOT HIM JUST AS HE LEFT THE HOUSE WHICH WAS RIGHT NEAR A PARK ... SEEMS THAT WE FOUGHT AND FOUGHT... HE KEPT SHOOTING AT ME...

LOOK!!

8-10

YO' DONE HAVE BLOOD ON YO' SHOULDER! YO' BEEN WOUNDED!!!

BY GOD-FREY!! A BULLET WOUND !!

THE SPIRIT

ACTION Mystery ADVENTURE

THE SPIRIT

BY Will Eisner

BEFORE WE BEGIN THIS STORY WE WANT TO MAKE ONE POINT VERY CLEAR..

THIS IS NOT A FUNNY STORY!!

...AND WHILE THE AUTHOR DOES NOT EXPECT YOU TO BELIEVE ALL OF THIS..HE FEELS BOUND TO ASSURE YOU THAT HE CANNOT GUARANTEE A COMPLETE ABSENCE OF RESEMBLANCE BETWEEN PERSONS LIVING OR DEAD AND THE CHARACTERS HERE PORTRAYED.

WE MEAN TO GIVE YOU A SIMPLE ACCOUNT OF GERHARD SHNOBBLE... BEGINNING AT THE POINT WHEN HE FIRST DISCOVERED HE COULD **FLY**.

PLEASE.... NO LAUGHTER....

WHILE GERHARD SHNOBBLE BLUNDERS SADLY THROUGH THE STREETS...A MANHUNT FOR THE BANK ROBBERS TAKES FORM.

EVERY STREET AND TRAIN DEPOT IS BLOCKED.. THEY CAN'T GET OUT.

THEY **COULD** ESCAPE BY **HELICOPTER**, DOLAN..

HOLY SMOKE, SPIRIT..YOU GOT SOMETHING THERE..WE HAD A REPORT THAT A HELICOPTER LANDED ON THE ELECTRIC BUILDING LATE LAST NIGHT!

WELL..WHAT ARE WE WAITING FOR? LET'S GET THERE AT ONCE!!

EEEEEEEE

A FAILURE... THAT'S WHAT I AM.. A **NOBODY** WITH NO TALENT.. IF ONLY I COULD DO SOMETHING **BIG**..THAT'D SHOW THEM!

POLICE

EEO...

SCREEECH

DO SOMETHING.. HMF..IF ONLY..IF ONLY I COULD.. **YES..WHY NOT?** I CAN FLY... NOW IT COMES BACK TO ME.. **I CAN FLY !!**

SURROUND THE BUILDING,MEN.. ~THE SPIRIT IS GOING UP AFTER THEM.

HOLD THAT ELEVATOR !!

I'LL SHOW THE WORLD.. I'LL BE FAMOUS.. I'LL FLY..**FLY!**

ROOF, PLEASE.

YES...TODAY I'LL DO IT.. TODAY THE WORLD WILL SEE...

YES, SIR.

4

ROOF.

ROOF

39

38

·OOF!
..PARDON
ME, SIR.

SLAM

PING

LOOK OUT...
THOSE MEN ARE
DESPERATE..THEY'RE
SHOOTING.

BANG

THE
SPIRIT!

HEY, LEFTY..
TUMBLERS..
WAIT FOR ME!

USE THE
HELICOPTER,
KNIFFS..IT
WUZ YOUR
IDEA!

IT'S EVERY
MAN F'HISSELF
NOW, BOYS!

NO YOU DON'T...
THAT HELICOPTER
STAYS HERE, KNIFFS.

THERE'S
A BIG CROWD
BELOW..THEY'LL
SEE ME..AND
I'LL BE
FAMOUS!!
HEH HEH

COPS BELOW...THE
BUILDING'S SURROUNDED!
..©×¢¢¢⅓★☆÷#!!

5

284

AND SO... LIFELESS...GERHARD SHNOBBLE FLUTTERED EARTHWARD..**BUT** DO NOT WEEP FOR SHNOBBLE...

RATHER SHED A TEAR FOR ALL MANKIND...
FOR NOT ONE PERSON IN THE ENTIRE CROWD THAT WATCHED HIS BODY BEING CARTED AWAY... NOT ONE OF THEM KNEW OR EVEN SUSPECTED THAT ON THIS DAY GERHARD SHNOBBLE HAD FLOWN.

THE SPIRIT

ACTION
Mystery
ADVENTURE

It will take you ten minutes to read this story...

...a very short time in any man's lifetime.

But these ten minutes that you will spend here are an eternity for one man.

For they are the last ten minutes in Freddy's life.

287

The time is now 10:31

TICK
TICK TICK
TICK TICK
TICK TICK
TICK TICK
TICK

...AND THAT'S THE BALL GAME! FOR THE BADGERS, FOUR RUNS, TEN HITS, AND NO ERRORS... FOR THE ORIOLES, ONE RUN, SIX HITS, AND ONE ERROR... THERE WERE *CLICK*

NUTS! I GOT THE ORIOLES THIS WEEK, SO ALL THEY GET IN SIX DAYS IS THREE RUNS!

BELIEVE ME, FREDDY, Y'CAN'T WIN ON THESE POOLS! ALWAYS I SAID FREDDY IS A SMART BOY... HE DON'T GAMBLE! HMM...STILL PLAYIN' THE PIN-BALL MACHINE?

WHAT'S IT *LOOK* LIKE I'M DOIN'?

A CHOCOLATE SUGAR CONE, MAX.

SO DON'T GET SORE! IN THIS HEAT Y'DON'T WANNA EXERT Y'SELF! WHEW...IMAGINE... IN SEPTEMBER, HEAT LIKE NOW!

@X&©©=#!

TILT!

TILT... *TILT!* ON AND OFF LIKE NEON LIGHTS... FREDDY'S LIFE STORY... ONE BIG TILT!

GIMME AN EGG CREAM, MAX! I'LL PAY YA TUESDAY.

HEY, LOOK! TH' LATEST TRUE HORROR ROMANCES!

OH BOY! LOOKA THIS TRUE LOVE STUFF!

FREDDY... THE GOOD BOY... THAT'S ME! "LOOKIT FREDDY..SEE, *HE* TAKES CARE OF *HIS* FAMILY... A *NICE* BOY!"

BING BING

I'M BURNIN' UP! I'M *CHOKIN'*! I CAN'T TAKE THIS NO MORE! I DON'T HAVE TO... AND... *I WON'T!*

HELLO...

RING, RING

BINK

YEH... O.K... HOLD THE WIRE...

HEY, YOU KIDS... GET MRS. SCHMIDT IN THE NEXT HOUSE.. SHE'S WANTED ON THE PHONE!

WE'RE ALL ALONE NOW... IT'LL TAKE 'EM FIVE MINUTES TO GET MRS. SCHMIDT... *IT'S TIME, MAX... THIS IS IT, MAX !!*

MOVE OVER, HUH, FREDDY? I WANNA SWEEP...

2

The time is now 10:33

TICK TICK
TICK
TICK TICK
TICK TICK
TICK

WOW!..AIN'T THIS HEAT MURDER? I'M TELLIN' YA, HEAT LIKE THIS CAN KILL YA...CAN Y" IMAGINE HEAT LIKE THIS IN SEPTEMBER?

MAX!

OH... NICE GUN, FREDDY...WHERE'DJA PICK IT UP? I ONCE HAD A .45....PICKED IT UP IN TH' FIRST WAR...I...

EMPTY OUT THE TILL, MAX.

FREDDY!..WHAT IS THIS, A JOKE 'R SUMPIN'? CUT TH' COMEDY!

O.K. I'LL DO IT MYSELF!

NO..NO... DON'T TOUCH THAT, YOU BUMMER!!

BANG

FREDDY!...YOU ARE ONE OF THE NEIGHBORHOOD BOYS...I...KNEW YOU... SINCE...YOU WAS...A KID... UGH...

MAX...I DIDN'T MEAN IT...BELIEVE ME, MAX...

I NEEDED DOUGH TO LEAVE TOWN...I'M SICK O" THIS BLOCK...A FRESH START...THAT'S ALL I WANT...

MAX....GET UP...
HA HA...
STOP KIDDIN..MAX...
F'HEAVEN'S SAKE GET UP!

I'M MRS. SCHMIDT...WHERE'S MY PHONE CALL... WHICH BOOTH?

HELLO..HELLO... WHO? CHARLIE? OH, HELLO CHARLIE...YEAH... CHARLIE...

HIYA, FREDDY! WHAT'RE YOU DOIN" BEHIND THE COUNTER? WHERE'S MAX?

289

The time now is 10:35

The time now is 10:39

TICK TICK TICK TICK TICK TICK TICK TICK **TICK TICK**

HOW DID IT ALL HAPPEN ??..I NEVER DID NOTHIN'... I'M TIRED... THE COPS... O.K... **TAKE ME!** ..I WON'T RUN ANY MORE..

HEY YOU!

SCREE

WHERE'S MAX'S CANDY STORE LOCATED AROUND HERE?

T..TWO... TWO BLOCKS DOWN...

I TELL YA, SPIRIT... THIS NEIGHBORHOOD IS LIKE A LIT FIRECRACKER... EVERY TWO WEEKS, A MURDER...

HOWDYA LIKE THAT? I MUST BE CHARMED! HA HA .. **HA HA HA..!!**

TOO BAD, COPS... YOU HAD YOUR CHANCE.

I...I'LL GO TO FLORIDA, LIKE I PLANNED... IT'S ALL WORKIN' OUT! MAX'S DOUGH WILL LAST TILL I FIND A JOB... THEN I'LL BE HONEST AGAIN!

SORRY, PAL... WE CAN'T CASH A TWENTY!

OH... OH, YEAH... SORRY... CHANGE... CHANGE... HERE, I... **OOPS**... ©#*#&¢#..!!

..YOUR MONEY?

YEH..THANKS..

6

292

The time now is
10:40

TICK TICK
TICK TICK
**TICK
TICK
TICK**

THAT WAS THE SPIRIT... HE'S PROBABLY CHECKIN' THE STATIONS... HE SAW ME BEFORE! HE CAN'T SUSPECT NOTHIN'!

13TH STREET

I'D LIKE TO TALK TO YOU... FREDDY!

THERE HE GOES!

OPEN THE DOOR, OPE...

LET GO, MISTER!

EEEEK!

TOO BAD... HE WAS ONLY A KID!

SO MANY OF THEM ARE KIDS, DOLAN! THEY BREAK THEM IN YOUNG AROUND HERE! ...I WONDER JUST WHEN IT WAS THAT FREDDY STARTED ON HIS CRIME CAREER...

SOME GUY YOU ARE! LATE... LATE... **LATE!!** ALWAYS LATE!!

BUT HONEY... IT'S ONLY 10:41! TEN MINUTES LATE... WHAT'S TEN MINUTES IN A MAN'S LIFE?

About E.C.

The initials "E.C." on comic-book covers stood at first for "Educational Comics." When M. C. Gaines started E.C. in the mid-1940s, the company was indeed "educational," publishing comic-book versions of the Bible and American history. After Gaines died in a boating accident in 1947, his son William M. Gaines took over the company and shifted its emphasis toward more commercial fare—westerns, romance comics, and crime titles (E.C. came to stand for "Entertaining Comics"). In 1949, horror stories—told by the Vault Keeper and the Crypt Keeper—edged into E.C.'s crime comics, and in 1950, E.C. began publishing three unabashed horror titles. The success of these comic books spawned the flood of horror comics, from many publishers, in the early 1950s.

Also in 1950, E.C. began publishing two science-fiction comic books, *Weird Science* and *Weird Fantasy.* Earlier science-fiction comics were "space operas," along the lines of *Buck Rogers,* but the E.C. comic books tried to approximate, in comics form, the work of serious science-fiction writers. The science-fiction comic books did not sell well, but William Gaines kept them alive with the profits from the horror comics—a rare and probably unique instance of a publisher's supporting comic books because he cared about them.

Al Feldstein was the principal editor of the horror and science-fiction comic books. Unlike the editors of most comic books, Feldstein and the other E.C. editors wrote most of their own stories—and illustrated some of them, too. Like Will Eisner, they worked in the short-story form (E.C.'s stories were only six to eight pages long), but unlike Eisner, the E.C. editors had no need to incorporate continuing characters into their stories; except for the "hosts" of the horror comics, very few E.C. characters made more than one appearance.

Feldstein relied on literary models: he adhered to the idea that short stories had to have surprise endings, and he used captions to tell his stories, rather than to add meaning to the drawings that the captions accompanied. Harvey Kurtzman, the other major E.C. editor, did not lean on literary devices to the same extent. More important, he brought to his work as editor and writer a particularly valuable trait: in a field dominated by fantasies, he tried never to lose sight of reality.

Kurtzman, who was born in Manhattan in 1924, illustrated a number of science-fiction stories for E.C. before he began editing E.C.'s war comic books, *Two-Fisted Tales* and *Frontline Combat.* In the war comics, Kurtzman tried to depict the life of men in combat with a realism that was missing from other comic books. He engaged in orgies of research, spending countless hours in the New York Public Library. In one of the most famous examples of Kurtzman's desire for authenticity, he sent his assistant Jerry De Fuccio down in a submarine so that the onomatopoeic words he would use to represent the sounds made by a submerged submarine would be accurate.

Kurtzman relied heavily on such artists as Jack Davis and John Severin, but he illustrated some of his best war stories himself. His drawings were never slick, but his brushwork was flowing, direct, and energetic—qualities that were perfect for the subject matter—and the two war stories we have chosen for this book, *Air Burst* and *Corpse on the Imjin,* were illustrated as well as written by Kurtzman. *Air Burst,* published while the Korean war was still being fought, is notable for its sympathetic depiction of the Chinese enemy. *Corpse on the Imjin* gives war a psychological as well as a physical reality (in a caption, the American soldier's mind returns to childhood and "dunking" as he struggles in the water with the enemy soldier).

The war comics required so much work that they wore Kurtzman out, and in 1952, while recovering from a bout with jaundice, he decided he wanted to try something less demanding. This turned out to be *Mad*—which was, in its original incarnation as a comic book, a vigorous satirical assault on popular culture.

In *Mad,* Kurtzman spoofed movies, comic strips, and even "classic" popular fiction like *Frankenstein* and the Sherlock Holmes stories, but he may have felt a little uneasy about poking fun at artifacts that were more widely accepted as worthwhile than comic books were. In any case, Kurtzman was probably at his best when he was going after other comic books and "kiddie" TV shows like *Captain Video* and *Howdy Doody.* In *Superduperman,* Kurtzman ridicules the idea that within our unimpressive exteriors there lurk "supermen"—that one day those who scorn us will see our true worth and confess their error. (And along the way, he points out that an all-powerful hero's altruism cannot be taken for granted.) Similarly, Kurtzman bears down on *Howdy Doody,* where he finds a veneer of patronizing jollity that cannot camouflage a hard sell to a particularly vulnerable audience. On *Mad,* Kurtzman collaborated with several fine artists, two of whom, Wallace Wood and Bill Elder, are represented here. Wood and Elder themselves invented many of the bizarre details that enriched *Mad*'s panels.

All of the E. C. artists were encouraged to work freely in their own styles (some publishers wanted their artists to squeeze themselves into an anonymous "house style"), but the editors always remained firmly in control. For example, when an artist named Bernard Krigstein was assigned by Al Feldstein to a story called *Master Race* in 1954, he was given six sheets of illustration board with the captions and the dialogue already lettered and in place; his job was to provide illustrations that matched this script. Instead, he expanded the story to eight pages (with the wary approval of Feldstein and William Gaines), by cutting up the lettering and pasting it on new boards. E.C.'s stories typically had six or seven panels per page; Krigstein added panels not just by making the story longer but by using more panels per page. Krigstein told John Benson and Bhob Stewart in an interview that where the script called for three panels, "I might have put in nine panels. Because it's what happens between these panels that's so fascinating." As Krigstein revised and expanded *Master Race,* he created one of the most interesting and admired of all comic-book stories.

Krigstein, who was born in Brooklyn in 1919, came late to E.C. (his work first appeared in issues with 1954 dates) after free-lancing for other comics publishers. He was greatly intrigued by the comics form, and particularly by the way stories are broken down into panels. More than most comic-book illustrators, he was aware of the effects possible by changing the shapes and arrangements of panels. In *Master Race,* Krigstein sometimes seems to be borrowing from film techniques, as many other cartoonists did, but he is up to something different. In the panels on the last page of *Master Race,* Krigstein has not imitated the flurry of images in a film with rapid cutting. He has instead dissected the action, giving his drawings a dreadful clarity that film could not match. His work has a cool objectivity that is unique in the work of the leading comic-book creators. Compare, for example, the death in the subway that comes on the last page of *Master Race* with the one that occurs on the last page of the 1949 *Spirit* story earlier in this book.

In 1954, a public outcry against comic books drove E.C.'s best sellers—the horror and crime comics—from the newsstands, and *Master Race* was published in the first issue of *Impact,* one of a half dozen "New Direction" titles that E.C. introduced late in 1954 and early in 1955 to take their place. The "New Direction" titles grasped desperately for a mature audience (one of the new titles was *Psychoanalysis*) and could not find it. The E.C. line—caught between declining sales and the new Comics Code—struggled for a year, until Gaines finally gave up and discontinued all of his comic books.

Mad survived. Gaines and Kurtzman had converted it into a twenty-five-cent, black-and-white magazine; as such, it was not subject to the Comics Code. Kurtzman and Gaines quarreled and Kurtzman left *Mad* after a few issues of the new magazine; he was replaced by Al Feldstein. *Mad* continues, as one of the great success stories in American publishing.

Kurtzman, after editing several new satire magazines that failed to catch on, did the *Little Annie Fanny* stories in *Playboy*. Bernard Krigstein worked for a time in commercial art, and more recently has been a teacher and a painter.

M.B.

From *Frontline Combat* No. 4, Jan.-Feb. 1952.
© 1981 William M. Gaines.

304

IT IS A DARK DAY IN MAY! LIGHTNING FLICKERS IN THE SOUTH KOREAN HILLS, AND A STORM WIND ROARS OVER THE IMJIN RIVER! OUT IN THE MIDDLE OF THE RAIN SWOLLEN IMJIN, A LONELY CORPSE FLOATS WITH THE RUBBLE DOWN TO THE SEA! FOR THIS IS WHAT OUR STORY IS ABOUT! A...

CORPSE ON THE IMJIN!

BUT MANY THINGS FLOAT ON THE IMJIN! DRIFTWOOD, AMMUNITION BOXES, RATION CASES, SHELL TUBES!

...WE IGNORE THE FLOATING RUBBLE! WHY THEN, DO WE FASTEN OUR EYES ON A LIFELESS CORPSE?

...THOUGH WE SOMETIMES FORGET IT, LIFE IS PRECIOUS, AND DEATH IS UGLY AND NEVER PASSES UNNOTICED!

1

From *Two-Fisted Tales* No. 25, Jan.-Feb. 1952.
1981 William M. Gaines.

THERE GOES ANOTHER ONE! THAT'S THE THIRD IN THE LAST HALF HOUR... FLOATING THERE LIKE A DEAD FISH!

GEE! WE MUST HAVE KILLED THOUSANDS OF THEM IN THIS OFFENSIVE! WONDER HOW THAT ONE GOT IT?

PROBABLY GOT HIT BY THE BOMBERS WHEN HE WAS TRYING TO CROSS FARTHER UPSTREAM THERE!

MAYBE IT WAS THE F-51'S! I SURE WOULDN'T LIKE TO BE CAUGHT SITTING BY F-51'S... WITH THEM 5 INCH ROCKETS!

THEN AGAIN, IT COULD HAVE BEEN THE 155 MM CANNONS! THEM SELF-PROPELLED 'LONG TOMS' ARE MURDER!

OR DID A RIFLEMAN CATCH HIM? COULD'VE BEEN A SHARP SHOOTER WITH A TELESCOPIC SIGHT SPRINGFIELD!

COULD'VE EVEN BEEN HAND TO HAND COMBAT... ALTHOUGH I DOUBT IT! THE WAY THEY TALK ABOUT HAND TO HAND COMBAT, YOU'D THINK IT HAPPENS ALL THE TIME, AND YET I'VE NEVER HEARD OF ANYONE WHO GOT CLOSE ENOUGH TO THE ENEMY TO USE A BAYONET!

I GUESS HAND TO HAND COMBAT WAS STRICTLY FOR THE OLDEN DAYS WHEN EVERYONE FOUGHT WITH SWORDS AND KNIVES! NOW WITH ALL THE LONG RANGE WEAPONS, WE CAN KILL PRETTY GOOD BY REMOTE CONTROL! AND WE NEVER GET CLOSER'N A MILE TO THE ENEMY!

CORRECTION, SOLDIER! NOT CLOSER THAN *FIFTEEN FEET*... FOR THE ENEMY IS WATCHING YOU EAT YOUR RATIONS NOT FIFTEEN FEET FROM YOUR RIFLE!

HE IS WET AND SCARED AND HUNGRY, AND HIS EYES GO FROM YOUR C-RATION CAN TO YOUR RIFLE! THE WIND HIDES ALL SOUND AS *HE SPRINGS!*

YOU SEE HIM OUT OF THE CORNER OF YOUR EYE AND YOU KICK OUT WITH BOTH YOUR FEET!

YOU KICK CLUMSILY AT YOUR RIFLE, BECAUSE THAT IS ALL YOU CAN DO TO GET IT OUT OF HIS REACH!

THE RIFLE TUMBLES OVER THE BANK AND INTO THE IMJIN RIVER! AND THEN THERE'S JUST THE SOUND OF THE WIND!

WHERE ARE THE WISECRACKS YOU READ IN THE COMIC BOOKS? WHERE ARE THE FANCY RIGHT HOOKS YOU SEE IN THE MOVIES? HE PICKS UP A BROKEN STICK!

HE'S A LITTLE FELLOW AND HE GRINS AS HE CIRCLES YOU WITH HIS STICK! YOU WIPE AT YOUR NOSE, AND THEN YOU REMEMBER YOUR BAYONET!

YOU GRIP YOUR BAYONET TIGHT... *TIGHT!* DEEP INSIDE, YOU DON'T *REALLY* BELIEVE YOU CAN STICK A KNIFE INTO A HUMAN BEING! IT'S ALMOST SILLY...

THEY SAY THE MAN WHO MOVES FIRST HAS WON HALF THE BATTLE, AND THE LITTLE GUY STRIKES OUT AT YOU·WITH THE STICK... *CRACKS YOUR FINGERS!*

YOU'VE LOST THE BAYONET AND NOW YOU'RE HURT! HE CLUBS YOU ON THE ARMS, THE SHOULDERS...

BUT THE PAIN MAKES YOU *REACT...* YOU FEEL A SURGE OF *FEAR... HATE...* ENERGY...TINGLING IN YOUR MUSCLES...

YOU SHRIEK AND CHARGE LIKE A CRAZY BULL TO ESCAPE THE STINGING CLUB! YOU CLUTCH AT HIM

HE'S REALLY HURT YOU AND YOUR LEGS ARE WOBBLY AND HE STRIKES AND STRIKES AND STRIKES!

YOU OUTWEIGH HIM THOUGH, AND WITH ALL THE STRENGTH YOU CAN MUSTER, YOU PUSH HIM TO THE RIVER...

...AND YOU BOTH FALL! YOU RELAX AND YOU FALL! YOU NEVER KNEW FALLING COULD BE SO PLEASANT!

HE KICKS TO STAY UP, BUT YOU ARE HEAVIER AND YOU *PRESS HIM UNDER!*

IT REMINDS YOU OF SOMETHING...AND YOU *PRESS HIM UNDER!*

LIKE DUNKING, WHEN YOU WENT SWIMMING! YOU *PRESS HIM UNDER!*

YES...YES...LIKE DUNKING AT THE SWIMMING HOLE... YOU DUNK...*DUNK*... *DUNK*...

HIS HANDS HAVE STOPPED CLAWING AT THE AIR...HIS FEET HAVE STOPPED THRASHING...

...BLOOD AND BUBBLES ARE COMING TO THE SURFACE AND THE MAN YOU ARE HOLDING RELAXES!

IT SEEMS LIKE HOURS HAVE GONE BY! THE BUBBLES ARE BARELY TRICKLING UP AND ALL IS STILL!

SUDDENLY, YOUR MIND IS QUIET, AND YOUR RAGE COLLAPSES! THE WATER IS VERY COLD!

YOU'RE TIRED... YOUR BODY IS GASPING AND SHAKING WEAK... AND YOU'RE ASHAMED!

YOU STUMBLE AND SLOSH OUT OF THE RIVER AND RUN...RUN AWAY FROM THE BODY IN THE WATER!

THE WIND IS RUSHING FITFULLY OVER THE IMJIN! IT STIRS THE HAIR ON THE BACK OF THE DEAD MAN'S HEAD!

THE WATER RIPPLES BEFORE THE WIND... LAPS AT THE SHORE...SWAYS THE BODY FROM SIDE TO SIDE!

THE FLOWING RIVER GENTLY SWINGS THE BODY OUT, AWAY FROM THE BANK AND INTO THE CURRENT!

AND NOW THE CURRENT, WEAK NEAR THE SHORE, SLOWLY TURNS THE BODY AROUND AND AROUND...

...AND IT IS AS IF NATURE IS TAKING BACK WHAT IT HAS GIVEN! HAVE PITY! HAVE PITY FOR A DEAD MAN!

FOR HE IS NOW NOT RICH OR POOR, RIGHT OR WRONG, BAD OR GOOD! DON'T HATE HIM! HAVE PITY...

...FOR HE HAS LOST THAT MOST PRECIOUS POSSESSION THAT WE ALL TREASURE ABOVE EVERYTHING... HE HAS LOST HIS *LIFE!*

LIGHTNING FLASHES IN THE KOREAN HILLS, AND ON THE RAIN SWOLLEN IMJIN, A CORPSE FLOATS OUT TO SEA.

LITTLE DO THOSE LADIES IN THE POWDER ROOM ACROSS THE HALL KNOW THAT I AM IN REALITY SUPERDUPERMAN, FASTER THAN A SPEEDING BULLET... *KAPWEENG*... WITH LI'L OL' X-RAY VISION!

ASSISTANT COPY BOY!

COMING, SIR! ON THE DOUBLE, SIR! CLARK BENT, ASSISTANT TO THE COPY BOY, ALL PRESEN AND ACCOUNTED FOR, SIR!

BLAST IT ALL, MAN! HOW MANY TIMES HAVE I TOLD YOU TO SALUTE WITH YOUR *RIGHT* HAND!

SODDY, YOU MISERABLE OL' WRETCH! LOST MY TEMPER! COPY BOY WORK DOES THINGS TO A MAN!... *COME* ON! *SNAP* TO! *COME* ON, BOY!

SMEK SMEK SMEK

I'LL TELL YOU WHY I CALLED YOU, OLD MAN! IT'S PAYROLL TIME! HERE ARE YOUR WEEK'S WAGES! SEVENTY-FIVE CENTS, AND A GOOD BUS TOKEN! SPEND IT WISELY! ... *DISMISSED!*

SEVENTY-FIVE WHOLE CENTS! AT LAST! AFTER SCRIMPING AND SAVING MY EARNINGS FOR 10 YEARS, I NOW HAVE A THOUSAND DOLLARS ... ENOUGH TO MAKE A DOWN PAYMENT ON THAT PEARL NECKLACE FOR LOIS PAIN, GIRL REPORTER!

WELL... HERE I AM WITH THE PEARL NECKLACE! LOIS SAYS I'M A CREEP! HAH, BOY! IF SHE KNEW MY *REAL* IDENTITY, BOY, SHE WOULDN'T CALL ME A CREEP!... OOP! THERE'S LOIS AT A BIG MEETING WITH THE MANAGING EDITOR!

HOKAY, BOYS! THAT CARBON STEEL BLOCK WE'VE CAST CAPTAIN MARBLES IN OUGHT TO HOLD 'IM! NOW GET OUT THE WAY 'CAUSE I THINK I MIGHT LEAP A TALL BUILDING AT A SINGLE BOUND!

AND AS FOR YOU, HAH, LOIS PAIN, GIRL REPORTER... I JUST SO HAPPENS MY TRUE IDENTITY IS CLARK BENT... MAN ASSISTANT TO THE COPY BOY! WHATA BURNER ON YOU, HUH?

HAH! AND I SUPPOSEN'T NOW YOU'D GIVE YOUR BOTTOM DOLLAR FOR ME TO SNIFF YOUR PERFUME I SUPPOSEN'T!

WHERE'ZAT OL' BOTTOM DOLLAR?

HANDS OFF!

SO YOU'RE SUPER-DUPERMAN INSTEAD OF CLARK BENT! ... BIG DEAL!

YER STILL A CREEP!

UP IN THE FIGHTING NEWSPAPER OFFICE OF THE 'DAILY DIRT'... GOING FROM SPITOON TO SPITOON...

...SHUFFLES AN INCREDIBLY WRETCHED AND MISERABLE LOOKING CREEP... CLARK BENT, ASSISTANT COPY BOY...

WHO IS IN REALITY, SUPERDUPERMAN SO WHAT DOES IT ALL PROVE? IT PROVES ONCE A CREEP, ALWAYS A CREEP!

KOF

KOF

POST NO BILLS

CHUGA CHUGGA CHUGGA CHUG

From *Mad* No. 18, December 1954.
© 1954 E.C. Publications, Inc.

3

...IS YOU A WOMAN?

KOWABUNGA! HIM GOT WOMAN'S *NAME*! IF HIM *MAN*, WHY HIM GOT WOMAN'S *NAME*? ALL I WANT IS THE *FACK'S*... WHICH REMIND ME... HOW'S YOUR MOM, ED?

LET'S GET OUT OF HERE! YOU KNOW WHAT CLARABELLA'S GOT IN THAT BOX HE CARRIES! ...YOU KNOW WHAT CLARABELLA'S ABOUT TO DO!

IT'S NO USE! HE'S ALREADY WHIPPING THOSE THINGS OUT OF THAT BOX!... HERE COMES THE SELTZER BOTTLE!... WE MIGHT AS WELL STAND AND MEET OUR FATE!

...GOSH... WHAT'S GOING TO HAPPEN NEXT? WELL, KIDS! IT'S ME, *HOWDY DOOIT* AGAIN AND THIS TIME I'M ADVERTISING *SKWUSHY'S* SLICED WHITE-BREAD! NOW LISTEN, KIDS... THE NEXT TIME YOUR MOTHER GOES TO THE STORE, I WANT YOU TO ASK HER TO BUY A LOAF OF *SKWUSHY'S*!

HALF-BAKED WHILE YOU SLEEP!
SKWUSHY'S
A WONDER PRODUCT: "IF IT'S GOOD BREAD-IT'S A WONDER!"

NOW IN CASE YOUR MOTHER REFUSES TO BUY YOU A LOAF OF *SKWUSHY'S*, HERE'S WHAT TO DO! NOW MAKE BELIEVE I'M YOU AND MAKE BELIEVE THAT'S YOUR MOTHER SHOPPING IN THE SUPER-MARKET AND SHE DOESN'T WANT TO BUY BREAD TODAY!

...YOU JUST WAIT TILL HER BACK IS TURNED AND SLIP A LOAF OF SWUSHY'S INTO THE SHOPPING BASKET!...HIDE IT WAY UNDER WHERE SHE CAN'T NOTICE IT!... THEN AGAIN... IF MOM HAPPENS TO BUY ANOTHER BRAND OF BREAD...

...WAIT TILL SHE GETS STUCK ON THE LINE AT THE CASHIER'S COUNTER AND QUICK SUBSTITUTE A LOAF OF *SKWUSHY'S!* SHE'LL *HAVE* TO BUY IT!... BESIDES *SKWUSHY'S* WHITE BREAD, TRY *SKWUSHY'S* GREEN AND PURPLE BREAD!

4

OF COURSE... ADVERTISING AND ENTERTAINMENT ARE LUCRATIVE FIELDS IF ONE HITS THE TOP BRACKETS... MUCH LIKE *HOWDY DOOIT* HAS! IN OTHER WORDS... WHAT I WANT TO DO WHEN I GROW UP, IS TO BE A HUSTLER LIKE *HOWDY DOOIT!* I WANT TO BE WHERE THE *CASH* IS... THE *GREEN* STUFF... MOOLAH... *POUND NOTES*... GET IT? ...MONEY!

BUT CHILD... *HOWDY DOOIT* IS NO "HUSTLER"! HE NEEDS NO MONEY! NO DOLLAR BILLS TO SMILE... NO MERCENARY INCENTIVE TO PASS OUT HAPPINESS!

AWW COME OFF IT, BUFFALO BILL!

NO, CHILD... *HOWDY DOOIT* IS A HAPPY WOODEN MARIONETTE, MANIPULATED BY STRINGS! *HOWDY DOOIT*, CHILD, IS NO MERCENARY, MONEY GRUBBING HUSTLER...

...I, BUFFALO BILL, AM THE MERCENARY, MONEY GRUBBING HUSTLER!

I'LL SHOW YOU WHO THE HUSTLER IS!

WHAT ARE YOU DOING, CHILD?

WAIT!

SOMEONE GRAB HIM!

STOP HIM, SOME-ONE!

HOLD HIM!

SNAP SNIP SNOP

WHAT DID HE DO?... WHAT'S WRONG WITH BUFFALO BILL?

...CUT THE SCENE! ...CUT THE SCENE! ...CUT! CUT!

...THAT KID!... HE HAD A PAIR OF SCISSORS!

CLIK CLIK CLIK

...HE CLIPPED BUFFALO BILL'S STRINGS!

WHY -TV?

CHANÉL NO. 5

MASTER ⌖ RACE

YOU CAN *NEVER FORGET*, CAN YOU, CARL REISSMAN? EVEN *HERE*...IN *AMERICA*...TEH YEARS AND THOUSANDS OF MILES AWAY FROM YOUR NATIVE GERMANY....YOU CAN NEVER FORGET THOSE *BLOODY WAR YEARS.* THOSE MEMORIES WILL HAUNT YOU FOREVER...AS EVEN NOW THEY HAUNT YOU WHILE YOU DESCEND THE SUBWAY STAIRS INTO THE QUIET SEMI-DARKNESS...

YOUR ACCENT IS STILL THICK ALTHOUGH YOU HAVE MASTERED THE LANGUAGE OF YOUR NEW COUNTRY THAT TOOK YOU IN WITH OPEN ARMS WHEN YOU FINALLY ESCAPED FROM BELSEN CONCENTRATION CAMP. YOU SLIDE THE BILL UNDER THE BARRED CHANGE-BOOTH WINDOW...

TWO TOKENS, PLEASE.

YOU MOVE TO THE BUSY CLICKING TURNSTILES...SLIP THE SHINY TOKEN INTO THE THIN SLOT...AND PUSH THROUGH...

THE TRAIN ROARS OUT OF THE BLACK CAVERN, SHATTERING THE SILENCE OF THE ALMOST DESERTED STATION...

YOU STARE AT THE ONRUSHING STEEL MONSTER...

YOU BLINK AS THE FIRST CAR RUSHES BY AND ILLUMINATED WINDOWS FLASH IN AN EVER-SLOWING RHYTHM...

From *Impact* No. 1, Mar.-Apr. 1955

AND THE TRAIN GRINDS TO A HISSING STOP...

YOU MOVE TO THE DOOR AS IT SLIDES OPEN. A PASSENGER EMERGES AND YOU FEEL HIS EYES UPON YOU AND YOU SHUDDER. WHY ARE YOU FRIGHTENED, CARL? THAT WAS A *LONG TIME AGO!* THIS IS *AMERICA.* YOU'RE *SAFE* NOW! YOU'RE *FREE*...

EXCUSE ME...

BUT YOU *ARE* AFRAID, *AREN'T* YOU, CARL? YOU'LL *ALWAYS* BE AFRAID. YOU'LL *KEEP REMEMBERING*... REMEMBERING THE *HORROR*... THE *HATE*... THE *SUFFERING*... AND YOU'LL *STAY* AFRAID. YOU STEP INTO THE ALMOST-EMPTY CAR AND YOU SIGH INTO A SEAT...

THE DOORS SLAM SHUT. THE TRAIN LURCHES AND ROLLS AHEAD, THUNDERING OUT OF THE STATION AND BACK INTO THE BLACK CHASMS TUNNELING BENEATH THE CITY. YOU UNFOLD YOUR PAPER...

YOU TRY TO READ, BUT THE WORDS ARE MEANINGLESS. NOTHING HAS MEANING ANY MORE... NOTHING BUT THE SICKENING SENSATION THAT HAS PLAGUED YOU FOR OVER TEN LONG YEARS. THE CONCENTRATION CAMP HAS LEFT ITS MARK UPON YOU, HASN'T IT, CARL REISSMAN?

YOU LOOK AROUND AT YOUR FELLOW PASSENGERS SITTING ALONE IN THEIR OWN LITTLE WORLDS OF FEAR. YOU STUDY THEIR FACES... THEIR FEATURES... THEIR EYES... LOOKING... ALWAYS LOOKING. WHAT ARE YOU *LOOKING* FOR CARL? WHO *IS* IT YOU'RE *AFRAID* OF?

THE TRAIN GROANS INTO ANOTHER STATION AND JERKS TO A STOP. THE DOORS HUM WIDE. YOU LOOK DOWN AT YOUR PAPER, ONLY *SENSING* PEOPLE GETTING OFF...

...SOMEONE GETTING ON...

AND THEN... DOWN DEEP INSIDE YOU... YOU FEEL THE CHILL... THE COLD CHILL ... THE CHILL OF DEATH. YOU STARE AT THE PAPER ON YOUR LAP, UNABLE TO RAISE YOUR EYES... AFRAID TO SEE WHAT YOU KNOW IS THERE. BUT, AFTER A FEW TERRORIZED MOMENTS, YOU CAN'T STAND IT! YOU *DO* LOOK UP! AND YOU *SEE* HIM...

CHOKE!

2

HE SITS STIFFLY, READING HIS PAPER, NOT LOOKING AT YOU, NOT NOTICING YOU. BUT *YOU'VE* SEEN *HIM*, CARL! YOU'VE SEEN HIS *FACE*... THE ONE YOU *KNEW* SOMEDAY YOU'D SEE AGAIN...THE FACE YOU'VE BEEN *AFRAID* TO SEE FOR *TEN LONG YEARS*. YOUR MOUTH TWITCHES. YOUR HANDS OPEN AND CLOSE, WET WITH PERSPIRATION...

NO! *NO!* HE *CAN'T* HURT ME NOW! HE *CAN'T!* HE *WOULDN'T!*

THE TRAIN SCREAMS AROUND A CURVE IN ITS SUBTERRANIAN ROUTE ...AND THE SCREAM IS SHRILL AND SHARP...SETTING YOUR TEETH ON EDGE...REACHING BACK INTO THE PAST...

...TO ANOTHER SHRILL SCREAM...THE SCREAM OF A LITTLE MAN WITH WILD EYES AND BLACK HAIR AND A SMALL BLACK MOUSTACHE...

SIEG HEIL...SIEG HEIL...SIEG HEIL!

REMEMBER, CARL? REMEMBER THE LITTLE MAN IN THE UNIFORM WHO STOOD FIRST BEFORE SMALL GROUPS... THEN BEFORE CROWDS...AND FINALLY BEFORE MULTITUDES...AND SCREAMED AND SCREAMED THEM INTO AN HYSTERICAL MISSION OF WORLD CONQUEST. *YOU* WERE THERE...IN ONE OF THOSE CROWDS. REMEMBER?

SIEG HEIL!

AND WHEN THE LITTLE MAN HAD STOPPED SCREAMING AND THE CROWD HAD DISPERSED, REMEMBER THE SICKENING FEELING YOU HAD,...THE REVULSION AND NAUSEA YOU FELT AS YOU TRUDGED HOME?...

THERE WERE *OTHERS* LIKE YOU, CARL...

...*OTHERS* WHO WERE *SICK* AND *REVOLTED* AND *NAUSEATED*, AT THE SCREAMING PROPOSALS OF THIS LITTLE MAN. BUT *THEY* COULDN'T STOP THE TIDE, *COULD* THEY, CARL? *THEY* COULDN'T STEM THE FLOW OF HATE THAT POURED THROUGH THE STREETS WITH CLUBS AND GUNS AND THE ECHOES OF THE LITTLE MAN'S SCREAMS URGING IT ON...

3

NO ONE COULD STOP THE BOOKS FROM BEING BURNED...

...OR THE SHOP WINDOWS FROM BEING SMASHED AND THEIR CONTENTS RANSACKED...

...OR THE SANCTITY OF HOMES FROM BEING VIOLATED...

IT WAS A MADNESS... A WAVE THAT SWEPT THROUGH YOUR HOMELAND LIKE A PLAGUE... A TIDAL WAVE OF FRENZIED HATE-FEARS AND BLOOD-LETTING AND EXPLODING VIOLENCE... A WILD UNCONTROLLED WAVE THAT SWEPT YOU AND YOUR KIND ALONG WITH IT...

WHAT HAPPENED TO YOU, CARL? WHEN WERE YOU CAUGHT UP IN THIS TIDE? WHEN DID YOU FIRST SEE BELSEN CONCENTRATION CAMP AND THE HUMAN MISERY THAT SOBBED WITHIN ITS BARBED-WIRE WALLS?...

DO YOU REMEMBER, CARL? DO YOU REMEMBER THE AWFUL SMELL OF THE GAS CHAMBERS THAT HOURLY ANNIHILATED HUNDREDS AND HUNDREDS OF YOUR COUNTRYMEN?...

DO YOU REMEMBER THE STINKING ODOR OF HUMAN FLESH BURNING IN THE OVENS... MEN'S... WOMEN'S... CHILDREN'S... PEOPLE YOU ONCE KNEW AND TALKED TO AND DRANK BEER WITH?...

DO YOU REMEMBER THE UNMERCIFUL TORTURES...THE SCREAMS IN THE NIGHT...THE PITIFUL WAILING OF THE DOOMED? DO YOU REMEMBER THE MAD EXPERIMENTS WITH HUMAN GUINEA PIGS...THE WANTON WASTE OF HUMAN LIFE?...

...THE BULBS THAT BURNED IN LAMPS ON DESKS IN THE CONCENTRATION CAMP OFFICES...GLOWING THROUGH THEIR HUMAN-SKIN-SHADES?...

LOOK, CARL! LOOK AT THE FACE OF THIS MAN SITTING ACROSS FROM YOU IN THIS NOW DESERTED SUBWAY CAR! LOOK...AND REMEMBER! REMEMBER THE GUARDS THAT GLEEFULLY CARRIED OUT THE SADISTIC ORDERS OF THE MASTER RACE...WHIPPING...KICKING...BEATING!...THE GUARDS THAT EAGERLY DRAGGED THE WOMEN AND CHILDREN TO THE WAITING, SMOKING OVENS!...

REMEMBER THE GUARDS THAT PUSHED AND SHOVED...HEAPING THE HELPLESS CAMP INMATES INTO THE FRESH DUG MASS GRAVES...

...LAUGHING WILDLY AS THEY BURIED THEIR VICTIMS ALIVE...SHOVELING THE DIRT DOWN UPON THEM, MUFFLING THEIR PATHETIC SCREAMS ...MUFFLING THEIR PATHETIC LIVES!...

LOOK AT THIS MAN AND REMEMBER, CARL! REMEMBER HIS FACE... THE LOOK THAT CAME INTO HIS EYES WHEN THE NEWS CAME THAT THE RUSSIANS WERE ONLY A FEW KILOMETERS AWAY! IT WAS OVER FOR YOU, THEN, CARL! THE KILLING AND MAIMING AND TORTURING WAS SUDDENLY OVER FOR YOU!

AND YET IT *WASN'T* OVER, BECAUSE HE LOOKED AT YOU AND *SWORE*...

SOMEDAY, *REISSMAN!* I'LL *GET* YOU... IF IT'S THE *LAST THING I DO!*

AND THEN YOU WERE *FREE*...RUNNING *PELL-MELL ACROSS EUROPE*, HIDING YOUR *CLOTHES*, LOSING YOURSELF IN AMONG THE STREAMS OF REFUGEES THAT CHOKED THE ROADS AND HIGHWAYS BEFORE THE ADVANCING ALLIED ARMIES ...

AND YET YOU *WEREN'T* FREE, CARL! EVEN THOUGH YOU SOMEHOW *GOT* TO AMERICA, YOU *NEVER FORGOT!* YOU NEVER FORGOT HIS *PROMISE!* SO YOU CARRIED THE FEAR *WITH* YOU FOR *TEN YEARS* AND *NOW* IT'S *CAUGHT UP* WITH YOU! HE'S *THERE*...SITTING *OPPOSITE* YOU...FEELING YOUR FRIGHTENED STARING EYES UPON HIM ...

AND NOW HE'S *LOOKING* AT YOU. HE'S LOOKING AT YOUR *HAIR*...AT YOUR *LIPS*...YOUR *NOSE*...DEEP INTO YOUR *FRIGHTENED EYES*. AND A SPARK OF *FAR-AWAY, LONG-AGO RECOGNITION* IGNITES HIS FACE...

YOU!

CHOKE...

HE RISES SLOWLY, HIS MOUTH SET IN A GRIM TAUT LINE, HIS EYES CLOUD WITH HATE, HIS FISTS CLENCH...

REISSMAN!...

...IT'S YOU!

NO! NO! GOTT IN HIMMEL!

THE TRAIN GRINDS TO A STOP. THE DOORS SLIDE OPEN. HE'S COMING *TOWARD* YOU, CARL! *RUN! THIS IS YOUR CHANCE! RUN!...*

RUN... AS YOU *RAN FROM BELSEN,* CARL! *RUN...* AS YOU *RAN ACROSS EUROPE,* FLEEING THE LIBERATING ALLIED ARMIES! RUN, *NOW,* CARL... AS YOU *REFUSED* TO RUN WHEN THAT *MAD WAVE SWEPT OVER GERMANY...SWEEPING YOU ALONG IN ITS BLOODY WAKE!...*

I SWORE...

I SWORE I'D GET YOU, REISSMAN!

NO!

HAVE PITY!

RUN DOWN THE LONG, EMPTY, DESERTED STATION PLATFORM, CARL! *RUN FROM THIS PERSONIFICATION OF THE MILLIONS OF YOUR COUNTRYMEN* WHO *COULDN'T* RIDE THE TIDE *YOU* CHOSE TO RIDE... WHO WERE *CAUGHT* IN ITS *UNDERTOW...*

IT'S *NO USE,* REISSMAN!

PLEASE...

...WHO WERE *PERSECUTED* AND *JAILED* AND *BURNED IN OVENS* AND *GASSED* AND *BURIED ALIVE* IN MASS GRAVES...

RUN FROM THIS SURVIVOR OF A HUMAN HELL ON EARTH...THIS SURVIVOR OF A GERMAN CONCENTRATION CAMP... *BELSEN CONCENTRATION CAMP...*

THE CAMP THAT YOU COMMANDED!

WHAT *HAPPENED?*

I DON'T *KNOW!* HE GOT OUT *AHEAD* OF ME AND BEGAN TO *RUN!*

HE *RAN UP THE PLATFORM* AND THEN *JUMPED* UNDER THE WHEELS OF THE TRAIN COMING IN THE *OTHER WAY...*

EVER *SEE* HIM BEFORE?

NO! HE...

HE WAS A *PERFECT STRANGER...*

THE END

333

A Selective, Annotated Bibliography

Most of the best research and writing about comic books has been published in comics "fanzines"—obscure magazines, with tiny circulations, that are devoted to discussions of comic books and related fields. We have cited a selection of those writings in this bibliography, along with some of the books and articles that have received more general distribution. Some "fanzines" can be found in large libraries, and in some cases back issues are available from the publishers or from University Microfilms. The addresses of the publishers are given when appropriate. And here are the addresses for the comics "fanzines" we will be listing several times below:

Fanfare (formerly *Graphic Story Magazine*)—Bill Spicer, 329 N. Avenue 66, Los Angeles, California 90042.

Funnyworld—University Microfilms International, 300 N. Zeeb Road, Ann Arbor, Michigan 48106.

Panels, Squa Tront—John Benson, 205 W. 80th Street, Apartment 2E, New York, New York 10024.

Please note: Inquiries about the price and availability of a publication should always be accompanied by a stamped, self-addressed envelope.

General

Bails, Jerry, and Hames Ware, eds. *The Who's Who of American Comic Books,* 4 vols., 1973–1976. (Jerry Bails, 21101 E. 11 Mile, Saint Clair Shores, Michigan 48081.) Biographical entries for more than 2,500 artists, writers, and editors.

Becker, Stephen. *Comic Art in America.* New York: Simon & Schuster, 1959. Chapter VII is about comic books.

Feiffer, Jules. *The Great Comic Book Heroes.* New York: Dial Press, 1965. Includes a dozen stories from super-hero comic books, in addition to Feiffer's nostalgic text.

Horn, Maurice, ed. *The World Encyclopedia of Comics.* New York: Chelsea House, 1976. This book remains the only comprehensive reference to the field (but reviewers have cited errors and omissions).

Lupoff, Dick, and Don Thompson, eds. *All in Color for a Dime.* New Rochelle, N. Y.: Arlington House, 1970. A collection of essays on comic books, some of which are listed individually below.

Overstreet, R. M. *The Comic Book Price Guide.* Tenth ed., 1980–1981. (Distributed by Harmony Books.) Some of the prices in this annual compilation may be taken with a grain of salt, but it contains reliable information about the publishing histories of many hundreds of titles.

Thompson, Don, and Dick Lupoff, eds. *The Comic-Book Book.* New Rochelle, N.Y.: Arlington House, 1974. A successor volume to *All in Color for a Dime,* and likewise composed of essays on comic books.

Waugh, Coulton. *The Comics.* New York: Macmillan, 1947. Chapter 20 is about comic books, and draws on interviews with M. C. Gaines and other pioneers.

On "Superman"

Kobler, John. "Up, Up and Awa-a-y! The Rise of Superman, Inc." *Saturday Evening Post,* June 21, 1941, p. 14.

White, Ted. "The Spawn of M. C. Gaines." In Lupoff and Thompson, eds., *All in Color for a Dime.*

On "Captain Marvel"

Lupoff, Dick. "The Big Red Cheese." In Lupoff and Thompson, eds., *All in Color for a Dime.*

On "Plastic Man" and Jack Cole

Thompson, Don. "The Rehabilitation of Eel O'Brian." In Thompson and Lupoff, eds., *The Comic-Book Book.*

On Basil Wolverton

Graphic Story Magazine No. 12, Fall 1970, and No. 14, Winter 1971–1972. Both issues are made up entirely of material by and about Wolverton.

On George Carlson

Ellison, Harlan. "Comic of the Absurd." In Lupoff and Thompson, eds., *All in Color for a Dime.*

On "Little Lulu" and John Stanley

Phelps, Don. "John Stanley." In the program book for the "Newcon" comics-fan convention, Boston, 1976.

Thompson, Maggie. "The Almost-Anonymous Mr. Stanley." *Funnyworld* 16 (Winter 1974–1975): 34.

On "Donald Duck" and Carl Barks

Barrier, Michael. "The Duck Man." In Thompson and Lupoff, eds., *The Comic-Book Book.*

Barrier, Michael. "Screenwriter for a Duck: Carl Barks at the Disney Studio." *Funnyworld* 21 (Fall 1979): 8.

Barrier, Michael. "Starting Out in the Comics: Carl Barks Becomes the Duck Man." *Funnyworld* 22 (1981): 12.

Boatner, E. B. "Carl Barks—From Duckburg to Calisota." In R. M. Overstreet, *The Comic Book Price Guide* 7 (1977–1978).

Summer, Edward. "Of Ducks and Men: Carl Barks Interviewed." *Panels* 2 (Spring 1981): 3.

On "Pogo" and Walt Kelly

Kelly, Walt. *Ten Ever-lovin' Blue-eyed Years with Pogo.* New York: Simon & Schuster, 1959.

The Okefenokee Star. (Swamp Yankee Studios, P.O. Box 2311, Bridgeport, Connecticut 06608.) Issued with the cooperation of Kelly's estate, this magazine has published a great deal of rare material by and about Walt Kelly.

Robinson, Murray. "Pogo's Papa." *Collier's,* March 8, 1952, p. 20.

On "The Spirit" and Will Eisner

Benson, John. "An Interview with Will Eisner." *Witzend* 6 (Spring 1969).

Eisner, Will (with John Benson). "Art & Commerce: An Oral Reminiscence." *Panels* 1 (Summer 1979): 5.

Feiffer, Jules (with John Benson). "Jules Feiffer Talks About the Spirit." *Panels* 1 (Summer 1979): 22.

Kyle, Richard. "Graphic Story Review." *Fantasy Illustrated (Graphic Story Magazine)* 6 (Summer/Fall 1966): 3.

Thompson, Maggie. "Blue Suit, Blue Mask, Blue Gloves—and No Socks." In Thompson and Lupoff, eds., *The Comic-Book Book.*

On E.C.

Benson, John. "Is War Hell? The Evolution of an Artist's Viewpoint." *Panels* 2 (Spring 1981): 18. On Harvey Kurtzman's war comic books.

Bray, Glenn. *The Illustrated Harvey Kurtzman Index.* 1976. (Glenn Bray, P.O. Box 4482, Sylmar, California 91342)

Durwood, Tom. "Harvey Kurtzman." *Crimmer's* (No. 3) (Spring 1976): 23. An interview.

Jacobs, Frank. *The Mad World of William M. Gaines.* Secaucus, N.J.: Lyle Stuart, Inc., 1972.

Spiegel, Ed. *"Fanfare* Interview: Editor of *Mad* Magazine, Al Feldstein." *Fanfare* 1 (Spring 1977): 16.

Squa Tront 6 (1975). An issue devoted to Bernard Krigstein. All issues of *Squa Tront* consist of material related to the E.C. comic books.

Thompson, Don. "The Spawn of the Son of M. C. Gaines." In Thompson and Lupoff, eds., *The Comic-Book Book.*

Reprints

Comic-book features have been reprinted in books with increasing frequency in recent years. Considering only the features represented in this book, *Superman, Batman,* and *Captain Marvel* (under the title of its 1970s revival, *Shazam!*) have been the subjects of collections published by Crown. Two collections of Carl Barks's *Donald Duck* and *Uncle Scrooge* have been published by Abbeville Press, but take warning that in these books substantial alterations were made in Barks's drawings and in his original dialogue. A collection of Barks's *Uncle Scrooge*—lovingly prepared and quite expensive—was published by Celestial Arts in 1982.

Will Eisner's *The Spirit* is being reprinted, in black and white, in a handsome bimonthly magazine, *The Spirit;* the magazine also publishes new work by Eisner. (Kitchen Sink Enterprises, Box 7, Princeton, Wisconsin 54968)

All E.C. comic books from 1950 to 1955 are being reprinted in slipcased sets; each set reprints, in several volumes, the complete run of an E.C. title in black and white, from the original artwork. To date, five sets— *Weird Science, Tales from the Crypt, Two-Fisted Tales, Weird Fantasy,* and *Shock SuspenStories*—have been published. (Russ Cochran, P.O. Box 469, West Plains, Missouri 65775)